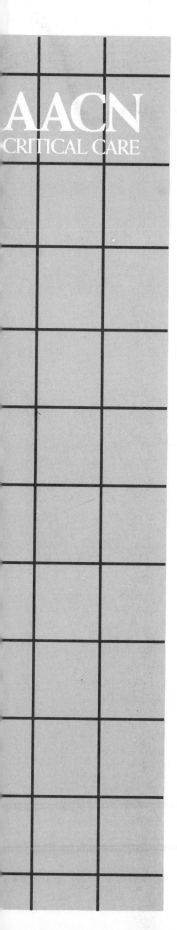

AMERICAN ASSOCIATION OF CRITICAL-CARE NURSES

Core Curriculum for Critical Care Nursing

Edited by

JoAnn Grif Alspach, RN, MSN, EdD
Nursing Education Consultant, Critical Care,
Editor, *Critical Care Nurse*
Annapolis, Maryland

W.B. SAUNDERS COMPANY
A Division of Harcourt Brace & Company
Philadelphia   London   Toronto   Montreal   Sydney   Tokyo

W.B. SAUNDERS COMPANY
A Division of
Harcourt Brace & Company

The Curtis Center
Independence Square West
Philadelphia, Pennsylvania 19106

Library of Congress Cataloging-in-Publication Data

Core curriculum for critical care nursing / [the American
Association of Critical-Care Nurses].—4th ed. / editor, JoAnn
Grif Alspach.

   p.   cm.

Includes bibliographical references.

ISBN 0–7216–3074–X

1. Intensive care nursing.   I. Alspach, JoAnn.   II. American
   Association of Critical-Care Nurses.
[DNLM: 1. Critical Care—nurses' instruction.   2. Critical
Care—outlines.   3. Curriculum—nurses' instruction.
4. Education, Nursing—United States. WY 18 C7966]

RT120.I5C63 1991

610.73'61—dc20

DNLM/DLC   90-9161

Editor: Thomas Eoyang
Designer: Joan Wendt
Production Manager: Ken Neimeister
Manuscript Editor: Jeanne M. Carper
Illustration Coordinator: Walt Verbitski
Indexer: Ruth Low
Cover Designer: Ellen M. Bodner

Listed here is the latest translated edition of this book together with the language of
the translation and the publisher.
Spanish—2nd ed., NEISA, Cedro 512, Apartado 26370, 06450 Mexico, Mexico

Core Curriculum for Critical Care Nursing, 4th Edition   ISBN   0–7216–3074–X

Printed in United States of America.

Last digit is the print number: 9   8   7   6   5   4

Contributors

Tess L. Briones, R.N., M.S.N., CCRN
Clinical Associate Faculty, University of Michigan School of Nursing; Clinical Nurse Specialist, Surgical Intensive Care Unit, University of Michigan Medical Center, Ann Arbor, Michigan
The Gastrointestinal System

John L. Carty, R.N., D.N.Sc.
Nurse Methods Analyst, U.S. Army, San Antonio, Texas
Psychosocial Aspects

Richard DeAngelis, R.N., M.S.
Nurse Consultant, Critical Care Nurse Educator, San Diego, California
The Cardiovascular System

Pamela Miller Gotch, R.N., M.S.N., CDE
Endocrine/Diabetes Clinical Nurse Specialist, Findling-Norton-Shaker SC, Milwaukee, Wisconsin
The Endocrine System

Bonnie Mowinski Jennings, R.N., D.N.Sc., LTC, AN
Nurse Researcher, U.S. Army Health Services Command, Health Care Studies Division, Ft. Sam Houston, Texas
The Hematologic System

Sara R. Neagley, R.N., M.A.
Research Nurse, The Milton S. Hershey Medical Center, The Pennsylvania State University, Hershey, Pennsylvania
The Pulmonary System

Diana L. Nikas, R.N., M.N., CCRN, CNRN, FCCM
Assistant Clinical Professor, School of Nursing, University of California, Los Angeles; Assistant Clinical Professor, School of Nursing, California State University, Long Beach; Neurosurgical Clinical

Nurse Specialist, Department of Neurosurgery, Harbor–UCLA Medical Center, Torrance, California
The Neurologic System

June L. Stark, R.N., B.S.N., M.Ed.
Associate Director of Critical Care Education, New England Medical Center Hospitals, Boston, Massachusetts
The Renal System

Ginger Schafer Wlody, R.N., M.S., CCRN, FCCM
Assistant Clinical Professor, School of Nursing, University of California, Los Angeles; Nursing Quality Assurance Director, Wadsworth Veterans Administration Medical Center, Los Angeles, California
Legal and Ethical Aspects of Critical Care Nursing

Chapter Reviewers

1. Pulmonary System

Mary Kathryn Reeves-Hoche, R.N., M.A., M.S.
Pulmonary Clinical Nurse Specialist, Pulmonary Division of Medicine, The Milton S. Hershey Medical Center, University Hospital, The Pennsylvania State University, Hershey, Pennsylvania

Leon W. Sweer, M.D.
Pulmonary Division of Medicine, The Milton S. Hershey Medical Center, University Hospital, The Pennsylvania State University, Hershey, Pennsylvania

2. Cardiovascular System

M. Lindsay Lessig, R.N., M.S.Ed.
Lieutenant Colonel (Retired), U.S. Army Nurse Corps; Director of Hospital Education, Avista Hospital, Louisville, Colorado

Paul M. Lessig, M.D.
Lieutenant Colonel, U.S. Army Medical Corps; Chief, Cardiology Service, Fitzsimons Army Medical Center, Aurora, Colorado

3. Neurologic System

Susan Johnson, R.N., M.N., CCRN
Nurse Manager, Neurosciences, UCLA Medical Center, Los Angeles, California

Connie Walleck, R.N., M.S., CCRN
Associate Director, Maryland Institute for EMS Systems, Baltimore, Maryland

Maurene Harvey, R.N., M.P.H., CCRN
Critical Care Educator, Glendale, California

Duncan McBride, M.D.
Chief, Neurosurgery, Harbor–UCLA Medical Center, Torrance, California

Mark Goldberg, M.D.
Chief, Neurology, Harbor–UCLA Medical Center, Torrance, California

4. Renal System

Charold L. Baer, R.N., Ph.D.
Professor, School of Nursing, The Oregon Health Sciences University, Portland, Oregon

Gennaro Carpinito, M.D.
Director of Urology, Boston City Hospital, Boston, Massachusetts

5. Endocrine System

Mary Ann Carr, R.N., M.S., CCRN, CS
Lieutenant Colonel, U.S. Army Nurse Corps, Nursing Research Service; Formerly Head Nurse, Kyle Metabolic Research Unit, Walter Reed Army Medical Center, Washington, D.C.

James W. Findling, M.D.
Director, Endocrine-Diabetes Center, St. Luke's Medical Center; Associate Clinical Professor of Medicine, Medical College of Wisconsin, Milwaukee, Wisconsin

6. Hematologic System

Stephanie Marshall, R.N., M.S.
Major, U.S. Army Nurse Corps; Oncology Clinical Nurse Specialist, Letterman Army Medical Center, San Francisco, California

Charles F. Miller, M.D., FACP
Colonel, U.S. Army Medical Corps; Chief, Department of Medicine, Letterman Army Medical Center, San Francisco, California

7. Gastrointestinal System

J. Keith Hampton, R.N., M.S.N.
Clinical Nurse Specialist—Medical Intensive Care Unit, University of Michigan Medical Center, Ann Arbor, Michigan

M. Michael Shabot, M.D., FACS
Associate Director of Surgery and Director, Surgical Intensive Care

Unit, Cedars Sinai Medical Center; Clinical Associate Professor of Surgery and Anesthesiology, University of California, Los Angeles, California

8. Psychosocial

Barbara Ann Erickson, R.N., M.S.
Psychiatric/Mental Health Clinical Nurse Specialist, Sacramento Veterans Administration Medical Center, Sacramento, California

Robb Imonen, M.D.
Colonel, U.S. Army Medical Corps; Chief, Department of Psychiatry, Tripler Army Medical Center, Honolulu, Hawaii

9. Legal/Ethical

June Levine, R.N., M.S.N.
Assistant Administrator, Patient Care Services, St. Luke's Medical Center, Pasadena, California

John Clochesy, R.N., M.S., CS
Instructor—Frances Payne Bolton School of Nursing, Case Western Reserve University, Cleveland, Ohio

Preface

The American Association of Critical-Care Nurses (AACN) has adopted the following definition of critical care nursing: "In *Nursing: A Social Policy Statement*[1] the American Nurses' Association defines nursing as 'the diagnosis and treatment of human responses to actual or potential health problems.' Critical care nursing is that specialty within nursing which deals specifically with human responses to life-threatening problems."[2] The purpose of the *Core Curriculum for Critical Care Nursing* is to enunciate the knowledge base of critical care nursing.

AACN's Conceptual Model for Critical Care Nursing (Figure 1) contains five components that we have attempted to exemplify in this fourth edition of the *Core Curriculum:* the AACN Scope of Practice Statement, the Principles of Practice Statement, the *Standards for Nursing Care of the Critically Ill,* the nursing process, and the provision of quality care for the critically ill patient.

The scope of critical care nursing practice embraces the critically ill patient–family unit, the critical care nurse, and the environment in which critical care nursing is provided. Throughout each chapter of the *Core Curriculum,* the patient with life-threatening health problems is the focus of coverage. The patient's family is considered in the data base the nurse obtains about the patient, in making relevant nursing diagnoses, in planning and providing nursing care, and in evaluating the effectiveness of that care. The critical care nurse and critical care environment are addressed in chapters devoted to psychosocial aspects of care and the legal and ethical aspects of critical care nursing.

The AACN Principles of Practice Statement considers the professional conduct of the critical care nurse when faced with practice and ethical dilemmas involving nurse–patient relationships. Previous editions of the *Core Curriculum* have neglected this area. The present edition dedicates Chapter 9 to these concerns.

In order to operationalize and fulfill the *Standards for Nursing Care of the Critically Ill,* the critical care nurse must possess knowledge of these quality statements as well as knowledge of the art and science of critical care nursing. The *Core Curriculum* continues to serve as a major reference in providing this content for both the neophyte and experienced critical care nurse.

Care is delivered to the critically ill patient and family through the interactive elements of the nursing process: assessment, diagnosis, planning, intervention, and evaluation. The present edition of the *Core Curriculum* integrates application of the nursing process more fully and adds the nursing diagnosis element as a major organizing theme for describing nursing care.

Each of these components contributes to the provision of quality care for the critically ill patient and family. This last component represents the ultimate aim of its counterparts and reminds us that the *Core Curriculum* is only one, albeit an essential one, of a number of AACN initiatives that help to ensure the highest quality of care for the critically ill.

AACN verifies clinical competency in critical care nursing through its CCRN certification program. In 1984, the AACN Certification Corporation completed its Role Delineation Study to validate the certification process and define the knowledge and skills requisite for competent critical care nursing practice. Two outcomes of this study were the revised CCRN examination blueprint and the *Critical Care Nursing Practice Task Statements.*[3] The examination blueprint lists the percentage of CCRN examination questions that should be apportioned for each content area. The Task Statements list the tasks defined as essential for critical care nursing practice.

In developing the fourth edition of the *Core Curriculum,* both of these competency elements were taken into account. The distribution of content in the *Core Curriculum* approximates as closely as possible the distribution of the knowledge base for critical care nursing as outlined

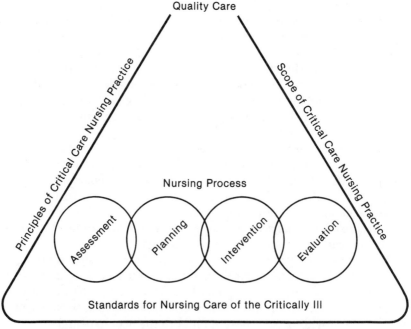

Figure 1. Conceptual Model of Critical Care Nursing.

in the CCRN examination blueprint. The third edition of the *Core Curriculum* also provided this feature, but because the findings of the Role Delineation Study were not available when that edition went to press, it reflected the examination blueprint used prior to 1985 rather than the revised blueprint. In addition, each of the over 300 task statements is included within its appropriate chapter. The blueprint and task statements assisted in determining the scope of content to be included in the present edition of the *Core Curriculum*.

Readers of this most recent edition will find both similarities and changes from the third edition. Similarities to earlier editions include the overall organization of content by body systems and the inclusion of subsections on physiologic anatomy and pathophysiology. These elements and the associated medical diagnoses have been retained because critical care nurses must be able to speak the language of the health care system and language of medicine in order to work collaboratively with other health care professionals.

The most notable differences in coverage in the current edition are its nursing-oriented approach and the emphasis on nursing process and nursing diagnosis. The medical nomenclature of patient history, physical examination, and diagnosis has been replaced with the Nursing Assessment Data Base. The nurse's data base includes the findings of a nursing history, a client examination, and the results of diagnostic tests. After the assessment phase of the nursing process, there is now a new subsection for identifying commonly encountered nursing diagnoses. These nursing diagnoses represent problems common to a majority of patients with health deviations in the body system discussed in that chapter. This segment is followed by a planning section, which identifies the expected patient outcomes for these diagnoses; an implementation section, which describes the nursing interventions necessary to attain those outcomes; and an evaluation section, which establishes the criteria by which attainment of the outcomes can be determined.

In order to move away from the disease model of medical care, the specific clinical entities are now characterized as patient health problems rather than as pathologic conditions. Because hospitals, physicians, and other health care professional groups communicate about patient populations by means of medical diagnoses, these labels are retained to designate particular groups of patients. Once the associated medical diagnosis is identified, however, the organizing theme returns to the nursing process. For each patient health problem, the nursing diagnoses related to this problem are used to organize all elements of planning, implementing, and evaluating care.

The last two chapters deviate from this organizational framework in different ways. The psychosocial chapter is organized entirely on the basis of nursing diagnosis, and the legal and ethical aspects chapter is organized by issues that relate more appropriately to each of these areas. Although some of the content of these chapters is integrated throughout the text, their separate consideration reflects the fact that this material pervades the entire scope of critical care nursing practice such that it cannot be arbitrarily assigned to one chapter alone.

We have attempted to provide you with the latest and most validated knowledge base for critical care nursing that is available and welcome your comments and suggestions.

JoAnn Grif Alspach

References

1. American Nurses' Association, Congress on Nursing Practice: *Nursing: A Social Policy Statement.* American Nurses' Association, Kansas City, Mo., 1980.
2. American Association of Critical-Care Nurses: *Definition of Critical Care Nursing.* American Association of Critical-Care Nurses, Newport Beach, Calif., 1984.
3. American Association of Critical-Care Nurses Certification Corporation: *Critical Care Nursing Practice Task Statements.* American Association of Critical-Care Nurses Certification Corporation, Newport Beach, Calif., 1984.

Acknowledgments

This fourth edition of the *Core Curriculum* represents a culmination of the efforts of many people over the course of many years. I would like to take this opportunity to thank some of them here.

From its inception as a proposal, this book has been guided in its development by the AACN Board of Directors and the AACN Professional Media Committee. Ellen French, AACN's Manager of Publications, provided continuing support and assistance throughout the course of this process as the staff liaison for this project.

Each of the chapter contributors afforded both their content expertise and their commitment to revisions and schedules necessary for preparing a book of high quality. We were greatly aided in this endeavor by a cadre of expert nurse and physician reviewers, who offered recommendations for improvements in the manuscript. We are indebted to each of these professionals for their time and dedication to this publication.

On a personal level, I would like to thank my husband Rodger Alspach, M.D., for designing the data base management system used throughout this project and for rescuing chapters "lost" by other computer operators. His diligence and expertise were invaluable over the years required to produce this book.

Contents

CHAPTER 3

THE NEUROLOGIC SYSTEM 315

Diana L. Nikas, R.N., M.N., CCRN, CNRN, FCCM

CHAPTER 4

THE RENAL SYSTEM 472

June L. Stark, R.N., B.S.N., M.Ed.

CHAPTER 5

THE ENDOCRINE SYSTEM 609
Pamela Miller Gotch, R.N., M.S.N., CDE

PSYCHOSOCIAL ASPECTS 836
John L. Carty, R.N., D.N.Sc.

CHAPTER 9

LEGAL AND ETHICAL ASPECTS OF
CRITICAL CARE NURSING 905
Ginger Schafer Wlody, R.N., M.S., CCRN, FCCM

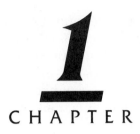

CHAPTER

The Pulmonary System

Sara R. Neagley, R.N., M.A.

PHYSIOLOGIC ANATOMY

The Respiratory Circuit

1. **The pulmonary system** exists for the purpose of gas exchange. Oxygen (O_2) and carbon dioxide (CO_2) are exchanged between the atmosphere and alveoli, between the alveoli and pulmonary capillary blood, and between the systemic capillary blood and all the cells of the body
2. **Atmospheric oxygen** is consumed by the body through cellular aerobic metabolism, which supplies the energy for life
3. **Carbon dioxide,** a by-product of aerobic metabolism, is eliminated through lung ventilation
4. **The respiratory circuit** includes all processes involved in the transfer of oxygen between room air and the individual cell and in the transfer of carbon dioxide between the cell and room air
5. **Cellular respiration** cannot be directly measured but is estimated by the amount of carbon dioxide produced ($\dot{V}_{CO_2}$) and the oxygen consumed ($\dot{V}_{O_2}$). The ratio of these two values is called the respiratory quotient (RQ). The RQ is normally about 0.8 but changes according to the nutritional substrate being burned (i.e., protein, fats, or carbohydrates). Patients fully maintained on intravenous glucose alone will have an RQ approaching 1.0 owing to the metabolic end product carbon dioxide
6. **The exchange of oxygen and carbon dioxide** at the alveolar-capillary level (external respiration) is called the respiratory exchange ratio (R) and is the ratio of carbon dioxide produced to oxygen taken up per minute. In homeostasis the respiratory exchange ratio is the same as the respiratory quotient, 0.8

7. **Proper functioning of the respiratory circuit** requires efficient interaction of the respiratory, circulatory, and neuromuscular systems
8. **In addition to its primary function of oxygen and carbon dioxide exchange,** the lung also carries out metabolic and endocrine functions as a source of hormones and a site of hormone metabolism. Additionally, the lung is a target of hormonal actions from other endocrine organs

Steps in the Gas Exchange Process

1. **Step 1—Ventilation:** the process of moving air between atmosphere and alveoli and distributing air within the lungs to maintain appropriate concentrations of oxygen and carbon dioxide in the alveoli
   a. Structural components involved in ventilation
      i. Lung
         (a) Anatomic divisions—right lung (three lobes), left lung (two lobes), bronchopulmonary segments (ten on right side, nine on left side), lobules
         (b) Lobule—contains primary functional units of lung (terminal bronchioles, alveolar ducts and sacs, pulmonary circulation). Lymphatics surround lobule, keep lung free of excess fluid, and remove inhaled particles from distal areas of lung
         (c) Bronchial artery circulation—systemic source of circulation for tracheobronchial tree and lung tissue down to the level of the terminal bronchiole. Alveoli receive their blood supply from the pulmonary circulation
      ii. Conducting airways: The entire area from nose to terminal bronchioles where gas flows, but is not exchanged, is called the anatomic dead space ($V_{D_{anat}}$). The approximate amount is calculated as 2 ml/kg body weight. The airways are a series of rapidly branching tubes of ever-diminishing diameter that eventually terminate in the alveoli
         (a) Nose
            (1) Passageway for movement of air into lung
            (2) Preconditions air by action of cilia, mucosal cells, and turbinate bones
               a) Warms air to within 2% to 3% of body temperature and humidifies it to full saturation before it reaches lower trachea
               b) Filters by trapping particles greater than 4 to 6 μm in size
            (3) Voice resonance, olfaction, sneeze reflex functions
         (b) Pharynx
            (1) Separation of food from air controlled by local nerve reflexes

(2) Opening of eustachian tube regulates middle ear pressure

(3) Lymphatic tissues control infection

(c) Larynx—incomplete rings of cartilage

  (1) Vocal cords—speech function

    a) Narrowest part of conducting airways in adults

    b) Contraction of muscles of larynx causes vocal cords to change shape

    c) Vibration of vocal cord produces sound. Speech is a joint function of vocal cords, mouth, and respiration, with control by temporal and parietal lobes of cerebral cortex

    d) Glottis—the opening between vocal cords

  (2) Valve action by epiglottis helps to prevent aspiration

  (3) Cough reflex—cords close and intrathoracic pressure increases to permit coughing or Valsalva maneuver

  (4) Cricoid cartilage

    a) Only complete rigid ring

    b) Narrowest part of child's airway; eliminates need for cuffed endotracheal tube

(d) Trachea—incomplete rings of cartilage

  (1) Conducting air passage

  (2) Warms and humidifies air

  (3) Mucosal cells trap foreign material

  (4) Cilia propel mucus upward through airway

  (5) Cough reflex present, especially at bifurcation (carina)

  (6) Smooth muscle innervated by parasympathetic branch of autonomic nervous system

(e) Terminal bronchioles

  (1) Smooth muscle walls (no cartilage); bronchospasm may narrow lumen and increase airway resistance

  (2) Ciliated mucosal cells become flattened, with progressive loss of cilia toward alveoli

  (3) Sensitive to carbon dioxide levels: increased levels induce bronchiolar dilation; decreased levels induce bronchiolar constriction

iii. Gas exchange airways: semipermeable membrane permits movement of gases according to pressure gradients. These airways do not contribute to air flow resistance but do contribute to distensibility of the lung. Acinus (terminal respiratory unit) is composed of respiratory bronchiole and its subdivisions (Fig. 1–1)

(a) Respiratory bronchioles and alveolar ducts

  (1) Terminal branching of airways

  (2) Distribution of inspired air

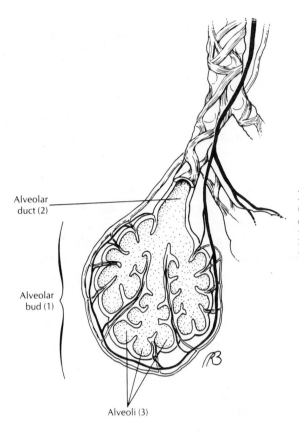

Alveolar
duct (2)

Alveolar
bud (1)

Alveoli (3)

Figure 1–1. Components of the acinus. (From Eubanks, D.H., and Bone, R.C.: Comprehensive Respiratory Care: A Learning System. C.V. Mosby Co., St. Louis, 1985, p. 160.)

    (3) Smooth muscle layer diminishes
  (b) Alveoli and alveolar bud
    (1) Most important structures in gas exchange
    (2) Alveolar surface area is large and depends on body size. It is about 1 m^2/kg body weight and is less than 1 μm in thickness. This fulfills the need to distribute a large quantity of perfused blood into a very thin film to ensure near equalization of oxygen and carbon dioxide
    (3) Alveolar cells
      a) Type I—squamous epithelium; adapted for gas exchange; sensitive to injury by inhaled agents; structured to prevent fluid transudation into alveoli
      b) Type II—large secretory; highly active metabolically; origin of surfactant synthesis and type I cell genesis
      c) Alveolar macrophages phagocytize foreign materials
    (4) Pulmonary surfactant
      a) Phospholipid monolayer at alveolar air–liquid in-

terface that has the property of varying surface tension with alveolar volume

   b) Enables surface tension to decrease as alveolar volume decreases during expiration, thus preventing alveolar collapse

   c) Decreases work of breathing, permits alveoli to remain inflated at low distending pressures, and reduces net forces causing tissue fluid accumulation

   d) Reduction of surfactant makes lung expansion more difficult (the greater the surface tension, the greater the pressure needed to overcome it)

   e) Surfactant also detoxifies inhaled gases and traps inhaled and deposited particles

(5) Alveolar-capillary membrane (alveolar epithelium, interstitial space, capillary endothelium)

   a) Bathed by interstitial fluid; lines respiratory bronchioles, alveolar ducts, alveolar sacs; forms walls of alveoli

   b) About 1 μm in thickness (less than one erythrocyte); permits very rapid diffusion of gases; any increase in thickness diminishes gas diffusion

   c) Total surface area in adult of about 70 m^2 is in contact with 60 to 140 ml of pulmonary capillary blood at any one time

(6) Gas exchange pathway (Fig. 1–2): alveolar epithelium → alveolar basement membrane → interstitial space → capillary basement membrane → capillary endothelium → plasma → erythrocyte membrane → erythrocyte cytoplasm

b. Alveolar ventilation ($\dot{V}_A$): that part of total ventilation taking part in gas exchange and therefore the only part useful to the body

   i. Alveolar ventilation is one component of minute ventilation

   (a) Minute ventilation ($\dot{V}_E$)—the amount of air exchanged in 1 minute. Equal to exhaled tidal volume (V_T) multiplied by respiratory rate (RR or F). Normal resting $\dot{V}_E$ in an adult is about 6 L/min

   $$V_T \times RR = \dot{V}_E \ (500 \text{ ml} \times 12 = 6000 \text{ ml})$$

   Tidal volume is easily measured at bedside by hand-held devices or on the ventilator. Minute ventilation is a routinely measured parameter

   (b) Minute ventilation is composed of both alveolar ventilation ($\dot{V}_A$) and physiologic dead space ventilation ($\dot{V}_D$)

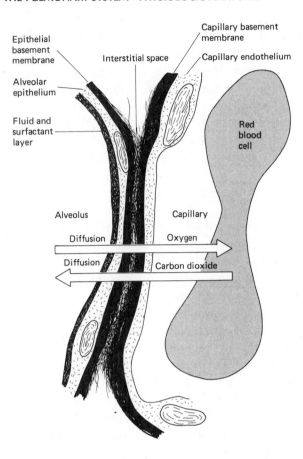

Epithelial basement membrane

Interstitial space

Capillary basement membrane

Capillary endothelium

Alveolar epithelium

Fluid and surfactant layer

Red blood cell

Alveolus

Capillary

Diffusion

Oxygen

Diffusion

Carbon dioxide

Figure 1–2. Ultrastructure of the respiratory membrane. (From Guyton, A.C.: Textbook of Medical Physiology, 7th ed. W.B. Saunders Co., Philadelphia, 1986, p. 488.)

$$\dot{V}_E = \dot{V}_D + \dot{V}_A$$
$$\dot{V} = \text{volume of gas per unit of time}$$

Physiologic dead space ventilation is that volume of gas in the airways that does not participate in gas exchange. It is composed of both anatomic dead space ventilation ($\dot{V}_{D_{anat}}$) and alveolar dead space ventilation ($\dot{V}_{D_A}$)

(c) Dead space to tidal volume ratio (V_D/V_T) is measured to determine how much of each breath is wasted (i.e., does not contribute to gas exchange). Normal values for spontaneously breathing patients range from 0.2 to 0.4 (20% to 40%)

ii. Alveolar ventilation cannot be directly measured but is inversely related to arterial carbon dioxide pressure (Pa_{CO_2}) in a steady state by this formula

$$\dot{V}_A = \frac{\dot{V}_{CO_2} \times 0.863}{Pa_{CO_2}}$$

where
$\dot{V}_A$ = alveolar ventilation

$\dot{V}_{CO_2}$ = carbon dioxide production

Pa_{CO_2} = arterial carbon dioxide pressure

0.863 = correction factor for differences in measurement units and conversion to STPD (standard temperature [0° C] and pressure [760 mm Hg], dry)

iii. Since $\dot{V}_{CO_2}$ remains the same in a steady state, measurement of the patient's Pa_{CO_2} reveals the status of the alveolar ventilation

iv. Pa_{CO_2} is the only adequate indicator of effective matching of alveolar ventilation to metabolic demand. Assessment of ventilation requires measurement of the Pa_{CO_2}

v. If Pa_{CO_2} is low, alveolar ventilation is high and hyperventilation is present

$$\downarrow Pa_{CO_2} = \uparrow \dot{V}_A$$

vi. If Pa_{CO_2} is within normal limits, alveolar ventilation is adequate

$$\text{Normal } \dot{V}_A = \text{normal } Pa_{CO_2}$$

vii. If Pa_{CO_2} is high, alveolar ventilation is low and hypoventilation is present

$$\uparrow Pa_{CO_2} = \downarrow \dot{V}_A$$

c. Defense mechanisms of the lung
   i. Although an internal organ, the lung is unique in that it has continuous contact with particulate and gaseous materials inhaled from the external environment. In the healthy lung, defense mechanisms successfully defend against these natural materials by the following means
      (a) The structural architecture of the upper respiratory tract, which reduces deposited and inhaled materials
      (b) The processing system, including respiratory tract fluid alteration and phagocytic activity
      (c) The transport system that removes material from the lung
      (d) The humoral and cell-mediated immune responses that augment bronchopulmonary defense mechanisms
   ii. Loss of normal defense mechanisms may be precipitated by disease, injury, surgery, insertion of endotracheal or tracheostomy tubes, or smoking
   iii. The upper respiratory tract warms and humidifies the inspired air, absorbs selected inhaled gases, and filters out particulate matter. Soluble gases and particles larger than 10 μm are aerodynamically filtered out. Normally no bacteria are present below the level of the larynx in the respiratory system
   iv. Inhaled and deposited particles reaching the alveoli are coated by surface fluids (surfactant and other lipoproteins) and rapidly phagocytized by pulmonary alveolar macrophages

    v. Macrophages and particles are transported in mucus by bronchial cilia beating toward the glottis and moving the materials along in a mucus–fluid layer eventually to be expectorated or swallowed. This process is referred to as the mucociliary escalator. Pulmonary lymphatics also drain and transport some cells and particles from the lung

    vi. Antigens activate humoral and cell-mediated immune systems, which add immunoglobins to the surface fluid of alveoli and activate alveolar macrophages

    vii. Disruption or injury to these defense mechanisms predisposes to acute or chronic pulmonary disease

  d. Lung mechanics

    i. Muscles of respiration: the act of breathing is accomplished through muscular actions that alter intrapulmonary and intrapleural pressures, thus changing intrapulmonary volumes

      (a) Muscles of inspiration. During inspiration the chest cavity enlarges. This enlargement is an active process brought about by contraction of

        (1) Diaphragm—the major inspiratory muscle

          a) Normal quiet breathing is accomplished almost entirely by this muscle

          b) Downward contraction increases superior-inferior diameter of chest and elevates lower ribs

          c) Innervation is from C3 to C5 level

          d) Normally accounts for 70% of tidal volume

        (2) External intercostals

          a) These muscles increase anteroposterior diameter of thorax by elevating ribs

          b) Anteroposterior diameter is about 20% greater during inspiration than during expiration

          c) Innervation is from T1 to T11

        (3) Accessory muscles in neck—scalene and sternocleidomastoid

          a) These muscles pull upward on sternum and ribs and increase anteroposterior diameter

          b) These muscles are not used in normal resting ventilation

      (b) Muscles of expiration. During expiration the chest cavity decreases in size. This is a passive act unless forced, and the driving force is derived from lung recoil. Muscles used when increased levels of ventilation are needed are the

        (1) Abdominals—force abdominal contents upward to elevate diaphragm

        (2) Internal intercostals—decrease anteroposterior diameter by depressing ribs

ii. Pressures within the chest: movement of air into the lungs requires a pressure difference between the airway opening and the alveoli sufficient to overcome the resistance to air flow of the tracheobronchial tree

EXAMPLE OF CHANGES IN PRESSURES THROUGHOUT
VENTILATORY CYCLE

Pressures	At Rest (No Air Flow)	Inspiration	Expiration
Atmospheric (P_B)	760 mm Hg	760	760
Intrapulmonary or intra-alveolar (P_{alv})	760 mm Hg	757	763
Intrapleural (P_{pl}) or intrathoracic	756 mm Hg	750	756

(a) Air flows into lungs when intrapulmonary air pressure falls below atmospheric pressure
(b) Air flows out of lungs when intrapulmonary air pressure exceeds atmospheric pressure
(c) Intrapleural pressure is normally negative with respect to atmospheric pressure due to the elastic recoil of the lungs tending to pull away from the chest wall. This "negative" pressure prevents collapse of the lung
(d) Increased effort (forced inspiration or expiration) may produce much greater changes in intrapulmonary and intrapleural pressures during inspiration and expiration

iii. Structural components of thorax
  (a) For protection: sternum, spine, ribs
  (b) Pleura
    (1) Visceral and parietal layers
    (2) Pleural fluid between layers—allows smooth movement of visceral over parietal layers
    (3) Adherence—normally the pleural space is a potential space or vacuum and, because of a constant "negative" pressure (less than atmospheric pressure by 4 to 8 mm Hg), any change in the volume of the thoracic cage is reflected by a similar change in the volume of the lungs
    (4) Nerve supply—parietal pleura has fibers for pain transmission but visceral pleura does not

iv. Resistances
  (a) Elastic resistance (static properties)
    (1) The lung, if removed from the chest, collapses to a smaller volume because of lung elastic recoil. This tendency of the lungs to collapse is normally counter-

acted by the chest wall tendency to expand. The volume of air in the lungs depends on the equal and opposite balance of these forces
  (2) Compliance is an expression of the elastic properties of the lung and is the change in volume accomplished by a change in pressure

$$C_L = \frac{\Delta V}{\Delta P}$$

  If compliance is high, the lung is more easily distended; if it is low, the lung is stiff and difficult to distend
  (b) Flow resistance (dynamic properties)
  (1) Airway resistance must be overcome to generate flow through the airways
  (2) Changes in airway caliber will affect airway resistance. Examples of changes would be those due to bronchospasm or secretions
  (3) Flow through the airway depends on pressure differences between the two ends of the tube, as well as resistance. The driving pressure for flow in the airways is the difference between atmospheric and alveolar pressures
  v. Work of breathing
  (a) The body automatically changes the respiratory pattern in order to minimize the work required to maintain a given level of ventilation
  (b) The work performed must be sufficient to overcome the elastic resistance and the flow resistance
  (c) In diseased states, the work load increases
e. Control of ventilation: although the process of breathing is a normal rhythmic activity that occurs without conscious effort, it involves an intricate controlling mechanism at the level of the central nervous system. The basic organization of the respiratory control system is outlined in Figure 1–3
  i. The respiratory generator is located in the medulla and composed of two groups of neurons
  (a) One group initiates respiration and regulates its rate
  (b) One group controls "switching off" inspiration, thus the onset of expiration
  ii. Input from other regions of the central nervous system
  (a) Pons—input is necessary for a normal, coordinated breathing pattern
  (b) Cerebral cortex—exerts a conscious or voluntary control over ventilation
  iii. Chemoreceptors—contribute to an important feedback loop that

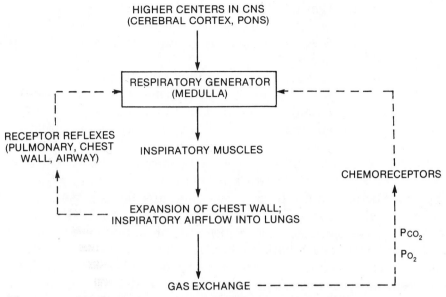

HIGHER CENTERS IN CNS
(CEREBRAL CORTEX, PONS)

RESPIRATORY GENERATOR
(MEDULLA)

RECEPTOR REFLEXES
(PULMONARY, CHEST
WALL, AIRWAY)

INSPIRATORY MUSCLES

CHEMORECEPTORS

EXPANSION OF CHEST WALL;
INSPIRATORY AIRFLOW INTO LUNGS

P_{CO_2}

P_{O_2}

GAS EXCHANGE

Figure 1–3. Schematic diagram depicting organization of the respiratory control system. The dotted lines show feedback loops affecting the respiratory generator. (From Weinberger, S.E.: Principles of Pulmonary Medicine. W.B. Saunders Co., Philadelphia, 1986, p. 200.)

exists to adjust respiratory center output if blood gases are not maintained within normal range

(a) Central chemoreceptor—located near ventrolateral surface of medulla (but is clearly separate from the medullary respiratory center)

(1) Responds not directly to blood P_{CO_2} but rather to the pH of the extracellular fluid (ECF) surrounding the chemoreceptor. The feedback loop for carbon dioxide can be summarized as follows

$\uparrow$ arterial $P_{CO_2} \rightarrow \uparrow$ brain ECF $P_{CO_2} \rightarrow \downarrow$ brain ECF pH $\rightarrow \downarrow$ pH at chemoreceptor $\rightarrow$ stimulation of central chemoreceptor $\rightarrow$ stimulation of medullary respiratory center $\rightarrow$ increased ventilation $\rightarrow$ decreased arterial P_{CO_2}

(b) Peripheral chemoreceptors—located in carotid body and aortic body

(1) Sensitive to changes in P_{O_2}, with hypoxemia stimulating chemoreceptor discharge

(2) Minor role in sensing P_{CO_2}

iv. Other receptors

(a) Stretch receptors in bronchial wall (Hering-Breuer reflex) respond to changes in lung inflation

(1) As lung inflates, receptor discharge increases

(2) Contributes to the start of expiration
(b) Irritant receptors located in lining of airways
(1) Respond to noxious stimuli, such as irritating dust or chemical
(c) "J" receptors (juxtacapillary) in alveolar interstitial space
(1) Cause tachypnea in response to deformation from accumulation of fluid or inflammation
(d) Receptors in chest wall (in the intercostal muscles)
(1) Involved in fine tuning of ventilation
(2) Adjust output of respiratory muscles for the degree of muscular work required

2. **Step 2—Diffusion:** the process by which alveolar air gases are moved across the alveolar-capillary membrane to the pulmonary capillary bed and vice versa. Diffusion occurs down a concentration gradient from a higher to lower concentration. No active metabolic work is required for diffusion of gases to occur. The work of breathing is accomplished by the respiratory muscles and heart, which produce the gradient across the alveolar-capillary membrane

a. The ability of the lung to transfer gases is called the diffusing capacity of the lung (D_L). The diffusing capacity measures the amount of gas (O_2, CO, CO_2) diffusing between alveoli and pulmonary capillary blood per minute per millimeter of mercury (mm Hg) mean gas pressure difference

b. Carbon dioxide is 20 times more diffusible across the alveolar-capillary membrane than is oxygen. If the membrane is damaged, its decreased capacity for transporting oxygen into the blood is usually more of a problem than its decreased capacity for transporting carbon dioxide out of the body. Thus the diffusing capacity of the lungs for oxygen is of primary importance

c. Diffusion is determined by several variables
   i. Surface area available for gas exchange
   ii. Integrity of alveolar-capillary membrane
   iii. Amount of hemoglobin in the blood
   iv. Diffusion coefficient of gas
   v. Driving pressures: the difference between alveolar gas tensions and pulmonary capillary gas tensions. This is the force that causes gases to diffuse across membranes

Alveolar Gas	Alveolar-Capillary Membrane	Pulmonary Capillaries
PA_{O_2} 104 mm Hg	$\xrightarrow{\text{diffusion}}$	$P\bar{v}_{O_2}$ 40 mm Hg
Pa_{CO_2} 40 mm Hg	$\xleftarrow{\text{diffusion}}$	$P\bar{v}_{CO_2}$ 45 mm Hg

(a) During breathing of 100% oxygen, the PA_{O_2} (alveolar oxygen tension) becomes so large that the difference between PA_{O_2} and mixed venous oxygen tension ($P\overline{v}_{O_2}$) significantly increases, proportionately increasing the driving pressure

   (b) Therefore, hypoxemia due solely to diffusion defects is improved by breathing 100% oxygen

d. The A–a gradient ($PA_{O_2} - Pa_{O_2}$) is the alveolar-arterial oxygen pressure difference, that is, the difference in partial pressure of oxygen in the alveolar gas spaces and the pressure in the systemic arterial blood. This gradient is always a positive number

   i. The normal gradient in young adults is less than 10 mm Hg (on room air) but increases with age and may be as high as 20 mm Hg in persons older than age 60

   ii. The A–a gradient provides an index of how efficient the lung is in equilibrating pulmonary capillary oxygen with alveolar oxygen. It indicates whether gas transfer is normal

   iii. A large A–a gradient generally indicates that the lung is the site of dysfunction (except when cardiac right-to-left shunting is present)

   iv. Formula for calculation (on room air)

$$A\text{–a gradient} = PA_{O_2} - Pa_{O_2}$$
$$PA_{O_2} = PI_{O_2} - (Pa_{CO_2} \div 0.8)$$
$$PI_{O_2} = (P_B - 47) \times FI_{O_2}$$

where

47 mm Hg = vapor pressure of water at 37° C
PI_{O_2} = pressure of inspired oxygen
0.8 = assumed respiratory quotient (ratio of CO_2 produced to O_2 consumed per unit time)
FI_{O_2} = fraction (percent) of inspired oxygen

Therefore

$$FI_{O_2} \ (P_B - 47) - (Pa_{CO_2} \div 0.8) - Pa_{O_2} = A\text{–a gradient}$$

Example of calculation

$$0.21 (760 - 47) - \quad (40 \div 0.8) - \quad 90 \ = 10$$

   v. Normally, values for A–a gradient increase with age and with increased FI_{O_2}

   vi. Pathologic conditions causing increased A–a gradient
      (a) Ventilation–perfusion ($\dot{V}/\dot{Q}$) mismatching
      (b) Shunting
      (c) Diffusion abnormalities

3. **Step 3—Transport of gases in the circulation**
   a. Approximately 97% of oxygen is transported in chemical combination with hemoglobin (Hb) in the erythrocyte and 3% is carried dissolved in the plasma. Pa_{O_2} is a measurement of the oxygen carried in the

plasma and is a reflection of the driving pressure that causes oxygen to dissolve in the plasma and combine with hemoglobin. Thus oxygen content is related to Pa_{O_2}

b. Oxyhemoglobin dissociation curve (Fig. 1–4)

    i. The relationship between oxygen saturation (and content) and the Pa_{O_2} is expressed in an S-shaped curve that has great physiologic significance. It describes the ability of hemoglobin to bind oxygen at normal arterial oxygen tension levels and release it at lower P_{O_2} levels

    ii. The relationship between content and pressure of oxygen in the blood is not linear

        (a) The upper flat portion of the curve is the arterial-association portion. This protects the body by enabling hemoglobin to load oxygen despite large decreases in Pa_{O_2}

        (b) The lower steep portion of the curve is the venous-dissociation portion. This protects the body by enabling the tissues to withdraw large amounts of oxygen with small decreases in P_{O_2}

    iii. Hemoglobin–oxygen binding is sensitive to oxygen tension. The binding is reversible; affinity of hemoglobin for oxygen changes as the P_{O_2} changes

        (a) When P_{O_2} is increased (as in pulmonary capillaries), oxygen binds readily with hemoglobin

        (b) When P_{O_2} is decreased (as in tissues), oxygen unloads from hemoglobin

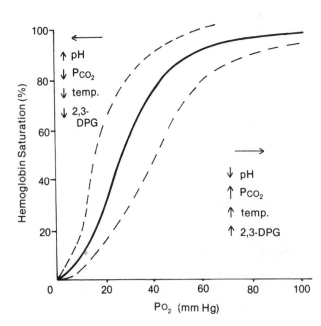

Figure 1–4. The oxyhemoglobin dissociation curve, relating percent hemoglobin saturation and P_{O_2}. The normal curve is shown with a solid line; the curves shifted to the right or left (along with the conditions leading to them) are shown with dotted lines. (From Weinberger, S.E.: Principles of Pulmonary Medicine. W.B. Saunders Co., Philadelphia, 1986, p. 12.)

      iv. Increase in rate of oxygen use by tissues causes an automatic increase in rate of oxygen release from hemoglobin

      v. Shifts of the oxyhemoglobin dissociation curve

        (a) Shifts to the right—more oxygen unloaded for a given P_{O_2}, thus increasing oxygen delivery to tissues. These shifts are caused by

          (1) pH decrease (acidosis), the Bohr effect

          (2) P_{CO_2} increase

          (3) Increase in body temperature

          (4) Increased levels of 2,3-diphosphoglycerate

        (b) Shifts to the left—oxygen not dissociated from hemoglobin until tissue and capillary oxygen levels are very low, thus decreasing oxygen delivery to tissues. These shifts are caused by

          (1) pH increase (alkalosis), the Bohr effect

          (2) P_{CO_2} decrease

          (3) Temperature decrease

          (4) Decreased levels of 2,3-diphosphoglycerate

          (5) Carbon monoxide poisoning

        (c) 2,3-diphosphoglycerate (2,3-DPG) is an intermediate metabolite of glucose that facilitates dissociation of oxygen from hemoglobin at tissues. Decreased levels of 2,3-DPG impair oxygen release to tissues. This may occur with massive transfusions of 2,3-DPG–depleted blood

  c. Hemoglobin's ability to release oxygen to the tissues is commonly assessed by the P_{50}

      i. P_{50}—the partial pressure of oxygen at which the hemoglobin is 50% saturated.

      ii. Normal P_{50} is about 26.6 mm Hg with variability based on disease process

  d. Each gram of normal hemoglobin can maximally combine with 1.34 ml of oxygen when fully saturated (the value 1.39 ml is also used)

  e. The amount of oxygen transported per minute in the circulation is a factor of both the oxygen content (Ca_{O_2}) and the cardiac output (CO). This amount reflects how much oxygen is delivered to the tissues per minute and is dependent on the interaction of the circulatory system (delivery of arterial blood), erythropoietic system (hemoglobin in erythrocyte), and respiratory system (gas exchange) according to the following equations

      i. Oxygen content (Ca_{O_2}) is calculated from oxygen saturation, oxygen capacity, and the dissolved oxygen

        (a) Oxygen capacity is the maximal amount of oxygen the blood can carry. It is expressed in milliliters of oxygen per deciliter of blood and is calculated by multiplying the hemoglobin in grams by 1.34

   (b) Oxygen saturation is the per cent of hemoglobin actually saturated with oxygen (Sa_{O_2} or $S\bar{v}_{O_2}$) and is usually measured directly. It is equal to the oxygen content divided by the oxygen capacity times 100

   (c) Oxygen content is the actual amount of oxygen the blood is carrying (oxyhemoglobin + dissolved oxygen)

$$O_2 \text{ content} = (O_2 \text{ capacity} \times O_2 \text{ saturation}) + (0.0031 \times Pa_{O_2})$$

ii. Systemic oxygen transport (ml/min) = arterial oxygen content (ml/dl) × cardiac output (L/min) × 10 (conversion factor)

   (a) Normal cardiac output = about 6 L/min (range of 4–8)

   (b) Normal arterial oxygen content = about 20 ml/dl

   (c) Therefore, systemic oxygen transport averages 1000 to 1200 ml/min

f. Focusing only on the oxygen tension of the blood is unwise because an underestimation of the severity of hypoxemia may result. Oxygen content and transport are more reliable parameters because they consider hemoglobin values and cardiac output

g. Arterial–mixed venous differences in oxygen content ($Ca_{O_2} - C\bar{v}_{O_2}$) is the difference between arterial oxygen content (Ca_{O_2}) and mixed venous oxygen content ($C\bar{v}_{O_2}$) and reflects the actual amount of oxygen extracted from the blood during its passage through the tissues

   i. Of the 1000 to 1200 ml of oxygen delivered per minute to the tissues, the cells use only 250 to 300 ml ($\dot{V}_{O_2}$ or oxygen consumption). If $\dot{V}_{O_2}$ remains constant, changes in cardiac output can be related to changes in $Ca_{O_2} - C\bar{v}_{O_2}$. Mixed venous oxygen values are measured from pulmonary artery catheters

   (a) Normal $Ca_{O_2} - C\bar{v}_{O_2}$ is 4.5 to 6 ml/dl

$$(Hb \times 1.34)(Sa_{O_2} - S\bar{v}_{O_2}) + (Pa_{O_2} - P\bar{v}_{O_2})(0.0031)$$

   (b) A fall in $C\bar{v}_{O_2}$ resulting in a rise in $Ca_{O_2} - C\bar{v}_{O_2}$ signifies decreased cardiac output and inadequate tissue perfusion

   (c) These values are average values because the actual oxygen use changes with different tissues. The heart uses almost all the oxygen it receives

h. Carbon dioxide transport: carbon dioxide is carried in the blood in three forms

   i. Physically dissolved carbon dioxide (Pa_{CO_2}), which accounts for 7% to 10% of carbon dioxide transported in the blood

   ii. Chemically combined with hemoglobin as carbaminohemoglobin. This reaction occurs rapidly, and reduced hemoglobin can bind more carbon dioxide than oxyhemoglobin. Thus unloading of oxygen facilitates loading of carbon dioxide (Haldane effect) and accounts for about 30% of carbon dioxide transport

iii. As bicarbonate through a conversion reaction

$$CO_2 + H_2O \overset{CA}{\longleftrightarrow} H_2CO_3 \longleftrightarrow H^+ + (\text{Hb buffer}) + HCO_3^-$$

(a) This reaction accounts for 60% to 70% of carbon dioxide in the body

(b) The reaction is slow in the plasma and fast in the erythrocyte, owing to the enzyme carbonic anhydrase

(c) When the concentration of these ions increases in the erythrocyte, bicarbonate (HCO_3^-) diffuses but hydrogen (H^+) remains

(d) In order to maintain electrical neutrality, chloride diffuses from the plasma—the "chloride shift"

i. Pulmonary circulation (pulmonary artery, arterioles, capillary network, venules, and veins)

i. Pulmonary vessels are peculiarly suited to maintaining a delicate balance of flow and pressure distribution that optimizes gas exchange. They are richly innervated by the sympathetic branch of the autonomic nervous system

ii. The pulmonary circulation is a low resistance system when compared with systemic circulation. Pulmonary arteries have far thinner walls than do systemic arteries, and vessels distend to allow for increases in volume from systemic circulation. Intrapulmonary blood volume increases or decreases of approximately 50% occur with changes in the relationship between intrathoracic and extrathoracic pressure

iii. In upright positions, the volume of blood within the pulmonary capillaries is normally equal to the stroke volume of the heart

iv. Pulmonary arteries accompany bronchi within the lung and give rise to a rich capillary network within the alveolar walls. Pulmonary veins are not situated contiguously with the bronchial tree

v. The primary function of the pulmonary circulation is to act as a transport system

(a) Transport of blood through the lung

(1) Flow resistance through vessels is defined by Ohm's law

$$R = \frac{\Delta P}{F}$$

where ΔP is the difference between upstream and downstream pressures and F is flow. The driving pressure for flow in the pulmonary circulation is the difference between the inflow pressure in the pulmonary artery and the outflow pressure in the left atrium

(2) In the lung the measurement of flow resistance is the pulmonary vascular resistance (PVR). PVR = mean pulmonary arterial pressure minus mean left atrial (or pulmonary wedge) pressure divided by cardiac output

(3) About 12% of the total blood volume of the body is in the pulmonary circulation at any one time

(4) Normal pressures in pulmonary vasculature
   a) Mean pulmonary artery pressure is 10 to 15 mm Hg
   b) Mean pulmonary venous pressure is 4 to 12 mm Hg
   c) Mean pressure gradient is therefore about 10 mm Hg (considerably less than systemic gradient)
   d) Pressures are higher at the base of the lung than at the apex

(5) A unique characteristic of the pulmonary arterial bed is that it constricts in response to hypoxia. Diffuse alveolar hypoxia causes generalized vasoconstriction, resulting in pulmonary hypertension. Localized hypoxia causes localized vasoconstriction that does not increase pulmonary hypertension. This localized vasoconstriction directs blood away from poorly ventilated alveoli, thus improving overall gas exchange

(6) Chronic pulmonary hypertension (↑ PVR) can result in right ventricular hypertrophy (cor pulmonale)

(b) Transvascular transport of fluids and solutes
   (1) Transvascular fluid filtration in the lung (and in all other organs) is described by the Starling equation. Simply stated, this means that fluid and solutes move because of increases or decreases in hydrostatic or osmotic filtration pressures or because of changes in the permeability of the vessel walls to fluids or proteins
   (2) Thus, excess fluid in lung (pulmonary edema) can occur due to a net increase in pressure forces favoring filtration or a decreased resistance to filtration

(c) Metabolic transport
   (1) All cardiac output passes through the lung prior to reaching the systemic circulation. Therefore, the pulmonary circulation can influence the composition of the blood supplying all organs
   (2) Several humoral substances are added, extracted, or metabolized in the lung. Examples are the inactivation

Figure 1–5. Diffusion of oxygen from a tissue capillary to the cells. (From Guyton, A.C.: Textbook of Medical Physiology, 7th ed. W.B. Saunders Co., Philadelphia, 1986, p. 494.)

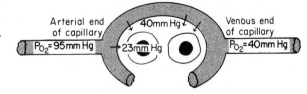

of vasoactive prostaglandins, conversion of angiotensin I to angiotensin II, and inactivation of bradykinin

4. **Step 4—Diffusion between systemic capillary bed and body tissue cells**
   a. Pressure gradients allow for diffusion of oxygen and carbon dioxide among systemic capillaries, interstitial fluid, and cells (Figs. 1–5 and 1–6)
   b. Within the mitochondria of each individual cell, oxygen is consumed through aerobic metabolism. This process produces the energy bonds of adenosine triphosphate (ATP) and the waste products of carbon dioxide and water

Hypoxemia: A state in which the oxygen pressure or saturation of oxygen in arterial blood or both is lower than normal values. Hypoxemia is generally defined as an Sa_{O_2} below 90 mm Hg at sea level in an adult breathing room air. Disorders that lead to hypoxemia do so through one or more of the following processes

1. **Low inspired oxygen tension**
   a. Because of reduced ambient pressure (P_B) or reduced oxygen concentration of inspired air (FI_{O_2})
   b. If lungs are normal, A–a gradient will be normal
   c. This is rarely a clinically important cause of arterial hypoxemia. It occurs at high altitudes among normal humans
2. **Alveolar hypoventilation ($\uparrow Pa_{CO_2}$)**
   a. A decrease in alveolar ventilation from disorders of the respiratory center, peripheral nerves that supply muscles of respiration, respiratory muscles of chest wall, or lungs
   b. This causes an increase in Pa_{CO_2}, resulting in a fall in PA_{O_2}
   c. If the lungs are normal, the A–a gradient will be normal. Hypoxemia will improve with ventilation
3. **Mismatching of ventilation ($\dot{V}$) to perfusion ($\dot{Q}$): ($\dot{V}/\dot{Q}$ abnormalities)**

Figure 1–6. Uptake of carbon dioxide by the blood in the capillaries. (From Guyton, A.C.: Textbook of Medical Physiology, 7th ed. W.B. Saunders Co., Philadelphia, 1986, p. 495.)

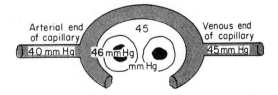

a. This is the most common cause of hypoxemia. A–a gradient will be increased
b. Ideally, ventilation of each alveolus is accompanied by a comparable amount of perfusion, yielding a $\dot{V}/\dot{Q}$ ratio of 1.00. Usually, however, there is relatively more perfusion than ventilation, yielding a normal $\dot{V}/\dot{Q}$ ratio of 0.8. The normal amount of blood perfusing alveoli ($\dot{Q}$) is 5 L/min, and the normal amount of air ventilating the alveoli ($\dot{V}$) is 4 L/min. Figure 1–7 represents a simplification of possible relationships between ventilation and perfusion in the lung
c. When the $\dot{V}/\dot{Q}$ ratio is decreased (less than 0.8), a decrease of

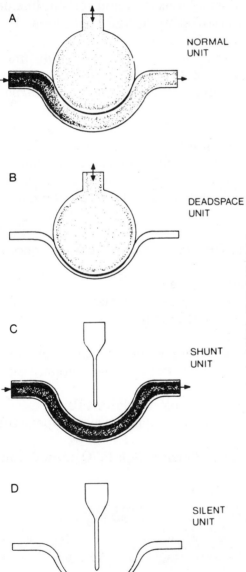

A

NORMAL
UNIT

B

DEADSPACE
UNIT

C

SHUNT
UNIT

D

SILENT
UNIT

Figure 1–7. The theoretical respiratory unit. *A.* Normal ventilation, normal perfusion. *B.* Normal ventilation, no perfusion. *C.* No ventilation, normal perfusion. *D.* No ventilation, no perfusion. (Reproduced with permission from Shapiro, B.A., et al.: Clinical Application of Blood Gases, 3rd ed., Year Book Medical Publishers, Inc., Chicago, 1982, p. 65.)

ventilation in relation to perfusion has occurred. This is similar to a right-to-left shunt because more deoxygenated blood is returning to the left side of the heart. Low $\dot{V}/\dot{Q}$ ratios and hypoxemia occur together, since good areas of the lung cannot be overventilated to compensate for the underventilated areas (hemoglobin cannot be saturated more than 100%). Atelectasis is an example of such a condition

d. When the $\dot{V}/\dot{Q}$ ratio is increased (greater than 0.8), a decreased perfusion in relation to ventilation has occurred, the equivalent to dead space or wasted ventilation. Examples of such disease states are pulmonary emboli and cardiogenic shock

e. Hypoxemia that is due to $\dot{V}/\dot{Q}$ mismatch may be corrected by giving the patient 100% oxygen for 10 to 15 minutes (all nitrogen is washed out, leaving only oxygen and carbon dioxide in alveoli)

4. **Shunting**

a. Shunting occurs when a portion of the venous blood does not participate in gas exchange. An anatomic shunt may occur (a portion of right ventricular blood does not pass through pulmonary capillaries) or a portion of pulmonary capillary blood flow may pass adjacent to airless alveoli

b. Normal physiologic shunting amounts to 2% to 5% of cardiac output (this is bronchial and thebesian vein blood)

c. Shunting occurs in arteriovenous malformations, adult respiratory distress syndrome, atelectasis, pneumonia, pulmonary edema, pulmonary embolus, vascular lung tumors, and intracardiac right-to-left shunts

d. Breathing 100% oxygen will not correct shunting, since all blood does not come into contact with open alveoli, and the shunted blood passes directly from the pulmonary veins to the arterial blood (venous admixture). The lack of improvement of hypoxemia with oxygen therapy is a hallmark of shunting. Shunting is the only cause of hypoxemia that cannot be corrected by the administration of 100% oxygen

e. Usually, shunting does not result in elevated Pa_{CO_2}, even though shunted blood is rich in carbon dioxide. Brain chemoreceptors sense elevated Pa_{CO_2} levels and respond by increasing ventilation

f. Shunting is measured by comparing mixed venous oxygen (from pulmonary artery catheter) to arterial oxygen ($Ca_{O_2} - C\bar{v}_{O_2}$). The amount of true shunt can be estimated by having patient breathe 100% oxygen for 15 minutes, thus eliminating effects of abnormal ventilation–perfusion and diffusion defects. Normal shunt is 5 ml/dl

5. **Diffusion defects**

a. Seen in patients with thickened alveolar-capillary membrane, as in pulmonary fibrosis, so that a larger distance between alveolar gas and pulmonary capillaries exists

   b. May be overcome by diffusion because rate of diffusion always
      depends on the pressure gradient
   c. Is rarely a cause of hypoxemia by itself but may contribute to
      hypoxemia in patients with ventilation–perfusion and/or shunting

Acid–Base Physiology and Blood Gases

1. **Terminology**
   a. Acid: a donator of hydrogen ions (H^+); any substance with a pH of
      less than 7.0
   b. Acidemia: the condition of the blood with a pH below 7.35
   c. Acidosis: the process, be it metabolic or respiratory, that causes the
      acidemia
   d. Base: an acceptor of hydrogen ions; any substance with a pH of
      greater than 7.0
   e. Alkalemia: the condition of blood with a pH above 7.45
   f. Alkalosis: the process, be it metabolic or respiratory, that causes the
      alkalemia
   g. pH: the negative logarithm of hydrogen ion concentration
        i. Increase in $[H^+]$ = lower pH, more acidic
       ii. Decrease in $[H^+]$ = higher pH, more alkaline
2. **Buffering:** a normal body mechanism that occurs rapidly in response to
   acid–base disturbances in order to prevent changes in $[H^+]$ concentration
   a. Bicarbonate (HCO_3^-) buffer system

$$(H^+) + HCO_3^- \longleftrightarrow H_2CO_3 \longleftrightarrow CO_2 + H_2O$$

   This system is very important because bicarbonate can be regulated
   by the kidneys and carbon dioxide by the lungs
   b. Phosphate system
   c. Hemoglobin and other proteins
3. **Henderson-Hasselbalch equation:** defines relationship between pH,
   P_{CO_2}, and bicarbonate. Arterial pH is determined by the logarithm of
   the ratio of bicarbonate concentration to arterial P_{CO_2}. Bicarbonate is
   regulated mainly by the kidney, and P_{CO_2} is regulated by alveolar
   ventilation

$$pH = pK + \log \frac{[HCO_3^-]}{Pa_{CO_2}}$$

$$pK = \text{a constant (6.1)}$$

   a. As long as the ratio of bicarbonate to carbon dioxide is about 20:1,
      the pH of the blood will be normal. It is this ratio that determines
      blood pH, rather than the absolute values of each
   b. The pH must be maintained within a narrow range of normal because
      the functioning of most enzymatic systems in the body is dependent
      on the hydrogen ion concentration (Fig. 1–8)

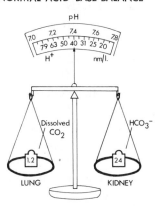

NORMAL ACID-BASE BALANCE

Figure 1–8. The balance between bicarbonate (24) and dissolved CO_2 (1.2 of $Pa_{CO_2} = 40$) is normally 20:1, and this is usually associated with a pH of about 7.40 and a H^+ concentration of about 40 nmol/L. (From Cherniack, R.M., and Cherniack, L.: Respiration in Health and Disease, 3rd ed. W.B. Saunders Co., Philadelphia, 1983, p. 85.)

4. Normal adult blood gas values (at sea level)

	Arterial	**Mixed Venous**
pH	7.40 (7.35–7.45)	7.36 (7.31–7.41)
P_{O_2}	80–100 mm Hg	35–40 mm Hg
S_{O_2}	95% or more	70%–75%
P_{CO_2}	35–45 mm Hg	41–51 mm Hg
HCO_3^-	22–26 mEq/L	22–26 mEq/L
Base excess	−2 to +2	−2 to +2

Note: Knowledge of blood gas values neither supersedes nor replaces sound clinical judgment

5. Effect of altitude on blood gas values

a. P_{O_2} and Sa_{O_2} are lower at high altitudes because of a lower ambient oxygen tension

b. Normal for 5280 ft (Denver) = Pa_{O_2} of 65–75 mm Hg, Sa_{O_2} of 94%–95%

6. Respiratory parameter (Pa_{CO_2}). If the primary disturbance is in the P_{CO_2}, the patient is said to have a respiratory disturbance

a. Pa_{CO_2} is a reflection of alveolar ventilation

    i. if Pa_{CO_2} is elevated, hypoventilation is present

    ii. If Pa_{CO_2} is decreased, hyperventilation is present

    iii. If Pa_{CO_2} is normal, adequate ventilation is present

    iv. Measurements of Pa_{CO_2} should be accompanied by measurements of minute ventilation to assess relationships

b. Respiratory acidosis (elevated Pa_{CO_2}), caused by hypoventilation of any etiology (may be acute or chronic). Treatment generally consists of improving alveolar ventilation

    i. Obstructive lung disease and other lung disease

    ii. Oversedation, head trauma, anesthesia and drug overdose

      iii. Neuromuscular disease

      iv. Inappropriate mechanical ventilation

  c. Respiratory alkalosis (low Pa_{CO_2}) caused by hyperventilation of any etiology. Treatment consists of correcting the underlying cause

      i. Hypoxemia from any cause

      ii. Nervousness and anxiety

      iii. Pulmonary embolus

      iv. Pregnancy

      v. Hyperventilation with mechanical ventilator

      vi. Restrictive lung disease

      vii. Response to metabolic acidosis (diabetic ketoacidosis)

      viii. Bacteremia or fever

      ix. Central nervous system disturbances

      x. Respiratory stimulant drugs

7. Nonrespiratory (renal) parameter (bicarbonate). If the primary disturbance is in the bicarbonate level, the patient is said to have a metabolic disturbance

  a. Concentration influenced by metabolic processes

      i. When bicarbonate is elevated, metabolic alkalosis occurs

        (a) Loss of nonvolatile acid

        (b) Or, bicarbonate is gained

      ii. When bicarbonate is decreased, metabolic acidosis occurs

        (a) Hydrogen is added in excess of capacity of kidney to excrete it

        (b) Or, bicarbonate is lost at rate exceeding capacity of kidney to regenerate it

  b. Causes of metabolic alkalosis (elevated bicarbonate)

      i. Chloride depletion (vomiting, prolonged nasogastric suctioning, diarrhea, diuretic therapy)

      ii. Cushing's syndrome, aldosteronism, potassium deficiency, administration of antacids

  c. Causes of metabolic acidosis (decreased bicarbonate)

      i. Increase in unmeasurable anions (acids that accumulate in certain diseases and poisonings); high anion gap

        (a) Diabetic ketoacidosis, starvation

        (b) Drugs

          (1) Salicylates

          (2) Ethylene glycol

          (3) Methyl alcohol

          (4) Paraldehyde

        (c) Lactic acidosis due to anaerobic metabolism (shock, sepsis)

        (d) Renal failure, uremia

      ii. No increase in unmeasurable anions; normal anion gap

        (a) Diarrhea

        (b) Drainage of pancreatic juices

(c) Ureterosigmoidostomy
(d) Rapid intravenous infusion
(e) Renal tubular acidosis
(f) Certain drugs
(g) Hyperalimentation

8. **Compensation for acid–base abnormalities:** a physiologic response of the body to minimize pH changes by maintaining a normal bicarbonate to P_{CO_2} ratio
   a. pH is returned to near normal by changing the component that is not primarily affected
   b. Respiratory disturbances result in kidney compensation, which may take several days to become maximal
      i. Compensation for respiratory acidosis
         (a) Kidneys excrete more acid
         (b) Kidneys increase bicarbonate reabsorption
         (c) Compensation is slow (days)
      ii. Compensation for respiratory alkalosis
         (a) Kidneys excrete bicarbonate
         (b) Compensation is slow (days)
   c. Metabolic disturbances result in pulmonary compensation, which begins within minutes but takes several hours to become maximal
      i. Compensation for metabolic acidosis
         (a) Hyperventilation to decrease Pa_{CO_2}
         (b) Compensation is rapid (minutes to hours)
      ii. Compensation for metabolic alkalosis
         (a) Hypoventilation (limited by fall in Pa_{CO_2})
         (b) Compensation is rapid (minutes to hours)
   d. The body does not overcompensate. Therefore, the acidity or alkalinity of the pH will identify the primary abnormality, if there is only one. Abnormalities may be multiple; each is not a discrete entity. Mixed acid–base disturbances occur commonly

9. **Correction of acid–base abnormalities:** caused by a physiologic or therapeutic response
   a. pH returned to normal by altering component primarily affected; blood gas values are returned to normal
   b. Correction for respiratory acidosis—increase ventilation; treat cause
   c. Correction for respiratory alkalosis—decrease ventilation; treat cause
   d. Correction for metabolic acidosis
      i. Treat cause
      ii. Administer bicarbonate intravenously or orally
   e. Correction for metabolic alkalosis
      i. Treat cause
      ii. Administer chloride (isotonic saline or potassium chloride)

      iii. Arginine monohydrochloride, ammonium chloride, or acetazol-amide are used in rare circumstances

10. Arterial blood gas analysis
  a. Purpose of analysis
      i. Shows end result of what occurs in lung
      ii. Confirms presence of respiratory failure and indicates acid–base status
      iii. Absolutely necessary in monitoring patients in acute respiratory failure and patients on ventilators
  b. Main components: Pa_{O_2}, Pa_{CO_2}, pH, base excess, bicarbonate, Sa_{O_2}, oxygen content, hemoglobin. Both FI_{O_2} and body temperature must be measured for interpretation

11. Guidelines for interpretation of arterial blood gases and acid–base balance
  a. Examine the pH first
      i. If pH is reduced (below 7.35), patient is acidemic
        (a) If Pa_{CO_2} is elevated, the patient has a respiratory acidosis
        (b) If bicarbonate is reduced, patient has a metabolic acidosis
        (c) If Pa_{CO_2} is elevated and bicarbonate is reduced, the patient has combined respiratory and metabolic acidosis
      ii. If pH is elevated (above 7.45), patient is alkalemic
        (a) If Pa_{CO_2} is decreased, patient has respiratory alkalosis
        (b) If bicarbonate is elevated, patient has metabolic alkalosis
        (c) If Pa_{CO_2} is decreased and bicarbonate is elevated, patient has a combined metabolic and respiratory alkalosis
      iii. Expected change in pH for changes in Pa_{CO_2}: a commonly used rule is that the pH will rise or fall 0.08 (or 0.1) in the appropriate direction for each change of 10 mm Hg in the Pa_{CO_2}
      iv. If the pH is normal (7.35–7.45), alkalosis or acidosis may still be present as a mixed disorder
  b. Assess hypoxemic state and tissue oxygenation state
      i. If patient is breathing room air and Pa_{O_2} is below 80 mm Hg, patient is hypoxemic. If Pa_{O_2} is below 40, hypoxemia is severe and should be corrected
      ii. If patient is receiving oxygen therapy, Pa_{O_2} values must be interpreted in terms of minimally predicted limits for the FI_{O_2} administered. Multiplying the FI_{O_2} in percent by 5 will generally give a rough approximation of the P_{O_2} expected for that oxygen therapy. A better way to assess the oxygen therapy is to use the following formula to calculate alveolar P_{O_2}

$$PA_{O_2} = [(P_B - 47) \times FI_{O_2}] - Pa_{CO_2} \times 1.25$$

where

$$PA_{O_2} = \text{alveolar } P_{O_2}$$

P_B = barometric pressure

47 = vapor pressure of water at 37°C

Although as discussed earlier in the section on A–a gradient, PA_{O_2} differs from Pa_{O_2}, the above equation still gives one an estimate of expected Pa_{O_2} for a given oxygen therapy

iii. Excessive Pa_{O_2} (above 100 mm Hg) is generally not warranted and oxygen delivery should be reduced

iv. Assessment of cardiac output and oxygen transport will determine tissue oxygenation. $P\overline{v}_{O_2}$ is the best guide to adequacy of tissue oxygenation

v. Effectiveness of oxygen transport may be judged clinically by examining the patient carefully for mental status, skin color, urine output, and heart rate

NURSING ASSESSMENT DATA BASE

Nursing History: The sequence and length of the standard history-taking process is modified as needed for acutely ill patients

1. **Client health history:** the patient's interpretation of his signs and symptoms and his emotional response to them play a significant role in the development or exacerbation of symptoms

   a. Common symptoms

      i. Dyspnea: the subjective feeling of shortness of breath or breathlessness

         (a) Difficult to quantify objectively

            (1) Count the average number of words the patient is able to speak between breaths

            (2) Ask the patient to rate his breathing comfort on a visual analog scale or on a scale from 1 to 10

         (b) Emotional problems may cause an increased awareness of respirations and complaints of inability to get enough air, despite normal blood gas values

         (c) Dyspnea due to increased work of breathing accompanies both obstructive and restrictive lung diseases, as well as accompanying dysfunction of nerves, respiratory muscles, or thoracic cage

         (d) Question patient regarding his exercise tolerance; some dyspnea is normal with exercise but abnormal if exercise tolerance is decreased

         (e) Assess whether patient's dyspnea is acute or chronic, and determine if it has increased or decreased lately

         (f) Determine all circumstances under which dyspnea occurs (activities such as walking, stair climbing, eating) as well as how long patient has experienced dyspnea with those activities

      (g) To assess orthopnea (dyspnea when lying supine), question patient as to how many pillows he usually sleeps on when in bed

      (h) Assess for paroxysmal nocturnal dyspnea by questioning patient if dyspnea has ever awakened him from sleep

      (i) Determine if dyspnea is accompanied by other symptoms, such as cough, wheezing, or chest pain

      (j) Differentiation of cardiac versus pulmonary dyspnea is difficult in some patients

  ii. Cough: a normal occurrence in some circumstances, as a lung defense mechanism

      (a) Determine if cough is acute and self-limiting or chronic and persistent

      (b) Note change in character and frequency

      (c) Determine timing (both daily and seasonal), and whether accompanied by sputum production, hemoptysis, wheezing, chest pain, or dyspnea

      (d) Most common etiologies

         (1) Inhaled irritants

         (2) Aspiration

         (3) Airways diseases (i.e., asthma, acute or chronic bronchitis)

         (4) Lung diseases (i.e., pneumonia, lung abscess, tumor)

         (5) Left ventricular failure

 iii. Sputum production

      (a) Quantify amount by asking in terms of how many teaspoons or shot glasses of sputum are coughed up daily

      (b) Determine aggravating and alleviating factors

      (c) Grossly assess character of sputum, noting color, odor, and consistency

      (d) Determine if sputum's current characteristics (quantity and quality) are changed from usual

  iv. Hemoptysis: the expectoration of blood from the lungs or airways

      (a) Determine if material coughed up is grossly bloody, blood streaked, or blood tinged (pink colored)

      (b) Try to differentiate from hematemesis. Hemoptysis is often frothy, alkaline, and accompanied by sputum, whereas hematemesis is nonfrothy, acidic, and dark red or brown, with food particles

      (c) Determine approximate amount of hemoptysis, using a reasonable measurement guideline such as how many teaspoons or shot glasses per day. Assess whether all expectorated specimens contained blood or whether this was an isolated event

       (d) Blood may originate from the nasopharynx, the airways, or the lung parenchyma; blood from these sites remains red due to the contact with atmospheric oxygen

       (e) The etiologies of hemoptysis fall into three categories by location: airways, pulmonary parenchyma, and vasculature

          (1) Airways disease—most common: bronchitis, bronchiectasis and bronchogenic carcinoma

          (2) Parenchymal causes—often infectious: tuberculosis, lung abscess, pneumonia

          (3) Vascular lesions—pulmonary embolism, pulmonary edema, arteriovenous malformation

       (f) Suspect neoplasm if hemoptysis occurs in patient without prior respiratory symptoms

    v. Chest pain: as a reflection of the respiratory system it does not originate in the lung, since the lung is free of sensory nerve fibers

       (a) Chest wall pain—arises from the parietal pleura, intercostal muscles, ribs, or overlying skin

          (1) Well localized

          (2) Often exacerbated by deep inspiration

       (b) Diaphragm pain—often caused by inflammatory process

          (1) Pain is often referred to the ipsilateral shoulder

       (c) Mediastinal pain—caused by mass or air under the mediastinum (pneumomediastinum)

          (1) Pain is substernal and dull

b. Miscellaneous symptoms of respiratory disease: nasal symptoms, postnasal drip, sinus pain, epistaxis, hoarseness, general fatigue, weight loss, fever, sleep disturbances, night sweats, anxiety and nervousness, appetite depression

c. Past medical history

    i. Question patient regarding presence of any allergies to either medications or food. Obtain description of type and severity of reaction

    ii. Determine past instances of present illness, with the treatment and outcome. Assess for previous episodes of, or exposure to, tuberculosis or positive skin tests. Record the treatment given (if any) and length of time patient stayed on medications

    iii. Past surgeries or hospitalizations: record dates, hospital, diagnosis, and complications and previous use of oxygen or mechanical ventilation

    iv. Previous chest x-ray films

       (a) Date of last examination

       (b) Reason for last examination and findings

    v. Previous pulmonary function tests, and results if known

2. **Family history** (extremely important)
    a. Assess for similar illness or signs and symptoms in patient's parents, siblings, and grandparents
    b. Determine current state of health or cause of death for parents, siblings, and grandparents
    c. There is often a familial history of diseases such as asthma, cystic fibrosis, bronchiectasis, and alpha$_1$-antitrypsin deficiency (emphysema)
    d. Determine if family member ever had tuberculosis, with consequent exposure to patient
3. **Social history and habits**
    a. Assess personal status: education, socioeconomic class, marital status, general life satisfaction, interests
    b. Health habits
        i. Smoking: tobacco
            (a) Determine if patient is a current or past smoker
                (1) Calculate pack-year history: number of packs per day × number of years = pack-years
                (2) Determine if patient has tried to stop smoking, and if so, the methods used. Assess patient's desire for information on smoking cessation resources available in the area
            (b) Question if patient has smoked marijuana. If so, quantify how many joints per day
            (c) Determine if patient chews tobacco. Quantify type chewed and amount per day
            (d) If patient is a former smoker, determine the following
                (1) Time since last cigarette
                (2) Pack-year history of habit when patient did smoke
        ii. Drinking habits: determine frequency and amount of consuming the following
            (a) Alcoholic beverages (which type)
            (b) Caffeine-containing beverages
        iii. Eating habits: assess quality of meals, adequacy, or excess
            (a) Determine if any respiratory symptoms occur with eating (i.e., meal-induced dyspnea, cough)
        iv. Drug history: assess intake of any recreational drugs
        v. Sexual history: question patient as to his sexual activity and preference
    c. Home conditions—economic conditions, housing, any pets and their health
        i. Some respiratory symptoms are exacerbated by allergic response to pet dander and house mite debris found in carpeting and bedding
    d. Occupational history—assess past and present work conditions

      i. Determine if there were exposures to heat and cold, industrial toxins, and pollutants. Assess the duration of exposure and whether protective devices were used

4. **Medication history** (both prescription and over-the-counter or home remedy)
   a. Current and recent medications, with their dose and reason for prescribing
   b. Assess if patient is using any inhaled medications
      i. Determine device used: canister inhaler, rotohaler, spinhaler, or nebulizer
      ii. Assess frequency of use: as needed or on a regular schedule
      iii. If possible, have patient demonstrate his technique for inhaling medication
         (a) Many patients with obstructive lung disease use incorrect technique when inhaling their medication. This results in reduced deposition of the drug in the lung, with consequent reduced efficacy. Patients should inhale drug *slowly and deeply* followed by breath holding of at least 10 seconds

Nursing Examination of Patient

1. **Inspection**
   a. Requirements for good inspection
      i. Patient be undressed to the waist and in the seated position, if possible
      ii. Warm room and good lighting
      iii. Thorough knowledge by the examiner of anatomic landmarks and lines
         (a) Manubrium, body and xiphoid process of sternum, right and left sternal borders
         (b) Angle of Louis, point of maximal impulse, suprasternal notch
         (c) Interspaces, ribs, costal margins, costal angle, and spinous processes
         (d) Pulmonary lobes and areas of contact with chest wall
         (e) Lines: midclavicular, midsternal, anterior axillary, midaxillary, posterior axillary, vertebral, and midscapular
   b. Observe the general condition and musculoskeletal development
      i. State of nutrition, debilitation, and evidence of chronic disease
      ii. Pectus carinatum: the sternum protrudes instead of being lower than the adjacent hemithoraces
      iii. Pectus excavatum: the sternum is abnormally depressed between the anterior hemithoraces
      iv. Kyphosis: an exaggerated anteroposterior curvature of the spine
      v. Scoliosis: lateral curvature of the spine, causing widened inter-

costal spaces on the convex side and crowding of the ribs on the concave side; when accompanied by kyphosis, it is called kyphoscoliosis. This condition can result in restrictive lung disease if severe

c. Observe the anteroposterior diameter of the thorax. Normal anteroposterior diameter is approximately one third of the transverse diameter

    i. In patients with obstructive lung disease, the anteroposterior diameter may be as great as or greater than the transverse diameter. This finding is referred to as *barrel chest*

d. Observe the general slope of the ribs

    i. In normal subjects, the ribs are at a 45° angle in relation to the spine; in patients with emphysema, the ribs are more nearly horizontal

e. Observe for asymmetry

    i. One side may be larger because of tension pneumothorax or pleural effusion

    ii. One side may be smaller because of atelectasis or unilateral fibrosis

    iii. If asymmetry is present, the abnormal side will move less than the other

f. Look for retraction or bulging of interspaces

    i. Retraction of the interspaces, which can be observed during inspiration, indicates more negative intrapleural pressure due to obstruction of inflow of air or increased work of breathing

    ii. Bulging of interspaces may result from a large pleural effusion or pneumothorax. It is often seen during a forced expiration in patient with asthma or emphysema

g. Observe the ventilatory pattern

    i. Assess level of dyspnea and work of breathing

        (a) Position in which patient can breathe most comfortably. Patients with obstructive pulmonary disease often assume a forward leaning position, resting arms on knees or a bedside table

        (b) Look for use of accessory muscles of breathing

        (c) Note if patient is using pursed lip breathing

        (d) Observe for flairing of ala nasi during inspiration, which is a common sign of air hunger

        (e) Paradoxic movement of diaphragm

    ii. Assess for presence of inspiratory stridor—low-pitched or crowing inspiratory sounds that occur when the trachea or major bronchi are obstructed because of

        (a) Tumor (intrinsic or extrinsic)

        (b) Foreign body

        (c) Severe laryngotracheitis

      (d) Crushing injury

      (e) Goiter

      (f) Scar or granulation tissue

  iii. Observe for expiratory stridor—low-pitched crowing sound heard on expiration. Possible causes include

      (a) Intrathoracic tracheal or mainstem tumor

      (b) Foreign body

  iv. Observe for unusual movements with breathing; on inspiration the chest and abdomen should expand or rise together

      (a) Paradoxical breathing occurs with respiratory muscle fatigue. On inspiration, the chest rises and the abdomen is drawn in, owing to the fatigued diaphragm not descending on inspiration as it should. Instead the diaphragm is drawn upward by the negative intrathoracic pressure during inspiration

   v. Observe and assess ventilatory pattern

      (a) Eupnea—normal quiet respirations

      (b) Bradypnea—abnormally slow ventilation

      (c) Tachypnea—rapid rate of ventilation

      (d) Hyperpnea—increase in the depth and perhaps the rate of ventilation. The overall result is increased tidal volume and minute ventilation

      (e) Apnea—complete or intermittent cessation of ventilation

      (f) Biot's breathing—two to three short breaths with long irregular periods of apnea

      (g) Cheyne-Stokes respiration—periods of increasing ventilation followed by progressively more shallow ventilations, until apnea occurs. May sometimes occur in normal persons when asleep, it usually indicates

        (1) Central nervous system disease

        (2) Heart failure

  vi. Note splinting of respirations—the act of resisting full inspiration of one or both lungs due to pain

h. Other observations

   i. General state of restlessness, pain, mental status, fright, or acute distress

      (a) Hypoxemia's earliest signs often include change in mental status and restlessness

  ii. If oxygen is being administered, record the amount and method of delivery

  iii. Inspect extremities

      (a) Clubbing of fingers is a sign of a chronic pulmonary or cardiac disease

      (b) Cigarette stains on fingers indicate current smoking habit

      (c) Lower extremity edema may indicate right-sided heart

failure from possible chronic pulmonary disease and hypoxemia-induced pulmonary hypertension

iv. Observe for cyanosis

    (a) The fundamental mechanism of cyanosis is an increase in the amount of reduced (deoxygenated) hemoglobin in the vessels of the skin brought about by

        (1) A decrease in the oxygen saturation of the capillary blood or

        (2) An increase in the amount of venous blood in the skin as a result of the dilation of venules and capillaries

    (b) Visible cyanosis is dependent on the presence of at least 5 g of reduced hemoglobin per deciliter of blood

        (1) This is an absolute, not a relative value. It is not the percentage of deoxygenated hemoglobin that causes cyanosis but the amount of deoxygenated hemoglobin without regard to the amount of oxyhemoglobin. The presence or absence of cyanosis may be an unreliable clinical sign

        (2) In anemia, cyanosis may be difficult to detect because the absolute amount of hemoglobin is too low

        (3) Conversely, patients with marked polycythemia tend to become cyanotic at higher levels of arterial oxygen saturation than do patients with normal hematocrit levels

    (c) Discoloration suggestive of cyanosis may occur in situations of abnormal blood or skin pigments (e.g., methemoglobinemia, sulfhemoglobinemia, argyria)

    (d) Factors influencing cyanosis

        (1) Rate of blood flow, perfusion

        (2) Skin thickness and color

        (3) Amount of hemoglobin

        (4) Cardiac output

        (5) Perception of examiner

    (e) Central versus peripheral cyanosis

        (1) Central cyanosis implies arterial oxygen desaturation or abnormal Hb derivative. Both mucous membrane and skin are affected

        (2) Peripheral cyanosis without central cyanosis may result from slowing of perfusion to body area as in cold exposure, shock, obstruction, and decreased cardiac output. Oxygen saturation may be normal

    (f) In carbon monoxide poisoning, the oxygen saturation may be dangerously low without obvious cyanosis because carboxyhemoglobin may give a cherry-red color to the skin

      v. Assess for neck vein distention, neck masses, and enlarged nodes

      vi. Look for signs of superior vena caval syndrome: distention of neck veins, edema of neck, eyelids, hands. It is often seen in lung cancer

2. Palpation

  a. Palpate thoracic muscles and skeleton, feeling for any of the following

      i. Pulsations, tenderness, bulges, or depressions in chest wall

  b. Expansion of the chest wall

      i. Examiner's hands should be placed over lower lateral aspect of the chest with the thumbs along the costal margin anteriorly or meeting posteriorly in the midline. Note movement of the hands on inspiration and expiration. Asymmetry of movement is abnormal. Reduced chest wall movement is often seen in patients with barrel chests and emphysema

  c. Position and mobility of trachea

      i. Deviations of trachea toward the defect are seen in atelectasis, unilateral pulmonary fibrosis, pneumonectomy, paralysis of hemidiaphragm, and inspiratory phase of flail chest

      ii. Deviations of the trachea to the side opposite the lesion are seen in neck tumors, thyroid enlargement, tension pneumothorax, mediastinal mass, pleural effusion, and expiratory phase of flail chest

  d. Point of maximal impulse—location may indicate mediastinal shift

  e. Palpation of ribs and chest for tenderness, pain, or air in the subcutaneous tissue (crepitus)

  f. Vocal fremitus—a palpable vibration of the chest wall, produced by phonation

      i. Patient should be instructed to say the word "ninety-nine" loud enough so that the fremitus can be felt, and with uniform intensity. In clinical practice, some soft-spoken women may need to falsely lower their voice so the fremitus can be felt. The examiner should place his hands on the chest wall

      ii. Diminished fremitus is a result of any condition that interferes with the transference of vibrations through the chest

        (a) Pleural effusion or thickening

        (b) Pleural tumors or masses

        (c) Pneumothorax with lung collapse

        (d) Obstruction of bronchus (i.e., due to sputum plugs or tumors)

        (e) Emphysema

      iii. Increased fremitus is a result of any condition that increases transmission of vibrations through the chest

        (a) Pneumonia, consolidation

        (b) Atelectasis (with open bronchus)

        (c) Pulmonary infarction

        (d) Pulmonary fibrosis

  g. Pleural friction fremitus

     i. Is produced when inflamed pleural surfaces rub together during respiration

     ii. Produces a "grating" sensation that occurs with the respiratory excursion

    iii. May be palpable during both phases of respiration but sometimes only felt during inspiration

  h. Rhonchal fremitus

     i. Produced by passage of air through thick exudate, secretions, or an area of stenosis in the trachea or major bronchi

     ii. Unlike friction fremitus, rhonchal fremitus can be relieved by coughing, suctioning, or clearing the secretions from the tracheobronchial tree

  i. Subcutaneous emphysema—indicates leak of air under skin from communication with airway, mediastinum, or pneumothorax

     i. May be palpated over area

     ii. On auscultation, may be mistaken for crackles

3. Percussion: the tapping or thumping of parts of the body to produce sound. The nature of the sound produced depends on the density of the structures immediately under the area percussed

  a. Sound vibrations produced by percussion probably do not penetrate more than 4 to 5 cm below the surface; therefore solid masses deep in the chest cannot be outlined with percussion. In addition, since a lesion must be several centimeters in diameter to be detectable by percussion, only large abnormalities can be located

  b. Procedure: percussion is done by striking the dorsal distal third finger of one hand that is held against the thorax with the distal tip of the flexed middle finger of the other hand

     i. The striking finger must strike the stationary finger only instantaneously; it must be withdrawn immediately

     ii. All movement is executed at the wrist

    iii. The examiner must be sensitive to the sounds that are received from the chest wall

    iv. Compare one side of the chest with the other side

     v. For percussion of the posterior chest, the patient should incline his head forward and rest his forearms on his thighs. This posture moves the scapulae laterally

    vi. Percussion begins at the apices and continues downward to the bases, alternating side to side

  c. Percussion sounds over the lung

     i. Resonance: the sound heard normally over lungs

     ii. Hyperresonance: the sound heard over lungs of normal children, in the apices of the lungs relative to the base in an upright adult, and throughout lung fields in adults with emphysema or pneumothorax

    (a) Lower in pitch than normal resonance

    (b) Relatively intense and easy to hear

    (c) Indicates increased air (less dense)

  iii. Tympany: produced by air in an enclosed chamber; it does not occur in the normal chest, except below the dome of the left hemidiaphragm, where it is produced by air in the underlying stomach or bowel

    (a) Relatively musical sound

    (b) Usually higher pitched than that of normal resonance; the higher the tension within the viscus, the higher the pitch

  iv. Dullness: the sound heard with lung consolidation, atelectasis, masses, pleural effusion, or hemothorax

    (a) Short and not sustained

    (b) Soft, not loud

    (c) Similar to a dull "thud"

    (d) Indicates more dense material (fluid or solid) is present in the underlying thorax; dullness is normally heard over the liver and heart

d. Percussion for diaphragmatic excursion: the range of motion of the diaphragm may be estimated with percussion by the following

  i. Instruct the patient to take a deep breath and hold it

  ii. Determine the lower level of resonance to dullness change (the level of the diaphragm) by percussing downward until a definite change in the percussion note is heard. Mark this spot with a pen

  iii. After instructing the patient to exhale and breath hold, repeat the procedure

  iv. The distance between the levels at which the tone change occurs is the diaphragmatic excursion

    (a) Normal diaphragmatic excursion is 3 to 4 cm; partial descent, or hemi-descent of the diaphragm may be related to paralysis of the diaphragm. Suspect nerve injury in postoperative patients with these signs following thoracic surgery

    (b) Diaphragm is normally higher on the right as compared with the left

    (c) The diaphragm is high in

      (1) Conditions that cause an increased intra-abdominal pressure (e.g., pregnancy, ascites)

      (2) Any condition that causes decreased thoracic volume (e.g., atelectasis)

(d) The diaphragm is fixed and lower than normal in emphysema

(e) It is difficult to differentiate between an elevated diaphragm and disease of the thorax that causes dullness to percussion (e.g., pleural effusion)

4. **Auscultation**: listening to sounds produced within the body
   a. Basic points
      i. Always compare one lung with the other by moving the stethoscope back and forth across chest starting at the top of the thorax and moving downward
      ii. The patient should be asked to breathe through the mouth a little deeper than usual. Breathing through an open mouth minimizes turbulent flow sound produced in the nose and throat
      iii. The diaphragm of the stethoscope is more sensitive to higher-pitched tones and thus is best for most lung sounds
      iv. Stethoscope earpieces should fit snugly to exclude extraneous sounds but not be so tight that they are uncomfortable
      v. The stethoscope tubing should be no longer that 20 inches (the shorter the better). Optimal length is 12 to 14 inches
      vi. Place stethoscope firmly on the chest to exclude extraneous sounds and eliminate sounds that may result from light contact with skin or air. Confusing sounds may be produced by
         (a) Movement of stethoscope on skin or hair
         (b) Breathing on the tubing
         (c) Sliding fingers on tubing or chest piece
         (d) Listening through clothing
   b. Normal breath sounds vary according to the site of auscultation
      i. Vesicular (always normal)
         (a) Soft sounds heard over fields of anterior, lateral, and posterior chest
         (b) Heard primarily during inspiration
      ii. Bronchial (may be normal or abnormal depending on location of sounds)
         (a) Heard normally over the trachea
         (b) High-pitched, harsh sound with long and loud expirations
         (c) When heard over lung fields, it is abnormal and suggests consolidation
      iii. Bronchovesicular (may be normal or abnormal depending on location)
         (a) Heard over large bronchi (near sternum, between scapulae, over right upper lobe apex)
         (b) Abnormal when heard over lung fields; signifies consolidation
   c. Abnormalities of breath sounds
      i. Absent or diminished sounds due to decreased air flow (airway

obstruction, chronic obstructive pulmonary disease, muscular weakness, splinting due to pain) or increased insulation blocking the transmission of the sounds to the stethoscope (obesity, pleural disease and fluid, pneumothorax)

   ii. Bronchial sounds heard over lung fields suggesting consolidation or increased density of lung tissue (atelectasis, pulmonary infarction, pneumonia, large tumors with no airway obstruction)

d. Adventitious sounds: abnormal sounds that are superimposed on underlying breath sounds

   i. Evaluate how position and coughing affect adventitious sounds

   ii. Terminology

     (a) Crackles (rales)—signify the opening of collapsed alveoli and small airways

       (1) Described as fine or coarse

       (2) Heard as small pops or crackles; the sound of fine crackles can be mimicked by rubbing a few pieces of hair together near one's ear. The sound of coarse crackles can be mimicked by pulling open Velcro

       (3) Fine crackles occurring late in inspiration imply conditions that cause restrictive ventilatory defect

       (4) Fine crackles heard early in inspiration are often atelectatic and caused by small airway closure

       (5) Coarse early inspiratory crackles are associated with bronchitis or pneumonia

     (b) Wheeze—indicates obstruction to air flow or air passing through narrowed airways

       (1) Continuous high-pitched sound with musical quality; also called sibilant wheeze

       (2) Commonly heard during expiration but may be heard during inspiration

       (3) Causative conditions—asthma, bronchitis, foreign bodies or tumors, mucosal edema, pulmonary edema, pulmonary emboli, poor mobilization of secretions

     (c) Gurgles or rhonchi result from air passing through secretions in large airways

       (1) Low-pitched continuous sounds

       (2) May have snoring quality when very large airways are involved; also called sonorous wheezes

       (3) Rhonchi tend to disappear after coughing

     (d) Pleural friction rub—indicates inflammation and loss of pleural fluid

       (1) Grating harsh sound in inspiration and expiration; disappears with breath holding. One can mimic the pleural friction rub sound by cupping a hand over one's

ear and rubbing the fingers of the other hand over the cupped hand
    (2) Heard with pleural infections, infarction, pulmonary emboli, and fractured ribs. Located in area of most intense chest wall pain
  (e) Mediastinal crunch—indicates air in pericardium and/or mediastinum
    (1) Heard synchronous with systole often associated with pericardial friction rubs
  (f) Pericardial friction rub
    (1) Occurs at atrial and ventricular systole, and there may be a diastolic component
    (2) Sounds persist with breath holding; heard most clearly at left lower sternal border

e. Voice sounds: spoken words are modified by disease in similar manner as breath sounds, resulting in increased or decreased conduction of sound
  i. Increased conduction occurs where normal lung tissue is replaced with denser, more solid tissue; associated with bronchial breathing
    (a) Bronchophony—when spoken word ("ninety-nine") is heard distinctly; the normal sound is muffled
    (b) Egophony—"e" sound changes to "a"; sound has the quality of sheep bleating
    (c) Whispered pectoriloquy—whispered sounds are heard with clarity, as if the patient is speaking into the diaphragm of one's stethoscope; the normal sound is muffled
  ii. Decreased conduction of sound occurs in the presence of obstructed bronchi, pneumothorax, or large collections of fluid or tissue between the lung and the chest wall
    (a) Decreased ability to hear the voice sounds
    (b) Is accompanied by decreased fremitus

Diagnostic Studies

1. Laboratory findings
a. Sputum examination
  i. Obtain specimen through voluntary coughing and expectoration, induction of sputum by inhaling aerosol, nasotracheal or endotracheal suctioning, transtracheal aspiration, or bronchoscopy
  ii. Assess important characteristics
    (a) Color and consistency
    (b) Volume—greater than 50 ml/day is excessive
    (c) Odor—should be odorless

(1) Foul-smelling sputum may indicate anaerobic putre-factive process

(2) Musty odor may indicate *Pseudomonas* infection

(d) Microscopic examination

(1) Cytologic study for malignant cells

(2) Smear to identify bacteria (e.g., Gram's stain) or fungi

(3) Sputum cultures to diagnose infection and assess drug resistance

(4) Special stains on cultures are required for mycobac-teria (acid-fast bacilli), fungi, *Pneumocystis carinii,* and *Legionella pneumophila*

b. Pleural fluid examination

   i. Diagnostic thoracentesis or pleural biopsy is performed to ob-tain specimen

   ii. Determination of transudate vs. exudate is based on protein and lactate dehydrogenase levels in pleural fluid and blood

   iii. Specimen is examined for cell counts, protein and lactate dehydrogenase, glucose, amylase, pH, Gram's stain for bacteria, and cytology for malignant cells and microorganisms

   iv. Frequently, a biopsy of the parietal pleura is also performed and the tissue specimen examined by microscopy

c. Skin tests

   i. For type I hypersensitivity (mediated by IgE): as in pollens, molds, dusts, grasses

   ii. For type II hypersensitivity (mediated by T lymphocytes): pur-ified protein derivative (PPD) test for tuberculosis

   iii. For fungal diseases

d. Serologic tests are used to determine causative pathogen in bacterial, viral, mycotic, and parasitic diseases

2. Radiologic findings

a. Chest x-ray films precede all other studies

   i. Posteroanterior and lateral views are most common

   ii. Portable anteroposterior films are used in the intensive care unit when the patient cannot be moved. These are generally of lesser quality than erect posteroanterior film because of

(a) Difficulty in positioning patient

(b) Short film distance from chest; also variable distance in serial films

(c) Less powerful x-ray generator

(d) Interference from tubes, lines, equipment attached to pa-tient

   iii. Lateral decubitus films are used if fluid levels need to be identified (as in pleural effusions and abscesses)

   iv. Oblique views are useful for localization of lesions, infiltrates

   v. Lordotic views enable evaluation of apical portion of lung and middle lobe or lingula and for determining whether lesion is anterior or posterior

vi. Expiratory films are used for visualizing pneumothorax or air trapping

b. Fluoroscopy

i. Useful for examining movement of pulmonary and cardiac structures, localizing pulmonary lesions, and examining diaphragmatic motion

ii. Also used for monitoring during special procedures: catheter insertion, bronchoscopy, thoracentesis, chest tube placement

iii. Exposure of patients to x-rays is greater during fluoroscopy than during standard x-ray examination

c. Tomography: provides views at different planes through the lungs

i. Gives better definition of small or questionable lesions and is particularly useful for determining if a lesion has calcification within it. However, since the advent of computed tomography, plain tomography is done less frequently than in the past

ii. Computed tomography (CT scan)

(a) Used for scanning axial cross sections of body

(b) Particularly useful in detecting subtle differences in tissue density

d. Magnetic resonance imaging

i. Used to distinguish tumors from other structures, such as blood vessels and bronchial walls

ii. Pleural thickening, pleural fluid, and chest wall tumors can be differentiated from each other

e. Pulmonary angiography: technique of visualizing the pulmonary arterial tree through the injection of radiopaque dye

i. Useful in investigating thromboembolic disease of the lung, congenital abnormalities of the circulation, and delineation of masses

ii. Procedure has some risks and is dangerous to perform in the presence of pulmonary hypertension; oxygen desaturation has occurred in some patients with injection of contrast media. Hemodynamic parameters should be measured prior to procedure

f. Ventilation–perfusion lung scanning uses injection or inhalation of radioisotopes to obtain information about pulmonary blood flow and ventilation

i. Used for detection of pulmonary emboli and assessment of regional lung function preoperatively

g. Ultrasonography

i. Is useful in evaluating pleural disease; can detect small amounts of pleural fluid and loculations within the pleural space and can distinguish fluid from pleural thickening

l detect disease immediately
scess
enetrates air poorly, it is not
lesions within the pulmonary

nction as normal or exhibiting
ive defect

hysiologic terms; permits de-
ndition to others
titative terms for future com-

n of risk of surgery
ies are performed in upright
position and are compared with predicted ones (Fig. 1–9)
(1) Volumes: there are four discrete and nonoverlapping
lung volumes
a) Tidal volume (V_T)—volume of gas inspired and
expired during each respiratory cycle
b) Inspiratory reserve volume (IRV)—maximal vol-

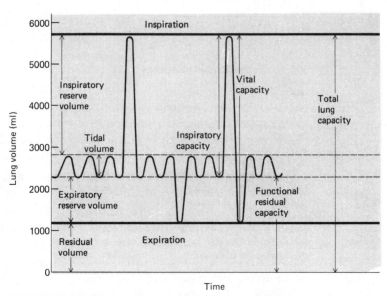

Figure 1–9. Diagram showing respiratory excursions during normal breathing and during maximal inspiration and maximal expiration. (From Guyton, A.C.: Textbook of Medical Physiology, 7th ed., W.B. Saunders Co., Philadelphia, 1986, p. 470.)

ume of gas that can be inspired after a tidal breath is taken

c) Expiratory reserve volume (ERV)—maximal volume of gas that can be expired from end-expiratory position

d) Residual volume (RV)—volume of gas remaining in lungs at end of a maximal expiration

(2) Capacities: there are four, each of which includes two or more of the primary volumes

a) Total lung capacity (TLC)—volume of gas contained in lung at end of a maximal inspiration

$$TLC = V_T + IRV + ERV + RV$$

b) Vital capacity (VC)—maximal volume of gas that can be expelled from lungs by a forceful effort following a maximal inspiration

$$VC = V_T + IRV + ERV$$

c) Inspiratory capacity (IC)—maximal volume of gas that can be inspired from resting expiratory level

$$IC = V_T + IRV$$

d) Functional residual capacity (FRC)—volume of gas remaining in the lungs at resting end-expiration

$$FRC = ERV + RV$$

(c) Ventilatory mechanics: provide information about dynamic lung function. Subjects perform forced breathing maneuvers

(1) Forced expiratory spirograms

a) Forced vital capacity (FVC), reduced in restrictive disease or in obstructive disease if there is air trapping

b) Forced expiratory volume in seconds (FEV_t), usually measured at 0.5, 1, and 3 seconds. Reduced in obstructive disease. Most common measure is FEV_1

c) Forced expiratory volume as a percentage of vital capacity with t representing time in seconds ($FEV_t/VC\%$). Evaluates obstruction to flow
   □ $FEV_1/VC\%$—normally > 75% in adults
   □ $FEV_3/VC\%$—normally > 95% in adults

d) Forced expiratory flows (FEF_{25-75}, FEF_{75-85}, and $FEF_{200-1200}$). These tests assess flows over a range of lung volumes

e) Values for timed flow studies are decreased out of proportion to vital capacity in obstructive disease

(2) Flow–volume loop studies
  a) Volume and flow during inspiration and expiration are plotted graphically
  b) Obstructive and/or restrictive disease produces abnormal flow–volume loops
(3) Maximum voluntary ventilation (MVV)
  a) Volume of air ventilated with maximal effort over short period of time
  b) May be used to predict patient's ability to undergo procedures that require ventilatory reserve (e.g., surgery)
(d) Lung compliance assesses the distensibility of the lungs and is the reciprocal of elastance
(1) Expressed as increase in volume per increase in transpulmonary pressure

$$C_L = \frac{\Delta V}{\Delta P}$$

where
V = volume
P = pressure

(2) Static compliance (C_{st}) is measured in the absence of air flow
  a) In the patient on a ventilator, C_{st} is measured by dividing V_T by plateau pressure (minus positive end-expiratory pressure) and is called the effective static compliance
  b) Normal values are around 100 ml/cm H_2O
(3) Dynamic compliance (C_{dyn}) is measured under conditions of flow
  a) In the patient on the ventilator, C_{dyn} is measured by dividing V_T by peak inspiratory pressure (minus positive end-expiratory pressure) and is called the effective dynamic compliance
  b) Normal values are between 40 and 50 ml/cm H_2O
(4) Compliance is decreased in conditions that make the lungs and/or thorax stiffer or reduce expansibility. Such conditions include atelectasis, pneumonia, pulmonary edema, fibrotic changes, pleural effusion, pneumothorax, kyphoscoliosis, obesity, abdominal distention, flail chest, and splinting due to pain
(5) Increases in compliance occur with age and/or emphysema
(6) Compliance curves (serial changes in volume plotted against changes in pressure) are useful in monitoring

patients on volume ventilators. Determinations of the best pressure–volume combinations for the patient may be made. Comparisons of static and dynamic pressure–volume curves help determine which component (airways, lungs, or chest wall) is contributing to changes in compliance

(e) Gas transfer and exchange studies
   (1) Blood gas and acid–base analysis
      a) Fundamental to diagnosis and management of pulmonary problems
      b) Refer to discussion under Physiologic Anatomy
   (2) Diffusing capacity (D_L)
      a) Measures the amount of functioning alveolar-capillary surface area available for gas exchange
      b) Values decrease with ventilation–perfusion mismatching, membrane problems, and decreases in pulmonary capillary blood volume

(f) Guidelines for interpretation of pulmonary function testing
   (1) Values are compared with predicted values for age, height, and sex
   (2) Restrictive pulmonary impairment generally results in decreased volumes and capacities
   (3) Decreased lung compliance indicates parenchymal disease
   (4) Obstructive defect generally results in decreased tests of dynamic ventilatory function. This may be reversible with use of bronchodilators
   (5) Chronic obstructive pulmonary disease with long-term air trapping and destruction of parenchyma results in increased functional residual capacity, residual volume, and total lung capacity
   (6) Patient preparation and cooperation are necessary to obtain reliable and valid data for most pulmonary function tests

b. Invasive tests
   i. Lung biopsy
      (a) Needle biopsy is used for diagnosis of malignancy or infection. Pneumothorax may be a complication
      (b) Open-lung biopsy requires a thoracotomy but has better diagnostic yields
   ii. Bronchoscopy: insertion of a fiberoptic scope into the airways for direct visualization and possible obtaining of specimens
      (a) Indicated for diagnosis of lung malignancy, evaluation of hemoptysis, removal of foreign body and/or secretions, and

sampling an area of lung through either washings, brushings, or biopsies

    (b) Patients must be observed post procedure for respiratory depression (from drugs used for sedation), decreased ventilation, and hypoxemia

    (c) Supplemental oxygen should be administered during the procedure

    (d) If transbronchial biopsy is performed, hemoptysis and/or pneumothorax are possible complications

  iii. Mediastinoscopy is performed for diagnostic exploration of mediastinum and to obtain biopsy specimens

COMMONLY ENCOUNTERED NURSING DIAGNOSES

Ineffective Airway Clearance: Related to Secretions

1. Assessment for defining characteristics
  a. Abnormal breath sounds
  b. Altered rate or depth of respiration
  c. Tachypnea
  d. Cough, effective or ineffective
  e. Cyanosis
  f. Dyspnea
  g. Fever
2. Expected outcomes
  a. Breath sounds clear bilaterally
  b. Absence of adventitious sounds
  c. Able to expectorate secretions
3. Nursing interventions
  a. Assist patient to breathe deeply
    i. Position patient to maximize inspiratory muscle length to maximize ventilation (semi-Fowler's to high Fowler's position, depending on patient comfort. Ask patient to take slow deep breaths and assess volume for adequacy (i.e., from functional residual capacity to total lung capacity) and sustain breath for several seconds before expiration. Provide patient with cues/devices to motivate independent deep breathing exercises
  b. Position patient to facilitate coughing
    i. Assist patient to assume a comfortable cough position (i.e., high Fowler's with knees bent and a lightweight pillow over abdomen to augment the expiratory pressures and minimize discomfort). Teach patient alternate cough techniques (huff or quad) if patient is having difficulty with the above technique

   c. Provide artificial airway and ventilation if indicated
   - i. Oropharyngeal airway
     - (a) Purpose—to maintain airway by holding tongue anteriorly
     - (b) Complications—vomiting and aspiration; malposition due to improper length
   - ii. Nasopharyngeal airway
     - (a) Purpose—useful in facial and jaw fractures when oral airway cannot be used. Patients tolerate it more readily than oropharyngeal airway
     - (b) Complications—nosebleed
     - (c) Adequate humidification is essential to ensure patency of narrow lumen
   - iii. Cricothyroidotomy: restricted to extreme emergencies when other methods fail or are unavailable. It involves making an incision through cricothyroid membrane
   - iv. Esophageal obturator airway
     - (a) For temporary emergency use only
     - (b) Usually easier to insert than endotracheal tube, requiring less training and skill. Reduces risk of aspiration while tube is in place
     - (c) Disadvantages
       - (1) Suctioning is difficult
       - (2) Stimulates vomiting; do not use if patient is conscious
       - (3) If patient vomits during or before passage of tube, device can be flooded
       - (4) Vomiting usually follows removal of tube. Place patient on his side before removing tube, and be prepared to suction
       - (5) Esophagus may be perforated
       - (6) Trachea may inadvertently be intubated
     - (d) Esophageal gastric obturator airway—allows for gastric suctioning
   - v. Endotracheal intubation
     - (a) Thorough training and retraining in this procedure is an absolute necessity for competency
     - (b) Key principles of procedure
       - (1) Preoxygenate with 100% oxygen for at least 2 minutes, if possible
       - (2) After insertion check for correct placement of tube by
         - *a)* Air movement felt through tube opening
         - *b)* Bilateral chest excursion during inspiration and expiration
       - (3) Auscultate both sides of chest peripherally
       - (4) Obtain chest x-ray film. The end of the tube should be about 3 cm above the carina

(c) Nasotracheal intubation is used when the oral route is not available and also for long-term intubations

(d) Nursing care considerations for intubated patient

(1) Frequent mouth care is mandatory

(2) Placement of tube should be checked often

(3) Tube should be secured carefully to prevent movement and decrease tracheal damage

(4) Adequate humidity is required

(5) Oral tubes should be moved from one side of mouth to the other at least daily

(6) Infection resulting from contaminated equipment or unsterile procedures may develop

(7) Suction as indicated. Pre- and post-suctioning oxygenation should be provided

(8) For prolonged intubation procedure, lidocaine may be instilled into tube or injected into vocal cords to increase patient tolerance

(e) Tracheal tube cuffs—principles and guidelines

(1) Quality of good cuff design

a) Low sealing pressure. Intracuff pressure should not exceed capillary filling pressure of trachea (25 cm H_2O or 20 mm Hg) to avoid tracheal necrosis

b) Cuff pressure distributed over large contact area

c) Large volumes of air accepted with minor increases in balloon tension

d) Maintains enough pressure to keep a good seal during inspiration and expiration (necessary to prevent aspiration)

e) Does not distort tracheal wall

(2) Low-pressure cuffs generally meet desired qualities and have replaced rigid hard cuffs in most situations

(3) Principles of cuff inflation and deflation

a) Inflation of low-pressure cuffs—inflate with sufficient air to ensure no leak, or only minimal leak, during peak inspiration. If increasing amounts of air are needed to obtain a seal, this may be due to tracheal dilation or to a leak in cuff. Condition should be corrected

b) Routine deflation is not necessary with good quality low-pressure cuffs

☐ Routine deflation during tracheal suctioning may be useful so that patient can breathe around tube during suctioning, but aspiration is a possible consequence so oropharynx must be suctioned first

        ☐ Periodic deflation is not necessary if minimal leak technique is used

    c) Regardless of cuff design or pressure characteristics, all cuff pressures should be routinely measured at least every 4 to 8 hours and whenever cuff is reinflated, and the cuff pressure must be readjusted as patient's peak inspiratory pressure changes

(f) Key points for extubation

    (1) Criteria for extubation will depend on purposes for which tube was originally inserted. Generally accepted criteria include

        a) Stable vital signs and hemodynamic parameters

        b) Patient is awake and oriented and/or able to keep airway open

        c) Blood gas levels are within acceptable limits, following trial of 30 minutes on nebulizer T tube at 40% oxygen

        d) Ventilatory measurements are within acceptable limits

    (2) Postextubation monitoring

        a) Repeat blood gas studies 20 minutes after extubation or sooner as indicated and periodically thereafter

        b) Observe for laryngospasm. Auscultate trachea with stethoscope for stridor and breathing difficulties. Treatment may consist of high humidity, corticosteroids to reduce laryngeal edema, and positive-pressure breathing with oxygen

        c) Monitor patient's tolerance to extubation by clinical observation, ventilatory measurements, and blood gas studies

vi. Tracheostomy

  (a) Purposes and indications

    (1) To remove secretions from tracheobronchial tree

    (2) To decrease dead space ventilation

    (3) To bypass upper airway obstruction

    (4) To prevent aspiration of oral or gastric secretions

    (5) To deliver assisted or controlled ventilation over an extended period of time

  (b) Principles of care

    (1) Stoma is kept clean and dry

    (2) Frequency of tube change remains controversial. Be prepared for complications during procedure

        a) Have self-inflating bag and mask, adequate suc-

tion, oxygen, intubation materials, and tracheal spreader ready
  b) Be prepared to intubate or otherwise support ventilation
    (3) Uncuffed tubes are used in children and patients with laryngectomies
    (4) Cuffed tubes are used when patient is receiving artificial ventilation
    (5) Suctioning is a sterile procedure
  (c) Weaning from tube
    (1) Criteria (refer to extubation criteria for endotracheal tube)
    (2) Patient must demonstrate physiologic and psychologic independence of artificial airway. Techniques include use of
      a) T tube
      b) Tracheostomy button
      c) Fenestrated tubes
      d) Progression from original-sized tube to smaller one of same type
      e) Breathing with cuff deflated or through fenestration
    (3) Patient is monitored carefully to see how weaning is tolerated. Blood gas studies and clinical observations are used
    (4) Complete sealing of tracheostomy incision may occur in 72 hours. Patients cannot produce adequate coughing pressure until this is accomplished
  d. Prevent complications of airway intubation
    i. Physiologic alterations caused by airway diversion
      (a) Inspired air is inadequately conditioned and is irritating to delicate pulmonary membranes
      (b) Plastic or metal tubes are foreign bodies. Body responds by increasing production of mucus; ciliary movement is impaired
      (c) Accumulated secretions are good medium for bacterial growth
      (d) Bypassing larynx produces aphonia
      (e) Eliminating glottis from air route prevents patient from developing increased intrathoracic pressures, thus making effective coughing difficult
    ii. Complications during placement in airway
      (a) Endotracheal tube
        (1) Mucous membrane disruption and tooth damage or dislodgment

       (2) With nasotracheal route, one may see

          a) Nosebleed

          b) Submucosal dissection

          c) Introduction of polyp or plug from nose into lungs, resulting in infection or obstruction

          d) Sinusitis

    (b) Tracheostomy (problems are fewer and less severe if this is an elective procedure done in the operating room)

       (1) Cardiac arrest

       (2) Hemorrhage

       (3) Pneumothorax

       (4) Damage to adjacent structures in neck

       (5) Mediastinal emphysema

  iii. Complications occurring while tube is in place

    (a) Obstruction due to

       (1) Plugging with secretions that have become dried and inspissated. This is entirely preventable by proper use of humidification and suctioning

       (2) Herniation of cuff over end of tube

       (3) Kinking of tube

       (4) Cuff overinflation

    (b) Displacement or dislodgment out of trachea

       (1) Especially hazardous during first 48 hours of tracheostomy. Avoid by using tube of proper length and fixing it securely to patient

       (2) Dislodgment out of trachea into tissue causes mediastinal emphysema, subcutaneous emphysema, and pneumothorax. Diagnosis is determined by poor blood gas values, poor chest excursion, inability to introduce suction catheter properly, and poor air movement

       (3) Low tube placement into one bronchus or at level of carina, resulting in obstruction or atelectasis of non-ventilated lung. Check placement of endotracheal tube by auscultation, followed by x-ray film or use of fiberoptic scope

          a) Displacement into one bronchus. Signs and symptoms are

            ☐ Decreased or delayed motion on one side of chest

            ☐ Unilateral diminished breath sounds

            ☐ Excessive coughing

            ☐ Localized expiratory wheeze

          b) Placement at level of carina. Signs and symptoms are

            ☐ Excessive coughing

      □ Localized expiratory wheeze
      □ Difficulty in introducing suction catheter
      □ Bilateral diminished breath sounds

(c) Poor oral hygiene. Mouth care is mandatory

(d) Local infection of tracheostomy wound, tracheal tissue, or lungs. Tracheostomy should be treated as a surgical wound and cultures obtained routinely

(e) Massive hemorrhage resulting from erosion of tracheostomy tube into the innominate vessels. May be fatal. Occurs most often with low placement of tube, excessive "riding" of tube within trachea, or pulling torsion on tube

(f) Disconnection between tracheal tube and ventilator
    (1) Most likely to occur when patient is being turned
    (2) Adequate alarms on all ventilators are necessary
    (3) Frequent checking of all connections should be routine

(g) Leaks due to broken cuff balloon
    (1) Diagnosis by ability of previously aphonic patient to talk, air movement felt at nose and mouth, pressure changes on ventilator, and decreased exhaled volumes as measured with Wright respirometer or ventilator spirometer
    (2) It is necessary to remove and replace tube. Always check cuff for leaks before inserting. Note amount of air required to fill cuff and compare with later values

(h) Tracheal ischemia, necrosis, dilation
    (1) Owing to oval shape of trachea and round shape of tube, there is a tendency for erosion in anterior and posterior trachea
    (2) Diagnosed by the necessity to use larger and larger amounts of air to inflate balloon
    (3) May progress to tracheoesophageal fistula; this is indicated if food is aspirated through the trachea or air is in the stomach, or a methylene blue dye test may be done
    (4) Prevention through use of low pressure cuffs and frequent monitoring of cuff pressures

iv. Early postextubation complications
  (a) Acute laryngeal edema
    (1) Most frequently seen in children
    (2) In adults, edema is commonly associated with the use of oversized tube with preexisting inflammation of upper airway
    (3) Prevention

a) Close observation for several hours after extubation

b) Patient should receive well-humidified air or oxygen after prolonged intubation

(4) Treatment

    a) Humidified oxygen, corticosteroids

    b) Smaller endotracheal tube introduced or tracheostomy performed

    c) Epinephrine administered to larynx with intermittent positive-pressure breathing

(b) Hoarseness

    (1) Almost universal after long endotracheal intubation

    (2) Usually disappears during first week

(c) Aspiration of food, saliva, and gastric contents

    (1) Presence of tube over long period results in loss of usual protective reflexes of larynx

    (2) Monitor patient carefully during feedings: watch for excessive coughing; start with clear liquids after tube removal

(d) Difficult removal of tracheostomy tube

    (1) More frequently seen in infants

    (2) Related to narrow lumen of trachea, which is further narrowed by swelling

v. Late postextubation complications

(a) Fibrotic stenosis of trachea

    (1) Cause—prolonged use of any tube with rigid inflatable cuff

    (2) Follows earlier ulceration and necrosis of site

    (3) Lesions may become advanced before clinical evidence (dyspnea, stridor) appears. Tracheoesophageal fistula may form

    (4) Prevention—use of low-pressure cuffs and frequent monitoring of cuff pressures

(b) Stenosis of larynx

    (1) Cause—discrepancy between anatomy of larynx and site and shape of tube

    (2) Treatment

        a) Dilation or surgical intervention

        b) Permanent tracheostomy

4. Evaluation of nursing care

  a. On auscultation, there is absence of adventitious sounds

  b. Patient is able to expectorate secretions

  c. Blood gas values and ventilatory parameters are within acceptable limits

Ineffective Breathing Pattern

1. **Assessment for defining characteristics**
   a. Dyspnea
   b. Tachypnea
   c. Fremitus
   d. Abnormal arterial blood gases
   e. Cyanosis
   f. Cough
   g. Nasal flaring
   h. Respiratory depth changes
   i. Assumption of three-point position
   j. Pursed lip breathing and prolonged expiratory phase
   k. Increased anteroposterior diameter
   l. Use of accessory muscles
   m. Altered chest excursion
2. **Expected outcomes**
   a. Respiratory rate, tidal volume, inspiratory-expiratory ratio within normal limits for patient
   b. Decreased dyspnea at rest and with exertion
3. **Nursing interventions**
   a. Teach pursed lip breathing, abdominal stabilization, and controlled coughing techniques to minimize energy expenditure of respiratory muscles
   b. Provide appropriate ventilatory support if necessary
      i. Major modes of mechanical ventilation
         (a) Negative external pressure ventilators: attempt to duplicate spontaneous breathing
            (1) The entire body up to the neck is placed within an "iron lung" or tank respirator, while the head and neck protrude to the atmosphere. Beneath the tank, electrically powered bellows create subambient pressure within the tank
            (2) Intermittently applied negative pressure creates a pressure gradient that promotes air entry into the lungs. Minute ventilation ($\dot{V}_E$) can be altered by changing the negative pressure (and thus the tidal volume) or the respiratory rate, but it is not possible to adjust the inspiratory flow rate
            (3) Use is restricted to patients with respiratory failure who have normal lung parenchyma (e.g., patients with poliomyelitis)
            (4) Disadvantages—unable to provide adequate support to those patients with lung disease; only available in controlled mode; adequate nursing care in tank is difficult; negative pressure can cause pooling of blood in the abdomen, termed *tank shock*

(5) Modified approach to negative pressure ventilation is the cuirass ventilator, consisting of a rigid shell placed around the rib cage, with an attached hose to a vacuum pump. This set-up avoids the problem of blood pooling in abdomen but is less efficient because adequate negative pressure is less reliably generated

(b) Positive-pressure ventilators: the most important types used in critical care. All apply positive pressure to the airway during inspiration

   (1) Ventilators are classified according to preset factors responsible for cessation of inspiratory flow

      a) Volume-cycled—deliver inspiratory flow until preset volume is met. This is the most widely used type of ventilator

      b) Pressure-cycled—deliver inspiratory flow until preset airway pressure is reached. Intermittent positive-pressure breathing (IPPB) therapy is the most common use for pressure-cycled ventilators

      c) Ventilators less commonly used include time-cycled ventilators in which gas flows to the patient until a preset inspiratory time is reached

      d) High-frequency ventilation—provides a faster respiratory rate and lower tidal volume than other ventilator systems, for the purpose of reducing barotrauma and cardiac depression. Three mechanical systems are capable of delivering high-frequency ventilation

        ☐ High-frequency positive-pressure ventilation (HFPPV)—time-cycled, volume-controlled ventilator that delivers a V_T 60 to 100 times per minute

        ☐ High-frequency jet ventilation (HFJV) delivers high-pressure gas through a small catheter in the trachea or endotracheal tube at frequencies of 60 to 200 times/min

        ☐ High-frequency oscillation moves a volume of gas to and fro in the airway, without bulk flow at rates of 600 to 3000 cycles/min

   (2) Additional classifications according to the initiation of the inspiratory cycle (Fig. 1–10)

      a) Spontaneous respiration—with certain ventilators, the patient is allowed to breath spontaneously through the ventilator circuit when the ventilator is set at zero. Positive airway pressure can be applied when breathing through such a circuit

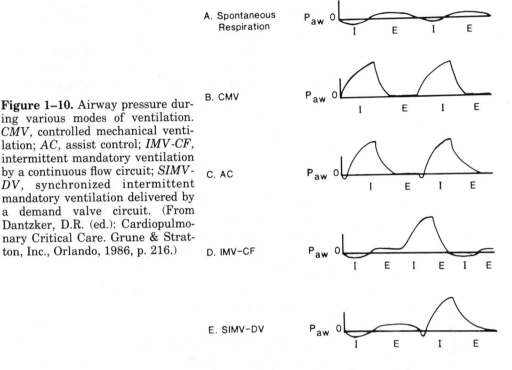

Figure 1–10. Airway pressure during various modes of ventilation. *CMV*, controlled mechanical ventilation; *AC*, assist control; *IMV-CF*, intermittent mandatory ventilation by a continuous flow circuit; *SIMV-DV*, synchronized intermittent mandatory ventilation delivered by a demand valve circuit. (From Dantzker, D.R. (ed.): Cardiopulmonary Critical Care. Grune & Stratton, Inc., Orlando, 1986, p. 216.)

A. Spontaneous Respiration

B. CMV

C. AC

D. IMV–CF

E. SIMV–DV

b) Controlled (CMV)—the ventilator delivers a preset number of breaths per minute of a predetermined volume. Additional breaths cannot be triggered by the patient. The patient can achieve a spontaneous breath by opening a valve in the system. However, it requires high negative inspiratory pressures to do so, and this leads to patient apprehension and air hunger. CMV is usually restricted to patients who are apneic as a result of sedation, paralysis, or brain damage

c) Assist-control (AC)—the ventilator delivers a breath either triggered by the patient's inspiratory effort or independently if such an effort does not occur within a preselected time period

d) Intermittent mandatory ventilation (IMV) allows the patient to breathe spontaneously but in addition provides periodic positive-pressure breaths at a preset volume and rate from the ventilator. A subtype of this mode is synchronized IMV (SIMV) in which a demand valve is incorporated into the IMV constant flow system that senses the start of a patient breath. A demand valve opens, and a positive-pressure breath is delivered in synchrony with the patient's breath *e)* Pressure support ventilation (PSV)—application of an amount of positive pressure to supplement the patient's spontaneous ventilatory efforts. This augmentation to inspiratory effort usually starts at the initiation of inhalation and ends at a minimum inspiratory flow rate. There are two applications for this mode

   ☐ As assistance to IMV to improve patient tolerance and decrease the work of spontaneous breaths, especially from demand-flow systems

   ☐ As a stand-alone ventilatory mode for patients under consideration for weaning

(c) Comparison of pressure-cycled and volume-cycled ventilators. (Models and their capabilities are continually changing. Refer to instructions supplied by the manufacturer for specifics.)

 (1) Pressure-cycled ventilators—advantages:

  a) Relatively inexpensive

  b) Mobility

  c) May be run on compressed air or oxygen

  d) Can usually be repaired on site

 (2) Pressure-cycled ventilators—disadvantages

  a) Tidal volume delivered varies with changes in airway resistance, lung compliance, and integrity of the ventilator unit

  b) Airway obstruction results in a low V_T and premature cycling of the ventilator circuits

  c) Inspired oxygen concentrations may be variable and unreliable; must use gas mixer

  d) Unable to generate airway pressures above 40 to 50 cm H_2O and do not achieve adequate ventilation in patients with low lung compliance

  e) Lack of adequate alarm systems may be a problem

  f) Ventilators cannot compensate for leak in system or around tube. Will have a continuous inspiratory phase if pressure limit is not reached

 (3) Volume-cycled ventilators—advantages

  a) More reliable in delivering the volume of air wanted despite varying airway resistance and compliance. Deliver a measured amount of air at whatever pressure is required, up to peak pressure capabilities of the machine

  b) Better delivery of accurate oxygen concentrations

  c) Built-in monitoring alarms

  d) Allow modifications of pressure delivered to chest

        e) Equipped or modified to deliver positive end-expiratory pressure (PEEP) and intermittent mandatory ventilation (IMV)

    (4) Volume-cycled ventilators—disadvantages

        a) Expensive, large, difficult to transport

        b) May deliver excessive pressures

        c) Will not deliver tidal volume if there is a leak in the system

(d) Intermittent positive-pressure breathing (IPPB) treatments—application of moderate pressure above ambient air pressure during patient's inspiratory phase

    (1) Purpose—primarily used as temporary therapy in spontaneously breathing patient. Widespread use is no longer justified by data

        a) To provide greater expansion of lungs and even distribution of gases and aerosol medications throughout lungs

        b) To prevent or correct atelectasis by deep lung inflations

        c) To deliver medications and humidity in order to provide bronchodilatation and to aid in loosening bronchial secretions

        d) To decrease work of breathing

    (2) Possible indications for IPPB treatments

        a) Hypoventilation in acute or chronic obstructive pulmonary diseases and, postoperatively, due to anesthetic gases, pain, and depressant drugs

        b) Retention of secretions

        c) Preoperative training

        d) Administration of aerosol medications

    (3) Contraindications to the use of IPPB

        a) Absolute contraindications

           ☐ Massive pulmonary hemorrhage

           ☐ Massive subcutaneous emphysema of unknown etiology

           ☐ Pneumothorax

        b) Relative contraindications: use IPPB with caution

           ☐ Hypovolemia

           ☐ Severe cardiac diseases

           ☐ Acute tuberculosis

           ☐ Hemoptysis

           ☐ Sensitivities to various drugs that may be used

    (4) Use and benefits remain controversial. Teaching patients to take deep breaths and cough is equally effective and clearly less expensive

ii. Guidelines for adjusting ventilator controls and settings for volume- and pressure-cycled ventilators. All are adjusted according to patient's primary disease and results of arterial blood gas analysis
  (a) Minute ventilation: usually 6 to 10 L/min but may be much higher depending on patient needs
    (1) Governed by estimated tidal volume of 10 to 15 ml/kg body weight and respiratory rate of 8 to 12 breaths/ min. The use of intermittent sighs during mechanical ventilation is no longer recommended
    (2) Respiratory rate varies according to ventilator flow rate, inspiratory-expiratory time ratio (usually 1:2), and whether ventilator is on control, assist, or IMV mode
    (3) Compliance curves are used to establish volume–pressure relationships
  (b) Oxygen concentration
    (1) Initially the FI_{O_2} is deliberately set at a high value (often 1.0) to ensure adequate oxygenation. An arterial blood gas sample is obtained and the FI_{O_2} is adjusted according to the patient's Pa_{O_2}. Adjust inspired partial pressure of oxygen so that arterial P_{O_2} is acceptable for patient's condition. This is usually between 60 and 90 mm Hg
    (2) Excessively high levels cause oxygen toxicity. Use the lowest FI_{O_2} that achieves the desired Pa_{O_2}
  (c) Continuous humidification is mandatory, with inspired air warmed to body temperature. Nebulizers must be emptied and refilled at least every 8 hours to reduce the risk of infection. Water condensed in ventilator tubing should be emptied from the system frequently
  (d) Established parameters concerning sensitivity settings (when patient can trigger machine for "assistance"); adjusted so that minimal patient effort is required
  (e) Flow rate
    (1) Adjusted so that inspiratory volume can be completed in time allowed, based on desired respiratory rate and inspiratory-expiratory ratio. An inspiratory flow rate of about 60 L/min is most commonly employed. Slow flow rates are preferred for optimal air distribution in normal lungs, while faster flow rates are beneficial in patients with obstructive pulmonary disease
    (2) Altering the flow rate may increase the comfort of patients who are restless while receiving mechanical ventilation

(f) Adjust amount of positive end-expiratory pressure and expiratory resistance or retard, if appropriate

(g) Pressure limits should be used during continuous ventilation

(h) Check that alarms are working and on at all times

(i) Optimal orders for ventilator settings and parameters

  (1) Require considerable technical knowledge of machines, combined with awareness of pathophysiology of each patient

  (2) Necessitate consultation of technical manual that accompanies each machine

c. Assess the effectiveness of mechanical ventilation on the patient

  i. General measures

    (a) Do not leave the patient unattended or unobserved

    (b) When medications are to be used, specific orders must be written. A bronchodilator cannot be administered continuously by aerosol

    (c) Many patients will have an arterial line, cardiac monitor, intravenous line, and urinary catheter if on continuous ventilation

  ii. General monitoring for patient on continuous ventilatory support

    (a) Pressure monitoring (arterial and venous, pulmonary artery, and wedge if pulmonary artery catheter is inserted)

    (b) Cardiac monitoring, heart sounds, pulses, pulse pressures, electrocardiogram as needed

    (c) Pulmonary function studies—vital capacity, minute ventilation, maximum voluntary ventilation

    (d) Biochemical, hematologic, and electrolyte studies

    (e) Cardiac output, blood volume status

    (f) Intake/output, body weight

    (g) Respiratory patterns, breath sounds, chest movement, vital signs

    (h) Dressings and drainages, tubes, and suction apparatus

    (i) Neurologic state, level of consciousness, pain, level of anxiety

    (j) Response to treatments, medications

  iii. Ventilatory monitoring of any patient on continuous ventilation

    (a) Ventilation checks performed routinely

      (1) When blood gases are drawn

      (2) When changes are made in ventilator settings

      (3) Frequently on any unstable patient

      (4) Routinely throughout each shift

    (b) Components of ventilator sheet to be recorded on flow sheet

(1) Blood gas values—record source (e.g., arterial, mixed venous) along with ventilator settings and measurements so that the decisions about changes may be made. It often is valuable to document patient position at time of blood gas drawing, since position changes (side lying, upright, supine) influence ventilation–perfusion relationships, and hence blood gas results. End tidal P_{CO_2} (E_{CO_2}) may correlate with arterial P_{CO_2} in a steady state. However, this is true only if a good expiratory plateau is achieved in the carbon dioxide tracing from the end-tidal carbon dioxide monitor. If this is not the case, the end tidal carbon dioxide value is generally regarded as a worthless measurement. Transcutaneous P_{O_2} and P_{CO_2} monitors may also be used, as well as ear or pulse oximetry

(2) Ventilator settings to be read from machine
   a) Ventilator mode (control/assist)
   b) Tidal volume, rate, flow rates
   c) Temperature of humidification device, temperature of inspired gas
   d) Oxygen concentration
   e) Inflation hold, expiratory time (only on some machines)
   f) Inspiratory pressure, positive end-expiratory pressure
   g) Alarms on

(3) Ventilator measurements to be taken on patients
   a) Peak, plateau, and end-expiratory pressures
   b) Partial pressure of inspired oxygen, fraction of inspired oxygen, A–a gradient, shunt fractions
   c) Minute ventilation, respiratory rate, tidal volume
   d) Effective compliance, static and dynamic; compliance curves
   e) Inspiratory/expiratory ratio and dead space/tidal volume (V_D/V_T) ratio

d. Prevent development of complications associated with the use of positive-pressure ventilation
   i. Cardiac effects
      (a) Decreased cardiac output—caused by decreased venous return to the heart and reduced transmural pressures (intracardiac minus intrapleural pressures). In addition, there is an increase in pulmonary vascular resistance and increased juxtacardiac pressure from the surrounding distended lungs

      (1) Pulse changes, decrease in urine output and blood pressure

      (2) Treatment—Trendelenburg position, fluids to increase preload, adjustment of volumes delivered by ventilator, careful positive end-expiratory pressure adjustment

  (b) Dysrhythmias are common

      (1) Causes—hypoxemia and pH abnormalities

      (2) Patients on ventilators should have cardiac monitoring

ii. Pulmonary effects

  (a) Barotrauma (pneumothorax, pneumomediastinum, subcutaneous emphysema) occurs when a high pressure gradient between the alveolus and the adjacent vascular sheet causes the overdistended alveolus to rupture. Gas is forced into the interstitial tissue of the underlying perivascular sheet. The gas may dissect centrally along the pulmonary vessels to the mediastinum and into the fascial planes of the neck and upper torso

      (1) Positive-pressure ventilation, especially with positive end-expiratory pressure, subjects patients to pneumothorax, particularly if high pressures and volumes are used

      (2) Barotrauma often occurs with adult respiratory distress syndrome and chronic obstructive pulmonary disease

      (3) Diagnosis—rises in airway peak pressure, decreased breath sounds and chest movement on the affected side, restlessness, changes in vital signs, cyanosis, chest x-ray changes

  (b) Atelectasis—collapse of lung parenchyma from occlusion of air passage, with reabsorption of gas distal to occlusion

      (1) Cause—obstruction, also possible lack of periodic deep inflations in patients ventilated with small tidal volumes

      (2) Diagnosis

         a) Diminished breath sounds or bronchial breath sounds, rales, or crackles

         b) Chest x-ray evidence

         c) A–a gradient increases

         d) Compliance decreases

      (3) Prevention

         a) Use of large tidal volumes or periodic sighing

         b) Humidity, vigorous tracheal suctioning

         c) Chest physical therapy repositioning

  (c) Tracheal damage, tracheoesophageal fistula, vessel rupture

      (d) Oxygen toxicity

          (1) Pathology—impaired surfactant activity, progressive capillary congestion, fibrosis, edema and thickening of interstitial space

          (2) Etiology—prolonged administration of high oxygen concentrations

          (3) Prevention—frequent monitoring of blood gases with administration of oxygen in lowest possible concentration to maintain adequate Pa_{O_2} and oxygen saturation

      (e) Inability to wean

          (1) Occurs in patients with chronic obstructive pulmonary disease, cystic fibrosis, debilitation, musculoskeletal disorders

          (2) Mechanical ventilation eases the work of breathing for these patients, making weaning difficult

      (f) Hypercapnea—respiratory acidosis

          (1) Due to inadequate ventilation leading to retention of carbon dioxide and decreased pH

          (2) Treated by increasing alveolar ventilation

      (g) Hypocapnea—respiratory alkalosis

          (1) Due to hyperventilation, causing increased diffusion, decreased carbon dioxide and increased pH

          (2) If lowering of carbon dioxide is too rapid, it may cause shock or seizures, particularly in children. Ventilation should be maintained to produce a normal pH, not necessarily a normal P_{CO_2}

          (3) Treated by decreasing respiratory rate, decreasing tidal volume if inappropriately high, or adding mechanical dead space

   iii. Fluid imbalance

      (a) Fluid retention—due to overhydration by airway humidification and decreased urinary output because of possible antidiuretic hormone effects. Symptoms include

          (1) Increased A–a gradient

          (2) Decreased vital capacity

          (3) Weight gain

          (4) Intake greater than output

          (5) Decreased compliance

          (6) Increased dead space/tidal volume (V_D/V_T) ratio

          (7) Hemodilution (decreased hematocrit and decreased sodium)

          (8) Increased bronchial secretions

      (b) Dehydration related to decreased enteral or parenteral intake in relation to urinary and/or gastrointestinal out-

put. In addition, insensible losses average 300 to 500 ml/day and increase with fever. Symptoms include
   (1) Decreased skin turgor
   (2) Intake less than combined outputs
   (3) Decreased body weight
   (4) Hemoconcentration
   (5) Thick, inspissated secretions
   (c) Parameters to be monitored
   (1) Daily weight changes (often more accurate than intake and output)
   (2) Skin turgor, moistness of oral mucosa
   (3) Hemoglobin/hematocrit
   (4) Character of pulmonary secretions
   (5) Maintain airway humidification
iv. Infection
   (a) Patients at risk: debilitated, aged, immobile, early postoperative patients and those who are immunocompromised
   (b) Intubation bypasses normal upper airway defense mechanisms
   (c) Ventilatory equipment/therapy may be carrier, particularly aerosols
   (d) Suctioning technique may not be sterile
   (e) Cross-contamination between patients and staff and/or autocontamination
   (f) Pulmonary patients frequently have indwelling catheters of all types
   (g) Unsterile solutions left out in open containers
   (h) Improper positioning of patients so that aspiration is encouraged
   (i) Preventative measures
   (1) Rigorous handwashing
   (2) Isolation techniques as needed
   (3) Routine cultures of patients and machines
   (4) Antibiotics as indicated
   (5) Bronchial hygiene, chest physical therapy
   (6) Restriction of number of patient contacts (staff and visitors)
   (7) Early recognition and response to clinical and laboratory signs of infection
   (8) Aseptic airway and tracheostomy technique
   (9) Ventilator tubing including humidifier reservoirs should be changed every 24 hours
   (10) Reservoir water should be emptied and changed every 8 hours; water in tubing should be emptied into a waste receptacle every 1 to 2 hours

(11) Sterile suction technique with infrequent use of suction catheter rinsing solutions or tracheal instillation

v. Gastrointestinal effects

(a) Complications

(1) Stress ulcer and bleeding

(2) Adynamic ileus

(3) Gastric dilatation from loss of adequate nerve supply. May lead to shock from fluid shifts

(b) Prevention and treatment

(1) Routinely auscultate bowel sounds

(2) Administer antacids, histamine antagonists

(3) Obtain Hematest and pH for stomach aspirate, and check stools for blood

vi. Patient "fighting" the respirator; displays agitation and distress

(a) Causes

(1) Incorrect ventilator set-up for patient's needs

(2) Acute change in patient status

(3) Obstructed airway

(4) Ventilator malfunction

(5) Acute anxiety

(b) Management

(1) Rapid bedside check of patient and ventilator

(2) Disconnect patient from ventilator and provide manual ventilation via self-inflating bag

(3) Check vital signs, chest, bedside monitoring equipment

(4) Suction airway, check patency of endotracheal or tracheostomy tube

(5) Obtain arterial blood gas studies

(6) Sedate patient if ordered, for acute anxiety. Observe for hypoventilation and adjust ventilator setting to meet patient's needs

(c) Principles for matching ventilator to patient's needs

(1) Do not assume patient will adjust to ventilator; the reverse is desirable

(2) Vary cycle frequency, tidal volume, triggering sensitivity, and inspiratory flow rate until correct combination is achieved

(3) Provide calm reassurance and moderate sedation as indicated

e. Provide optimal methods for weaning patients from continuous ventilation

i. Generally accepted indications for weaning (the term *weaning* is usually reserved for those patients who have been on ventilatory support for more that 12 hours prior to the initiation of weaning)

  (a) Resolution of underlying disease process and signs that disease process is manageable
  (b) Patient's strength, vigor, and nutritional status are adequate
  (c) Patient does not require more than 5 cm of positive end-expiratory pressure or an FI_{O_2} greater than 0.5 to maintain an acceptable Pa_{O_2} (usually at least 55 mm Hg)
  (d) Stable and acceptable hemodynamic parameters and hemoglobin
  (e) Stable and acceptable measurements of arterial blood gases, tidal volume, vital capacity, respiratory rate, minute ventilation, maximum inspiratory and expiratory airway pressures, A–a gradient, and compliance; V_D/V_T ratio is within minimal acceptable range (less than 0.6)
  (f) Level of consciousness is acceptable
  (g) Patient is psychologically prepared, emotionally ready, and cooperative
  (h) Predictors of successful weaning and criteria for weaning trial
    (1) Resting minute volume of less than 10 L and ability to double this value during maximum voluntary effort
    (2) Maximum inspiratory pressure more negative than minus 20
    (3) Vital capacity above 10 ml/kg body weight
    (4) Pa_{O_2} above 55 mm Hg (with maximal positive end-expiratory pressure of 5 cm H_2O and maximal FI_{O_2} of 0.5)
    (5) Static compliance is greater than 30
ii. Principles of weaning process
  (a) Explain to patient what will take place. Place in upright position if possible for better lung expansion. Obtain baseline vital signs
  (b) To assess ability to ventilate adequately without mechanical assistance, perform ventilatory measurements and obtain vital signs frequently while patient is off ventilator. Measurements include minute ventilation, respiratory rate, tidal volume, peak inspiratory pressure (P_{insp}), peak expiratory pressure (P_{exp}), and vital capacity
  (c) Be prepared to give periodic manual ventilation as needed. Have all equipment at bedside and in working order
  (d) Consider putting patient back on ventilator if signs of poor response to weaning or tiring occur, such as
    (1) Decreased tidal volume, increased respiratory rate

(2) Increasing Pa_{CO_2}

(3) Patient apprehension

(4) Diaphoresis, fatigue, decreasing level of consciousness

(5) Cardiac dysrhythmias, blood pressure changes, hemodynamic changes

(e) Mechanisms producing a failure to wean may include insufficient ventilatory drive, hypoxemia, high ventilatory requirement, respiratory muscle weakness, low compliance, or excessive work of breathing. The longer the mechanical ventilation is continued, the more difficult it is to wean

(f) If patient tolerates being off ventilator for 20 to 30 minutes, obtain blood gas measurements

(g) Progress slowly with increasing periods of spontaneous breathing off ventilator. Monitor respiratory and hemodynamic parameters frequently

(h) Schedules for weaning will vary with patient response. There are no rigid timetables. Patient is extubated when able to remain off ventilator

iii. Intermittent mandatory ventilation (IMV)—control mode ventilation with spontaneous breathing in between

(a) Used in support and weaning of patients from mechanical ventilation. Delivers mechanical ventilation at preset rate while allowing spontaneous ventilations of patient, with controlled $F_{I_{O_2}}$. Synchronized IMV (SIMV) is similar, but the respirator breath is synchronized with the spontaneous breath of the patient. The terms *intermittent demand ventilation* (IDV) and *intermittent assisted ventilation* (IAV) are also used interchangeably with SIMV. In all these modes the machine will deliver the mandatory breath in response to the patient's effort

(b) Indications for IMV

(1) Patients who fail to meet previously established criteria for attempting a trial of spontaneous ventilation; for example, those placed on the ventilator because of respiratory failure due to chronic obstructive pulmonary disease

(2) Patients who have been on a ventilator for extended periods and require a slower, less stressful weaning process

(3) Patients with abnormal ventilatory measurements

(4) IMV or SIMV is often used as the initial ventilatory mode of support for some patients

(c) Advantages of IMV

       (1) Can start early in phase of controlled ventilation, as soon as respiratory parameters have stabilized

       (2) Provides for exercise of ventilatory musculature

       (3) More physiologic Pa_{CO_2} may be achieved with IMV than with assisted or controlled breathing (this may reduce weaning time). Allows patient to adjust ventilation for maintenance of arterial blood gas values

       (4) Safer than trial-and-error method of complete removal from ventilator because it prevents precipitous fall in Pa_{O_2} and rise in Pa_{CO_2}

       (5) Good acceptance by patients when procedure is carefully explained, as in any weaning process. Helps avoid psychologic dependence on ventilator

       (6) Can effect rapid changeover from spontaneous ventilation to ventilatory support if patient's condition warrants it

       (7) Decreased risk of contamination from switching machines and equipment

       (8) Good control of Fi_{O_2} and reliable humidification

       (9) Same positive end-expiratory pressure valve on ventilator serves for both ventilator and spontaneous breaths

    (d) Disadvantage of IMV—may cause respiratory muscle fatigue if used improperly, resulting in delay of weaning process

  f. Evaluate individual patient's inspiratory muscles for training and, if appropriate, initiate inspiratory muscle training

    i. Monitor oxygen saturation with ear oximeter during training session to verify that patient does not demonstrate desaturation

  g. Monitor color, consistency, and volume of sputum. A change in sputum characteristics may indicate infection, which could increase the work of breathing

  h. Induce periodic hyperinflation of the lungs with a series of slow deep breaths. Shallow respirations can result in progressive atelectasis and reduced lung compliance. Intermittent lung hyperinflation will reinflate collapsing small airways and promote increased lung compliance

  i. Position patient in upright position as needed (to increase vital capacity)

  j. Continue to monitor rate and depth of respiration, breath sounds, use of accessory muscles of respiration, and sensation of dyspnea

    i. Clinical manifestations of respiratory muscle fatigue include

      (a) Shallow rapid breathing in the early stages

      (b) Increased Pa_{CO_2} and decrease in respiratory rate in late stages

  (c) Use of accessory muscles

  (d) Magnified sensation of dyspnea

 k. Monitor ratio of inspiratory time/total duration of respiration. (An increase in the ratio of inspiratory time to total duration of respiration indicates a decrease in respiratory muscle endurance.)

 l. Observe for abnormal chest wall motion as an indication of respiratory muscle dysfunction

  i. Paradoxic motion of the chest wall is characterized by expansion of the rib cage and inward motion of the abdomen during inspiration

  ii. Asynchronous chest wall motion is characterized by disorganized and uncoordinated respiratory motion

 m. Administer appropriate drug therapy for maintenance of ventilation

  i. Narcotics: morphine sulfate, meperidine

   (a) Respiratory depressants; good euphoric agents and excellent analgesics

   (b) Provide sedation and good control of ventilation without adverse side effects in well-ventilated, well-oxygenated, acid–base-balanced patient

   (c) Reduces the sensation of dyspnea

   (d) Large doses may cause increased venous capacitance

  ii. Narcotic antagonists—used in narcotic overdoses to reverse the effects of the narcotics. They are not stimulants but compete with narcotic molecules for cellular receptors in drug-depressed neurons

  iii. Benzodiazepines

   (a) Diazapam causes alveolar hypoventilation and respiratory acidosis in patients with chronic obstructive pulmonary disease

   (b) Severe respiratory depression and apnea can result if used with other central nervous system depressant drugs

  iv. Paralyzing agents—pharmacologic intervention at myoneural junction, resulting in muscle paralysis. When used in conscious patients, the patients must also be sedated

   (a) Nondepolarizing muscle relaxants

    (1) Compete with acetylcholine at receptor site

    (2) D-tubocurarine—may cause hypotension

    (3) Pancuronium bromide—may cause tachycardia

    (4) Given as initial loading doses followed by maintenance doses, with careful monitoring

   (b) Depolarizing muscle relaxant (succinylcholine)

    (1) Attaches to muscle-cell wall and causes depolarization

    (2) Used primarily for inducing muscle relaxation in anesthesia and endotracheal intubation

  v. Bronchodilators

(a) Methylxanthines—theophylline, aminophylline (80% theophylline)

    (1) Actions—stimulate the central nervous system, act on the kidney to produce diuresis, stimulate cardiac muscle, and relax bronchial smooth muscle

    (2) Serum levels—therapeutic range 10 to 20 μg/ml

(b) Beta-agonists—stimulate beta receptors in the bronchial smooth muscle, resulting in bronchial smooth muscle relaxation. They are the most potent bronchodilators currently available

    (1) Epinephrine—stimulates $beta_1$ and $beta_2$ receptors; given by inhalation or parenterally, with rapid action either way; duration of action is 1 to 3 hours

    (2) Isoproterenol—stimulates $beta_1$ and $beta_2$ receptors; given intravenously or sublingually or inhaled; duration of action is 1 to 2 hours

    (3) Metaproterenol has more $beta_2$ than $beta_1$ effects; given in inhaled or oral form; duration of action is 3 to 6 hours

    (4) Isoetharine—mainly $beta_2$ effects; inhaled, with a duration of action of 2 to 4 hours

    (5) Terbutaline—mainly $beta_2$ actions; given subcutaneously or orally or inhaled; duration of action is 2 to 4 hours for subcutaneous route, 3 to 6 hours inhaled; 5 to 8 hours orally; however, side effects are worse with oral doses

    (6) Albuterol—$beta_2$ selective; inhaled and oral forms; duration of action is 3 to 6 hours if inhaled and 5 to 8 hours for oral form

    (7) Bitolterol—$beta_2$ selective; given in inhaled form only; duration of action is 4 to 8 hours

(c) Anticholinergic bronchodilators—block cholinergic constricting influences on bronchial muscle

    (1) Atropine, ipratropium—given in inhaled forms

(d) Antiallergy medications—block IgE-dependent mast cell release of mediators of bronchoconstriction

    (1) Cromolyn sodium—does not actively bronchodilate but prevents bronchoconstriction; inhaled liquid by nebulizer or inhaled powder by spinhaler

vi. Corticosteroids—augment the effects of beta agonist bronchodilators and are anti-inflammatory; often start with high dose, then taper off; doses should be kept low to minimize adrenocortical and pituitary suppression and side effects

(a) Prednisone—oral dose, often is given once daily, in early morning to minimize systemic side effects

(b) Hydrocortisone, methylprednisolone given intravenously

(c) Inhaled corticosteroids (i.e., beclomethasone) given after inhaled beta agonists. Provide beneficial pulmonary corticosteroid effects with minimal systemic absorption

n. Assist the patient in maintaining adequate nutrition

   i. Assess nutritional status

(a) Anthropometric measurements (i.e., weight/height ratio, skinfold thickness, mid-arm circumference, mid-arm muscle circumference, and creatinine/height index) are all reduced in patients with malnutrition

(b) Biochemical markers (i.e., albumin, transferrin, prealbumin, retinol binding protein, total lymphocyte count, and reaction to skin tests) are all reduced in malnutrition

  ii. Administer appropriate nutritional therapy to meet the following goals

(a) Replenish depleted stores of somatic and visceral protein

(b) Promote wound healing

(c) Restore patient to pre-illness weight

(d) Restore patient's immunocompetence and normal nitrogen balance

(e) In certain patients, successfully wean from the ventilator

 iii. Methods of nutritional support

(a) Oral feedings with high calorie supplements; high fat mixtures provide increased calories with less carbon dioxide production

    (1) Often small frequent feedings are more tolerable for dyspneic patients

(b) Enteral feedings via nasogastric or gastric feeding tubes of high calorie liquids for patients who are unable to eat but have functional gastrointestinal tracts

    (1) Patients with endotracheal tubes are not able to take oral feedings

    (2) Precautions must be taken to avoid pulmonary aspiration

(c) Peripheral total parenteral nutrition (TPN)—amino acids (3.5%), glucose (5%), and fat (10% to 20%) solutions via peripheral infusions

(d) Central TPN—higher concentrations of nutrients are given for patients with severe stress, fluid restriction, previous nutritional deficits, or nonfunctioning gastrointestinal tract

 iv. General patient care and personal hygienic measures (especially meticulous oral care) will improve patient's appetite

4. Evaluation of nursing care

a. Rate, depth, and inspiratory-expiratory ratio of respirations remain within normal limits for patient

b. Patient reports decreased dyspnea at rest and with exertion

c. Increases maximal inspiratory pressure

Impaired Gas Exchange

1. **Assessment for defining characteristics**
   a. Confusion
   b. Somnolence
   c. Restlessness
   d. Irritability
   e. Inability to move secretions
   f. Hypercapnea
   g. Hypoxia
   h. Dyspnea
   i. Cyanosis
   j. Decreased mental acuity
   k. Tachycardia/dysrhythmias
   l. Anxiety
   m. Clinical evidence of abnormal blood oxygen levels
2. **Expected outcomes**
   a. Resolution or improvement of hypoxemia with or without oxygen supplement or mechanical ventilation
   b. Patient performs techniques that maximize ventilation–perfusion matching
   c. Performs activities of daily living with or without supplemental oxygen
   d. Patient is able to conserve energy by adjusting activities for self-care
   e. Patient expresses feelings of comfort in maintaining air exchange
3. **Nursing interventions**
   a. Assess oxygenation status
      i. Hypoxia–hypoxemia relationships
         (a) Definition of hypoxia: decrease in tissue oxygenation (a clinical diagnosis). Must be corrected, but in some cases oxygen therapy alone may not correct tissue hypoxia
         (b) Definition of hypoxemia—decrease in arterial blood oxygen tension (a laboratory diagnosis). A good Pa_{O_2} alone does not guarantee tissue oxygenation
         (c) Organs most susceptible to lack of oxygen—brain, adrenal glands, heart, kidneys, liver, retina of eye
         (d) Factors governing effective oxygenation of blood and tissues
            (1) Sufficient oxygen supply in inspired air

(2) Sufficient ventilation to provide gas exchange between atmosphere and alveoli of lungs

(3) Ready diffusion of gases across the alveolar-capillary membrane

(4) Adequate circulation of blood from lungs to tissues; volume of blood and hemoglobin levels must be adequate. A decreasing cardiac output will cause a compensatory rise in oxygen extraction at the tissue level

(5) Oxygen brought to tissues must be readily released from hemoglobin molecule and readily diffused into and taken up by various tissues

ii. Assessment of hypoxemia/hypoxia

(a) Clinical signs and symptoms—restlessness, anxiety, dysrhythmias, apprehension, headache, angina, confusion, disorientation, impaired judgment, hypotension, tachycardia, abnormal respirations, hypoventilation, dyspnea, yawning, cyanosis

(b) Arterial blood gas analysis—including arterial oxygen tension, saturation, and content; hemoglobin; arteriovenous oxygen content and pressure differences

(c) Noninvasive oxygen monitoring

(1) Transcutaneous oxygen tension (TCP_{O_2}): measures oxygen concentration at the skin. Skin blood flow, thickness, temperature, and skin oxygen consumption are important variables in readings. Heat is applied to improve blood flow, and burns may result. Careful monitoring of electrode temperature is imperative, as is site rotation

(2) Pulse or ear oximetry—measures oxygen saturation by using light waves to detect differences between saturated and reduced hemoglobin in the tissue of the ear lobe or finger. Is accurate in Sa_{O_2} range of 70% to 100% but is inaccurate in low blood flow states. This device also reads carboxyhemoglobin and thus is not a reliable instrument in patients who recently smoked a cigarette or in situations of carbon monoxide poisoning. May be used for monitoring patients with chronic obstructive pulmonary disease and sleep-disordered breathing with episodic oxygen desaturation

b. Provide oxygen therapy

i. Areas in nursing care where periodic administration of oxygen may benefit patient

(a) Before, during, and after tracheal suctioning

(b) When ambulatory patient who is intubated or tracheostomized has inadequate tidal volume, a self-inflating bag and oxygen are indicated

  (c) Before any activity or nursing care given to cardiac patients

  (d) When transferring an unstable patient

ii. Rationale for use of low flow oxygen in patient with chronic obstructive pulmonary disease and chronic carbon dioxide retention

  (a) Because of decreased sensitivity of central chemoreceptors to blood carbon dioxide levels, carbon dioxide no longer serves as a respiratory stimulus, and the only remaining stimulus is hypoxemia. Therefore, high flow concentrations of oxygen depress the hypoxic drive, leading to depressed respiration and apnea

  (b) Nursing implications

    (1) Administer only enough oxygen to raise Pa_{O_2} to adequate levels for that patient (usually around 50 to 60 mm Hg)

    (2) Safety lies in controlled low flow rates, frequent monitoring of blood gases, and careful observation

iii. Principles of oxygen therapy

  (a) Remember the airway—no oxygen treatment is of any use without an adequate airway

  (b) Oxygen is a drug and as such should be administered in a prescribed dose (the $F_{I_{O_2}}$ is the dose)

  (c) Response to oxygen administration should be interpreted in terms of its effect on tissue oxygenation rather than its effect on the arterial blood gas values alone

  (d) The pathology of the patient's disease is the major determinant of the effectiveness of oxygen therapy

  (e) Delivered concentration of gas from any appliance is subject to the condition of the equipment, technique of application, cooperation of the patient, and ventilatory pattern of the patient

  (f) Low-flow oxygen systems do not provide the total inspired gas (patient is breathing some room air) and therefore are adequate only if tidal volume is adequate, respiratory rates are not excessive, and ventilator pattern is stable. Variable oxygen concentration of 21% to 90+% is provided, but the $F_{I_{O_2}}$ varies greatly with changes in tidal volume and ventilatory pattern

  (g) High-flow oxygen systems provide the entire inspired gas (patient is breathing only the gas supplied by the apparatus) and are adequate only if flow rates exceed inspiratory flow rate and minute ventilation. Both high and low oxygen concentrations may be delivered by high-flow systems (24% to 100% O_2)

iv. Hazards of oxygen therapy
   (a) Oxygen-induced hypoventilation
      (1) Prevent by use of low flow rates of 1 to 2 L/min
      (2) Greatest risk is when the patient's Pa_{CO_2} is greater than 50 mm Hg
      (3) Oxygen therapy should be used with special caution in
         a) Patient with chronic obstructive pulmonary disease and carbon dioxide retention
         b) Respiratory center depression caused by sedatives or narcotics
   (b) Microatelectasis, caused by elimination of nitrogen (nitrogen washout) and effect of oxygen on pulmonary surfactant
   (c) Retrolental fibroplasia in newborns
      (1) Fibrotic process behind lens caused by retinal vasoconstriction resulting from high Pa_{O_2}
      (2) Oxygen concentration should be kept as low as necessary to maintain adequate Pa_{O_2}
   (d) Oxygen toxicity
      (1) Caused by too high a concentration (usually considered to be an FI_{O_2} over 0.4 to 0.5) over too long a time (from 6 to 30 hours)
      (2) May be mild or fatal
      (3) Early signs and symptoms of oxygen toxicity
         a) Retrosternal distress
         b) Paresthesias in extremities
         c) Nausea, vomiting
         d) Fatigue, lethargy, malaise
         e) Dyspnea, coughing
         f) Anorexia
         g) Restlessness
      (4) Late signs and symptoms
         a) Progressive respiratory difficulty
         b) Cyanosis
         c) Dyspnea
         d) Asphyxia
      (5) Pathologic process
         a) Local toxicity to alveolar epithelial cells and pulmonary capillaries with exudative response (adult respiratory distress syndrome)
         b) Nitrogen washout and absorption atelectasis
      (6) Both oxygen concentration and duration of oxygen

administration are critical (40% oxygen or greater over several days is potentially dangerous)

(7) Changes seen in oxygen toxicity

    a) Decreased compliance and vital capacity

    b) Increasing A–a oxygen gradient

(e) Guidelines for prevention of complications caused by oxygen therapy

(1) Oxygen is a potent drug that should be used with reason and according to indications

(2) If high concentrations are necessary, the duration of administration should be kept to a minimum and reduced as soon as possible

(3) The objective is to maintain a Pa_{O_2} of at least 50 to 60 mm Hg to produce an acceptable Sa_{O_2} of 85% to 90% without damaging lungs or causing carbon dioxide retention

(4) Frequent arterial blood gas monitoring is a mandatory safety measure when concentrations above 40% are used

(5) Exact concentration of inspired oxygen should be measured with an oxygen analyzer

(6) Patient should never be exposed to dangerous levels of hypoxia for fear of developing oxygen toxicity. Hypoxia is far more common than oxygen toxicity and must be corrected. Pure oxygen has no contraindications in emergency situations

v. Methods of oxygen delivery (low-flow and high-flow systems)

(a) Masks

(1) General points

    a) Useful if oxygen needed quickly and for short periods

    b) Concentrations of 24% to 100% oxygen are delivered, depending on device

(2) Disadvantages

    a) Uncomfortable and hot

    b) Necrosis of skin caused by tight fit

    c) Difficult to control FI_{O_2} precisely, except when using Venturi mask

    d) Must be removed to eat, thus losing oxygen delivery

(3) Possible complications

    a) Patients who are prone to vomit may aspirate

    b) Obstruction by flaccid tongue may occur in comatose patient. Use oral airway and stay with patient

    c) May cause carbon dioxide retention and hypoventilation if flow is too low and exhalation ports are too small

    (4) Types of masks

       a) Simple—35% to 60% oxygen at 6- to 10-L flows. $F_{I_{O_2}}$ varies considerably with changes in tidal volume, ventilatory pattern, and inspiratory flow rate

       b) Rebreathing—used for administration of anesthesia

       c) Partial rebreathing

         ☐ Delivers 35% to 60% or higher at 6- to 10-L flows

         ☐ Flows must be adjusted so that reservoir bag does not collapse during inspiration, otherwise carbon dioxide retention may occur

       d) Nonrebreathing

         ☐ Delivers 90% to 100% concentration of gases, provided there are no leaks in system

         ☐ Is precise method of delivering a specific gas concentration for short-term purposes

         ☐ Reservoir bag must not collapse during inspiration

       e) Air entrainment (Venturi)

         ☐ Adjustments allow for delivery of precise oxygen concentrations of 24% to 40%

         ☐ Total air flow must be adequate for ventilatory needs of patient

         ☐ Is best suited to patient who must have a consistent $F_{I_{O_2}}$

  (b) Cannula (nasal)

    (1) Low oxygen concentrations delivered (below 40%) but depends on patient's tidal volume

    (2) Cooperative patient necessary

    (3) Advantages—easy to apply, light, economical, and disposable; allows patient mobility

    (4) Disadvantages—easily dislodged; high flow rates are uncomfortable

  (c) Nasal catheter

    (1) Low oxygen concentrations delivered (below 40%)

    (2) Better for less dependable and restless patients

    (3) Disadvantages—technique of insertion, gastric distention, nasopharyngeal injury

    (4) Data show that eventual delivery of oxygen to blood is not significantly different when either cannula or catheter is used and whether patient's mouth is open

or closed. Variability of FI_{O_2} is caused by oxygen flow-rate setting and patient's rate and depth of respiration

(d) Transtracheal catheter

(1) Small catheter inserted transtracheally through anterior neck for low-flow oxygen delivery

(2) Advantages—economical (less oxygen used to maintain a given Sa_{O_2} than other methods); very cosmetically appealing for patient (catheter may be concealed by clothing)

(3) Disadvantages—technique of insertion, risk of infection or subcutaneous emphysema if catheter dislodges

(e) Heated nebulizer

(1) Oxygen settings may not be accurate

(2) Flow rates should be run at flush

(f) Tracheal masks

(1) 35% to 70% oxygen concentrations

(2) Use with heated nebulizer, large-bore tubing

(g) T-piece

(1) 25% to 70% oxygen concentrations

(2) Use with heated nebulizer, large-bore tubing

(h) Hyperbaric oxygenation

(1) Administration of oxygen under greatly increased pressure

(2) Used in carbon monoxide poisoning, radiation therapy, gas gangrene, burns, decubiti

c. Administer positive end-expiratory pressure (PEEP): a major oxygenation treatment modality

i. Pressure above atmospheric is maintained at airway opening at end-expiration. Its purpose is to prevent alveolar collapse at end-expiration

ii. At end of quiet expiration, lung volume is increased; therefore, functional residual capacity (FRC) is increased. Increase in FRC is dependent on both the amount of PEEP used and the functional state of the lungs. Alveolar volume is increased and recruitment of alveoli occurs

iii. Major goal of PEEP is enhanced oxygen transport. PEEP serves to reduce the shunt effect of collapsed alveoli and may increase Pa_{O_2} dramatically. It raises Pa_{O_2} without requiring an increasing FI_{O_2}, which could lead to oxygen toxicity

iv. Clinical use

(a) Adult respiratory distress syndrome and pulmonary infiltrates (characterized by closure of airways or collapse of alveoli at end-expiration, resulting in hypoxemia and need for increased FI_{O_2})

(b) Acute respiratory failure that has caused a persistent

hypoxemia even though $F_{I_{O_2}}$ of 0.5 or greater has been maintained

(c) Cardiogenic pulmonary edema

(d) Avoidance of pulmonary oxygen toxicity from high $F_{I_{O_2}}$ levels

v. Amount of PEEP is tailored to patient's need. There is no arbitrary upper limit. Determination of optimal level requires accurate assessment of cardiopulmonary function, including lung compliance and cardiac output studies. PEEP levels above 15 cm H_2O are generally considered dangerous

vi. Side effects of PEEP

(a) Hemodynamic consequences of positive-pressure breathing are accentuated by PEEP. Patients with poor cardiovascular dynamics are at most risk. Adequate intravascular volume is essential

(1) Venous return may be impaired, resulting in decreased cardiac output

(2) Venous return, cardiac output, and oxygen delivery may be decreased even though Pa_{O_2} is increased

(3) Goal of increased oxygen transport cannot be met if cardiac output decrease is disproportionate to gain in arterial oxygenation (because oxygen transport is a product of oxygen content and blood flow)

(b) Barotrauma—rupture of lung tissue with high PEEP levels, especially in patients with lung disease

vii. Monitoring guidelines

(a) Essential to monitor those parameters that indicate status of cardiac output and tissue perfusion. These include blood pressure, urine output, pulse (central and peripheral), intake-output, mental status, skin color and temperature, arterial blood gases (specifically Pa_{O_2}), mixed venous oxygen content ($C\bar{v}_{O_2}$), mixed venous oxygen pressure ($P\bar{v}_{O_2}$), and mixed venous oxygen saturation ($S\bar{v}_{O_2}$). PEEP is adjusted gradually in small increments, with careful evaluation of side effects and patient response

(b) Ideally, patient should have arterial pressure monitoring catheter and pulmonary artery pressure catheter in place. Blood pressure, cardiovascular status, and urinary output must be closely monitored

(c) If significant drop in cardiac output occurs, PEEP may be reduced or Trendelenburg position may be indicated. Hypovolemia must be corrected when this is a contributing factor in decreased cardiac output. Short-term vasopressor therapy may sometimes be employed to correct decreased cardiac output in the normovolemic patient

        (d) PEEP is lost if patient is disconnected from ventilator for suctioning. Precipitous drop in Pa_{O_2} occurs in some patients. Adaptors for suctioning without disconnection are available and should be used

  d. Administer continuous positive airway pressure (CPAP)

     i. A nonventilator technique—a means of maintaining positive pressure during breathing. Similar to positive end-expiratory pressure but used on spontaneously breathing patient

     ii. Net result is improved arterial oxygen tensions. Technique allows for a reduction in inspired oxygen concentration

     iii. Used in weaning and pediatrics

  e. Encourage patients to take deep breaths (see Ineffective Airway Clearance, p. 47)

  f. Position patient to facilitate ventilation–perfusion matching ("good side down")

  g. Provide rest periods to minimize oxygen demands

  h. Alleviate or minimize fear/anxiety that may increase oxygen demands

  i. Monitor patient's response to self-care or any activity. If deterioration exists, provide physical care, including full assistance with turning and transfer and passive range of motion exercises

  j. Teach patient and significant others techniques of self-care that will minimize oxygen consumption

  k. Maintain body temperature at patient's normal level to avoid extremes, particularly shivering

4. Evaluation of nursing care

  a. Arterial blood gases within normal limits for patient with or without supplemental oxygen or mechanical ventilation

  b. Absence of cyanosis and dyspnea

  c. Patient performs techniques that maximize ventilation–perfusion matching

  d. Patient performs activities of daily living with or without supplemental oxygen

  e. Absence of fever, chills, and shivering

  f. Demonstrates energy conservation techniques for self-care

Ineffective Individual or Family Coping

1. Assessment for defining characteristics

  a. Verbalization of inability to cope or inability to ask for help

  b. Inability to meet role expectations

  c. Inability to meet basic needs

  d. Inability to problem-solve

  e. Alteration in societal participation

  f. Inappropriate use of defense mechanisms

g. Change in usual communication patterns
h. Destructive behavior toward self or others
i. Lack of appetite
j. Excessive smoking and/or drinking
k. Chronic fatigue
l. Insomnia
m. Sensory overload (i.e., noise)
n. Poor self-esteem
o. Chronic depression and/or worry
p. Patient expresses or confirms a concern or complaint about significant other's response to patient's health problem
q. Significant other describes preoccupation with personal reactions, (e.g., fear, anticipatory grief, guilt, anxiety regarding patient's illness or disability or to other situational or developmental crises)
r. Significant other describes or confirms an inadequate understanding or knowledge base that interferes with effective assistive or supportive behaviors
s. Significant other attempts assistive or supportive behaviors with less than satisfactory results
t. Significant other withdraws or enters into limited or temporary personal communication with patient at the time of need
u. Significant other displays protective behavior disproportionate to patient's abilities or need for autonomy

2. **Expected outcomes**
   a. Demonstrates increased independence
   b. Demonstrates increased functional activity
   c. Demonstrates decreased social isolation
   d. Appropriately expresses ideas, feelings, and needs
   e. Uses problem-solving skills
   f. Demonstrates assertiveness
   g. Completes everyday tasks involving social skills without the development of crises
   h. Communicates clearly
   i. Demonstrates decreased anxiety
   j. Demonstrates increased self-esteem
   k. Verbalizes need for more information or clearer understanding relating to situation
   l. Demonstrates understanding of information given
   m. Discusses changes in patient and family as result of health challenge
   n. Verbalizes feelings to health care professionals and other family members
   o. Identifies changes in family roles and processes as a result of patient's health challenges
   p. Recognizes roles to maintain family integrity
   q. Significant others participate in care of patient

r. Seeks help in adjusting to changes in family process from appropriate sources

3. **Nursing interventions**
   a. Provide adequate and correct information to patient and significant others
   b. Discuss "sick role" with patient and significant others
   c. Encourage family to have realistic perspective based on accurate information
   d. Discuss usual reactions to health challenges such as anxiety, dependency, and depression
   e. Provide opportunities for patient to discuss need for support with significant others
   f. Monitor areas in which knowledge or understanding is inadequate in relation to the patient's health challenge
   g. Maintain as much privacy as possible
   h. Minimize sensory overload as well as possible
   i. Provide an alternative to the patient's room for family discussion
   j. Encourage patient and significant others to verbalize feelings such as loss, guilt, anger, and relief
   k. Use communication techniques that confirm the legitimacy of both positive and negative feelings, such as reflecting feelings ("You seem frightened") and presenting reality ("Many persons feel angry in this situation")
   l. Assist the family to appraise the situation, including both strengths and weaknesses
   m. Assist the family to identify changes in relationships as a result of a patient's health challenge
   n. Provide opportunities for patient to control or make choices whenever appropriate
   o. Involve family members in care of patient as much as possible
   p. Encourage family members to seek help in adjusting to changes in family process from appropriate sources: friends, clergy, professional health care providers
   q. Provide alternative means for communication in patients who are intubated or have tracheostomy or laryngectomy
   r. Administer analgesics and/or mild sedatives if ordered to increase comfort
   s. Use nonpharmacologic pain relief measures (e.g., relaxation, distraction)

4. **Evaluation of nursing care**
   a. Verbalizes understanding of information given and of situation
   b. Displays decreased levels of anxiety and emotional discomfort
   c. Shows signs of successfully coping with changes in family dynamics related to patient's health challenge
   d. Communicates effectively through either verbal or nonverbal means

    e. Significant others are able to identify and provide appropriate support for the patient

    f. Patient is able to obtain adequate sleep

PATIENT HEALTH PROBLEMS

Acute Respiratory Failure: Failure of the respiratory system to carry out its two major functions: the delivery of an adequate amount of oxygen into the arterial blood and the removal of a corresponding amount of carbon dioxide from the mixed venous blood. As indicated by the designation *acute,* the onset must be relatively sudden; however the onset can be over days, as is particularly likely to occur in the patient with preexisting lung disease, or within minutes to hours, as often occurs in the patient without preexisting lung disease.

    Acute respiratory failure can be categorized according to the extent to which the arterial blood gases are abnormal. Abnormalities can exist in the P_{O_2}, P_{CO_2}, or both; the more severe the hypoxemia or hypercapnea, the greater the consensus about categorization. However, interpretation of arterial blood gases must take into consideration two important aspects of the clinical situation: the blood gas values *before* the onset of acute respiratory failure (which depend on whether previous lung disease was present) and the rapidity with which the abnormalities in the blood gases developed.

    As indicated above, the abnormalities in arterial blood gases may be in P_{O_2} (hypoxemic respiratory failure), in P_{CO_2} (hypercapneic respiratory failure), or both. The critical value for the diagnosis based on arterial hypoxemia is a Pa_{O_2} of 50 to 60 mm Hg; lower values can cause marked unsaturation of hemoglobin and a considerable drop in oxygen content because of the shape of the oxygen dissociation curve. The corresponding critical value for diagnosing acute hypercapneic respiratory failure is a value for Pa_{CO_2} greater than 50 to 55 mm Hg (with an accompanying acidemia: pH $<$ 7.30).

1. **Pathophysiology:** there are four pathophysiologic mechanisms that can cause acute respiratory failure—hypoventilation, ventilation–perfusion mismatching, shunt, and diffusion limitation. Of these, the first three mechanisms are by far the most common, since diffusion limitation is a relatively unimportant cause of clinically significant hypoxemia. These physiologic abnormalities result from structural processes that make up the pathologic background for the abnormalities of gas exchange. The two major processes involved are

    a. Increase in extravascular lung water

       i. Characterized by severe hypoxemia with normal to low Pa_{CO_2}

      ii. Occurs in patients with cardiogenic or noncardiogenic pulmonary edema and other parenchymal infiltrates

b. Impaired ventilation
   i. Characterized by elevated Pa_{CO_2} and decreased Pa_{O_2}
   ii. Occurs with intrapulmonary (airway disease) or extrapulmonary problems (neuromuscular disorders, chest wall diseases, or alterations in respiratory drive)

2. **Etiology or precipitating factors** (multiple)
   a. Increase in extravascular lung water
      i. Adult respiratory distress syndrome, pulmonary edema, aspiration, pneumonia, atelectasis
   b. Impaired ventilation
      i. Intrapulmonary problems: emphysema, chronic bronchitis, asthma, bronchiectasis; especially following sepsis or acute respiratory infection; pulmonary embolism, pneumothorax
      ii. Extrapulmonary problems: pleural effusion, kyphoscoliosis, multiple rib fractures, thoracic surgery, abdominal surgery, peritonitis; neuromuscular defects such as polio, Guillain-Barré syndrome, multiple sclerosis, myasthenia gravis, brain or spinal injuries, drugs or toxic agents; respiratory center damage or depression: narcotics, barbiturates, tranquilizers, anesthetics; cerebral infarction or trauma

3. **Nursing assessment data base**
   a. Nursing history
      i. Subjective findings
         (a) Patient's chief complaint—most often dyspnea or increased work of breathing
         (b) Other symptoms include
            (1) Increased secretions
            (2) Manifestations of hypoxemia—disorientation, confusion, restlessness, impaired intellectual functioning, tachypnea, tachycardia
            (3) Manifestations of hypercapnea with acidemia—headache, confusion, inability to concentrate, irritability, somnolence, dizziness
      ii. Objective findings
         (a) Etiologic or precipitating factors
            (1) Determine if patient has a past history of chronic airway obstruction, restrictive defects, neuromuscular defects, or respiratory center damage that could impair ventilation
            (2) Determine if patient has any of the conditions that impair gas exchange and diffusion
            (3) Assess for presence of ventilation–perfusion abnormalities
         (b) Family history—determine if any parents, grandparents, or siblings ever had significant pulmonary disease. One

form of emphysema caused by deficiency of the enzyme alpha$_1$-antitrypsin is an inherited disorder

    (c) Social history—determine if patient is a current or past smoker; calculate pack-year history of smoking

    (d) Medication history—obtain list of all prescribed and over-the-counter medications along with their doses and last time patient took the medication. Assess for evidence of noncompliance in taking prescribed medications (i.e., missed doses and/or overdoses)

b. Nursing examination of patient

  i. Inspection

    (a) Observe for thoracic abnormalities, such as

      (1) Increased anteroposterior diameter, or barrel chest

      (2) Retraction of thorax

      (3) Pectus carinatum or pectus excavatum

      (4) Spinal deformities

    (b) Inspect ribs and interspaces

      (1) Intercostal retractions indicate increased work of breathing

      (2) Bulging of interspaces on expiration occurs when there is obstruction to air outflow

    (c) Pattern of respiration

      (1) Evidence of increased work of breathing: use of accessory muscles

      (2) Rate, depth, rhythm of breathing

      (3) Inspiration/expiration ratio (normal ratio is 1:2)

      (4) Inspiratory and/or expiratory stridor, indicative of air flow obstruction

    (d) General observation

      (1) Patient's posture, state of comfort

      (2) Skin color and perfusion—presence of cyanosis, temperature of skin, presence of diaphoresis

      (3) Observe for signs of right-sided heart failure, such as pitting edema of lower extremities and presence of cardiac gallop

      (4) Observe for signs of hypercapnea with acidemia—muscle twitching, asterixis, miosis, papilledema, engorged fundal veins, diaphoresis, hypertension

  ii. Palpation

    (a) Evaluate lung expansion

    (b) Assess vocal fremitus

      (1) Increased fremitus is found with any condition that results in increased density of lung, such as consolidation

      (2) Decreased fremitus is found if there is obstructed major

bronchus or fluid in the pleural space or if patient has severe chronic obstructive pulmonary disease with air trapping

iii. Percussion

(a) Dullness is heard over more dense lung tissue, such as consolidation or pulmonary edema

(b) Hyperresonance is heard over chest with air trapping (chronic obstructive pulmonary disease) or pneumothorax

iv. Auscultation

(a) Decreased breath sounds are heard when there is less air movement and less dense lung tissue (chronic obstructive pulmonary disease)

(b) Bronchial and/or bronchovesicular breath sounds are heard over more dense lung tissue (consolidation, atelectasis, pulmonary edema)

(c) Adventitious sounds

(1) Crackles or rales

(2) Rhonchi or gurgles

(3) Wheezes

(d) Pleural friction rub—heard when inflamed pleural surfaces rub together

c. Diagnostic study findings

i. Arterial blood gases

(a) Respiratory failure is defined by arterial blood gas measurements as hypoxemic ($\downarrow$ Pa_{O_2}) and/or hypercapnic ($\downarrow$ Pa_{O_2} and $\uparrow$ Pa_{CO_2})

(b) Criteria—Pa_{O_2} below 50 to 60 mm Hg, Pa_{CO_2} above 50 mm Hg, or both

(1) Acute—acidosis, normal or mildly increasing blood buffers (bicarbonate)

(2) Chronic—relatively normal pH, elevated blood buffers

ii. Radiologic findings—depends on primary disease

iii. Intrapulmonary shunt greater than 15%

4. **Nursing diagnoses** (see Commonly Encountered Nursing Diagnoses, p. 47)

a. Ineffective airway clearance related to secretions

b. Ineffective breathing pattern

c. Impaired gas exchange

d. Ineffective individual and family coping

Adult Respiratory Distress Syndrome (ARDS): A group of manifestations of an evolving, severe diffuse lung injury, especially to the parenchyma. The acute form of ARDS nearly always occurs suddenly in the presence of certain identifiable risk factors. In some types of acute ARDS, if the patient survives, the injury resolves and recovery is complete. In other patients with acute ARDS, notably the form associated with sepsis, there is a high mortality even after the increased permeability pulmonary edema subsides. Instead of healing, the injured lung parenchyma rapidly undergoes organizational changes and a chronic phase evolves

1. **Pathophysiology**
    a. The acute phase is characterized by damaged integrity of the blood–gas barrier. There is extensive damage to the type I alveolar epithelial cells with increased endothelial permeability. Interstitial edema is found along with protein containing fluid leaking into the alveoli. This alveolar fluid also contains erythrocytes and leukocytes in addition to amorphous material comprising strands of fibrin. There also is impaired production and function of surfactant. The resultant physiologic abnormalities include the following
        i. Shunting of blood through atelectatic or fluid-filled lung units causes a widening of the alveolar to arterial difference in P_{O_2}; the resultant hypoxemia is resistant to high FI_{O_2} but is often responsive to positive end-expiratory pressure
        ii. The physiologic dead space is increased, frequently exceeding 60% of each breath; consequently very large minute ventilation may be required to maintain tolerable levels of arterial P_{CO_2}
        iii. The compliance of congested atelectatic lungs is reduced. The increased stiffness of the lungs is associated with a decrease in functional residual capacity and a requirement for high peak inspiratory pressures during mechanical ventilation
        iv. The resistance to blood flow through the lungs is increased by narrowing or obstruction of the pulmonary vessels. As a result, the pulmonary arterial pressure is often increased even though the capillary wedge pressure remains normal or low
    b. Chronic phase of ARDS is characterized by thickening of the endothelium, epithelium and the interstitial space. Type I cells are destroyed and replaced by type II cells, which proliferate but do not differentiate into type I cells as normal. The interstitial space is greatly expanded by edema fluid, fibers, and a variety of proliferating cells. Fibrosis commences after the first week. Within the alveoli, the protein-rich exudate may organize to produce the characteristic "hyaline membrane," which effectively destroys the structure of the alveoli. Resultant physiologic abnormalities are
        i. Increased vascular resistance
        ii. Hypoxemia from ventilation–perfusion mismatch or possible diffusion defect
        iii. Decreased tissue compliance
2. **Etiology or precipitating factors**—from direct or indirect injury
    a. Direct injury: pulmonary contusion, gastric aspiration, near-drowning, inhalation of toxic gases and vapors, some infections, fat embolus, amniotic fluid embolus, radiation, bleomycin

   b. Indirect injury: septicemia, shock or prolonged hypotension, nonthoracic trauma, cardiopulmonary bypass, head injury, pancreatitis, diabetic coma, multiple blood transfusions
3. **Nursing assessment data base**
   a. Nursing history
      i. Subjective findings
         (a) Patient's chief complaint—severe dyspnea
         (b) Other symptoms
            (1) Altered level of consciousness if hypoxemia is severe (i.e., confusion, somnolence, restlessness, irritability, anxiety, decreased mental acuity)
            (2) Production of frothy pink sputum
      ii. Objective findings
         (a) Etiologic or precipitating factors—determine if patient has a history of any of those listed above
         (b) Family history—ARDS is the lung's response to a stressful condition or event and is not an inherited disorder
         (c) Social history
            (1) Determine if there is a history of drug use, particularly heroin
            (2) Determine recent alcohol and food intake; assess for signs of aspiration
         (d) Medication history—determine the quantities of all medications recently taken by patient, both over-the-counter and prescription drugs
   b. Nursing examination of the patient
      i. Inspection
         (a) Assess work of breathing
            (1) Posture, if patient is seated
            (2) Nasal flaring
            (3) Intercostal retractions
            (4) Use of accessory muscles
         (b) Assess rate and depth of respiration
            (1) Tachypnea and hyperpnea
      ii. Palpation
         (a) Assess lung expansion—reduced due to low lung compliance
         (b) Assess vocal fremitus—increased due to increased density from diffuse pulmonary edema
      iii. Percussion
         (a) Dullness to percussion over all lung fields if substantial pulmonary edema is present
      iv. Auscultation
         (a) Bronchovesicular breath sounds over most lung fields due to the increased density of lung

(b) Adventitious sounds—diffuse crackles and rhonchi over all lung fields
c. Diagnostic study findings
  i. Arterial blood gases
    (a) Hypoxemia is the hallmark of this disease and is due to intrapulmonary shunting. Hypoxemia is refractory to oxygen therapy (i.e., Pa_{O_2} below 55 mm Hg with FI_{O_2} above 0.5)
    (b) Respiratory alkalosis occurs because of hyperventilation
    (c) Hypercapnea is usually not seen initially and is an ominous sign if present
  ii. Chest x-ray film: demonstrates diffuse bilateral interstitial and alveolar infiltrates in the acute phase, evolving into a fine or coarse reticular pattern in the chronic phase
  iii. Pulmonary function
    (a) Reduced pulmonary compliance
    (b) Reduced functional residual capacity, secondary to micro-atelectasis and edema
    (c) Shunt studies demonstrate large right-to-left shunt (usually greater than 20% of cardiac output) measured while patient is breathing 100% oxygen
    (d) Increased dead space ventilation ($\dot{V}_D/\dot{V}_T$)
    (e) Increased A–a gradient
  iv. Pulmonary capillary wedge pressure may be normal, but pulmonary arterial pressure is often elevated
4. **Nursing diagnoses** (see Commonly Encountered Nursing Diagnoses, p. 47)
  a. Impaired gas exchange
    i. Additional nursing interventions
      (a) Change patient's position every 2 hours to mobilize secretions and allow aeration of all lung fields
      (b) Observe for signs of fluid overload
      (c) Monitor arterial blood gas results; notify physician immediately if Pa_{O_2} drops and/or Pa_{CO_2} rises. Be prepared for the possibility of endotracheal intubation and mechanical ventilation
      (d) Teach patient such relaxation techniques as imagery, progressive muscle relaxation, and meditation to decrease demand for oxygen. Help and encourage patient to do relaxation techniques every 4 hours
  b. Ineffective individual and family coping

Chronic Obstructive Pulmonary Disease (COPD): Condition in which patients have chronic cough and expectoration and various degrees of exertional dyspnea with a significant and progressive reduction in expiratory air flow as measured by the forced expiratory volume in 1 second (FEV_1). This air flow abnormality does not show major reversibility in response to pharmacologic agents. Terms such as chronic obstructive airway disease (COAD), chronic obstructive lung disease (COLD), chronic air flow obstruction or chronic airway obstruction (CAO), and chronic air flow limitation (CAL) all mean the same thing. COPD is usually divided into two subtypes: chronic bronchitis and emphysema. The separate pathophysiology of these subtypes is described below; however, many patients exhibit signs and symptoms of both clinical conditions

1. Pathophysiology

a. Chronic bronchitis: a clinical diagnosis defined as the presence of chronic cough with sputum production on a daily basis for a minimum of 3 months per year for not less than 2 successive years. Patients with chronic bronchitis are sometimes referred to as "blue bloaters" because they are chronically hypoxemic with resultant episodes of cor pulmonale. The "blue bloater" has reduced responsiveness of his respiratory center to hypoxemic stimuli, a trait that is probably inherited. Some of the pathophysiologic findings of chronic bronchitis are

   i. Increase in size of the tracheobronchial mucus glands (increased Reid index) and goblet cell hyperplasia, resulting in increased sputum production

   ii. Epithelial mucus cell metaplasia, resulting in a decreased number of cilia. Hypersecretion of mucus and impaired cilia lead to a chronic productive cough

   iii. Increase in bronchial wall thickness with progressive obstruction to air flow (chronic obstructive bronchitis)

   iv. Exacerbations are usually due to infection, with the following clinical picture

      (a) Increased amount of sputum and retained secretions

      (b) Increased ventilation–perfusion abnormalities, which increase hypoxemia, carbon dioxide retention, and acidemia

      (c) Hypoxemia and acidemia increase pulmonary vessel constriction, raising pulmonary artery pressure and ultimately leading to right-sided heart failure (cor pulmonale)

b. Emphysema: an anatomic alteration of the lung characterized by an abnormal enlargement of the air spaces distal to the terminal, nonrespiratory bronchioles, accompanied by destructive changes in the alveolar walls. Emphysema patients are often referred to as "pink puffers" owing to an inherent increased responsiveness to hypoxemia, with resultant increased dyspnea and breathing effort. The resultant clinical picture is that of a pink (well oxygenated) and puffing (dyspneic) patient. The pulmonary abnormalities seen in the emphysema patient are

    i. Reduction of gas exchange surface of respiratory bronchioles, alveolar ducts, and alveoli

    ii. Increased air trapping caused by loss of elastic recoil and airway support structures (resulting in increased anteroposterior diameter)

    iii. Ventilation–perfusion inequality occurs and functional residual capacity is increased

    iv. Air sacs are replaced by bullae, and capillary area is proportionately diminished

    v. Increased work of breathing results in greater oxygen consumption

2. **Etiology or precipitating factors** for chronic bronchitis/emphysema
   a. Cigarette smoking: most important factor and major toxic stimulus
   b. Environmental pollution, occupational exposure
   c. Predisposition due to genetic makeup, especially if there is known deficiency of alpha$_1$-antitrypsin deficiency

3. **Nursing assessment data base**
   a. Nursing history
      i. Subjective findings
         (a) Patient's chief complaint: these diseases may present as pure entities, but it is common for patients to have a combination of symptoms of both
            (1) Chronic bronchitis—chronic cough and sputum production
            (2) Emphysema—dyspnea on exertion (early symptom) and eventual dyspnea at rest
         (b) Other symptoms
            (1) Chronic bronchitis—wheezing, peripheral edema
            (2) Emphysema—weight loss, an inability to do activities of daily living
      ii. Objective findings
         (a) Etiologic or precipitating factors—history of cigarette smoking and/or environmental or occupational exposure
         (b) Family history of emphysema
         (c) Social history—assess extent of cigarette smoking; calculate pack-year history
         (d) Medication history—determine doses and times of all medications, both over-the-counter and prescription drugs. Assess compliance in taking correct dose, adhering to correct schedule, and using proper inhalation technique for inhaled medications
   b. Nursing examination of patient: findings are described in terms of the pure entities chronic bronchitis and emphysema; however, most patients exhibit some symptoms of both conditions
      i. Inspection

    (a) Chronic bronchitis—observe for signs of right-sided heart failure: peripheral edema, distended neck veins. Skin color: dusky or cyanotic skin tone. Patients with chronic bronchitis show little sign of respiratory distress or dyspnea

    (b) Emphysema—observe thoracic cage for barrel chest appearance. Note posture and work of breathing; use of accessory muscles of respiration is commonly noted. Observe for use of pursed lip breathing. Note skin color (usually well oxygenated and thus pink)

  ii. Palpation

    (a) Chronic bronchitis—note chest expansion: may be normal. Assess vocal fremitus: may be normal or increased due to copious secretions in bronchial tree

    (b) Emphysema—chest excursion: reduced because patient's lungs are hyperinflated from chronic air trapping. Vocal fremitus will be reduced due to less dense, more hyperinflated lungs

  iii. Percussion

    (a) Chronic bronchitis—may demonstrate resonance if there are no areas of secretion retention/consolidation. Dullness to percussion is heard in areas of increased lung density (i.e., consolidation)

    (b) Emphysema—hyperresonance throughout all lung fields

  iv. Auscultation

    (a) Chronic bronchitis—coarse crackles and rhonchi. Expiratory wheezes heard commonly

    (b) Emphysema—distant, quiet breath sounds due to reduced air movement and air trapping. Wheezes heard on occasion

c. Diagnostic study findings

  i. Chronic bronchitis

    (a) Pulmonary function—reduction in FEV_1 with some reversibility following bronchodilator therapy

    (b) Arterial blood gases—hypoxemia and hypercapnea with compensated respiratory acidosis

    (c) Other laboratory findings

      (1) Polycythemia on complete blood cell count

  ii. Emphysema

    (a) Pulmonary function—increased functional residual capacity and total lung capacity. Reduced FEV_1 and nonreversibility with bronchodilators. Increased lung compliance and decrease in static recoil. Decreased diffusion capacity indicating a reduction in alveolar capillary gas exchange area

    (b) Arterial blood gases—may be normal. Hypoxemia may be

mild with normal Pa_{CO_2}. Hypoxemia is greatest during sleep

(c) Radiologic findings—hyperinflated lungs indicated by flattened diaphragms and increased retrosternal air space and costal angles greater than or equal to 90° (lateral)

4. **Nursing diagnoses** (see Commonly Encountered Nursing Diagnoses, p. 47)
   a. Ineffective airway clearance
   b. Ineffective breathing pattern
   c. Impaired gas exchange
      i. Additional nursing interventions
         (a) Careful administration of oxygen using lowest $F_{I_{O_2}}$ that produces adequate oxygenation; observe for carbon dioxide retention with oxygen administration
         (b) Observe for signs of fluid overload
         (c) Monitor arterial blood gases; notify physician immediately if Pa_{O_2} drops and/or Pa_{CO_2} rises. Be prepared for the possibility of endotracheal intubation and mechanical ventilation
         (d) Teach patient to avoid cigarette smoking and other irritants and pollutants
   d. Ineffective individual and family coping

Asthma and Severe Asthmatic Attack (Status Asthmaticus)

1. **Pathophysiology**
   a. Asthma: a chronic disease of variable severity characterized by airway hyperreactivity that produces airway narrowing of a reversible nature
      i. Increased responsiveness of airways to various stimuli
      ii. Widespread narrowing of airway with changes in severity; airway closure may occur
      iii. Cellular infiltration and mucosal edema
      iv. Airway hyperreactivity, with smooth muscle contraction and excessive mucus production and diminished secretion clearance
      v. Ventilation–perfusion abnormalities
      vi. Increased work of breathing and airway resistance
      vii. Hyperinflation of lung, with increase in residual volume
      viii. Host defect of altered immunologic state ("extrinsic" asthma)
   b. Status asthmaticus: severe asthma attack that is refractory to bronchodilator therapy, including beta-adrenergic agents and intravenous aminophylline
      i. Severely reduced spirometric values for peak expiratory flow, forced vital capacity, and forced expiratory volume

    ii. Hypoxemia is present with a widened A–a oxygen tension gradient

    iii. Airway narrowing from

      (a) Bronchial smooth muscle spasm—minor component

      (b) Inflammation of bronchial walls, which leads to increased mucosal permeability and basement membrane thickening

      (c) Mucus plugging from airways due to increased production and reduced clearance of secretions. The mucus plugging, mucosal edema, and inspissated secretions account for the apparent resistance to bronchodilator therapy in patients with status asthmaticus

2. **Etiology or precipitating factors** for development of an asthma attack
   a. Respiratory infection
   b. Allergic reaction to inhaled antigen
   c. Inappropriate bronchodilator management
   d. Idiosyncratic reaction to aspirin or other nonsteroidal anti-inflammatory agents
   e. Emotional stress
   f. Environmental exposure (air pollution, metabisulfite ingestion)
   g. Exercise
   h. Occupational exposure
   i. Nonselective beta-blocking agents (propranolol, timolol maleate)
   j. Mechanical stimulation (coughing, laughing, and cold air inhalation)
   k. Reflux esophagitis
   l. Sinusitis

3. **Nursing assessment data base**
   a. Nursing history
       i. Subjective findings
         (a) Patient's chief complaint is usually dyspnea and/or cough
         (b) Other symptoms commonly seen with asthma are
           (1) Wheezing
           (2) Physical exhaustion, inability to sleep or rest, anxiety
           (3) Thick tenacious sputum production
       ii. Objective findings
         (a) Etiologic or precipitating factors—determine the presence of one or more etiologic or precipitating factors
         (b) Family history—determine if there is a history of asthma in immediate family, grandparents, uncles, and aunts
         (c) Social history
           (1) Assess occupational exposure to dusts, industrial toxins, heat, or cold
           (2) Determine if patient smokes tobacco and/or marijuana, the amount, and whether any of the patient's symptoms relate to the cigarette consumption
           (3) Assess patient's recent eating habits for presence of

known allergens (i.e., metabisulfites used as food preservatives)

    (4) Evaluate home conditions for presence of potential allergens

       a) Pet dander

       b) Carpets, rugs, etc., containing house mite debris

       c) Smoker in the household

       d) Plants

       e) Type of humidification or air filtration system at home

  (d) Medication history—list all medications, both prescribed and over-the-counter drugs, that patient has taken in past week. Assess patient compliance in taking correct medications and doses at appropriate times. If patient is using any inhalers, assess inhalation technique if possible. Question patient regarding any change in symptoms in response to any of the medications

b. Nursing examination of patient

  i. Inspection

    (a) Observe the anteroposterior diameter of the chest—in severe asthmatics, chronic air trapping may result in barrel-chested appearance

    (b) Assess patient's work of breathing

      (1) Posture

      (2) Use of pursed lip breathing

      (3) Presence of nasal flaring

      (4) Bulging of interspaces on expiration

    (c) Assess breathing pattern

      (1) Prolonged expiration

      (2) Expiratory stridor

      (3) Rate of respirations—tachypnea and/or hyperpnea

    (d) Assess for signs of dehydration; dehydration is believed to predispose to mucus impaction secondary to increased bronchial secretion viscosity

  ii. Palpation

    (a) Assess chest expansion—asthmatic lungs are hyperinflated and often show minimal chest excursion with inspiration

    (b) Assess vocal fremitus—may be decreased due to decreased density (due to hyperinflation) of lungs. Rhonchal fremitus may be present if there are copious secretions

  iii. Percussion

    (a) Hyperresonance is usually heard throughout lung fields

    (b) Assessment of diaphragmatic excursion reveals low position of diaphragm and reduced excursion

iv. Auscultation
   (a) Prolonged expiration
   (b) Expiratory wheezes and/or rhonchi are heard when air and secretions move through narrowed airways
   (c) Decreased breath sounds throughout is an ominous sign. The asthmatic is then not moving enough air for it to be heard by the examiner

c. Diagnostic findings
   i. Laboratory
      (a) Evidence of infection (e.g., positive sputum cultures, elevated leukocyte count)
      (b) Arterial blood gases
         (1) May initially show normal or $\downarrow$ Pa_{CO_2}, $\uparrow$ pH, and $\downarrow$ Pa_{O_2}
         (2) In severe asthmatic attacks, there may be progression to carbon dioxide retention (an ominous sign)
   ii. Radiologic findings—chest x-ray film may be normal or hyperlucent
   iii. Pulmonary function—reduced FEV_1 and peak flow rates. Serial measurements of these parameters with the response to bronchodilators is the best means to establish the severity of the obstruction and assess adequacy of therapy. In status asthmaticus, peak expiratory flow may be less than 60 L/min and FEV_1 may be less than 600 ml. The FVC is often reduced to less than 1 L, thus yielding a normal FEV_1:FVC ratio

4. **Nursing diagnoses** (see Commonly Encountered Nursing Diagnoses, p. 47)
   a. Ineffective airway clearance
      i. Additional nursing interventions
         (a) Administer bronchodilators and monitor therapeutic ranges and clinical response
         (b) Administer fluids and humidification to keep airway secretions thin and easily expectorated
         (c) Patient education to avoid allergens and importance of taking medications properly
   b. Ineffective breathing pattern
   c. Impaired gas exchange
      i. Additional nursing interventions
         (a) Close objective monitoring of blood gas levels, acid–base status, and ventilatory parameters (especially FEV_1 and peak flow rates)
         (b) Careful monitoring for cardiopulmonary arrest in severe cases
   d. Ineffective individual and family coping

Pulmonary Embolism: Obstruction of the pulmonary arteries by emboli affects lung tissue, the pulmonary circulation, and the function of the right and left sides of the heart. The degree of compromise correlates with the extent of embolic vascular occlusion and the degree of preexisting cardiopulmonary disease

1. Pathophysiology

    a. Most emboli (more than 90%) originate in the popliteal or ileofemoral veins. Other sites include the right side of the heart and the pelvic area. Nonthrombotic emboli such as fat, air, and amniotic fluid also occur but are relatively uncommon

    b. Factors favoring venous thrombosis include the following (Virchow's triad)

        i. Blood stasis

        ii. Blood coagulation alterations

        iii. Vessel-wall abnormalities

    c. Distribution of emboli is related to size of emboli and flow. Very large emboli impact in a large artery; however, the thrombus may break up and block several smaller vessels. The lower lobes are frequently involved because thay have a high blood flow

    d. Pulmonary infarction, that is, death of the embolized tissue, occurs infrequently. More often there is distal hemorrhage and atelectasis but alveolar structures remain viable. Infarction is more likely if the embolus completely blocks a large artery or if there is preexisting lung disease. Infarction results in alveolar filling with extravasated erythrocytes and inflammatory cells and causes opacity on the x-ray film. Occasionally the infarct becomes infected, leading to an abscess

    e. Effects of acute pulmonary artery obstruction

        i. Altered gas exchange due to

            (a) Right-to-left shunting and ventilation–perfusion inequalities. Possible causes for these alterations include

                (1) Overperfusion of unembolized lung results in low ventilation–perfusion ratios

                (2) Eventual reperfusion of atelectatic areas distal to the embolic obstruction

                (3) Development of postembolic pulmonary edema

        ii. The degree of hemodynamic compromise correlates with the degree of vascular occlusion in patients with no underlying heart or lung disease

            (a) Initial hemodynamic consequence is acute reduction in pulmonary vascular cross-sectional area with a subsequent increase in the resistance to blood flow through the lungs

            (b) If cardiac output remains constant or increases, the pulmonary arterial pressure must rise

        iii. If cardiac or pulmonary disease exists and has already impaired the pulmonary vascular reserve capacity, a small degree of vascular occlusion will result in greater pulmonary artery hypertension and more serious right ventricular dysfunction

2. **Etiology or precipitating factors** for deep venous thrombosis and pulmonary embolism
   a. Congestive heart failure
   b. Acute myocardial infarction
   c. Shock (bacteremia or nonbacteremia)
   d. Obesity
   e. Estrogens
   f. Malignancy
   g. Polycythemia vera
   h. Dysproteinemia
   i. Surgery or anesthesia
   j. Immobility
   k. Diabetes mellitus
   l. Burns
   m. Trauma (especially fractures of spine, pelvis, or legs)
   n. Varicose veins
   o. Previous pulmonary embolus
3. **Nursing assessment data base**
   a. Nursing history
      i. Subjective findings
         (a) Patient's chief complaint varies considerably depending on severity and type of embolism. Dyspnea, tachypnea, and chest pain are three subjective complaints common to many clinical situations
         (b) Other symptoms
            (1) Massive pulmonary embolism (more than 50% vascular occlusion)
               a) Mental clouding, anxiety, feeling of impending doom and apprehension
            (2) Pulmonary embolism—symptoms may be vague and nonspecific
               a) Sensation of rapid heartbeat
               b) Pleuritic chest pain, diffuse chest discomfort
               c) Hemoptysis, if pulmonary infarction is present
               d) Anxiety, restlessness, apprehension
               e) Cough
      ii. Objective findings
         (a) Etiologic or precipitating factors—history of one of the precipitating factors
         (b) Family history—no familial tendencies for pulmonary emboli; may be familial history of some of the precipitating factors that increase the patient's risk for pulmonary embolism (i.e., obesity)

(c) Social history—assess patient's activity level to determine if immobility is a factor

(d) Medication history—determine if female patients are taking oral contraceptives

b. Nursing examination of patient

i. Inspection

(a) Assess chest expansion—may be reduced on affected side owing to pleuritic pain

(b) Observe for signs of increased work of breathing, tachypnea, and dyspnea

(c) Examine patient for petechiae over thorax and upper extremities

(d) Observe skin for diaphoresis, signs of shock, cyanosis

(e) Assess behavior and mental status for mental aberrations, agitation, anxiety, restlessness

ii. Palpation

(a) May elicit asymmetric chest expansion

(b) Increased fremitus with large hemorrhagic pulmonary infarct

(c) Pleural friction fremitus may be palpated in patients with pleural inflammation distal to infarct

iii. Percussion

(a) Resonance heard throughout lung fields except

(b) Dullness to percussion over area of infarction

iv. Auscultation

(a) Crackles (rales) may be heard

(b) Increased intensity of pulmonic second sound (P_2)

(c) Fixed splitting of the second heart sound (S_2) is an ominous finding owing to marked right ventricular overload

(d) Murmur heard over lung field, augmented by inspiration. This murmur is generated by flow through a partially obstructed pulmonary artery. It may be absent initially and then develop as an embolus resolves

(e) Pleural friction rub

c. Diagnostic study findings

i. Laboratory findings

(a) Arterial blood gases—may indicate respiratory alkalosis (due to hyperventilation) and hypoxemia; A–a gradient increased

ii. Radiologic findings

(a) Chest x-ray film—nonspecific, frequently normal

(b) Pulmonary angiography—most definitive test for pulmonary embolism

iii. Radionuclide testing

(a) Lung ventilation–perfusion scan—not definitive but

suggestive of pulmonary embolism; less risky than angi-ography

iv. Electrocardiogram is usually normal but in massive pulmonary embolism it may reveal P pulmonale, right axis deviation, incomplete right bundle branch block, or new right bundle branch block

4. **Nursing diagnoses** (see Commonly Encountered Nursing Diagnoses, p. 47)

a. Ineffective breathing pattern

i. Additional nursing interventions

(a) Early ambulation, turning, coughing, deep breathing

(b) Elastic stockings, leg elevation

(c) Adequate fluid intake

(d) Administer anticoagulants as ordered; monitor for signs of bleeding

(e) Administer thrombolytic therapy as ordered

(f) Administer analgesics to prevent splinting; monitor for respiratory depression

b. Impaired gas exchange

c. Ineffective individual and family coping

Chest Trauma

1. **Pathophysiology:** depends on type and extent of injury. Trauma to chest and/or lungs may interfere with any of the components involved in inspiration, gas exchange, and expiration

a. Blunt injuries—chest wall damage must be evaluated in conjunction with the accompanying intrathoracic and intra-abdominal visceral injuries. Injuries seen with blunt trauma include

i. Visceral injuries without chest wall damage

(a) Pneumothorax

(b) Hemothorax

(c) Lung contusion

(d) Diaphragmatic injury

(e) Aortic rupture

(f) Rupture of trachea or bronchus

(g) Cardiac injury

ii. Soft tissue injuries—may be a sign of severe underlying damage

(a) Cutaneous abrasion

(b) Ecchymosis

(c) Laceration of superficial layers

(d) Burns

(e) Hematoma

iii. Fracture of sternum occurs either as a result of direct impact or as the indirect result of overflexion of the trunk

     iv. Rib fractures occur as a result of overflexion or from straightening. Rib fractures can be unifocal or multifocal. Multiple fractures result in flail chest and are often complicated by injuries to the soft tissues and pleura

     v. Separation or dislocation of ribs and cartilages from an anterior blow to chest

  b. Penetrating injuries

     i. Pleural cavity as well as chest wall has been entered. Damage to deeper structures is a serious consequence

     ii. Generally able to predict the extent of injury and the organs injured by course of wound and nature of penetrating instrument. High velocity projectiles do more damage than is apparent from the surface

     iii. Injuries seen with penetrating trauma

       (a) Open sucking chest wounds with air entering pleural space during inspiration

       (b) Hemothorax or hemopneumothorax or chylothorax

       (c) Combined thoracoabdominal injuries (esophageal, diaphragmatic, or abdominal viscus injuries)

       (d) Damage to trachea and large airways

       (e) Wounds of heart or great vessels

2. Etiology or precipitating factors

  a. Blunt trauma: automobile accidents, falls, assaults, explosives

  b. Penetrating trauma: those as in blunt trauma and also bullets, knives, shell fragments, free flying objects, industrial accidents

3. Nursing assessment data base

  a. Nursing history

     i. Subjective findings

       (a) Patient's chief complaint will vary with specific injury. Tachypnea, dyspnea, pain, and respiratory distress may occur with any injury

       (b) Other symptoms are described according to type of trauma

         (1) Fractures of ribs, sternochondral junction, or sternum—pain accentuated by chest wall movement, deep inspiration, or touch

         (2) Flail chest—dyspnea and localized pain

         (3) Trauma to lung parenchyma, trachea, or bronchi—hemoptysis and respiratory distress

         (4) Contusion to heart—angina

         (5) Rupture of aorta and major vessels—dyspnea and backache, intense pain in chest or back unaffected by respirations

         (6) Open sucking chest wound—if opening in chest wall is smaller than diameter of trachea, patient may have minimal subjective symptoms. If opening is larger,

more air enters pleural space, collapsing the lung, resulting in ineffective gas exchange and dyspnea

ii. Objective findings

    (a) Etiologic or precipitating factors—a good history describing the traumatic incident is essential. If the patient is not able to answer questions, obtain information from witnesses on the incidence of the blow to chest, weapon used (if applicable), and position patient was in at the moment of impact

    (b) Family history—not applicable

    (c) Social history—assess recent use of alcohol and/or drugs, which may have been a causal factor in the trauma

    (d) Medication history—assess all medications taken, their doses and schedule. Determine if there is a lack of patient compliance with medications; the physiologic result of inadequate or excessive medication could influence level of consciousness, with resultant injury while operating machinery or motor vehicles

b. Nursing examination of patient

  i. Inspection

    (a) Observe skin for ecchymosis, hematomas, abrasions, burns, and lacerations

    (b) Observe work of breathing; use of accessory muscles of breathing; intercostal retractions

    (c) Observe depth and rate of respirations: patients with rib fractures, or any injury that causes pain, may breathe shallowly to minimize the pain. Tachypnea will often accompany pain and apprehension

    (d) Look for asymmetry—may be seen with tension pneumothorax or hemothorax. In flail chest, chest wall movement is paradoxical, sinking in on inspiration and flailing out on expiration

    (e) Examine wound in both respiratory phases

    (f) Try to determine intrathoracic/intra-abdominal trajectory of the offending instrument

  ii. Palpation

    (a) Evaluate chest expansion—often reduced due to pain; will be unequal with pneumothorax or hemothorax. With flail chest there is a fall in the chest cage on inspiration and rise of the cage on expiration

    (b) Palpate for subcutaneous emphysema—may be found in pneumothorax or rupture of trachea or bronchus

    (c) Assess for presence of vocal fremitus—will be reduced in conditions in which air or blood occupies the pleural space: pneumothorax, tension pneumothorax, or hemothorax.

Will be increased in conditions of increased lung density: pulmonary hemorrhage

(d) Palpate position of trachea—will be displaced toward the injured side in pneumothorax; will be displaced toward contralateral side in hemothorax or tension pneumothorax

iii. Percussion

(a) Ipsilateral tympany or hyperresonance is heard in pneumothorax and tension pneumothorax

(b) In rupture of diaphragm the left hemidiaphragm is usually involved, resulting in dullness (from fluid-filled bowel) or tympany (from gas-filled bowel) heard over left chest

(c) Dullness to percussion is heard with hemothorax, hemopneumothorax, or parenchymal hemorrhage

iv. Auscultation

(a) Reduced breath sounds are heard in any condition that causes shallow respirations

(b) Diminished or absent breath sounds are heard in pneumothorax, tension pneumothorax, flail chest, hemothorax, or hemopneumothorax

(c) Bronchial breath sound may be heard with parenchymal hemorrhage

(d) Bowel sounds in chest may be heard with rupture of diaphragm

c. Diagnostic study findings

i. Chest x-ray films are obtained for all injuries if patient's condition is stable

(a) Rib fractures, parenchymal hemorrhage, hemothorax, or hemopneumothorax are identifiable on chest x-ray films

(b) Pneumothorax—expiratory chest x-ray films are often used in diagnosis

(c) Tension pneumothorax—will show a shift in the mediastinum in addition to pneumothorax

(d) Rupture of diaphragm—findings show bowel loops in thorax

(e) Rupture of aorta or major vessels is revealed by widening of mediastinum

ii. Bronchoscopy may be used to confirm diagnosis of rupture of trachea or bronchus

iii. Aortography confirms the diagnosis of rupture of aorta or other major vessels

iv. Electrocardiogram is done to evaluate contusion to heart, when tachycardia, dysrhythmias, and electrocardiographic changes may be found

4. Nursing diagnoses (see Commonly Encountered Nursing Diagnoses, p. 47)

a. Ineffective airway clearance
  i. Additional nursing interventions
    (a) Use suctioning as needed to stimulate cough and clear the airways of blood and secretions
    (b) Symptomatic treatment for uncomplicated rib fractures to ensure ability to cough and breathe deeply as required
b. Ineffective breathing pattern
  i. Additional nursing interventions
    (a) Administer analgesia carefully to avoid compromise of ventilation
    (b) Monitor water seal chest drainage in treatment of pneumothorax or hemothorax
    (c) Apply petrolatum gauze for closure of sucking chest wound
    (d) Assist with emergency decompression of tension pneumothorax with large-bore needle into second anterior interspace or with insertion of chest tube
c. Impaired gas exchange
d. Ineffective individual and family coping

Acute Pneumonia: An inflammatory process of the alveolar spaces caused by infection
1. **Pathophysiology**
  a. Possible pathogenic mechanisms for development of pneumonia include
    i. Aspiration
    ii. Inhalation
    iii. Inoculation
    iv. Direct spread from contiguous sites
    v. Hematogenous spread
  b. Acquisition of infection depends on the nature of infecting organism, the immediate environment, and the defense status of the host
  c. Important constituents of pulmonary defense system
    i. Upper airway defenses—adversely affected by nasotracheal intubation, endotracheal intubation, tracheostomy suction catheters, and nasogastric tubes
      (a) Nasopharyngeal filtration
      (b) Mucosal adherence
      (c) Bacterial interference
      (d) Saliva
      (e) Secretory IgA
    ii. Lower airway defenses: may be impaired and/or inactivated by old age, underlying diseases such as diabetes or chronic bronchitis, hypoxia, pulmonary edema, malnutrition, and drug or oxygen therapy

    (a) Cough reflex

    (b) Mucociliary clearance

    (c) Humoral factors

    (d) Cellular factors

2. **Etiology or precipitating factors** can be categorized in the following way

  a. Normal host infected with usual organisms

    i. *Streptococcus pneumoniae:* most common cause, especially in elderly and patients with a variety of chronic diseases

    ii. *Mycoplasma pneumoniae:* spread by droplet nuclei and may occur in epidemics

    iii. *Hemophilus influenzae:* with encapsulated type B organisms is more likely to cause bacteremia; nontypable *H. influenzae* is seen more in the elderly

    iv. Viruses: relatively uncommon cause of pneumonia in adults, accounting for 25% to 50% of nonbacterial pneumonias. Influenza virus is most common cause

    v. Fungi: *Histoplasma capsulatum* inhalation results in acute severe pulmonary histoplasmosis. Similar reactions in patients with blastomycosis, cryptococcosis or coccidioidomycosis

  b. Normal host infected with unusual organisms

    i. *Legionella pneumophila:* may be sporadic or occur in localized outbreaks in institutions

    ii. *Bacillus anthracis:* infects humans who were in contact with anthrax-infected animals

    iii. *Yersinia pestis:* causes plague; transmitted from wild animals and their fleas or via the respiratory route

    iv. *Francisella tularensis:* causes pleuropulmonary tularemia, endemic in certain parts of the United States; transmitted by ticks or possible inhalation from infected animals

    v. Group A *Streptococcus* and *Meningococcus* bacteria that reside in the upper respiratory tract; pneumonia occurs in those housed in groups, such as found in military service. *S. pyogenes* causes pneumonia typically after outbreaks of viral infections

    vi. *Mycobacterium tuberculosis* or atypical tuberculosis can produce life-threatening pulmonary complications in hosts whose only risk factor is age

  c. Abnormal host infected with usual organisms: compromised states can result from chronic underlying disease, poor nutrition, trauma, or surgery or subsequent to immunosuppression

    i. Pneumococcal pneumonias are more severe in this population

    ii. Gram-negative bacilli, such as *Escherichia coli, Pseudomonas aeruginosa, Serratia, Proteus,* and *Acinetobacter*

    iii. Anaerobic bacteria cause severe pulmonary infections in the abnormal host

    d. Abnormal host infected with unusual organisms

        i. Enterococcal pneumonia: associated with the use of third-generation cephalosporins

        ii. Group B streptococcal pneumonia: reported in the elderly with underlying diseases

        iii. Hospital-acquired infection with *Legionella pneumophila:* in renal transplant patients and those with malignancies

        iv. *Legionella micadadei,* the Pittsburgh pneumonia agent: seen in renal transplant patients during corticosteroid therapy

        v. Fungi: *Aspergillus fumigatus* and *A. flavum:* seen mostly in patients who had received high doses of corticosteroids and broad-spectrum antibiotics

        vi. *Nocardia asteroides:* in renal transplant patients and patients with hematologic malignancies

        vii. *Pneumocystis carinii,* typical and atypical mycobacteria, and cytomegalovirus infections are seen in patients with acquired immunodeficiency syndrome (AIDS)

3. Nursing assessment data base

    a. Nursing history

        i. Subjective findings

            (a) Patient's chief complaint—varies depending on organism. Some of more common presentations include

                (1) Pneumococcal pneumonia—abrupt shaking chills or rigor, fever, dyspnea, pleuritic pain, and cough productive of rust-colored sputum

                (2) *Mycoplasma*—fever, myalgias, headache, minimally productive cough, and nonpleuritic chest pain

                (3) *H. influenzae*—fever, chills, cough with purulent sputum

                (4) *Klebsiella*—sudden onset, blood-tinged sputum, tachypnea

        ii. Objective findings

            (a) Etiologic or precipitating factors—determine if patient is normal or abnormal host. Assess for presence of above precipitating factors

            (b) Family history—usually not a familial tendency for pneumonia; may be familial tendency for some of the precipitating factors (e.g., diabetes, cystic fibrosis)

            (c) Social history—assess nutritional habits, smoking habits, and alcoholic intake

            (d) Medication history—assess all prescribed and over-the-counter medications, their doses, and their times of administration. Determine patient compliance, especially with antibiotics

    b. Nursing examination of patient

   i. Inspection
- (a) Observe posture and work of breathing. Assess use of accessory muscles of breathing
- (b) Inspect chest for intercostal retractions
- (c) Observe for signs of dyspnea (e.g., nasal flaring)
- (d) Assess respiratory patterns. Tachypnea and/or hyperpnea are often seen
- (e) Observe for signs of hypoxemia (e.g., duskiness or cyanosis, mental status changes)

  ii. Palpation
- (a) Assess chest expansion—expect to see asymmetric chest movement in unilateral pneumonias owing to pleuritic pain and reduced lung compliance on the affected side
- (b) Assess vocal fremitus—increased fremitus is found over area of consolidation as in lobar pneumonia

 iii. Percussion
- (a) Dullness to percussion is heard with lobar pneumonia

 iv. Auscultation
- (a) Fine early inspiratory crackles or bronchial breath sounds heard with lobar pneumonia
- (b) In atypical pneumonias, crackles may be heard but rarely signs of consolidation (bronchial breath sounds)

c. Diagnostic study findings
   i. Chest x-ray findings vary with involvement
- (a) Segmental or lobar consolidation
- (b) Multiple infiltrates
- (c) Pleural effusions

  ii. Sputum examination
- (a) Color and consistency typically vary with pathogen
- (b) Initial Gram's stain and microscopic examination
  - (1) Good sputum specimen is one that contains few squamous epithelial cells picked up in transit through the upper respiratory tract. When not expectorated by patient, other means of obtaining sputum include suctioning, transtracheal aspiration, fiberoptic bronchoscopy, needle aspiration of lung, and open-lung biopsy
  - (2) Staining demonstrates polymorphonuclear neutrophils (PMNs) and bacterial agent
  - (3) Large numbers of PMNs are seen in most bacterial pneumonias
  - (4) Fewer PMNs and more mononuclear inflammatory cells are seen in mycoplasma and viral pneumonias
- (c) Sputum cultures are done with initial Gram's stain and microscopic examination. However, some bacteria are rel-

atively difficult to grow, and in many cases initial Gram's stain is just as important in making the etiologic diagnosis

   iii. Blood cultures
- (a) Very important in evaluation of patient because of high specificity of a positive culture
- (b) Pneumonia patient with bacteremia has poor prognosis

   iv. Leukocyte counts
- (a) Often elevated in lobar pneumonias
- (b) May be normal with atypical pneumonia

   v. Arterial blood gases: may indicate hypoxemia and hypocapnia in lobar pneumonias

4. **Nursing diagnoses** (see Commonly Encountered Nursing Diagnoses, p. 47)
- a. Ineffective airway clearance
    - i. Additional nursing interventions
        - (a) Aseptic technique with handwashing to reduce cross contamination
        - (b) Administer appropriate antibiotic therapy and monitor response
- b. Impaired gas exchange

Pulmonary Aspiration: May result from vomiting or regurgitation. Vomiting is an active mechanism that interrupts breathing, causes the diaphragm to descend, contracts the anterior abdominal wall, elevates the pelvic diaphragm, closes the pylorus, and opens the esophageal sphincter, resulting in material ejected from the stomach. Regurgitation is completely passive and may occur even in the presence of paralyzed muscles. Powerful laryngeal and cough reflexes normally prevent aspiration of gastric contents into the tracheobronchial tree. Any impairment or depression of these normal reflexes increases the risk of pulmonary aspiration

1. **Pathophysiology:** varies with types of aspiration
- a. Large particles: can obstruct major airways and cause immediate asphyxia and death; requires immediate intervention
- b. Clear acidic liquid: the pH of aspirated material largely determines the extent of pulmonary injury. As the pH decreases below 2.5, the severity of lung injury increases
    - i. Chemical burn destroys type II alveolar cells, which produce surfactant, and increases alveolar capillary membrane permeability, with subsequent extravasation of fluid and blood into the interstitium and alveoli
    - ii. As fluid and blood accumulate in the alveolar space, lung volume diminishes; thus both functional residual capacity and compliance decrease. Reflex airway closure may also occur
    - iii. Alveolar ventilation decreases relative to perfusion, which re-

sults in intrapulmonary shunting. Hypoxia can occur minutes after acid aspiration

iv. Extensive irritation of the airways by acidic fluid may induce intense bronchospasm

v. Widespread peribronchial hemorrhage may occur along with pulmonary edema and necrosis

c. Clear nonacidic liquid: the nature and extent of pulmonary damage depends on the volume of the aspirate and its composition

i. Aspiration of less acidic or neutral pH liquids can induce hypoxia with acute respiratory decompensation. Reflex airway closure, pulmonary edema, and changes in the characteristics of surfactant may occur. There is little necrosis

ii. Sequelae are more frequently transient and more easily reversible

d. Food stuff or small particles: may produce a severe subacute inflammatory pulmonary reaction with extensive hemorrhage

i. Within 6 hours of aspiration there is extensive hemorrhagic pneumonia

ii. Extravasation of fluid from the intravascular space into the lungs usually occurs but is generally not as intense or rapid as after acid aspiration

iii. Severe intrapulmonary shunting may result and arterial P_{O_2} may be as low as or lower than that seen after the aspiration of acidic liquid

iv. Arterial P_{CO_2} is usually much higher after the aspiration of food. This may indicate a higher degree of hypoventilation

v. Aspiration of acidic foodstuff may produce even more tissue necrosis owing to the combined effects of acid and foodstuff

e. Contaminated material: aspiration of material grossly contaminated with bacteria (e.g., bowel obstruction) is often fatal

2. **Etiology or precipitating factors**

a. Aspiration usually occurs in association with specific predisposing conditions

i. Altered consciousness: drugs, alcohol, anesthesia, seizures, central nervous system disorders, shock, use of sedatives

ii. Altered anatomy: tracheostomy, esophageal or tracheal abnormalities, nasogastric tube, endotracheal tube, intestinal obstruction

iii. Protracted vomiting or coughing

iv. Improper positioning of patients, especially if receiving enteral hyperalimentation

3. **Nursing assessment data base**

a. Nursing history

i. Subjective findings

(a) Patient's chief complaint—cough, dyspnea, and wheezing

are seen with aspiration of solid objects. With gastric acid aspiration there is an abrupt onset of acute respiratory distress
   (b) Other symptoms
      (1) Symptoms of hypoxemia (e.g., mental status changes)
      (2) Increased respiratory secretions and fever in gastric acid aspiration

   ii. Objective findings
      (a) Etiologic or precipitating factors—determine presence of one or more of the above. Obtain detailed description of events leading to onset of symptoms
      (b) Family history—noncontributory
      (c) Social history—assess patient's recent oral intake; assess alcohol and drug intake
      (d) Medication history—assess recent intake of all prescription and over-the-counter medications and their doses and schedules of administration. Determine patient compliance with regard to excessive or inadequate dosing, especially with sedatives, analgesics, or anticonvulsants

b. Nursing examination of patient
   i. Inspection
      (a) Observe posture and work of breathing; assess use of accessory muscles of respiration
      (b) Look for retraction of interspaces indicating an obstruction of inflow of air into the airways
      (c) Observe for inspiratory stridor caused by foreign body obstruction to large bronchus
      (d) Observe respiratory rate—tachypnea is usually present
      (e) Assess for presence of cyanosis or other signs of hypoxemia
   ii. Palpation
      (a) Assess vocal fremitus—would find decreased or absent fremitus with foreign body obstruction of large bronchus
      (b) May find increased fremitus in area of dependent lobe infiltrates and atelectasis
   iii. Percussion
      (a) Dullness to percussion is found in area of infiltrates and atelectasis
   iv. Auscultation
      (a) Wheezing is heard with aspiration of solid objects
      (b) Crackles and possible wheezing are heard in affected lung with aspiration of gastric acid
      (c) Absent breath sounds with occluded bronchus

c. Diagnostic study findings
   i. Radiographic findings: dependent lobe infiltrates and atelectasis. Gravity-dependent areas of lungs most prone to aspiration

include superior segments of lower lobes and posterior segments of upper and lower lobes
  ii. Pulmonary function studies: may show decreased compliance and decreased diffusing capacity
  iii. Sputum examination: presence of anaerobes normally found in the oropharynx in culture of purulent sputum
  iv. Arterial blood gases: may demonstrate hypoxemia
4. **Nursing diagnoses** (see Commonly Encountered Nursing Diagnoses, p. 47)
  a. Ineffective airway clearance
    i. Additional nursing interventions
      (a) Avoid supine position or any position that predisposes to aspiration
      (b) Closely monitor characteristics of secretions suctioned or expectorated
  b. Impaired gas exchange
    i. Additional nursing interventions
      (a) Administer corticosteroids if ordered; they may be of benefit if given immediately after acid aspiration

Near-Drowning: Immersion that necessitates the victim's being transported to a hospital emergency department but is not severe enough to result in death within the first day
1. **Pathophysiology**
  a. Electrolyte change: there is a tendency toward hemoconcentration in salt water drownings and hemodilution in fresh water drowning; however, dangerous changes in plasma electrolytes are very unusual
  b. Pulmonary effects: 90% of victims aspirate fluid and most (85%) aspirate less than 25 ml/kg of body weight. But the water aspirated may contain mud, sand, algae, chemicals, and/or vomitus
    i. In fresh water aspiration, water rapidly enters the circulation, whereas in salt water aspiration the hypertonic sea water draws fluid from the circulation into the lungs. However, near-drowning victims of salt and fresh water immersion have the same initial pathophysiologic aberrations: hypoxemia, hypercapnia, and acidemia
    ii. Organic and inorganic contents of the aspirated fluid, regardless of the type of water, produce an inflammatory reaction in the alveolar-capillary membrane that leads to an outpouring of plasma-rich exudate into the alveolus, the displacement of air, and the deposition of proteinaceous material
    iii. There is destruction of surfactant by aspirated water and proteinaceous exudate, resulting in large areas of atelectasis
    iv. Regional hypoxia promotes hypoxic vasoconstriction, which raises pulmonary intravascular pressures, promoting further

interstitial fluid flux and frequently giving rise to pulmonary edema

    v. Some patients develop hyaline membranes on the wall of injured bronchioles, alveolar ducts, and alveoli. This results in reduced compliance and increased V_D/V_T ratio, respiratory work, and ventilation–perfusion mismatch.

2. **Etiology or precipitating factors**
   a. Fresh or salt water drowning
   b. Prior alcohol or drug ingestion may be associated with the near-drowning event
3. **Nursing assessment data base**
   a. Nursing history
      i. Subjective findings
         (a) Patient's chief complaint—respiratory distress, coughing
         (b) Other symptoms
            (1) Unconsciousness
            (2) Neurologic abnormalities if period of cerebral anoxia occurred
      ii. Objective findings
         (a) Etiologic or precipitating factors—determine presence of one or more of the above factors
         (b) Family history—noncontributory
         (c) Social history—assess for recent intake of alcohol or drugs; question the client's past level of expertise in swimming
         (d) Medication history—determine all recent prescription and over-the-counter medications and their doses and schedule of administration. Determine if any medications were taken in excessive doses, especially sedatives, analgesics, or mood-altering drugs
   b. Nursing examination of patient
      i. Inspection
         (a) Observe posture and work of breathing for signs of labored respirations
         (b) Assess level of consciousness
         (c) Observe for use of accessory muscles of breathing
         (d) Assess respiratory patterns
            (1) Tachypnea in the conscious patient
            (2) Apnea in the unconscious patient
         (e) Observe for intercostal retractions from more negative pleural pressures required to inflate less compliant lungs
         (f) Assess for presence of cyanosis and other signs of hypoxemia
         (g) Assess for presence of fever
      ii. Palpation

        (a) Assess chest expansion—often is decreased owing to low lung compliance

        (b) Assessment of vocal fremitus is difficult in dyspneic patient; would expect to see no change or slight increase bilaterally

    iii. Percussion: may find dullness to percussion over most lung zones owing to diffuse pulmonary edema

    iv. Auscultation: may hear diffuse crackles on inspiration bilaterally

  c. Diagnostic study findings

    i. Chest x-ray film: may demonstrate aspiration and/or pulmonary edema

    ii. Laboratory findings

        (a) Minimal electrolyte and hemoglobin changes

        (b) Arterial blood gas studies show hypoxemia and metabolic acidosis

        (c) Leukocytosis

        (d) Coagulation studies—because coagulation disorders, including disseminated intravascular coagulation, have been reported in near-drowning victims, screening studies of prothrombin time (PT), activated partial thromboplastin time (APTT), and platelet count are often done. If these results are abnormal, fibrinogen levels, fibrin split products, and euglobin clot lysis time should be determined

    iii. Electrocardiography: may show dysrhythmias and nonspecific changes. Few victims die of ventricular fibrillation; acidemia, carbon dioxide retention, and hypoxemia result in marked irregular bradycardia, which precedes asystole and cardiac arrest

4. Nursing diagnoses (see Commonly Encountered Nursing Diagnoses, p. 47)

  a. Ineffective airway clearance

    i. Additional nursing interventions

        (a) Monitor fluid intake to avoid fluid overload and worsening pulmonary edema

  b. Impaired gas exchange

    i. Additional nursing interventions

        (a) Monitor arterial blood gases; notify physician immediately if Pa_{O_2} drops and/or Pa_{CO_2} rises. Be prepared for the possibility of endotracheal intubation and mechanical ventilation and positive end-expiratory pressure

  c. Ineffective individual and family coping

Pulmonary Problems in Surgical Patients: Surgery represents a stress to the respiratory system. Pulmonary problems are the major cause of morbidity after surgery

1. **Pathophysiology**
   a. Changes in pulmonary function occur normally during the immediate postoperative period. These changes are most evident following abdominal or thoracic surgery
      i. Reduction in FVC consistent with a restrictive defect is significant but usually temporary
      ii. A reduction in lung volumes, especially functional residual capacity, also exists. These changes are due in part to
         (a) Pain
         (b) Supine position
      iii. Reduced lung compliance is present, resulting in reduced tidal volume and increased respiratory frequency
   b. Microatelectasis is the most common cause of hypoxemia; the increased respiratory frequency leads to respiratory alkalosis
   c. Bacterial invasion of lower airways and reduced clearance postoperatively predispose to respiratory infection
   d. Aspiration of gastric and oropharyngeal contents occurs postoperatively in patients who have a disturbance in consciousness
   e. Arterial hypoxemia due to ventilation–perfusion mismatch is common during postoperative period for normal patients and exaggerated for patients with chronic obstructive pulmonary disease

2. **Etiology or precipitating factors**
   a. History of chronic obstructive pulmonary disease or cigarette smoking is the most important risk factor. Preoperative hypercapnea is a serious risk factor
   b. Obesity—results in decreased vital capacity
   c. The very young and the elderly are at increased risk of postoperative pulmonary complications
   d. Those with underlying chronic diseases, with or without malnutrition, are at greater risk
   e. Prolonged anesthesia time increases risk
   f. Thoracic and abdominal surgery are especially hazardous to patients at risk. Maximal inspirations are voluntarily limited because of pain, thus increasing risk of atelectasis

3. **Nursing assessment data base**
   a. Nursing history
      i. Subjective findings
         (a) Patient's chief complaint—varies with the type of surgery but often is incisional pain
         (b) Other symptoms include cough with or without sputum production, fear, and reluctance to cough, breathe deeply, and move about after surgery
      ii. Objective findings

      (a) Etiologic or precipitating factors—determine patient's past medical history for smoking, chronic obstructive pulmonary disease, and cardiovascular disease. Determine type of surgery and anesthesia time

      (b) Family history—not applicable except in relation to contributing to past medical history

      (c) Social history—assess dietary habits to determine overall nutritional status; assess smoking habits and pack-year history

      (d) Medication history—determine all recent prescription and over-the-counter medications and their doses and administration schedule. Determine which medications must be resumed in the immediate postoperative period

  b. Nursing examination of patient

    i. Inspection

      (a) Observe for change in respiratory pattern (i.e., tachypnea, shallow respirations)

      (b) Assess lung expansion and observe for splinting of respirations due to incisional pain

      (c) Observe for asymmetry of chest expansion due to possible unilateral atelectasis

      (d) Observe for signs of respiratory distress, increased work of breathing

    ii. Palpation

      (a) Assess chest expansion for degree and symmetry
         Vocal fremitus—assess for increased fremitus over area of atelectasis or consolidation

      (c) Rhonchal fremitus—assess for presence of secretions in airways

   iii. Percussion

      (a) May find dullness to percussion in areas of consolidation or atelectasis

      (b) Assess diaphragm position and excursion to determine if patient is able to breathe deeply when instructed

    iv. Auscultation

      (a) Assess for presence of adventitious sounds

         (1) Crackles from small airway collapse due to shallow breathing

         (2) Rhonchi from secretions in airways

         (3) Wheezing indicating air flow obstruction

      (b) Assess breath sound's character

         (1) Bronchial breath sounds heard with consolidation

         (2) Decreased breath sounds with shallow breathing/splinting

    c. Diagnostic study findings

        i. Preoperative medical evaluation will include chest x-ray films, electrocardiogram, sputum examination, and pulmonary function tests

            (a) Maximal voluntary ventilation (MVV), maximal expiratory flow rate (MEFR), forced expiratory flow in 1 second (FEV$_1$), forced vital capacity (FVC), and peak expiratory flow rate (PEFR) are used to predict development of postoperative pulmonary complications

            (b) Split pulmonary function studies estimate amount of pulmonary function remaining postoperatively

            (c) Patients with abnormal results of pulmonary function studies will have specimens drawn for arterial blood gas analysis preoperatively. The presence of hypoxemia and/or carbon dioxide retention indicates postoperative blood gas levels should be followed closely

4. **Nursing diagnoses** (see Commonly Encountered Nursing Diagnoses, p. 47)

    a. Ineffective airway clearance

        i. Additional nursing interventions

            (a) Preoperatively

                (1) Encourage cessation of smoking at least 48 hours prior to surgery

                (2) Administer bronchodilators to patients with chronic obstructive pulmonary disease as ordered

                (3) Instruct patient in deep breathing, coughing techniques, ambulation and activity exercises, and active and passive range of motion

                (4) Familiarize patient with respiratory therapy equipment

            (b) Postoperatively

                (1) Encourage early ambulation and leg exercises

                (2) Provide chest/abdominal incision support when patient is coughing

    b. Ineffective breathing pattern, related to incisional pain

        i. Additional nursing interventions

             (a) Administer analgesics as needed, and closely monitor breathing pattern for hypoventilation/splinting

    c. Impaired gas exchange

        i. Additional nursing interventions

             (a) Monitor arterial blood gases; notify physician immediately if Pa$_{O_2}$ drops and/or Pa$_{CO_2}$ rises. Be prepared for the possibility of endotracheal intubation and mechanical ventilation and positive end-expiratory pressure

Acute Pulmonary Inhalation Injuries: Smoke inhalation, thermal burns, carbon monoxide poisoning

1. **Pathophysiology**
   a. Displacement of oxygen from the environment and inhalation of noxious agents and asphyxiant gases. Effects range from mild irritation of mucous membranes of upper airway to fatal respiratory failure. Toxic exposure causes edema of mucous membranes, inflammatory capillary damage, and bronchospasm
   b. Thermal injury to lung tissues produces mucosal sloughing, bronchorrhea, and pulmonary edema
   c. Systemic absorption of carbon monoxide or other chemical asphyxiants
      i. Carbon monoxide toxicity is related to dose, duration, alveolar ventilation (activity, cardiac output), and preexisting cardiovascular disease
      ii. Carbon monoxide is normally attached to hemoglobin at levels of about 1% but has an affinity for the hemoglobin molecule that is 200 to 250 times that of oxygen. Small amounts of inspired carbon monoxide have major effects on oxygen-carrying capacity of blood and cause severe tissue hypoxia. Elimination of carbon monoxide is via the lungs only
2. **Etiology or precipitating factors**
   a. Exposure to smoke or toxic gases
   b. Closed space injury
   c. Prolonged exposure
   d. Unconsciousness
   e. Preexisting respiratory or cardiovascular disease
   f. Solubility of gas
3. **Nursing assessment data base**
   a. Nursing history
      i. Subjective findings
         (a) Patient's chief complaint—varies with type of inhalation. Headache is often seen with carbon monoxide inhalation; Cough, wheezing, and dyspnea are seen with inhalation of smoke and other noxious agents
      ii. Objective findings
         (a) Etiologic or precipitating factors—determine presence of one or more of above. A carefully detailed description of events leading up to and during pulmonary inhalation injury is essential
         (b) Family history—noncontributory
         (c) Social history—assess living conditions, exposure to household product fumes if applicable, occupational inhalation exposures, smoking history, recent alcohol and/or drug

use, and history of depression and/or previous suicide attempts

    (d) Medication history—determine all prescription and over-the-counter medications and their doses and administration schedule. Assess for overdose or missed doses, especially in medications that influence level of consciousness (e.g., sedatives)

b. Nursing examination of patient

  i. Inspection

    (a) Observe for facial burns, singed nares, sooty tongue, and pharynx and mouth blistering

    (b) Inspect for edema of lips and face

    (c) Observe for depressed mentation

    (d) Observe for cyanosis

    (e) Observe for cherry-red color to the skin for carbon monoxide poisoning (a rare finding)

    (f) Assess work of breathing; use of accessory muscles of respiration

    (g) Assess respiratory patterns—tachypnea

  ii. Palpation

    (a) Assess chest expansion—rapid shallow breathing seen due to low compliance of lungs

  iii. Percussion: no notable changes

  iv. Auscultation: diffuse adventitious sounds heard bilaterally—wheezes, crackles, and rhonchi

c. Diagnostic findings

  i. Serial carboxyhemoglobin analysis for carbon monoxide poisoning. Normal nonsmoking persons have a carboxyhemoglobin level of less than 2%, while smokers may have a level of 5% to 10%. Severe carbon monoxide poisoning is present when levels are higher than 30% to 40%

  ii. Serial arterial blood gas analysis

    (a) Carbon monoxide poisoning does not cause a decrease in measured Pa_{O_2} but does impair the oxygen-carrying capacity of hemoglobin

    (b) Hypoxemia in thermal injury and toxic exposure

  iii. Chest x-ray studies

    (a) No change in carbon monoxide inhalation

    (b) Diffuse pulmonary edema in thermal injury and toxic inhalation

  iv. Fiberoptic bronchoscopy to assess upper airway edema

4. **Nursing diagnoses** (see Commonly Encountered Nursing Diagnoses, p. 47)

a. Ineffective airway clearance

  i. Additional nursing interventions

(a) Observe for signs of vocal cord edema and stridor
b. Impaired gas exchange
   i. Additional nursing interventions
      (a) Humidified 100% oxygen administration for carbon monoxide poisoning to shorten the half-life of carboxyhemoglobin
      (b) Hyperbaric oxygenation for carbon monoxide poisoning if readily available
      (c) Observation of carbon monoxide poisoning victim for cognitive, memory, visual, and personality changes

Neoplastic Lung Disease

1. **Pathophysiology**—almost all lung cancers fall within one of four histologic categories: squamous cell, small cell, adenocarcinoma, and large cell carcinoma. In addition to these, there are two other forms of neoplastic lung disease that will be discussed: bronchial carcinoids and malignant mesothelioma
   a. Squamous cell carcinoma: constitutes approximately one third of all bronchogenic carcinomas. These tumors originate in the epithelial layer of the bronchial wall. A series of progressive histologic abnormalities result from chronic or repetitive cigarette smoke–induced injury.
      i. Initially there is metaplasia of the normal bronchial columnar epithelial cells, which are replaced by squamous epithelial cells
      ii. Squamous cells become more atypical until there is development of a well-localized carcinoma (carcinoma in situ)
      iii. Tumors tend to be located in relatively large or proximal airways, most commonly at the subsegmental, segmental, or lobar level. With growth of tumor into the bronchial lumen, the airway may become obstructed and the lung distal to the obstruction frequently becomes atelectatic and may develop a postobstructive pneumonia
      iv. Sometimes the tumor develops a cavity within it; cavitation is much more common with squamous cell than with other types of bronchogenic carcinoma
      v. Spread of squamous cell carcinoma beyond the airway usually involves
         (a) Direct extension to the pulmonary parenchyma or to other neighboring structures
         (b) Invasion of lymphatics, with spread to local lymph nodes in the hilum or mediastinum
      vi. These tumors have a tendency to remain within the thorax and to cause problems by intrathoracic complications rather than by distant metastasis. The overall prognosis for 5-year survival

is better for patients with squamous cell carcinoma than for patients with any of the other cell types

b. Small cell carcinoma: comprises about 20% of all lung cancers and consists of several subtypes. Tumors generally originate within the bronchial wall, most commonly at a proximal level

    i. Oat cell carcinoma, the most common subtype, shows a submucosal growth pattern, but the tumor quickly invades lymphatics and submucosal blood vessels. Hilar and mediastinal nodes are involved early in the course of the disease and are frequently the most prominent aspect of the radiographic presentation

    ii. Metastatic spread to distant sites is a common early complication. Common sites for metastasis are brain, liver, bone (and bone marrow), and adrenal glands

    iii. This propensity for early metastatic involvement gives small cell carcinoma the worst prognosis among the four major categories of bronchogenic carcinoma

c. Adenocarcinoma: accounts for more than one third of all lung tumors, with the majority occurring in the periphery of the lung

    i. The characteristic appearance is the tendency to form glands and to produce mucus

    ii. Usually presents as a peripheral lung nodule or mass. Occasionally, tumors can arise within a relatively large bronchus and therefore may present with complications of localized bronchial obstruction

    iii. May spread locally to adjacent regions of the lung, to pleura, or to the hilar or mediastinal lymph nodes or may metastasize to distant sites: liver, bone, central nervous system, and adrenal glands. Compared with small cell carcinoma, adenocarcinoma is more likely to be localized at the time of presentation

    iv. Overall prognosis is intermediate between that of squamous cell and small cell carcinoma

d. Large cell carcinoma: accounts for 15% to 20% of all lung cancers. Defined by the characteristics that they lack (i.e., the specific features that would otherwise classify them as one of the other three cell types). It is difficult to pinpoint the cells of origin from which these tumors arise

    i. Behave similar to adenocarcinomas

        (a) Found in the periphery of the lungs, although tend to be somewhat larger than adenocarcinomas

        (b) Tumor spread and prognosis is the same as for adenocarcinoma

e. Bronchial carcinoid—are viewed as low-grade malignancies that constitute approximately 5% of primary lung tumors

    i. Arise in relatively central airways of the tracheobronchial tree from the neurosecretory Kulchitsky cells (K cells). In some carcinoid tumors, the histology has more atypical features suggestive of frank malignancy; these tumors have a poorer overall prognosis than those without such features

ii. Patients with bronchial carcinoids are younger than those with other pulmonary malignancies

iii. Treatment is surgical resection if possible, with an excellent prognosis. However in patients with atypical histology, metastatic disease is commonly found and prognosis is worse

f. Malignant mesothelioma: involves the pleura rather than the airways or pulmonary parenchyma. The tumor eventually traps the lung and spreads to mediastinal structures. No clearly effective form of therapy is available, and fewer than 10% of patients survive 3 years

2. **Etiology or precipitating factors**

a. Smoking is the single most important risk factor for development of carcinoma of the lung. The duration of the smoking history, the number of cigarettes smoked per day, the depth of inhalation, and the amount of each cigarette smoked all correlate with the risk for developing lung cancer. Each of the four major categories of carcinoma is associated with cigarette smoking. However, the statistical association between smoking and the individual cell types is greatest for squamous cell and small cell carcinomas, which are seen almost exclusively in smokers. Even though smoking increases the risk for developing adenocarcinoma and large cell carcinoma, these cell types are also observed in nonsmokers. In addition, smoking does not appear to be a risk factor for bronchial carcinoids and malignant mesothelioma

b. Occupational factors

i. Asbestos, a fibrous silicate used because of its properties of fire resistance and thermal insulation, is the most widely studied of the environmental or occupationally related carcinogens. Carcinoma of the lung is the most likely malignancy to complicate asbestos exposure, although other tumors, especially mesothelioma, are strongly associated with prior asbestos exposure. The risk for development of lung cancer is particularly high in a smoker exposed to asbestos, in which case the two risk factors have a multiplicative effect. There is a long time lapse (> 20 years) after exposure before the tumor becomes apparent

ii. Other occupational exposures have been implicated in the subsequent development of lung cancer. As with asbestos, there is usually a long latent period of at least 2 decades from time of exposure until presentation of the tumor. Examples of these exposures include

      (a) Arsenic—in the manufacture of pesticides, glass, pigments, and paints

      (b) Ionizing radiation—uranium miners

      (c) Haloethers—in chemical industry workers

      (d) Polycyclic aromatic hydrocarbons—in petroleum, coal tar, and foundry workers

3. Nursing assessment data base

  a. Nursing history

    i. Subjective findings

      (a) Patient's chief complaint—cough and hemoptysis are the most common symptoms developing in the patient with lung cancer

      (b) Other symptoms vary depending on region of tumor involvement

        (1) Dyspnea secondary to obstructed bronchus or large pleural effusion

        (2) Chest pain from pleural involvement

        (3) Dysphagia from tumor involvement of adjacent esophagus

        (4) Hoarseness from vocal cord paralysis

        (5) Edema of face and upper extremities from superior vena cava obstruction

        (6) Nonspecific symptoms—anorexia and weight loss

    ii. Objective findings

      (a) Etiologic or precipitating factors—assess for presence of one or more of the above

      (b) Family history—although there may be unidentified genetic factors that affect one's susceptibility to environmental carcinogens, there is no clear evidence that a familial tendency exists

      (c) Social history—carefully question patient regarding all previous occupational exposures, duration of time exposed, and what protective devices were used. Assess smoking history, calculating the number of pack-years

      (d) Medication history—document all prescription and over-the-counter medications

  b. Nursing examination of patient

    i. Inspection

      (a) Observe for overall nutritional status, weight loss, and wasting

      (b) Assess work of breathing and use of accessory muscles of breathing

      (c) Assess respiratory patterns—tachypnea

      (d) Observe for edema of the face and upper extremities

    ii. Palpation

(a) Evaluate chest expansion—may be decreased on the affected side

(b) Assess vocal fremitus

(1) May be increased if patent bronchus leads to parenchymal tumor or area of pneumonia

(2) Will be absent over area of pleural involvement

iii. Percussion

(a) Dullness heard over large tumor near chest wall or pleural mass

(b) May detect elevated diaphragm in patients with diaphragmatic paralysis

iv. Auscultation

(a) Bronchial breath sounds over area of large tumor or postobstructive pneumonia

(b) Decreased to absent breath sounds with pleural effusion or tumor

c. Diagnostic study findings

i. Radiologic evaluation

(a) Chest x-ray film may reveal a nodule or mass within the lung and involvement of hilar or mediastinal nodes or the pleura

(b) Tomography and CT scanning help to define the location, extent, and spread of tumor within the chest and can also reveal information about the densities of the lesions

ii. Bronchoscopy: allows direct examination of the airways intrabronchially and sampling from the lesion for later cytologic evaluation

iii. Microscopic examination: cytologic examination can be performed on sputum, washings or brushings obtained through a bronchoscope, or material aspirated from the tumor with a small-gauge needle

iv. Staging of lung cancer is based on

(a) Size, location, and local complications such as direct extensions to adjacent structures or obstruction of the airway lumen

(b) Mediastinal lymph node involvement

(c) Distant metastasis

4. Nursing diagnoses (see Commonly Encountered Nursing Diagnoses, p. 47)

a. Ineffective airway clearance: related to postobstructive pneumonia

i. Additional nursing interventions

(a) Suction airway only if secretions are reachable by catheter and patient is unable to cough

(b) Administer antibiotics as ordered and monitor clinical response

b. Ineffective breathing pattern: related to tumor progression or thoracotomy
c. Impaired gas exchange: related to altered oxygen supply
d. Ineffective individual and family coping
   i. Additional nursing diagnoses
      (a) Collaborate with social workers in getting another patient with similar diagnosis who has successfully coped with situation to visit patient to provide encouragement
      (b) Provide referral to hospice care or similar organization, if appropriate

References

Albert, W.M., Priest, G.R., and Moser, K.M.: The outlook for survivors of ARDS. Chest 84:272–274, 1983.

American Thoracic Society: Position Paper: Guidelines for fiberoptic bronchoscopy. Am. Thorac. Soc. News 9:4, 1983.

American Thoracic Society: Report of ATS subcommittee on definiton of asthma. Am. Thorac. Soc. News 8:5, 1982.

Arabian, A., Spangnolo, S., and Rohatgi, P.: Evaluation and treatment of pulmonary problems in surgical patients. Clin. Notes Respir. Dis. 21:3–14, 1982.

Askanazi, J., Weissman, C., Rosenbaum, S., Hyman, A., Milic-Emili, J., and Kinney, J.: Nutrition and the respiratory system. Crit. Care Med. 10:163–172, 1982.

Balk, R., and Bone, R.: Classification of acute respiratory failure. Med. Clin. North Am. 67:551–556, 1983.

Balk, R., and Bone, R.: The adult respiratory distress syndrome. Med. Clin. North Am. 67:685–699, 1983.

Banner, T., and Gibbs, T.: Risk of aspiration. Curr. Rev. Respir. Ther. 7:59–63, 1984.

Barbee, R.: The medical history in pulmonary disease. Am. Thorac. Soc. News 9:9–14, 1983.

Barrocas, A., Tretola, B.S., and Alonso, A.: Nutrition and the critically ill pulmonary patient. Respir. Care 28:50–61, 1983.

Bartlett, J.G.: Aspiration pneumonia. Clin. Notes Respir. Dis. 18:3–8, 1980.

Beale, P., McMickan, J., Marsh, H., Sill, J., and Southorn, P.: Continuous monitoring of mixed venous oxygen saturation in critically ill patients. Anesth. Analg. 61:513–517, 1982.

Bell, W., and Simon, T.: Current status of pulmonary embolism. Am. Heart J. 103:239–262, 1982.

Belshe, R.B.: Viral respiratory disease in the intensive care unit. Heart Lung 15:222–226, 1986.

Blodgett, D.: Manual of Respiratory Care Procedures, 2nd ed. J.B. Lippincott Co., Philadelphia, 1987.

Bodai, B.I.: A means of suctioning without cardiopulmonary depression. Heart Lung 11:172–176, 1982.

Bone, R.C.: Acute respiratory failure and chronic obstructive lung disease: Recent advances. Med. Clin. North Am. 65:563–578, 1981.

Bouvier, J.R.: Measuring tracheal cuff tube pressures: Tool and technique. Heart Lung 10:686–690, 1981.

Bowden, D.H.: Alveolar response to injury. Thorax 36:801–804, 1981.

Boysen, P.G.: Management of perioperative respiratory dysfunction: I. Curr. Rev. Respir. Ther. 8:163–167, 1986.

Boysen, P.G.: Management of perioperative respiratory dysfunction: II. Curr. Rev. Respir. Ther. 8:171–175, 1986.

Breslin, E.H.: Prevention and treatment of pulmonary complications in patients after surgery of the upper abdomen. Heart Lung 10:511–519, 1981.

Brodsky, J.: Oxygen: A drug. Int. Anesthesiol. Clin. 19:1–8, 1981.

Brown, S., Stansbury, D., Merrill, E., Linden, G., and Light, R.: Prevention of suctioning-related arterial oxygen desaturation: Comparison of off-ventilator and on-ventilator suctioning. Chest 83:621–627, 1983.

Burki, N., and Albert, R.: Noninvasive monitoring of arterial blood gases. Chest 83:666–670, 1981.

Carlon, C.: Monitoring in respiratory failure, based on pathophysiologic considerations. Respir. Care 27:696–699, 1982.

Cherniack, R.M., and Cherniack, L.: Respiration in Health and Disease, 3rd ed. W.B. Saunders Co., Philadelphia, 1983.

Clark, S.: Nursing diagnosis: Ineffective coping: I. A theoretical framework. Heart Lung 16:670–676, 1987.

Clark, S.: Nursing diagnosis: Ineffective coping: II. Planning care. Heart Lung 16:677–686, 1987.

Clemmer, T.: Oxygen transport. Int. Anesthesiol. Clin. 19:21–38, 1981.

Cohen, P.J.: Oxygen and intracellular metabolism. Int. Anesthesiol. Clin. 19:9–19, 1981.

Crapo, R.: Smoke inhalation injuries. JAMA 246:1694–1696, 1981.

Cunningham, C.A., and Sergent, J.B.: A preliminary view of the contamination of suction apparatus. Focus Crit. Care 10:10–14, 1983.

Dantzker, D.R. (ed.): Cardiopulmonary Critical Care. Grune & Stratton, Orlando, 1986.

Demers, R.: Complications of endotracheal suctioning techniques. Respir. Care 27:453–547, 1982.

Deneke, S., and Fanburg, B.: Oxygen toxicity of the lung: An update. Br. J. Anaesth. 54:737–749, 1982.

Derenne, J.P., Fleury, B., and Pariente, R.: Acute respiratory failure of chronic obstructive pulmonary disease. Am. Rev. Respir. Dis. 138:1006–1033, 1988.

Driver, A.G., McAlevy, M.T., and Smith, J.L.: Nutritional assessment of patients with chronic obstructive pulmonary disease and acute respiratory failure. Chest 82:568–571, 1982.

Dudley, D.L., and Sitzman, J.: Psychosocial and psychophysiologic approach to the patient. Semin. Respir. Med. 1:59–83, 1979.

Echenique, M.M.: Nutritional assessment and therapy of hospitalized patients: I. Curr. Rev. Respir. Ther. 7:42–47, 1984.

Echenique, M.M.: Nutritional support: II. Curr. Rev. Respir. Ther. 7:51–55, 1984.

Edelman, N.H., Rucker, R.B., and Peavy, H.H.: Nutrition and the respiratory system. Am. Rev. Respir. Dis. 134:347–352, 1986.

Emanuelsen, K.L., and Rosenlicht, J.M. (eds.): Handbook of Critical Care Nursing. John Wiley & Sons, New York, 1986.

Eubanks, D.H., and Bone, R.C.: Comprehensive Respiratory Care: A Learning System. C.V. Mosby Co., St. Louis, 1985.

Fein, A., Leff, A., and Hopewell, P.C.: Pathophysiology and management of the complications resulting from fire and the inhaled products of combustion. Crit. Care Med. 8:94–98, 1980.

Fein, A., Lippman, M., Holtzman, H., Eliraz, A., and Goldberg, S.: The risk factors, incidence, and prognosis of ARDS following septicemia. Chest 83:40–42, 1983.

Fernandez, E.: Beta-adrenergic agonists. Semin. Respir. Med. 8:353–365, 1987.

Fernandez, E., and Martin, R.: Treatment of acute, severe asthma. Semin. Respir. Med. 8:227–238, 1987.

Fishman, A.P.: Pulmonary Diseases and Disorders, 2nd ed. McGraw-Hill Book Co., New York, 1988.

Fitzgerald, J.M., and Hargreave, F.E.: The assessment and management of acute life threatening asthma. Chest 95:888–894, 1988.

Flenley, D.: Blood gas and acid–base interpretations. Respir. Care 27:311–317, 1982.

Fluck, R., Wagner, I., and Wiezalis, C.: The esophageal obturator airway: A review. Respir. Care 27:1373–1379, 1982.

Frame, P.T.: Acute infectious pneumonia in the adult. Am. Thorac. Soc. News 8:18–25, 1982.

Frownfelter, D.L.: Chest Physical Therapy and Pulmonary Rehabilitation: An Interdisciplinary Approach, 2nd. ed. Year Book Medical Publishers, Chicago, 1987.

Gallagher, T., and Civetta, J.: Goal-directed therapy of acute respiratory failure. Anesth. Analg. 59:831–834, 1980.

Gallagher, T.J., Klain, M.M., and Carlon, G.C.: Present status of high frequency ventilation. Crit. Care Med. 10:613–617, 1982.

Gallus, A.: Established venous thrombosis and pulmonary embolism. Clin. Haematol. 10:583–611, 1981.

Gee, J., and Smith, G.: Lung cell and disease. Am Thorac. Soc. News 7:42–47, 1981.

George, R.B., Light, R.W., and Matthay, R.A.: Chest Medicine. Churchill Livingstone, New York, 1983.

Gershan, J.A.: Effects of positive end expiratory pressure on pulmonary capillary wedge pressure. Heart Lung 12:143–148, 1983.

Gilbert, J., Puckett, J., and Smith, R.B.: Near-drowning: Current concepts of management. Respir. Care 30:108–120, 1985.

Glauser, F.L., Polatty, C., and Sessler, C.N.: Worsening oxygenation in the mechanically ventilated patient: Causes, mechanisms, and early detection. Am. Rev. Respir. Dis. 138:458–465, 1988.

Gold, M.: IPPB therapy: A current overview. Respir. Care 27:586–587, 1982.

Goldman, M.D.: Interpretation of chest movements during breathing. Clin. Sci. 62:7–11, 1982.

Grace, M.P., and Greenbaum, D.M.: Cardiac performance in response to PEEP in patients with cardiac dysfunction. Crit. Care Med. 10:358–360, 1982.

Granovetter, B.: Blunt chest trauma. In Brenner, B.E. (ed.): Comprehensive Management of Respiratory Emergencies. Aspen Publishers, Rockville, Md., 1985.

Grossbach, I.: Troubleshooting ventilator- and patient-related problems: I. Crit. Care Nurse 6(4):58–69, 1986.

Grossbach, I.: Troubleshooting ventilator- and patient-related problems: II. Crit. Care Nurse 6(5):64–79, 1986.

Grossman, G.D.: Nutritional assessment of critically ill patients. Respir. Care 30:463–470, 1985.

Guckian, J.C.: The Clinical Interview and Physical Examination. J.B. Lippincott Co., Philadelphia, 1987.

Guenter, C., and Braun, T.: Fat embolism syndrome: Changing progress. Chest 79:143–145, 1981.

Guyton, A.C.: Textbook of Medical Physiology, 7th ed. W.B. Saunders Co., Philadelphia, 1986.

Hansell, H.N.: The behavioral effects of noise on man: The patient with "intensive care unit psychosis". Heart Lung 13:59–66, 1984.

Harper, R.W.: A Guide to Respiratory Care. J.B. Lippincott Co., Philadelphia, 1981.

Harper, R.W.: Application of alveolar ventilation physiology. Dimens. Crit. Care Nurs. 1:80–86, 1982.

Harries, M.G.: Drowning in man. Crit. Care Med. 9:407–408, 1981.

Hauser, C.J., and Harley, D.P.: Transcutaneous gas tension monitoring in the management of intraoperative apnea. Crit. Care Med. 11:830–831, 1983.

Hectman, H., Utsunomiya, T., Krausz, M., and Shepro, D.: Management of cardiopulmonary failure in surgical patients. Adv. Surg. 15:123–156, 1981.

Hills, B.A., and Bryan-Brown, C.W.: Role of surfactant in the lung and other organs. Crit. Care Med. 11:951–956, 1983.

Hogg, J.C.: The pathophysiology of asthma. Chest 82:8S–12S, 1982.

Hoidal, J., and Niewoehner, D.: Pathogenesis of emphysema. Chest 83:679–685, 1983.

Hudson, L., and Pierson, D.: Comprehensive respiratory care for patients with COPD. Med. Clin. North Am. 65:629–645, 1981.

Janson-Bjerklie, S.: Defense mechanisms: Protecting the healthy lung. Heart Lung 12:643–649, 1983.

Johanson, W.G.: Infectious complications of respiratory therapy. Respir. Care 27:445–452, 1982.

Jung, R.C., and Newman, J.: Minimizing hypoxia during endotracheal airway care. Heart Lung 11:208–212, 1982.

Kafer, E. R., and Sugioka, K.: Respiratory and cardiovascular responses to hypoxemia and the effects of anesthesia. Int. Anesthesiol. Clin. 19:85–122, 1981.

Kennedy, S., and Wilson, R.: Oxygen measurement. Int. Anesthesiol. Clin. 19:201–236, 1981.

Kim, M.J., McFarland, G.K., and McLane, A.M.: Pocket Guide to Nursing Diagnoses, 2nd. ed. C.V. Mosby Co., St. Louis, 1987.

Kinaswitz, G.: Use of end-tidal capnography during mechanical ventilation. Respir. Care 27:169–171, 1982.

King, M.: Mucus and mucociliary clearance. Am. Thorac. Soc. News 8:17–23, 1982.

Kinsman, R., Yaroush, R.A., Fernandez, E., Dirks, J., Schocket, M., and Fukuhara, J.: Symptoms and experiences in chronic bronchitis and emphysema. Chest 83:755–761, 1983.

Kirby, R.R., and Smith R.A.: Current concepts in mechanical ventilation. Curr. Rev. Resp. Ther. 8:82–87, 1986.

Kirby, R.R., and Taylor, R.W.: Respiratory Failure. Year Book Medical Publishers, Chicago, 1986.

Koss, J.A., Conine, T.A., Eitzen, H.E., and LoSasso, A.M.: Bacterial contamination potential of sterile, prefilled humidifiers and nebulizer reservoirs. Heart Lung 8:1117–1122, 1979.

Kuhn, M.: Pneumonia: Pathogenesis, clinical and laboratory features. In Brenner, B.E. (ed.): Comprehensive Management of Respiratory Emergencies. Aspen Publishers, Rockville, Md., 1985.

Leitch, A.G.: Asthma: Mechanisms and management. Clin. Notes Respir. Dis. 21:2–9, 1982.

Leff, A.: Pathogenesis of asthma: Neurophysiology and pharmacology of bronchospasm. Chest 81:224–229, 1982.

Loudon, R.: Cough: A symptom and a sign. Am. Thorac. Soc. News 7:19–24, 1981.

Loudon, R.G.: Auscultation of the lung. Clin. Notes Respir. Dis. 21:3–7, 1982.

Luce, J., Tyler, M., and Pierson, D.: Intensive Respiratory Care. W.B. Saunders Co., Philadelphia, 1984.

Lucey, J.: Clinical use of transcutaneous oxygen monitoring. Adv. Pediatr. 28:27–56, 1981.

Miller, J., and Winter, P.: Clinical management of pulmonary oxygen toxicity. Int. Anesthesiol. Clin. 19:179–199, 1981.

Modell, J.: Biology of drowning. Annu. Rev. Med. 29:1–8, 1978.

Mohsenifar, Z., Goldbach, P., Tashin, D.P., and Campisti, D.J.: Relationship between O_2 delivery and O_2 consumption in the adult respiratory distress syndrome. Chest 84:267–271, 1983.

Montgomery, A.B., and Luce, J.M.: Infection monitoring. Respir. Care 30:489–499, 1985.

Moser, K., and Fedullo, P.: Venous thromboembolism, three simple decisions. Chest 83:117–121, 256–260, 1983.

Moser, K.M., and Spragg, R.G.: Respiratory Emergencies, 2nd ed. C.V. Mosby Co., St. Louis, 1982.

Mosley, S. Inhalation injury: A review of literature. Heart Lung 17:3–9, 1988.

Murray, J.F., Matthay, M.A., Luce, J.M., and Flick, M.R.: An expanded definition of the adult respiratory distress syndrome. Am. Rev. Respir. Dis. 138:720–723, 1988.

Murray, J.F., and Nadel, J.A.: Textbook of Respiratory Medicine. W.B. Saunders Co., Philadelphia, 1988.

Neagley, S.R., Vought, M., Weidner, W., and Zwillich, C.W.: The effect of radiographic contrast media on oxygenation. Arch. Intern. Med. 146:1094–1097, 1986.

Nicotra, M.B.: Newer insights into management and rehabilitation of the patient with pulmonary disease. Semin. Respir. Med. 8:113–122, 1986.

Nierenberg, R.: Respiratory failure: A pathophysiologic approach. In Brenner, B.E. (ed.): Comprehensive Management of Respiratory Emergencies. Aspen Publishers, Rockville, Md., 1985.

Nunn, J.F.: Applied Respiratory Physiology. Butterworth & Co., London, 1987.

Off, D., Braun, S., Tompkins, B., and Bush, G.: Efficacy of minimal leak technique of cuff inflation in maintaining proper intracuff pressures for patients with cuffed artificial airways. Respir. Care 28:1115–1120, 1983.

Parker, J., and Raffin, T.A.: Mechanical ventilatory support: Current techniques and recent advances. Curr. Rev. Resp. Ther. 29:26–31, 1986.

Patterson, A.R.: Pulmonary aspiration syndromes. In Kirby, R.R., and Taylor, R.W. (eds.): Respiratory Failure. Year Book Medical Publishers, Chicago, 1986.

Petty, T. (ed.): Chronic obstructive pulmonary disease, vol. 28. In Lenfant, C. (ed.): Lung Biology in Health and Disease, 2nd ed. Marcel Dekker, New York, 1985.

Petty, T.: The use, abuse, and mystique of positive end-expiratory pressure. Am. Rev. Respir. Dis. 138:475–478, 1988.

Petty, T., and Cherniack, R.: Comprehensive care of COPD. Clin. Notes Respir. Dis. 20:3–11, 1981.

Petty, T., and Fowler, A.: Another look at ARDS. Chest 8:98–104, 1982.

Pick, R.A., Handler, J.B., Murara, G.H., and Friedman, A.S.: The cardiovascular effect of PEEP. Chest 82:345–350, 1982.

Pierson, D.: Weaning from mechanical ventilation in acute respiratory failure: Concepts, indications, and techniques. Respir. Care 28:646–662, 1983.

Pingleton, S.K., and Hadzima, S.K.: Enteral alimentation and gastrointestinal bleeding in mechanically ventilated patients. Crit. Care Med. 1:13–16, 1983.

Podjasek, J.M.: Respiratory infection in the mechanically ventilated patient: An overview. Heart Lung 12:5–10, 1983.

Popovich, J.: The physiology of mechanical ventilation and the mechanical zoo: IPPB, PEEP, CPAP. Med. Clin. North Am. 67:621–631, 1983.

Procter, C.D.: Nutritional support. In Kirby, R.R., and Taylor, R.W. (eds.): Respiratory Failure. Year Book Medical Publishers, Chicago, 1986.

Quan, S.F., Otto, C.W., Calkins, J.C., Hameroff, S.R., Conahaw, T.J., and Waterson, C.K.: High frequency ventilation: A promising new method of ventilation. Heart Lung 12:152–155, 1983.

Raffin, T.: Oxygen toxicity: Etiology. Int. Anesthesiol. Clin. 19:169–177, 1981.

Rebuck, A., Braude, A., and Chapman, K.: Evaluation of the severity of the acute asthmatic attack. Chest 82:28S–29S, 1982.

Reischman, R.R.: Review of ventilation and perfusion physiology. Crit. Care Nurse 8:24–30, 1988.

Rinaldo, J., and Rogers, R.: Adult respiratory distress syndrome: Changing concepts of lung injury and repair. N. Engl. J. Med. 306:900–909, 1982.

Rindfleisch, S., and Tyler, M.: Duration of suctioning: An important variable. Respir. Care 28:457–459, 1983.

Roberts, S.L.: Pulmonary tissue perfusion altered: Emboli. Heart Lung 16:128–138, 1987.

Robotham, J., Cherry, D., Mitzner, W., Rabson, J., Lixfield, W., and Bromberger-Barnea, B.: A re-evaluation of the hemodynamic consequences of intermittent positive pressure ventilation. Crit. Care Med. 11:783–793, 1983.

Rosen, M.A.: Pulmonary embolism. In Brenner, B.E. (ed.): Comprehensive Management of Respiratory Emergencies. Aspen Publishers, Rockville, Md., 1985.

Roussos, C., and Macklem, P.: The respiratory muscles. N. Engl. J. Med. 307:786–797, 1982.

Safar, P.: Cardiopulmonary Cerebral Resuscitation. W.B. Saunders Co., Philadelphia, 1981.

Sahn, S.A.: Pulmonary Emergencies. Churchill Livingstone, New York, 1982.

Said, S.I.: The lung in relation to hormones: An update. Am. Thorac. Soc. News 7:14–18, 1981.

Said, S.I.: Metabolic functions of pulmonary circulation. Circ. Res. 50:325–333. 1982.

Shapiro, B., Cane, R., and Harrison, R.: Positive end-expiratory pressure in acute lung injury. Chest 83:558–563, 1983.

Shapiro, B.A., Harrison, R.A., and Walton, J.R.: Clinical Application of Respiratory Care, 3rd ed. Year Book Medical Publishers, Chicago, 1982.

Shoemaker W.C., Thompson, W.L., and Holbrook, P.R.: Textbook of Critical Care, 2nd ed. W.B. Saunders Co., Philadelphia, 1989.

Shoemaker W.C., and Vidyasagar, D.: Transcutaneous O_2 and CO_2 monitoring of the adult and neonate. Crit. Care Med. 9:689–760, 1981.

Simmons, B., and Wong, E.: Guidelines for prevention of nosocomial pneumonia. Respir. Care 28:221–232. 1983.

Sladen, R.N.: The oxyhemoglobin dissociation curve. Int. Anesthesiol. Clin. 19:39–70, 1981.

Slutsky, A.S.: Nonconventional methods of ventilation. Am. Rev. Respir. Dis. 138:175–183, 1988.

Sjostrand, U.: High frequency positive-pressure ventilation (HFPPV): A review. Crit. Care Med. 8:435–346, 1980.

Standard of nursing care of patients with COPD. Am. Thorac. Soc. News 7:31–38, 1981.

Staub, N.: Lung structure and function—1982. Am. Thorac. Soc. News 8:26–31, 1982.

Stauffer, J., Olson, D., and Petty, T.: Complications and consequences of endotracheal intubation and tracheostomy. Am. J. Med. 70:65–76, 1981.

Stevens, R.P., Lillington, G.A., and Parsons, G.H.: Fiberoptic bronchoscopy in the intensive care unit. Heart Lung 10:1037–1045, 1981.

Stratton, C.W.: Bacterial pneumonias: An overview with emphasis on pathogenesis, diagnosis, and treatment. Heart Lung 15:226–244, 1986.

Swearingen, P.L.: Manual of Nursing Therapeutics: Applying Nursing Diagnoses to Medical Disorders. Addison-Wesley Publishing Company, Reading, Mass., 1986.

Tahvanainen, J., Meretoja, O., and Nikki, P.: Can central venous blood replace mixed venous blood samples? Crit. Care Med. 10:758–761, 1982.

Taylor, R.W.: The adult respiratory distress syndrome. In Kirby, R.R., and Taylor, R.W. (eds.): Respiratory Failure. Year Book Medical Publishers, Chicago, 1986.

Tobin, M.: Respiratory monitoring in the intensive care unit. Am. Rev. Respir. Dis. 138:1625–1642, 1988.

Traver, G.A. (ed.): Respiratory Nursing: The Science and Art. John Wiley & Sons, New York, 1982.

Tyler, M.: Complications of positioning and chest physiotherapy. Respir. Care 27:458–466, 1982.

Unger, K., Snow, R., Mestas, J., and Miller, W.: Smoke inhalation in firemen. Thorax 35:838–842, 1980.

Vasbinder-Dillon, D.: Understanding mechanical ventilation. Crit. Care Nurse 8:42–56, 1988.

Vij, D., Babcock, R., and Magilligan, D.: A simplified concept of complete physiological monitoring of the critically ill patient. Heart Lung 10:75–82, 1981.

Wade, J.F.: Comprehensive Respiratory Care, 3rd ed. C.V. Mosby Co., St. Louis, 1982.

Warren, T.E., and Howell, C.: High-frequency jet ventilation: A nursing perspective. Heart Lung 12:432–437, 1983.

Weiberger, M., Hendeles, L., and Ahrens, R.: Pharmacologic management of reversible obstructive airways disease. Med. Clin. North Am. 65:579–613, 1981.

Weigelt, J.A.: Management of patients with adult respiratory distress syndrome. Semin. Respir. Med. 8 (suppl):54–65, 1986.

Weinberger, S.E.: Principles of Pulmonary Medicine. W.B. Saunders Co., Philadelphia, 1986.

Wilson, J.: Pulmonary embolism: Diagnosis and treatment: I. and II. Clin. Notes Respir. Dis. 19:3–11, 12–13, 1981.

Wilson, J., Bynum, L., and Parkey, R.: Heparin therapy in venous thromboembolism. Am. J. Med. 70:808–816, 1981.

Wittman, M.: Penetrating thoracic trauma. In Brenner, B.E. (ed.): Comprehensive Management of Respiratory Emergencies. Aspen Publishers, Rockville, Md., 1985.

Woolcock, A.J. (ed.): Asthma: What are the important experiments? Am. Rev. Respir. Dis. 138:730–744, 1988.

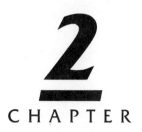

CHAPTER

The Cardiovascular System

Richard DeAngelis, R.N., M.S.

PHYSIOLOGIC ANATOMY

Skeletal Muscle

1. **Central nucleus**
2. **Sarcoplasma:** intracellular proteinaceous fluid
3. **Sarcolemma:** the membrane that surrounds the muscle fiber (a single cell)
4. **Fiber:** composed of many fibrils, each surrounded by a sarcotubular system
5. **Sarcotubular system:** a membranous continuation of sarcolemma
   a. T tubules function to transmit action potential rapidly from sarcolemma to all fibrils in muscle
   b. Sarcoplasmic reticulum houses calcium ions. Action potential in T tubules causes release of calcium from reticulum, resulting in a contraction
6. **Contractile unit:** sarcomere (Fig. 2–1). Muscle fiber composed of fibrils
   a. Each fibril is divided into filaments
   b. Each filament is made up of contractile proteins
   c. Contractile proteins consist of actin, myosin, troponin, and tropomyosin
      i. Myosin forms the thick filaments
      ii. Actin, troponin, and tropomyosin form the thin filaments

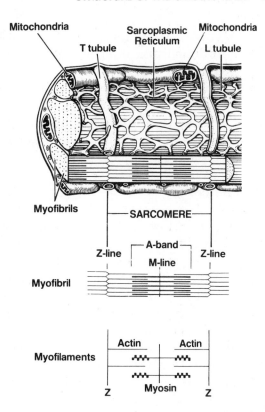

Figure 2–1. The sarcomere. (From Shepard, N., et al.: A guide to arrhythmia interpretation and management. Crit. Care Nurse 2[5]:59, 1982.)

Cardiac Muscle: Differs from skeletal muscle. It has more mitochondria and can provide more adenosine triphosphate (ATP) and energy for repetitive action

1. **Fibers:** connected to each other by intercalated discs forming a lattice arrangement called a functional syncytium
2. **Syncytium:** when one fiber is depolarized (see p. 145), the action potential spreads along the syncytium to all fibers, stimulating them also. Thus, the whole syncytium contracts, not just one fiber (all or none response)

Structure of the Cardiac Wall

1. **Pericardium:** a fibroserous membranous sac that encloses the heart and roots of great vessels in a fluid-lubricated (pericardial) space. It functions to protect heart from friction and is composed of two layers
   a. Fibrous pericardium: outermost layer
   b. Serous pericardium: lines the fibrous pericardium, covers the heart, and has two layers
      i. Parietal layer
      ii. Visceral layer: this is the outer surface of the heart (epicardium)
2. **Epicardium:** equivalent to visceral layer of serous pericardium; covers the heart and great vessels

3. **Myocardium:** muscular portion of heart
4. **Endocardium:** inner membranous surface of heart, lining chambers of heart
5. **Papillary muscles:** arise from the myocardial surface of ventricles and attach to chordae tendineae
6. **Chordae tendineae:** tendinous attachments from the papillary muscles to tricuspid and mitral valves; serve to prevent eversion of the valves into the atria during systole

Chambers

1. **Atria:** thin-walled, low-pressure–receiving chambers
   a. Right atrium (RA) and left atrium (LA) act as reservoirs of blood for their respective ventricles
   b. Right atrium receives systemic venous blood via superior vena cava, inferior vena cava, and coronary sinus
   c. Left atrium receives oxygenated blood returning to heart from lungs via the four pulmonary veins
   d. Seventy per cent of blood flows passively from atria into ventricles during early ventricular diastole (protodiastole)
   e. Atria contract forcefully ("atrial kick"), supplying another 10% to 20% of blood for ventricular output
2. **Ventricles:** the major "pumps" of the heart
   a. Right ventricle (RV)
      i. Contracts and propels deoxygenated blood into pulmonary circulation via pulmonary artery (PA) (the only artery in the body that carries deoxygenated blood)
      ii. A low-pressure system
   b. Left ventricle (LV): main "pump"
      i. Ejects blood into systemic circulation via aorta during ventricular systole
      ii. A high-pressure system

Cardiac Valves

1. **Atrioventricular (AV) valves**
   a. Located between the atria and ventricles; mitral valve on the left, tricuspid valve on the right
      i. Mitral valve is bicuspid, comprising posterior (mural) and anterior (aortic) leaflets
      ii. Tricuspid valve consists of three leaflets (anterior, posterior, and septal)
      iii. The cusps are joined at their edges near their base for 0.5 to 1.0 cm, termed a *commissure*
   b. Allow unidirectional blood flow from respective atrium to respective

ventricle during ventricular diastole and prevent retrograde flow during ventricular systole

    i. With ventricular diastole, the ventricles, and hence the papillary muscles, relax; valve leaflets open

    ii. With increased ventricular pressure and systole, valve leaflets close completely

    iii. Valve closure produces a sound that constitutes the first heart sound (S_1), consisting of a mitral and a tricuspid component (M_1T_1). M_1 is the initial and major component of S_1

2. Semilunar valves

  a. Location

    i. Pulmonary valve is situated between right ventricle and pulmonary artery. It consists of an annulus and three semilunar cusps that attach to the wall of the pulmonary trunk. The free borders of the cusps are directed upward into the lumen of the artery

    ii. Aortic valve is situated between the left ventricle and aorta. It consists of three valve cusps whose bases attach to a valve annulus

  b. Allow unidirectional blood flow from the outflow tract during ventricular systole and prevent retrograde blood flow during ventricular diastole

    i. Opening occurs when respective ventricle contracts: when pressure is greater than in the artery, the valve opens

    ii. After ventricular systole, pressure in artery exceeds pressure in respective ventricle. This and retrograde blood flow causes valve to close

    iii. Valve closure produces a sound that constitutes the second heart sound (S_2), consisting of an aortic and pulmonary component (A_2P_2). A_2 is the initial and major component of S_2

Systemic Vasculature

1. **Major functions:** to supply tissues with blood, nutrients, and hormones and to remove metabolic wastes
2. **Resistance to flow:** depends on diameter of vessels (especially the arterioles), viscosity of the blood, and elastic recoil in vessel walls
3. **Blood flow to tissues:** controlled via local control, nervous control, and humoral control mechanisms
4. **Major components of vasculature system**

  a. Arteries

    i. Strong, compliant, elastic-walled vessels that carry blood away from heart and distribute it to capillary beds throughout the body

    ii. This is a high-pressure circuit

       iii. Owing to elastic fibers located within arterial wall, arteries are able to stretch during systole and recoil during diastole

b. Arterioles

       i. Contain smooth muscle innervated by the autonomic nervous system (adrenergic fibers), the stimulation of which causes constriction of vessels. Decreased adrenergic discharge dilates vessels, thus controlling blood distribution to various capillary beds

       ii. Also controlled by autoregulation (see p. 140)

       iii. Comprise the major vessels controlling systemic vascular resistance and thus arterial pressure

       iv. May give rise directly to capillaries: regulation of flow is through constriction or dilation

       v. May first give rise to metarterioles (precapillaries), which then give rise to capillaries. They serve as thoroughfare channels to venules or conduits to supply capillary beds

       vi. In some instances precapillary sphincters (smooth muscle), located where the arterioles or metarterioles give rise to the capillaries, control blood flow through the cognate capillaries

c. Capillary system

       i. Nutritional flow: capillary blood flow allows for exchange of oxygen and carbon dioxide and solutes between blood and tissues and permits fluid volume transfer between plasma and interstitium

          (a) Caused by sum of hydrostatic and osmotic pressures across membrane

          (b) Increased hydrostatic pressure leads to movement of fluid from vessel to interstitium via osmosis

          (c) Greater capillary osmotic pressure leads to fluid movement from interstitium into vessels

       ii. Capillaries lack smooth muscle. Control of their diameter is passive owing to changes in precapillary and postcapillary resistance

       iii. Because of their narrow lumens, capillaries can withstand high internal pressures without rupturing. This can be explained by Laplace's law, which states that the tension in the wall of the vessel necessary to balance the distending pressure is lessened as the radius of the blood vessel decreases

       iv. Diffusion: the most important process in moving substrates and wastes between blood and tissues via the capillary system

d. Venous system

       i. Stores approximately 65% of the total volume of blood in the circulatory system

       ii. Venules

          (a) Receive blood from capillaries

(b) Conduct blood back to heart within a low-pressure system

(c) Venous pump (skeletal muscle pump)—veins are surrounded by skeletal muscles. When muscles contract, they compress veins, moving blood toward the heart. Valves in veins prevent retrograde blood flow

    (1) Under normal conditions, venous pump keeps venous pressure in lower extremities at 25 mm Hg or less

    (2) Gravity has profound effects on the erect, immobile extremities, which results in swelling and decrease in blood return to the heart caused by leakage of fluid from circulatory system into interstitium

Anatomy of the Cardiac Conduction System (Fig. 2–2)

1. Sinoatrial node (SA node)

  a. Normal pacemaker of the heart, because it possesses fastest inherent rate of automaticity (approximately 70 beats/min)

  b. Initiates a rhythmic impulse

2. Internodal atrial pathways

  a. Conduct the impulse from SA node through RA musculature to the atrioventricular (AV) node

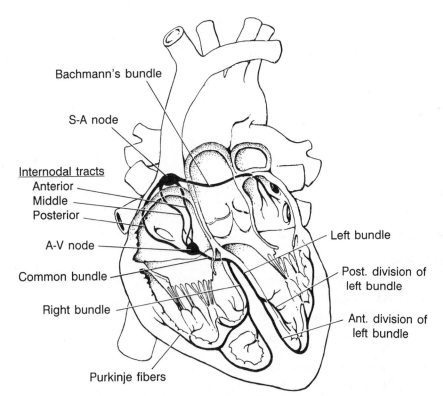

Figure 2–2. Anatomy of the cardiac conduction system.

    b. Consist of
       i. Anterior tract (Bachmann's)
      ii. Middle tract (Wenckebach's)
     iii. Posterior tract (Thorel's)

3. Bachmann's bundle: conducts impulses from SA node to LA

4. Atrioventricular node: (AV node or AV junction)
    a. Delays impulse from atria before it goes to ventricles. This allows time for both ventricles to fill prior to ventricular systole
    b. Inherent rate of automaticity is 40 to 60 beats/min

5. Bundle of His: arises from AV node and conducts impulse to bundle branch system

6. Bundle branch system: pathways that arise from bundle of His, composed of
    a. Right bundle branch (RBB): a direct continuation of the bundle of His
       i. Transmits impulse down right side of interventricular septum to the RV myocardium
      ii. The bundle divides into three parts—anterior, lateral, and posterior, which further divide, becoming parts of the Purkinje system (see below)
    b. Left bundle branch (LBB): separates into
       i. Left posterior fascicle—transmits impulse over posterior and inferior endocardial surface of LV
      ii. Left anterior fascicle—transmits impulse to anterior and superior endocardial surfaces of LV
     iii. Septal fascicle

7. Purkinje system
    a. Arises from distal portion of bundle branches
    b. Transmits impulse into subendocardial layers of both ventricles; provides for depolarization (from endocardium to epicardium), followed by ventricular contraction and ejection of blood out of ventricles
    c. Ventricles have their own inherent rate of less than 40 beats/min

Coronary Vasculature (Fig. 2–3)

1. Arteries
    a. Branch off at the base of aorta, supplying blood to the electrical conduction system and to the myocardium
    b. Right coronary artery (RCA), supplies
       i. SA node in 55% of hearts
      ii. AV node in 90% of hearts
     iii. RA and RV heart muscle
     iv. Inferoposterior wall of LV
      v. In 80% of hearts, the RCA provides a branch, the posterior

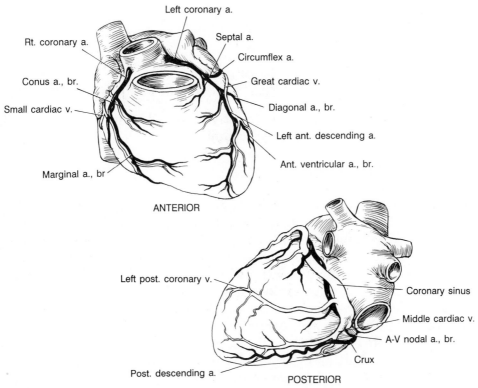

Figure 2–3. Coronary vasculature. Arteries are drawn in black; veins are drawn in white.

descending artery. (If so, the RCA system is considered "dominant.")
    (a) Located in the posterior interventricular groove
    (b) Supplies RV and inferior wall of LV and posterior part of the interventricular septum
  vi. RCA also gives off a marginal acute branch
    (a) Descends from lateral side of heart down to apex
    (b) Supplies inferior surface of RV
c. Left main coronary artery (LMCA), branches into
  i. Left anterior descending (LAD), supplying
    (a) Anterior part of the interventricular septum
    (b) Anterior wall of the LV
    (c) RBB
    (d) Anterosuperior division of the LBB
  ii. Circumflex (CF) also branches off from the LMCA (major branch of CF is the obtuse marginal branch—OMB). CF supplies
    (a) AV node in 10% of hearts
    (b) SA node in 45% of hearts
    (c) Lateral posterior surface of LV via the OMB

2. **Veins** (see Fig. 2–3)
   a. Return deoxygenated blood back to the heart
   b. Consist of
      i. Great cardiac vein
      ii. Small cardiac vein (both form the coronary sinus that drains into the RA)
      iii. Thebesian veins occur mostly in the RA and RV. They drain blood directly into these chambers

Control of Peripheral Blood Flow

1. **Local control mechanisms:** the ability of the tissues to control their own blood flow is known as autoregulation. This occurs in two phases: acute control (rapid changes in blood flow occurring in seconds to minutes) and long-term control (slow changes in blood flow taking days to months to occur). Acute control will be discussed. There are two major hypotheses that exist to explain how tissues control the flow of blood when the level of oxygen changes or the rate of metabolism changes
   a. Vasodilatory theory for control of local blood flow
      i. As rate of metabolism increases, oxygen is consumed at a higher rate, resulting in locally decreased partial pressure of oxygen
      ii. The decrease in oxygen increases the production of vasodilator substances (e.g., carbon dioxide, lactic acid, adenosine). This dilates metarterioles and arterioles, increasing blood supply
   b. Oxygen demand theory for control of local blood flow (nutrient demand theory)
      i. Oxygen is required to maintain vascular contraction
      ii. When the oxygen level (and that of other nutrients) decreases, dilation of the blood vessels occurs to increase blood flow and the subsequent level of oxygen
      iii. Also, as increased metabolism occurs at tissue level, oxygen use increases, decreasing the amount of oxygen availability and causing local vasodilation
   c. When arterial pressure acutely increases or decreases, there is an immediate increase or decrease in blood flow to adjust for the change and maintain homeostasis. This autoregulation of blood flow occurs based on the following two theories
      i. Myogenic theory: as arterial pressure rises, the vessels stretch. This stimulates the contraction of smooth muscles in the vessels (a feedback mechanism), reducing the blood flow back to normal. As tension decreases, smooth muscles relax
      ii. Metabolic theory: As the arterial pressure rises, the increased blood flow brings many nutrients to the tissues and removes vasodilator substances from the area. Both these effects cause the blood vessels to constrict. On the other hand, because of the

normal metabolic activity of the tissues, metabolites (carbon dioxide, potassium, prostaglandins, and phosphates) accumulate and cause vasodilation, which increases the blood to the area that flushes these waste products away

    iii. There is a delicate balance between these two mechanisms: myogenic response → vasoconstriction → decrease in blood supply → local increase in metabolites → vasodilation → wastes removed

2. **Autonomic regulation of vessels**
   a. Adrenergic sympathetic nervous system fibers secrete norepinephrine at nerve endings, producing vasoconstriction
      i. In arterioles, this mechanism helps to regulate blood flow and arterial pressure
      ii. In veins, this mechanism helps to vary the amount of blood stored; that is, venoconstriction causes an increase in venous return to the heart
   b. Parasympathetic nervous system fibers secrete acetylcholine at the endings (cholinergic effect), producing vasodilation
3. **Stretch receptors:** baroreceptors (pressoreceptors)
   a. Receptor sites located in aortic arch, carotid sinus, venae cavae, pulmonary arteries, and atria
   b. Sensitive to arterial pressures above 60 mm Hg
   c. Activated by elevated blood pressure or blood volume
      i. Respond to stretching of arterial walls
      ii. Impulse transmitted from aortic arch via vagus nerve to medulla and from carotid sinus via Hering's nerve to glossopharyngeal nerve to medulla
      iii. Sympathetic action inhibited
      iv. Vagal reflex dominates
      v. Result: decreased heart rate and contractility, dilation of peripheral vessels, decreased systemic vascular resistance, blood pressure lowered to normal
   d. Action with decreased blood pressure
      i. Vagal tone decreases
      ii. Sympathetic system becomes dominant
      iii. Result: increases heart rate and contractility, arterial and venous constriction (preserving blood flow to brain and heart) and blood pressure elevated to near normal
4. **Vasomotor center in medulla:** also called cardioaccelerator center or cardiac center. It consists of two areas: vasoconstrictor and vasodepressor
   a. Stimulation of vasoconstrictor area causes secretion of norepinephrine
      i. Increased heart rate, stroke volume, cardiac output, and, ultimately, arterial blood pressure
      ii. Venoconstriction, which decreases stores of blood in venous

system, increases venous return and thus increases blood pressure

b. Inhibition of vasoconstrictor area stimulates vasodepressor area, which causes vasodilation. There is an increase in storage of blood in venous system, thus decreasing stroke volume and cardiac output, and hence arterial blood pressure

c. Vasomotor center works with stretch receptors and chemoreceptors located in carotid sinus and aortic arch

   i. Rise in blood pressure stimulates carotid sinus, which in turn inhibits vasoconstrictor area. This induces vasodilation via stimulation of vasodepressor area, and sequence of events follows as listed previously

   ii. Fall in oxygen saturation, rise in carbon dioxide, or fall in pH stimulates chemoreceptors, which then stimulate vasoconstrictor center and cause a rise in arterial blood pressure

Arterial Pressure

1. **Regulation**

   a. Arterial pressure is controlled by various mechanisms outlined in section on control of peripheral blood vessels

   b. Arterial pressure is also controlled by hormonal mechanisms

      i. Renin–angiotensin–aldosterone system (see also Chapter 4, The Renal System)

         (a) Renin—a protease secreted by kidney; converts angiotensinogen to angiotensin I

         (b) Release of renin from kidney is stimulated by

            (1) Stretch receptors in juxtaglomerular cells that are sensitive to changes in blood pressure (as effected, for example, by hemorrhage, dehydration, diuretics, and sodium depletion)

               a) Decreased blood pressure → increased renin secretion

               b) Increased blood pressure → decreased renin secretion

            (2) Rise in sympathetic output causes increased renin secretion

            (3) Fall in sodium concentration causes increased renin secretion

         (c) Increased renin secretion stimulates the formation of angiotensin II, the most potent vasoconstrictor known; it produces arteriolar constriction with a resultant rise in systolic and diastolic pressures. Angiotensin II also stimulates the adrenal cortex to secrete aldosterone, which causes sodium and water retention. The extracellular fluid volume increases and shuts the stimulus off that initiated the renin secretion, and blood pressure is maintained at a normal level

c. Capillary fluid shift mechanisms

d. Local control mechanisms (see section on local control mechanisms, p. 140)

e. Renal: fluid volume process

    i. With rise in arterial pressure, kidneys excrete more fluid (causing reduction in extracellular fluid and blood volumes), which reduces circulating blood volume and cardiac output, leading to normalization of arterial pressure

    ii. With fall in arterial pressure, kidneys retain fluid and sodium, causing increased intravascular volume and cardiac output, which results in normalization of arterial pressure

2. **Factors affecting arterial blood pressure**

a. Cardiac output

b. Heart rate

c. Systemic vascular resistance

d. Arterial elasticity

e. Blood volume

f. Blood viscosity

g. Age

h. Body surface area

i. Exercise

j. Emotions

k. Sodium retention

3. **Pulse pressure**

a. Definition: arithmetic difference between systolic and diastolic pressures expressed as a numerical value in millimeters of mercury (mm Hg)

b. A function of stroke volume and arterial capacitance

4. **Mean arterial pressure (MAP):** Berne and Levy (1986) define the MAP as "the average pressure during a given cardiac cycle that exists in the aorta and its major branches . . . it is dependent on the mean volume of blood in the arterial system and the elastic properties of the arterial walls"

a. MAP is calculated by the following formula

$$\overline{Pa} = Pd + \frac{1}{3}(Ps - Pd)$$

where

$\overline{Pa}$ = Mean arterial pressure

Pd = Diastolic pressure

Ps = Systolic pressure

$Ps - Pd$ = Pulse pressure

Thus the MAP = diastolic pressure + $\frac{1}{3}$ pulse pressure

b. Example: Blood pressure of 120/60 mm Hg

$\overline{\text{Pa}}$ = Pd + ⅓ (Ps − Pd)
$\overline{\text{Pa}}$ = 60 + ⅓ (60)
$\overline{\text{Pa}}$ = 60 + 20
$\overline{\text{Pa}}$ = 80

c. Level of MAP is a function of cardiac output and systemic vascular resistance

Neurologic Control of the Heart

1. **Autonomic nervous system**
   a. Sympathetic stimulation: the release of norepinephrine elicits two types of effects
      i. Alpha-adrenergic: causes arteriolar vasoconstriction
      ii. Beta-adrenergic (beta$_1$)
         (a) Increases SA node discharge, thus increasing the heart rate (positive chronotropy)
         (b) Increases the force of myocardial contraction (positive inotropy)
         (c) Accelerates AV conduction time (positive dromotropy)
   b. Parasympathetic stimulation: occurs through action of right vagus (affecting SA node) and left vagus (affecting AV conduction tissue). It causes release of acetylcholine
      i. Decreases rate of SA node discharge, thus slowing heart rate (negative chronotropy)
      ii. May slow conduction through AV tissue (negative dromotropy)
2. **Chemoreceptors**
   a. Located in carotid and aortic bodies
   b. Sensitive to changes in P_{O_2}, P_{CO_2}, and pH, thus causing change in heart rate and respiratory rate via stimulation of vasomotor center in medulla
3. **Stretch receptors:** respond to pressure and volume changes
4. **Bainbridge reflex:** stretch receptors located in atria, large veins, and pulmonary artery
   a. Increase in venous return stretches the receptors
   b. Afferent nerve impulses transmit to the vasomotor center in medulla
   c. Medulla increases efferent impulses, increasing heart rate and cardiac output
   d. This enables the heart to pump all the blood returned to it
5. **Respiratory reflex**
   a. Inspiration decreases intrathoracic pressure, increasing venous return to the heart
   b. Inspiration stimulates stretch receptors in the lungs and thorax
   c. Impulses from stretch receptors are sent (via afferent fibers) to the vasomotor center in the medulla and inhibit this center

　　d. This inhibition decreases vagal tone, causing an increase in the heart rate, which allows the heart to pump out extra blood adequately

Electrophysiology

1. **Resting membrane potential (RMP) for cardiac muscle cell**
　　a. Sodium ion concentration greater outside cell than inside
　　b. Potassium ion concentration greater inside cell than outside
　　c. Unbound calcium ion concentration also greater outside cell
　　d. RMP for myocardial muscle fibers is -80 to -90 mV (Fig. 2–4)
2. **Stimulation of resting membrane**
　　a. Results from chemical, electrical, or mechanical stimulation
　　b. The stimulus reduces the RMP to a less negative value. This process is known as depolarization
　　c. Once the threshold potential (the voltage level where once reached, an action potential is produced) is reached, changes occur in the membrane
　　　　i. For all cardiac tissue except SA and AV nodes, the threshold potential is -60 to -70 mV
　　　　ii. For the SA and AV nodes, the threshold potential is -30 to -40 mV
　　d. The permeability of the cell membrane is altered, and specialized channels in the membrane open, permitting the passage of sodium and calcium ions into the cell
　　e. The events can be recorded graphically in the form of an action potential (AP) (see Fig. 2–4)
　　f. Excitability: all cardiac cells are excitable; that is, they have the

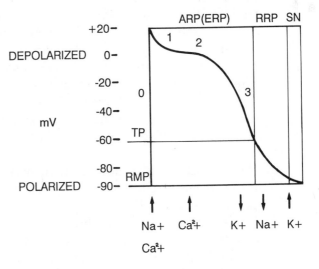

Figure 2–4. Diagram of the action potential of a ventricular muscle cell. *RMP*, resting membrane potential; *O*, depolarization; *1,2,3*, repolarization phases of the action potential; *TP*, threshold potential; *ERP*, effective refractory period; *RRP*, relative refractory period; *SN*, supernormal period. In phase 0, influx of Na^+ and Ca^{2+} produces plateau phase of repolarization; in phase 3, there is return of intracellular potential to -90 mV owing to efflux of K^+. At the termination of phase 3, the active transport system pumps K^+ into the cell and extrudes Na^+ from the cell.

ability to depolarize and form an action potential when sufficiently stimulated

g. Conductivity: all cardiac cells have the ability to conduct the electrical impulse to neighboring cells, thus spreading the impulse throughout the heart and achieving total depolarization

3. **The "gate theory":** it is believed that the fast channels of the membrane specific for sodium are controlled by two gates

   a. One gate (activation gate) opens fast channels as the RMP becomes less negative, allowing the sodium to diffuse rapidly into the cell, causing depolarization (phase 0 of the AP curve—the upstroke)

   b. The other gate (deactivation gate) tends to close the channels, impeding the influx of sodium into the cell

   c. Closure of the gates is complete in phase 1 of the AP curve, and sodium ceases to diffuse into the cell

   d. As the membrane potential begins to return to the RMP, an inward current of calcium (and to a lesser extent, sodium) via slow channels occurs, producing the plateau phase of the AP—phase 2. Also during this phase, potassium ions diffuse out of the cell

   e. As the slow, inward current of sodium and calcium decreases, the outward current of potassium increases. This causes the cell to rapidly repolarize—phase 3 of the AP curve

   f. After repolarization, the sodium–potassium pump regulates the concentration of the cations in the cell. The pump, found in the cell membrane, actively extrudes excess sodium out of the cell and pumps in the potassium that diffused out during phase 2

4. **Refractoriness of heart muscle** (see Fig. 2–4) (the temporary inability of depolarized cells to respond to another stimulus)

   a. Absolute refractory period (effective refractory period): encompasses phases 0, 1, 2, and part of 3 of the AP curve. During this period of time another stimulus to the cell will not produce another AP

   b. Relative refractory period (latter part of phase 3): during this period a stimulus stronger than the one that would elicit an AP when in the RMP state can initiate an AP response and cause depolarization

   c. Supernormal period (occurs at the end of phase 3): in this period, a very weak stimulus (one that would not normally elicit an AP) can evoke a response and cause depolarization

5. **Cardiac pacemaker cells** (SA and AV nodes) action potential (Fig. 2–5)

   a. Phase 0: there is a slow, inward movement of calcium and sodium into the cell, producing a slow-response AP curve different from the cardiac muscle cell

   b. Unlike other cells of the heart, which when having repolarized and attained phase 4 require another stimulus to depolarize them, the SA and AV nodes spontaneously depolarize in phase 4 without a stimulus. This spontaneous depolarization is due to the steady influx

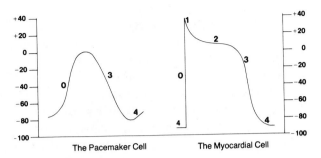

Figure 2–5. Comparison of the pacemaker cell and the myocardial cell action potential curves. (From Shepard, N., et al.: A guide to arrhythmia interpretation and management. Crit. Care Nurse 2[5]:62, 1982.)

of sodium and the efflux of potassium ions. This process raises the nodal tissues back to the threshold potential, initiating an AP. This phenomenon is known as automaticity

   i. The rate of automaticity may be altered by increasing or decreasing the slope of phase 4

  ii. Increasing the slope of phase 4 speeds the heart rate; decreasing the slope of phase 4 slows the heart rate

Excitation–Contraction Process of Muscle (Fig. 2–6)

1. **The AP produced during depolarization** is transmitted to the interior of the cell via T tubules, which transmit the AP to all myofibrils of muscle
2. **Calcium is stored in lateral sacs of sarcoplasmic reticulum** and is released when the AP reaches the sarcoplasmic reticulum

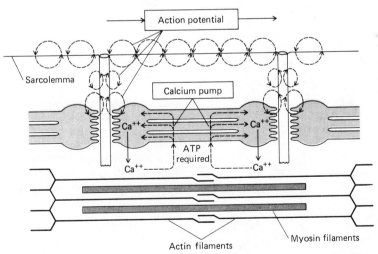

Figure 2–6. Excitation–contraction coupling in the muscle, showing an action potential that causes release of calcium ions from the sarcoplasmic reticulum and then reuptake of the calcium ions by a calcium pump. (From Guyton, A. C.: Textbook of Medical Physiology, 7th ed. W. B. Saunders Co., Philadelphia, 1986, p. 128.)

3. **Calcium enters interior of cell** and, through a complex interaction with enzymes, causes interaction between actin and myosin filaments

4. **Actin filaments move progressively inward on myosin filaments** as successive electrochemical interactions take place (interdigitation–sliding filament hypothesis)

5. **The result is a shortening of sarcomeres,** causing shortening of muscle fibers and thus myocardial contraction

6. **Free calcium is then pumped back into the sarcoplasmic reticulum,** resulting in relaxation of the muscle fibers (Fig. 2–7)

Events During the Cardiac Cycle Produced by Depolarization and Repolarization

1. **The electroactivity of the heart,** which ultimately produces contraction, is graphically described in Figure 2–8
   a. Electrical depolarization of the atria produces the P wave on the electrocardiogram (ECG), following which the pressure in the atria rises (the "a" wave)
   b. During this period, the pressure in the atria is higher than the diastolic pressure in the ventricles, forcing blood from the atria into the ventricles. The ventricles are in diastole at this time
   c. Electrical depolarization of the ventricles occurs, producing the QRS complex on the ECG

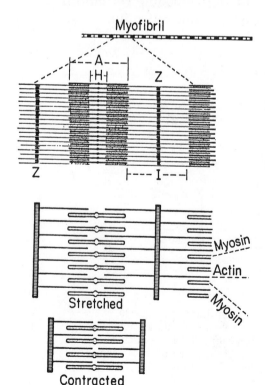

Figure 2–7. Muscular contraction. The myofibrils are composed of overlapping thick myosin filaments and thin actin filaments. The amount of overlap is diminished during stretching and increased during contraction. (From Rushmer, R. F.: Cardiovascular Dynamics, 3rd ed. W. B. Saunders Co., Philadelphia, 1970, p. 41.)

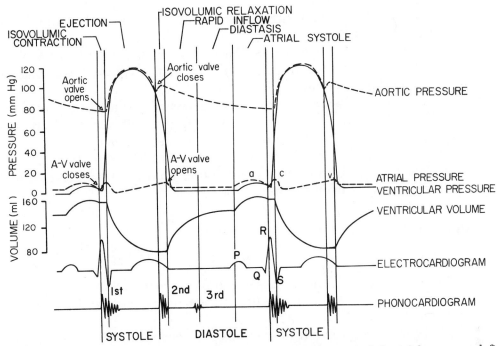

Figure 2–8. The events of the cardiac cycle showing changes in left atrial pressure, left ventricular pressure, aortic pressure, ventricular volume, the electrocardiogram, and the phonocardiogram. (From Guyton, A. C.: Textbook of Medical Physiology, 7th ed. W. B. Saunders Co., Philadelphia, 1986, p. 154.)

d. The first phase of ventricular contraction (systole) is called isometric or isovolumetric contraction, when pressure is increasing but no blood is entering or leaving the ventricles

e. As pressure rises in the ventricles the AV valves close, producing the first heart sound (S_1; composed of mitral and tricuspid components—M_1T_1). The "c" wave of the atrial pressure curve is produced because the AV valves are pushed backward toward the atria as the pressure in the ventricles builds

f. Once pressure in the LV exceeds the pressure in the aorta, the aortic valve opens (comparable events in RV occur with the pulmonic valve)

g. The blood flow is rapidly ejected into the aorta (systolic ejection)

h. As the outflow of blood from the LV decreases and ventricular ejection stops, the pressure in the LV also decreases, falling below the pressure in the aorta

i. This causes a back flow of blood from the aorta to the LV that forces the aortic valve closed and produces the second heart sound (S_2; composed of aortic and pulmonic components—A_2P_2). Comparable events occur in the pulmonary artery, closing the pulmonic valve. The closure of the aortic valve is indicated by the dicrotic notch in the aortic pressure waveform

j. Repolarization of the ventricles occurs at this time and produces the T wave on the ECG

k. As soon as the aortic valve closes, the pressure in the LV falls rapidly: isometric or isovolumetric relaxation phase—no blood is entering the ventricle

l. A "v" wave is produced on the atrial pressure curve during isometric relaxation, owing to the blood flowing into the atrium from the pulmonary and systemic circuit against closed AV valves

m. When pressure is lower in the ventricles than in the atria, the AV valves open to initiate the rapid filling phase during diastole and the cycle starts over again

Variables Affecting Left Ventricular Function

1. Preload

a. Resting force on the myocardium is determined by pressure in ventricles at end of diastole (left ventricular end-diastolic pressure, LVEDP)

b. Preload can be related to a number of variables (e.g., fiber length, stretch, volume)

c. Increase in preload is accomplished by increasing the volume returning to the ventricles

d. Increase in preload stretches myocardial fibers; this event causes more forceful subsequent ventricular contractions, increasing stroke volume and thus cardiac output (see p. 190) but also ventricular work

e. Muscle fibers can reach a point of stretch beyond which contraction is no longer enhanced; stroke volume decreases, leading to heart failure

f. These concepts are known as the Frank-Starling law of the heart (Fig. 2–9)

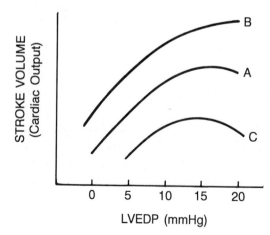

Figure 2–9. Ventricular function curves representing the Frank-Starling principle. The graph shows the relationship of left ventricular (LV) filling pressures (preload) to cardiac output (force) in the normal heart and in progressive left ventricular dysfunction. Curve A depicts the normal LV function, curve B depicts an increased contractile state (an improvement in LV function), and curve C depicts impairment of LV contractility (failure).

   g. Factors affecting preload
      i. Mitral insufficiency (increases)
      ii. Mitral stenosis (decreases)
      iii. Aortic insufficiency (increases)
      iv. Volume of circulating fluids
         (a) Increased volume increases preload
         (b) Decreased volume decreases preload
      v. Drugs
         (a) Vasoconstrictors increase preload
         (b) Vasodilators decrease preload
      vi. Atrial kick increases, loss of which decreases preload

2. Afterload
   a. The initial resistance that must be overcome by the ventricles in order to open the semilunar valves and to propel blood into the systemic and pulmonary circulatory systems
   b. Clinically reflected by arterial systolic pressure (systemic vascular resistance [SVR]—also called peripheral vascular resistance)
   c.

$$\text{SVR} = \frac{\text{MAP} - \overline{\text{CVP}}}{\text{CO (L/min)}} = \text{a value measured in resistance units}$$

   This number $\times$ 80 converts into dynes/sec/cm^{-5}
   d. A dyne is defined by Taber's (1981) as "a unit of force which would propel a mass of weight one gram with a velocity of one cm in a second"
   e. Normal SVR = 900 to 1400 dynes/sec/cm^{-5}
   f. Factors affecting afterload
      i. Aortic valvular stenosis (increases afterload)
      ii. Peripheral arteriolar vasoconstriction (increases afterload)
      iii. Hypertension (increases afterload)
      iv. Polycythemia (increases afterload)
      v. Drugs
         (a) Arteriolar vasodilators decrease afterload
         (b) Arteriolar vasoconstrictors increase afterload
   g. Excessive afterload will increase LV stroke work, decrease stroke volume, increase myocardial oxygen demands, and may result in LV failure

3. Contractility
   a. Factors that increase the contractile state of the myocardium, shifting the curve to the left and up (see Fig. 2–9, curve B)
      i. Positive inotropic drugs: digitalis, epinephrine, dobutamine
      ii. Increased heart rate (Bowditch's law)
      iii. Sympathetic stimulation (via beta$_1$ receptors)
      iv. Hypercalcemia

b. Factors that decrease the contractile state of the myocardium, shifting the curve to the right and down (see Fig. 2–9, curve C)
   i. Negative inotropic drugs: quinidine, barbiturates, propranolol
   ii. Hypoxia (O_2 saturation less than 50%)
   iii. Hypercapnia
   iv. Intrinsic depression: due to cardiac muscle disease or loss of functional myocardial tissue due to an infarct
   v. Parasympathetic stimulation (via vagus nerve) has a depressive effect on the SA node, atrial myocardium, and AV junctional tissue. Hence, decreased heart rate results in decreased contractility
   vi. Metabolic acidosis

NURSING ASSESSMENT DATA BASE

Nursing History

1. **Chief complaint:** consists of patient's own words as to why he is seeking help; one sentence is usually sufficient
2. **History of present illness:** determine
   a. Date of onset
   b. Description of complaint
   c. Mode of onset, course, duration
   d. Exacerbations, remissions of all signs and symptoms
      i. Pain: character, location, radiation, quality, duration, factors that aggravate or produce, factors that alleviate
      ii. Fatigue: with or without activity
      iii. Edema: location, degree
      iv. Syncope: with or without dizziness, time of occurrence
      v. Dyspnea: orthopnea, paroxysmal nocturnal dyspnea, dyspnea on exertion
      vi. Palpitations or dysrhythmias
      vii. Hemoptysis
      viii. Cyanosis (circumoral, extremities)
      ix. Intermittent claudication
      x. Clubbing
3. **Past medical history:** includes all previous illnesses, injuries, surgical procedures
4. **Family history:** determine
   a. State of health or cause of death of immediate family members
   b. Hereditary, familial diseases pertaining to cardiovascular system
      i. Diabetes mellitus
      ii. Hypertension

      iii. Cardiovascular disease (stroke, transient ischemic attacks, myocardial infarctions, peripheral occlusive disease)
      iv. Gout
      v. Obesity
      vi. Allergies
5. **Social history:** determine
    a. Present and past work experiences
    b. Smoking habits
    c. Drinking habits
    d. Daily living patterns
    e. Types of foods eaten
    f. Relationship with significant others
    g. Recreational habits
    h. Sex life
    i. Educational level
6. **Medication history:** note all medication prescribed or bought over the counter and dosages being taken. Also, determine why the patient is taking the drug

Nursing Examination of the Patient

1. **Inspection**
    a. Note general overall appearance
    b. Check skin and mucous membranes
      i. Color
      ii. Temperature
      iii. Moisture
      iv. Turgor
      v. Edema: usually found in extremities and sacrum but may also be found behind scapula or in periorbital area
      vi. Nail beds: color, clubbing, refill
      vii. Angiomas
      viii. Petechiae
    c. Observe neck veins: internal jugular veins are more reliable than external jugular veins. They reflect pressure and volume changes in RA
      i. Check for distention and pulsation
        (a) Place patient at 45° angle
        (b) Shine bright light tangentially to illuminate vessels
      ii. Determine central venous pressure (see p. 195)
        (a) Place patient at 45° angle
        (b) Sternal angle is roughly 5 cm above atrium
        (c) Measure distance in centimeters from sternal angle to top of distended neck vein

(d) Value obtained plus the 5 cm provides a rough estimate of central venous pressure

d. Check for hepatojugular reflux (HJR)

   i. Place patient at 45° angle

   ii. Compress upper right abdomen for 30 to 45 seconds

   iii. If HJR is present, jugular pulses will become more pronounced and the level of filling of the neck veins will rise

e. Extremities: note and compare both sides for the following

   i. Edema

   ii. Color, temperature changes

   iii. Hair distribution

   iv. Clubbing of nail beds

   v. Ulcerations

   vi. Peripheral pulses

   vii. Blood pressure

f. Thorax

   i. Observe for heaves, thrusts over the precordial area

   ii. Shape and contour of chest

   iii. Symmetry

   iv. Breathing pattern

   v. Pulses

   vi. Visible point of maximal intensity of cardiac impulse (PMI)

2. **Palpation:** check bilaterally and simultaneously (except for carotids)

a. Arteries

   i. Check rate, rhythm, contour, and volume

   ii. Rated on scale of 0 to 3

     (a) 0   = absent pulses

     (b) 1+ = palpable but thready, easily obliterated

     (c) 2+ = normal, not easily obliterated

     (d) 3+ = bounding, easily palpable, cannot obliterate

   iii. Most common sites for palpation

     (a) Carotid

     (b) Brachial

     (c) Radial

     (d) Femoral

     (e) Popliteal

     (f) Dorsalis pedis

     (g) Posterior tibialis

   iv. Pulses should be described as to their characteristics

     (a) Pulsus magnus—strong, bounding pulses with rapid upstroke and downstroke. Noted in

       (1) Essential hypertension

       (2) Thyrotoxicosis

       (3) Aortic insufficiency

       (4) Patent ductus arteriosus

(5) Arteriovenous fistula
(b) Pulsus parvus—small, weak pulse with a delayed upstroke and prolonged downstroke. Noted in
(1) Aortic stenosis
(2) Mitral stenosis
(3) Constrictive pericarditis
(4) Cardiac tamponade
(c) Pulsus alternans—alternating pulse waves, every other beat being weaker than the preceding beat owing to a weakened myocardium. Noted in severe LV failure
(d) Pulsus paradoxus—an exaggeration of normal physiologic response to inspiration. Inflate the sphygmomanometer until no Korotkoff sounds are heard. Slowly deflate the cuff until sounds are heard only on expiration; note the reading. Continue to deflate the cuff until sounds are heard in both expiration and inspiration; note this reading. Subtract the second reading from the first reading—this represents the pulsus paradoxus. Normally, on inspiration, there is a fall of less than 10 mm Hg in arterial systolic pressure. With pulsus paradoxus, arterial pressure drop on inspiration exceeds 10 mm Hg. To be significant, fall must occur during normal inspiratory effort. Noted in
(1) Pericardial effusion
(2) Constrictive pericarditis
(3) Severe pulmonary emphysema
(4) Cardiac tamponade
(5) Hemorrhagic shock
(e) Pulsus bisferiens ("double beating" pulse)—characterized by two pulses palpated during systole. Noted in
(1) Hypertropic cardiomyopathy
(2) Constrictive pericarditis
(3) Aortic stenosis and insufficiency
b. Precordium
  i. Palpate in order to note
    (a) Pulsations (e.g., the point of maximal intensity [PMI])
    (b) Thrills (palpable murmurs, analogous to sensation felt on throat of purring cat)
    (c) Friction rubs (analogous to sensation felt when rubbing two pieces of leather together)
  ii. Seven areas on the precordium should be palpated (Fig. 2–10)
  iii. Of particular importance is the apical impulse (the point of maximal intensity [PMI] in the normal heart)
    (a) Normally found in fifth left intercostal space, midclavicular line and is approximately 2 cm in size

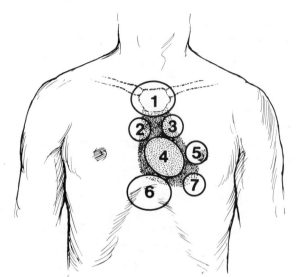

Figure 2–10. Inspection and palpation areas on the precordium.

1. Sternoclavicular area
2. Aortic area
3. Pulmonic area
4. Rt. ventricular area
5. Ectopic areas
   (location variable)
6. Epigastric area
7. Apical area

      (b) Lateral displacement of the apical impulse greater than 7 to 9 cm away from the left sternal border indicates
          (1) LV dilatation (aortic, mitral insufficiency)
          (2) Upward displacement of the diaphragm (pregnancy, tumor, ascites)
          (3) Right-to-left mediastinal shift (pleural effusion, right tension pneumothorax)
      (c) Medial displacement of apical impulse indicates
          (1) Downward displacement of diaphragm (chronic obstructive pulmonary disease)
          (2) Left-to-right mediastinal shift (left pleural effusion, left tension pneumothorax)
      (d) A forceful, sustained apical impulse indicates LV hypertrophy

3. Percussion
    a. Limited use in this system owing to extracardiac factors interfering with the technique
    b. Used to determine outer limits of cardiac dullness (i.e., heart size)

4. Auscultation
    a. Sound: an object is set in motion (vibration), initiating a sound wave cycle

b. Characteristics of sound
    i. Frequency/pitch: frequency (number of wave cycles per second) determines pitch of sound. The higher the frequency (rapid vibrations), the higher the pitch; the lower the frequency (slow vibrations), the lower the pitch. Inelastic, large masses such as the heart produce mainly low-pitched sounds. Small, elastic masses rapidly vibrate and produce high-pitched sounds
    ii. Intensity/loudness (will be considered synonymous): determined by amplitude of the vibrations. Amplitude depends on the energy producing the vibration—more energy produces higher amplitude of sound wave, and thus louder sound
    iii. Quality: pure tones are produced by one object emitting a single frequency. Most sources such as the heart produce vibrations of many frequencies at once, and these are perceived as noise
c. Auscultation recording instruments
    i. Stethoscope
        (a) Bell used to hear low-pitched sounds (heart sounds S_3 and S_4 and ventricular filling murmurs)
        (b) Diaphragm used to hear high-pitched sounds (heart sounds S_1 and S_2, ejection clicks, opening snaps and murmurs due to stenotic valves)
        (c) When using the bell of the stethoscope, do not press, otherwise the underlying skin functions as a diaphragm and you lose the low-pitched sounds
    ii. Phonocardiogram: used to demonstrate cardiac sounds graphically
    iii. Auscultate the following five areas on the chest
        (a) Aortic area (second intercostal space, right sternal border)
        (b) Pulmonic area (second intercostal space, left sternal border)
        (c) Erb's point (third intercostal space, left sternal border—murmurs of aortic and pulmonic origin are often heard here)
        (d) Tricuspid area (fifth intercostal space, left sternal border)
        (e) Mitral or apical area (fifth intercostal space, left midclavicular line)
d. Origin of heart sounds: opening and closing of valves (see Fig. 2–8) and muscular contraction can cause turbulent blood flow or rapid acceleration or deceleration of blood, producing either low- or high-frequency sounds
e. Normal heart sounds
    i. First heart sound (S_1) is produced when mitral and tricuspid valves close
        (a) Ventricles depolarize and hence contract asynchronously—left before right

(b) Component parts of S_1 may be heard (M_1 and T_1)

(c) Occurs at onset of ventricular systole

(d) Heard loudest at apex

  ii. Second heart sound (S_2) is produced when aortic and pulmonic valves close

(a) Due to asynchronous ventricular contraction, both component parts of S_2 may be heard (A_2 and P_2)

(b) Occurs at end of ventricular systole

(c) Heard loudest at the base

  iii. Third heart sound (S_3) may normally be heard in diastole

(a) Due to ventricular filling

(b) May be normal in children and young adults (physiologic S_3)

(c) If heard in older age groups or in association with disease states, it is probably abnormal

  iv. Variant splitting of heart sounds

(a) Split S_1 (M_1 T_1)

  (1) A normal and common finding

  (2) Must be distinguished from an atrial (presystolic) gallop preceding M_1, which indicates a disease state

(b) Physiologic (normal) split of S_2 (A_2 P_2)

  (1) P_2 is delayed on inspiration because the RV is slower to contract than the LV and there is an increased return of blood to the heart on inspiration. These factors prolong ejection of blood from the RV; thus pulmonic valve closure (producing P_2) occurs after aortic valve closure (producing A_2)

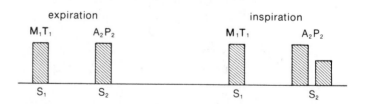

  (2) Aortic component (A_2) precedes pulmonic component (P_2) and is generally louder

  (3) Heard best over aortic and pulmonic areas

  (4) May be heard best in recumbent position and in young adults

  (5) Split S_2 may be heard transiently

 f. Abnormal heart sounds

  i. Fixed splitting of S_2

(a) Persistent splitting of S_2 that does not disappear with expiration (no respiratory variation)

   (b) Seen in
      (1) Atrial septal defect
      (2) Pulmonic stenosis/insufficiency
      (3) Right bundle branch block
      (4) Severe mitral insufficiency
      (5) Pulmonary hypertension
      (6) Ventricular septal defect
      (7) Sickle cell anemia

ii. Wide splitting of S_2—second heart sound is split on expiration and more widely split on inspiration (due to the increase in volume to RV on inspiration: increased volume→RV empties more slowly→closure of pulmonary valve is delayed); seen in
   (a) Atrial septal defect
   (b) Right bundle branch block
   (c) Pulmonary stenosis
   (d) Severe mitral insufficiency
   (e) Ventricular septal defect

iii. Paradoxic splits (reversed splitting of S_2)
   (a) When split widens on expiration and narrows on inspiration, implication is that P_2 came first, that is,

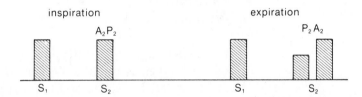

   (b) Second component of split will be louder and is A_2
   (c) Occurs when LV ejection time is prolonged, delaying aortic closure—thus pulmonic valve closes first, as in
      (1) Left bundle branch block
      (2) Severe aortic stenosis
      (3) Patent ductus arteriosus
   (d) Having patient sit or stand may help in detecting a paradoxic split (or any split)

iv. Ventricular (diastolic or S_3) gallop
   (a) Is pathologic counterpart of normal S_3
   (b) Occurs during rapid phase of ventricular filling and is caused by resistance to ventricular filling, resulting from increased volume load or decreased compliance
   (c) Sound is low pitched (heard best with bell)
   (d) When originating in LV, it is heard best at apex with patient in left lateral decubitus position and exhaling
   (e) When originating in RV, it is heard best along third to fourth intercostal space, left sternal border

(f) Heard transiently in mitral insufficiency, ischemia, advanced congestive failure, tricuspid insufficiency, left-to-right shunts

(g) Sounds like "Ken-tuc-ky"

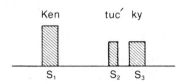

v. Atrial (presystolic or S_4) gallop

(a) Occurs with atrial contraction and just before S_1, during late phase of ventricular filling

(b) Occurs when there is an overload of either ventricle and diastolic pressure is increased

(c) Occurs in
   (1) Myocardial infarction
   (2) Pulmonary hypertension
   (3) Aortic or pulmonary stenosis
   (4) Heart failure
   (5) Hyperthyroidism

(d) Heard best
   (1) A right-sided S_4 is usually louder on inspiration
   (2) A left-sided S_4 is usually louder on expiration

(e) If heard over left lower sternal border, probably RV origin

(f) If heard over apex, probably LV origin

(g) Sounds like "Ten-nes-see"

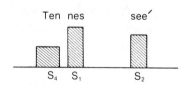

vi. Summation gallop

(a) Occurrence of an atrial and ventricular gallop simultaneously

(b) Heard with tachycardias or any situation causing shortening of diastole

(c) Summation sound is louder than S_1 or S_2

(d) Usually mid-diastolic and commonly found in advanced heart failure

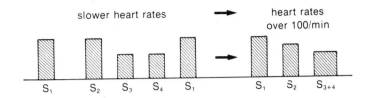

vii. Extracardiac sounds
   (a) Clicks
   (b) Pericardial friction rubs
   (c) Mediastinal crunch
   (d) Venous hum
viii. Murmurs
   (a) Sounds produced by turbulent blood flow. Examiner should note
      (1) If murmur is in systole or diastole
         a) First, listen in systole and examine all areas of precordium starting at the base and inching down the precordium to the apex. Listen closely to the five areas described on p. 157, in section on auscultation
         b) Second, listen in diastole, examining all five areas
         c) Listen to all areas with both bell and diaphragm
      (2) Site of maximal intensity
      (3) Radiation of sound (murmurs radiate in direction of blood flow)
      (4) Its duration and location in systole
         a) Pansystolic (holosystolic)—heard throughout systole

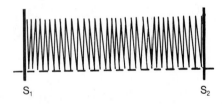

         b) Ejection murmur—starts after S_1 and ends before S_2

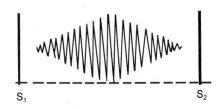

(5) Its duration and location in diastole
    a) Protodiastolic—a diastolic murmur in early diastole

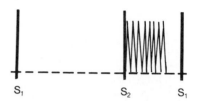

    b) Presystolic—a diastolic murmur in late diastole

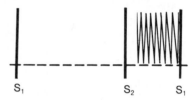

(6) Effect of ventilation on murmur—does it increase or decrease with either inspiration or expiration?
(7) Effect of patient position on the intensity of the murmur
(8) Characteristic pattern of murmurs
    a) Crescendo—builds up in intensity

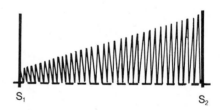

    b) Decrescendo—decreases in intensity

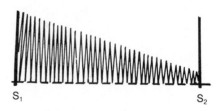

    c) Crescendo-decrescendo—peaks in intensity

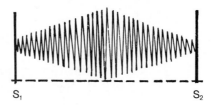

S₁   S₂

    (9) Intensity—based on grade of I to VI
        a) I—barely audible
        b) II—just easily audible
        c) III—hear well; not associated with a thrill
        d) IV—loud and may be associated with a thrill
        e) V—very loud; can be heard with the stethoscope partly off the chest (tilted); associated with a thrill
        f) VI—very loud; can be heard with stethoscope off the chest; associated with a thrill
        g) Recorded with grade over VI to show scale being used (i.e., II/VI)
   (10) Quality
        a) Blowing
        b) Musical
        c) Rough
   (11) Pitch
        a) High-pitched
        b) Low-pitched
 (b) Innocent murmurs (hemodynamically insignificant, physiologic)
    (1) Definition—murmurs that are not associated with cardiovascular disease
    (2) Common in children and pregnant women
    (3) Found in hyperthyroidism
    (4) Found in anemia
    (5) Example—physiologic S_3 ("functional murmur")
 (c) Abnormal murmurs (hemodynamically significant)
    (1) Systolic
        a) Mitral insufficiency (regurgitation)
          ☐ Pansystolic
          ☐ Loudest at apex
          ☐ Radiates to left axilla
          ☐ Intensity will vary, grades I–V
          ☐ May be associated with thrill at apex and axilla
          ☐ Blowing quality, high-pitched
        b) Tricuspid insufficiency (regurgitation)
          ☐ Pansystolic

☐ Loudest at lower left sternal border

☐ Variable in intensity (increases with inspiration)

☐ Blowing quality, high-pitched

☐ Radiates to right sternal border

c) Aortic stenosis (obstruction may be supravalvular or subvalvular or may involve the aortic valve itself)

☐ Valvular stenosis
  - Systolic ejection murmur
  - Crescendo-decrescendo murmur
  - Intensity varies—no relation to severity of murmur
  - Thrill may be found at second intercostal space, right sternal border
  - Radiates to neck and apex
  - Harsh in quality, medium- to high-pitched
  - Maximal intensity at base of heart, usually at second intercostal space, right sternal border

☐ Subvalvular aortic stenosis (idiopathic hypertrophic subaortic stenosis [IHSS])—occurs when septal wall just below aortic valve is hypertrophied
  - Maximal intensity at second through fourth intercostal spaces, right sternal border
  - May radiate to apex
  - Thrill may be found at lower left sternal border
  - Ejection murmur
  - Crescendo-decrescendo
  - Decreases during expiration and squatting; increases with Valsalva maneuver

☐ Supravalvular aortic stenosis
  - Ejection murmur
  - Maximal intensity at second intercostal space, right sternal border or in suprasternal notch
  - Radiates to neck
  - Thrill may be felt in suprasternal notch
  - Harsh
  - Crescendo-decrescendo

d) Pulmonary stenosis

☐ Maximal loudness at second intercostal space, left sternal border

□ Pulmonary systolic ejection sound (click)

□ Radiates to left side of neck

□ Thrill may be felt at second intercostal space, left sternal border

□ Harsh

□ Crescendo-decrescendo

□ Usually louder on inspiration

□ Usually grade III–IV intensity

□ Expiratory split of S_2—the more severe the stenosis, the more pronounced the split

□ Heard louder when patient is supine and during inspiration

   e) Interventricular septal defect

□ Maximal loudness along lower sternal border

□ Radiates widely

□ Thrill usually present at lower left sternal border

□ Pansystolic

(2) Diastolic

   a) Mitral stenosis

□ Mid-diastolic or presystolic rumble

□ Often very faint in intensity

□ May be heard only when patient is lying on left side at PMI

□ Maximal intensity at apex

□ If presystolic, usually crescendo

□ May be associated with an opening snap and accentuated S_1

□ Intensity not affected by inspiration

   b) Tricuspid stenosis

□ Maximal intensity at fourth intercostal space, left sternal border

□ Radiates to xiphoid area

□ Intensity should increase on inspiration

□ Protodiastolic

□ Rumbling decrescendo

□ May increase with hepatic compression

□ May have an opening snap

   c) Aortic insufficiency (regurgitation)

□ Maximal intensity at third to fourth intercostal space, left sternal border, and at second intercostal space, right sternal border

□ Blowing quality, high-pitched

□ Intensity varies with severity

□ Radiates to apex

☐ Thrill uncommon
☐ Pandiastolic
☐ Decrescendo
☐ Heard best when patient is sitting up and leaning forward and during exhalation

d) Pulmonary insufficiency (regurgitation)
☐ Maximal loudness along second intercostal space, left sternal border
☐ Radiates along left sternal border
☐ Decrescendo
☐ High-pitched
☐ Blowing quality
☐ Sometimes increases with inspiration

e) Patent ductus arteriosus
☐ Maximal intensity second intercostal space, left sternal border
☐ Radiates to neck
☐ Thrill at second intercostal space, left sternal border
☐ Usually continuous
☐ Intensity varies
☐ Harsh in quality

Diagnostic Studies

1. Laboratory
a. Serum
   i. Complete blood cell count (CBC), hemoglobin (Hb), hematocrit (HCT)
  ii. Clotting profile
    (a) Prothrombin time (PT)
    (b) Partial thromboplastin time (PTT)
    (c) Thrombin time (TT)
    (d) Bleeding time
    (e) Platelet count
  iii. Enzymes (see p. 224)
    (a) Serum glutamic oxaloacetic transaminase (SGOT)
    (b) Lactate dehydrogenase (LDH)
    (c) Creatinine phosphokinase (CPK)
    (d) Isoenzymes (CPK-MB, LDH-1)
  iv. Serum glucose
   v. Electrolytes
  vi. Lipid profile: type II A (elevated cholesterol levels with normal triglyceride levels) and type II B (elevated cholesterol and

triglyceride levels) hyperlipoproteinemia predisposes to development of coronary artery disease

    b. Urine

        i. Routine urinalysis

        ii. Electrolytes

2. Noninvasive methods of cardiac diagnosis

    a. Routine chest x-ray film to visualize the heart and great vessels

    b. Radiopharmaceuticals: patient is injected in a peripheral vein with the radioactive substance

        i. Blood clot indicators: radioactive tracers injected are used to detect

            (a) Pulmonary emboli

            (b) Venous obstruction, by measuring rates of peripheral venous emptying

            (c) Clot formation in peripheral circulation

        ii. Multiple-gated acquisition (MUGA) scan

            (a) Red blood cells are tagged with technetium

            (b) Sequential pictures of the ventricles (ventriculography) are taken (see pp. 192–193)

            (c) Images of cardiac volumes are collected in both systole and diastole

            (d) Analysis of these data reveals the ejection fraction (EF) and analysis of ventricular wall motion. Patients with coronary artery disease may have decreased wall motion (hypokinesis), systolic bulging (dyskinesis), or no wall motion (akinesis) to those areas supplied by the obstructed artery

               (1) EF is a measurement of the efficacy of ventricular contractility

               (2) The end-systolic volume (ESV) is subtracted from the end-diastolic volume (EDV); the result is divided by the EDV and multiplied by 100

$$EF = \frac{EDV - ESV}{EDV} \times 100$$

               (3) Normal EF is 50% or better

               (4) EF < 50% indicates ventricular dysfunction

        iii. Myocardial infarct indicators

            (a) Technetium-99 pyrophosphate is injected into a peripheral vein

            (b) Infarcted areas of the heart will show increased levels of radioactivity as "hot spots." These appear within 12 to 36 hours of infarct and remain positive for 4 to 7 days

            (c) Useful in those situations in which ECG changes are not

definitive or when enzyme levels may have already returned to normal

    iv. Myocardial perfusion imaging

        (a) Thallium-201 is injected

        (b) Normal myocardium will extract the thallium-201 from the bloodstream

        (c) Areas of decreased myocardial perfusion due to blocked coronary arteries will show decreased uptake; ischemic areas will show normal uptake at rest and decreased uptake ("cold spots") on exercise. Infarcted areas show no uptake in either condition

        (d) Technique may be used simultaneously with treadmill exercises in order to initiate the ischemic process

        (e) Is extremely useful in cases in which ECG changes are not definitive of ischemia and in patients who have false-positive or false-negative results of treadmill stress tests

    v. Positron emission tomography (PET scan)

        (a) New technique that few institutions use (very expensive)

        (b) Allows for the measurement of regional myocardial blood flow, fatty acid metabolism, glucose metabolism, and blood volume

        (c) PET scan provides an objective separation of normal myocardium, ischemic but viable tissue, and dead tissue in patients sustaining an acute myocardial infarction. This information will then objectively substantiate the need (or no need) for further treatment (i.e., thrombolysis, emergent coronary artery bypass grafting)

c. Phonocardiography

    i. The recording of heart sounds by microphone

    ii. Simultaneously recorded along with ECG

    iii. Allows for a more precise analysis of heart sounds in relation to the cardiac cycle

    iv. Less frequently used in recent times

d. Echocardiography: a transducer on the patient's chest emits high-frequency sound waves toward the heart and its structures. The waves are reflected back and converted into electrical signals, which are then recorded for interpretation. It is used to study structural cardiac abnormalities and blood flow dynamics

    i. M-mode echocardiography measures intracardiac structures using a single ultrasound beam. It provides a narrow segmental view of the heart

    ii. Two-dimensional echocardiography provides for real-time imagery of cardiac structures using a planar ultrasound beam. This method gives a wider view of the heart and its structures

    iii. Both methods are used to assess the heart and are complementary of each other. Echocardiography is used to evaluate/diagnose the following

  (a) Size of chambers

  (b) Valvular heart disease—provides information regarding the site, cause, and severity of the defect

  (c) LV wall motion (shows areas of hypokinesis, akinesis, dyskinesis), wall thickness, cavity size

  (d) Cardiomyopathy

  (e) Pericardial effusion, cardiac tamponade

  (f) Atrial size

  (g) Function of prosthetic ball valves

  (h) Papillary muscle function

  (i) Intracardiac masses to include tumors, thrombi, and valvular vegetations

  (j) Congenital defects

  iv. Doppler echocardiography: a combination of Doppler and echocardiographic techniques used to demonstrate the flow of blood through the heart. It complements findings from traditional echocardiographic methods. Information is provided on intracardiac pressures, valvular stenosis and incompetence, blood flow velocity (which provides cardiac output measurements), and intracardiac shunts, all of which help evaluate valvular function, congenital heart defects, pericardial disease, and cardiomyopathies

e. Magnetic resonance imaging (MRI): very safe diagnostic technique that does not use any ionizing radiation or contrast agents

  i. Provides a three-dimensional view

  ii. Detects changes in the chemistry of tissues before they become structural changes

  iii. Valuable in determining the anatomy of the heart

  iv. Is safe for children and pregnant women

  v. Since it is a magnetic device, it interferes with pacemaker function

f. Electrocardiography

  i. General information

    (a) Measures electrical activity of heart by measuring difference in electrical potential between two points on the body

    (b) Demonstrates or detects the following

      (1) Disturbance of rhythm and conduction

      (2) Ischemia or infarct

      (3) Electrolyte abnormalities

      (4) Drug toxicity

      (5) Hypertrophy of atria and ventricles

    (c) ECG paper

      (1) Vertical lines measure time

      a) Each small (1 mm) box = 0.04 second
      b) Each large (5 mm) box = 0.20 second
      c) Allows for measurement of the P wave, QRS complex, and T wave (in time), as well as PR and QT intervals

    (2) Horizontal lines measure voltage
      a) Each small box (1 mm) = 0.1 mV
      b) Each large box (5 mm) = 0.5 mV
      c) Allows for measurement of amplitude of P wave, QRS complex, and T wave and therefore determines voltage
      d) Useful in detection of atrial and ventricular hypertrophy

(d) Deflections—the waves (constituting an ECG tracing) are either above or below isoelectric line
    (1) Isoelectric line is a straight line on ECG indicating either no electrical forces or equivalent amounts of movement away from recording electrode during depolarization

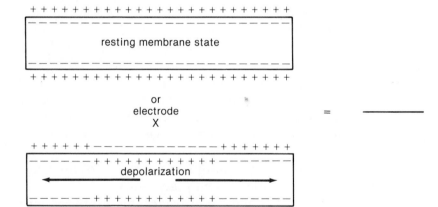

    (2) Positive deflections are produced when electrical forces of a depolarizing cell move toward the recording electrode

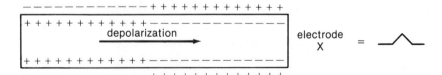

    (3) Negative deflections are produced when electrical forces of a depolarizing cell move away from the recording electrode

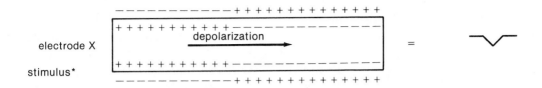

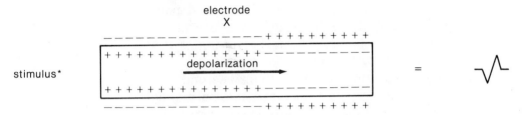

(4) Biphasic deflections are produced when electrical forces of a depolarizing cell move both toward and away from the recording electrode

ii. Cardiac conduction cycle (Fig. 2–11)
   (a) P wave represents atrial depolarization
       (1) First portion represents right atrial depolarization
       (2) Second portion represents left atrial depolarization
       (3) Normal amplitude of P wave < 3 mm. Abnormal if P wave > 3 mm in amplitude in any lead

Figure 2–11. Normal electrocardiogram (ECG) complex. The various waveforms and normal time intervals are indicated. The complex is superimposed on the standard electrocardiographic paper at customary amplitude (1 mm = 0.1 mV) and paper speed (25 mm/second). (From Sanderson, R. G., and Kurth, C. L.: The Cardiac Patient: A Comprehensive Approach, 2nd ed. W. B. Saunders Co., Philadelphia, 1983, p. 129.)

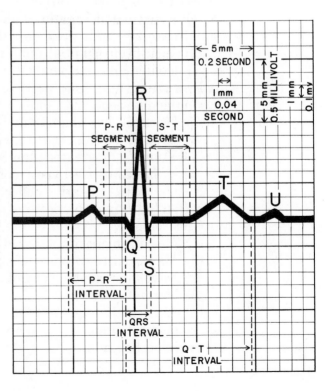

(4) Abnormalities
  a) Increased amplitude or width associated with atrial hypertrophy
  b) Tall, peaked P waves in leads II, III, and aVF and tall or diphasic P waves in V_1 are associated with RA hypertrophy
  c) Wide, notched P waves (P mitrale) in limb leads and V_{4-6} and biphasic P waves with a broad negative deflection in lead V_1 are associated with LA hypertrophy

(b) PR interval represents atrial depolarization and conduction through AV node—measures AV conduction time
  (1) Measured from beginning of P wave to beginning of QRS complex
  (2) Normal—0.12 to 0.20 second
  (3) PR segment represents normal delay of impulse in AV node—normally isoelectric
    a) With abnormalities this delay is prolonged, increasing the PR interval >0.20 second
      ☐ Indication of diseased AV node, ischemia, drug effects, or increased vagal tone
      ☐ Called first-degree AV block

(c) Q wave is the first negative deflection resulting from ventricular depolarization
  (1) Abnormal if greater than 0.04 second wide or more than 25% of R wave amplitude
  (2) Seen in myocardial infarction, left ventricular hypertrophy, and left bundle branch block

(d) R wave is the first positive deflection resulting from ventricular depolarization
  (1) Normal—less than 13 mm amplitude
  (2) Greater than 11 mm in aVL, greater than 27 mm in V_5 or V_6, or greater than 35 mm in V_5 plus S wave in V_1 indicates LV hypertrophy

(e) S wave is first negative deflection of ventricular depolarization following first positive deflection (R wave)

(f) QRS complex
  (1) Measurement of total ventricular depolarization
  (2) Measured from onset of Q wave (or R wave if no Q wave is present) to end of S wave
  (3) Normal—0.06 to 0.10 second
  (4) Abnormal if greater than 0.11 second; indicative of delayed impulse; seen in bundle branch blocks and hyperkalemia

(g) ST segment represents beginning ventricular repolarization
  (1) Measured immediately after QRS complex to beginning of T wave and is normally isoelectric
  (2) Prolonged ST segment indicative of hypocalcemia
  (3) Elevated ST segment may indicate pericarditis, infarcts, aneurysms (for exact leads refer to each particular entity in this chapter)
  (4) Depressed ST segment may indicate ischemia or digitalis toxicity or may be nonspecific
(h) T wave represents ventricular repolarization
  (1) Inverted T waves may indicate infarcts or ischemia
  (2) Tall, peaked T waves may indicate hyperkalemia, acute injury, or normal variant
(i) QT interval—summation of depolarization and repolarization representing electrical systole and diastole; varies with heart rate
  (1) The interval in seconds from the beginning of the Q wave to the end of the T wave
  (2) QT interval is affected by heart rate, gender, and age. The corrected QT interval (QTc) takes heart rate into account and provides various normal values based on the rates. In general, a QTc of 0.44 second or more is abnormal
  (3) Certain pathologic conditions such as ischemia, electrolyte imbalances, hypertrophy, and antidysrhythmic drugs (quinidine, amiodarone) prolong the QTc
  (4) Acute ischemia, hypercalcemia, and drugs such as digitalis shorten the QTc
  (5) Prolonged QTc interval is associated with a higher incidence of ventricular tachycardia and sudden death
iii. 12-lead ECG
  (a) Bipolar leads—standard limb leads (I, II, III)
    (1) Record electrical potential in frontal plane
    (2) Record difference in potential between two limb leads
      a) Lead I—R arm negative, L arm positive
      b) Lead II—R arm negative, L leg positive
      c) Lead III—L arm negative, L leg positive
    (3) Normally, all major waveforms are positive deflections in standard limb leads
  (b) Unipolar leads—augmented
    (1) aVR—R arm positive electrode; normally a negative deflection
    (2) aVL—L arm positive electrode; usually a positive deflection

(3) aVF—L leg positive electrode; usually a positive deflection

(c) Unipolar precordial (chest) leads

    (1) V_1—fourth intercostal space, right sternal border

    (2) V_2—fourth intercostal space, left sternal border

    (3) V_3—halfway between V_2 and V_4

    (4) V_4—fifth intercostal space, left midclavicular line

    (5) V_5—fifth intercostal space, left anterior axillary line

    (6) V_6—fifth intercostal space, left midaxillary line

    NOTE: Normally, in moving from V_1 toward V_6, R waves get progressively larger and S waves get progressively smaller (normal R wave progression)

(d) Miscellaneous leads

    (1) Lewis lead—used to amplify waves of atrial activity (P waves)

      a) A bipolar chest lead

      b) Negative electrode (RA) placed on second intercostal space, right of sternum

      c) Positive electrode (LA) placed on fourth intercostal space, right of sternum

      d) Ground electrode placed on fourth intercostal space, left of sternum

      e) Record tracing on lead I

    (2) Modified chest left arm 1 (MCL_1)

      a) Enables one to differentiate between right bundle branch block with aberrancy and LV ectopy

        ☐ If the first beat of a run of ectopics has a rSR′ pattern in this lead, then it favors a right bundle branch block with aberration

        ☐ LV ectopy—the "rabbit ears" configuration has a taller left peak than the right peak (Rsr′ pattern). Other configurations indicative of LV ectopy are R, QR, or qR in this lead

      b) The difference between RV and LV ectopy is apparent

        ☐ LV ectopy—the QRS deflection is above the isoelectric line and may have a monophasic or biphasic pattern (QR, qR, or R)

        ☐ RV ectopy—the QRS complex is below the isoelectric line, usually with an RS configuration

      c) Allows for the differentiation between right and left bundle branch blocks

        ☐ RBBB—classic rSR′ pattern

        ☐ LBBB—a mostly negative QS or rS pattern

      d) Lead placement (similar to lead V_1)

☐ Ground electrode—just below the right clavicle, midclavicular line

☐ Positive electrode—fourth intercostal space, right sternal border

☐ Negative electrode—just below left clavicle, midclavicular line

    e) Typical pattern of PQRST is negative

(3) Modified chest left arm 3 (MCL$_3$)

    a) P waves show up very well in this lead

    b) QRS complexes are positive

    c) Lead placement (similar to lead V$_3$)

☐ Ground electrode—just below right clavicle, midclavicular line

☐ Positive electrode—between fourth and fifth intercostal space, halfway between left sternal border and midclavicular line

☐ Negative electrode—just below left clavicle, midclavicular line

iv. Electrical axis: cardiac vectors*

v. ECG interpretation (*NOTE:* the following section on electrocardiography is not meant to be an all-encompassing discussion of dysrhythmias. Only the general characteristics of the dysrhythmias will be covered. There are many excellent books on the topic that discuss all aspects of the dysrhythmias to include treatment modalities and nursing interventions.)

(a) Analysis—each dysrhythmia should be analyzed in a systematic manner with particular attention to

(1) Rate—both atrial and ventricular

(2) Rhythm—regular, irregular

(3) Identification of P waves

    a) Relationship to QRS

    b) Consistency/normalcy of configuration/morphology

(4) Determine PR interval

(5) Determine QRS interval

(6) Identify origin of dysrhythmia if possible

(7) Identify possible implications for patient

(b) Categories of dysrhythmias

(1) Sinus origin

    a) Sinus arrhythmia

☐ Seen normally during sinus rhythm

☐ Varying PP intervals (or RR); all other aspects normal

---

*This aspect of electrocardiography will not be dealt with here. It is used to determine right and left axis deviations that result from abnormalities such as ventricular hypertrophies or hemiblocks. For more information, refer to any dysrhythmia/ECG textbook.

□ Usually related to respiration; PP interval shortens during inspiration (see respiratory reflex, p. 144)

b) Sinus bradycardia
  □ Normal PQRST complexes and intervals
  □ Essentially a regular rhythm
  □ Heart rate less than 60 beats/min

c) Sinus tachycardia
  □ Normal PQRST complex and intervals
  □ Regular rhythm
  □ Heart rate between 100 and 180 beats/min

d) Sinus block (sinus exit block)
  □ SA node initiates an impulse, but it is blocked within the SA node and does not activate the atrial tissue
  □ No PQRST complex is seen on the ECG rhythm strip
  □ Distinguishing characteristic of sinus block is that the rhythm remains regular. The interval before and after the pause is twice the normal interval

e) Sinus arrest
  □ SA node fails to initiate an impulse at the proper time; therefore, the atria are not stimulated to contract
  □ No PQRST complex is seen on the ECG
  □ There is a long pause after the preceding conducted beat
  □ RR intervals vary; hence the rhythm is not maintained (because the pause is not equal to two normal cycles)

f) Sick sinus syndrome: There may be various combinations of sinus block, sinus arrest, sinus bradycardia, and sinus tachycardia (bradytachy syndrome) that interfere with cerebral perfusion causing syncope or other cerebral dysfunction. There is also a failure of other escape pacemakers of the heart to initiate impulses when the SA node fails

(2) Atrial origin
  a) Premature atrial contractions (PAC)
    □ An ectopic focus in the atria outside the SA node initiates an early impulse, interrupting the inherent regular rhythm
    □ The P wave of the ectopic beat is morphologi-

cally different compared with the P wave of the normal sinus beat

☐ Conduction of the ectopic atrial beat through the AV junctional tissue may occur if the AV junction has repolarized enough; otherwise the beat may be blocked or delayed (prolonged PR interval)

☐ Conduction through the ventricles also depends on what stage of repolarization they are in. Because of this, you may see a normal QRS complex if repolarization was complete, an abnormal QRS complex if the beat is conducted aberrantly because the ventricle is partially repolarized, or no QRS complex if the beat arrived too early during the ventricle's absolute refractory period

b) Atrial tachycardia

☐ The atria discharge at a rate of 150 to 250 beats/min owing to the rapid firing of an ectopic area or to some intra-atrial reentry mechanism

☐ The reentrant type of atrial tachycardia is more common and classically occurs as a paroxysmal phenomenon (starts and stops abruptly), usually following a PAC. The mechanism for this dysrhythmia is a reentry phenomenon occurring in the AV node itself. Characteristically, the PP or RR interval is absolutely regular. If the rate is fast enough, the P waves may be buried in the preceding T waves

☐ Atrial tachycardia due to an ectopic focus in the atria is less common. RR interval may vary when the rhythm is associated with a block at the AV junction, which is often the case. (The junction protects the ventricles from the rapid impulses.)

c) Multifocal atrial tachycardia (chaotic atrial tachycardia)

☐ Several ectopic foci in the atria discharge impulses

☐ Rates vary from 100 to 150 beats/min

☐ Because of the different foci, PP and RR intervals vary widely, as will the P wave morphology

☐ Often associated with chronic pulmonary disease

d) Wandering atrial pacemaker

☐ The dominant pacemaker changes from SA node to atria to junction, producing P waves of varying shape

☐ Irregular PR interval that gradually shortens and RR intervals that lengthen causing an irregular rhythm

☐ Rates less than 100 beats/min

  e) Atrial flutter

☐ The impulse originates in the atria

☐ Characteristically, there are wide sawtooth waves called flutter waves (F waves)

☐ The F waves are used to count the atrial rates— from 250 to 350 beats/min

☐ Ventricular rates may be constant or more often vary, depending on the degree of block in the AV junction. Therefore, one may see 1, 2, 3, 4, or more F waves for each QRS complex (i.e., 2:1, 3:1 block, etc.)

☐ The flutter waves continue through the QRS complex and must be counted when determining flutter/atrial rate

☐ Ventricular rhythm will vary from regular to irregular depending on the conduction ratio

  f) Atrial fibrillation

☐ The impulse originates in the atria at extremely rapid rates, and conduction through the atria is very chaotic. There is no organized atrial activity

☐ Impulse is characterized by rapid, irregular atrial "f" waves instead of P waves on the ECG

☐ Impulses are randomly conducted through the AV junction, and hence the ventricular response varies and is usually grossly irregular. Rates vary between 100 and 160 beats/min

(3) AV junction origin

  a) Premature junctional beats/contractions (PJB or PJC)

☐ The impulse originates in the junctional tissue, spreading either antegrade or retrograde

☐ If the impulse spreads retrograde, the atria depolarize first (producing a P wave) and then the ventricles depolarize. The P wave will precede the QRS complex and usually be inverted (because of the retrograde conduction); the PR interval will be shortened (< 0.12 second)

      ☐ If the impulse travels antegrade and then retrograde, the ventricles depolarize first, producing a QRS complex, which is followed by a P wave—a "retrograde P wave." The P wave will be inverted in leads where it is normally positive (I, II, III)

      ☐ If antegrade conduction to the ventricles occurs simultaneously as retrograde conduction to the atria, the P wave will be buried in the QRS complex and the ECG complex will appear with no P wave

      ☐ QRS complex is usually normal

      ☐ Basic underlying rhythm is disrupted because of the ectopic beat

   b) Junctional escape rhythm

      ☐ If the SA node fails to initiate the impulses as normal, then the junctional tissue will take over this function. This tissue's inherent rate is 40 to 60 beats/min

      ☐ RR interval is regular

      ☐ P wave morphology as stated in section on premature junctional beats

      ☐ QRS complex is normal

   c) Accelerated junctional rhythm

      ☐ Enhanced automaticity within the AV junctional tissue discharges impulses at rates of 60 to 100 beats/min usually as a result of digitalis excess

      ☐ RR interval is regular

      ☐ P wave morphology as stated in section on premature junctional beats

      ☐ QRS usually normal

   d) Junctional tachycardia

      ☐ All salient features are the same as discussed for other junctional dysrhythmias except the ventricular rate is now 100 to 160 beats/min

   e) Accelerated junctional tachycardia

      ☐ All salient features are the same as discussed for other junctional dysrhythmias except the ventricular rate is now 160 to 220 beats/min

(4) Supraventricular tachycardia (SVT)

   a) A catch-all term used to describe any tachycardia originating above the bifurcation of the bundle of His for which P waves are not discernible

   b) Atrial tachycardia, atrial fibrillation, atrial flutter, and junctional tachycardia are examples of dysrhythmias that can be classified as SVTs

  c) The hemodynamic consequences of SVT can be significant because of the following

□ Ineffective atrial contraction/loss of atrial kick; this decreases about 15% of ventricular filling causing cardiac output decrease

□ Rapid rates decrease diastolic ventricular filling time; this decreases the stroke volume and cardiac output

□ Since the coronary arteries fill during diastole and diastole is shortened, the coronary circulation may be diminished—may induce angina

□ Rapid rates increase myocardial oxygen consumption, which may induce angina

(5) Paroxysmal supraventricular tachycardia (PSVT)—characteristically starts and ends abruptly. Due to a reentry mechanism an impulse activates some tissue once. Due to a return pathway and slow conduction properties, the same impulse is able to reactivate the tissue when the tissue is not refractory. This sets up a circuit mechanism. In order for this mechanism to exist, the pathway must also have two segments that depolarize and repolarize at different rates, otherwise the impulse would depolarize the tissue synchronously. Types include

  a) SA node reentry mechanism

□ Initiated by a sinus beat or a premature atrial complex

□ Perinodal fibers are believed to exist that act as the conduction barrier while they are refractory

□ This prepares the pathway for a return impulse from the atria

□ Once the perinodal fibers repolarize, they conduct the impulse back to the SA node

□ There now exists a reentry pathway between the SA node and atria

□ ECG features—one often notes a sinus rhythm with sudden onset and cessation of sinus tachycardia. P waves may be similar to the sinus P waves. The overall rhythm is irregular due to the paroxysms. Rates vary from 100 to 150 beats/min. Conduction through to the ventricles is normal

  b) AV node reentry mechanism

□ Confined to the AV junction itself. There are two separate pathways in the node (slow and fast pathways)

□ The slow pathway has the shortest refractory period. Thus, when an ectopic atrial beat arrives, it can only be conducted down the slow pathway (antegrade) toward the ventricles

□ Before the impulse leaves the AV junctional tissue totally, the fast channel fully repolarizes. This allows some of the impulse to travel retrograde to the atria. It then is conducted to the slow pathway again and the circus-type movement continues around and around

□ ECG features—impulse often begins abruptly with a PAC. Atrial and ventricular rates are 170 to 250 beats/min with regular rhythm. Inverted P waves are seen due to retrograde activation of the atria from the junction (seen in leads II, III, and aVF)

(6) Ventricular origin

   a) Premature ventricular contractions (PVC)

      □ Originate from various foci in the ventricles, outside the normal conduction system. Ventricular conduction is abnormal and delayed, producing wide (>0.12 second), bizarre QRS complexes with ST segment oriented opposite to T wave direction

      □ The sinus node continues to discharge impulses, depolarizing the atria and producing P waves as normal. The PVC occurs anywhere within the normal cycle. The next sinus beat is not conducted to the ventricles because the ventricles are still in the refractory period. This produces a pause following the PVC. The SA node rate is not altered so that the next sinus beat occurs at its normal time. The pause is considered a "full compensatory" pause because the RR interval surrounding the PVC is precisely equal to two sinus-cycle intervals. To measure for a full compensatory pause

        • On a piece of paper or using the calipers, mark off three normal cycles using their QRS complexes

        • Place the first mark on the QRS complex immediately preceding the PVC complex; if there is a true full compensatory pause, the third mark should fall on the QRS complex of the normal beat immediately following the PVC

☐ A PVC may be interpolated between two normal beats and not disrupt the rhythm nor be associated with a full compensatory pause

☐ More than six PVCs per minute, of different morphology (suggesting multiple irritable foci) occurring as consecutive PVCs or occurring in a pattern of bigeminy or trigeminy or PVCs that occur on the T wave of the preceding beat (which is the supernormal period of the action potential curve); in a diseased heart may lead to ventricular fibrillation and warrant closer monitoring

☐ In the MCL$_1$ lead, the QRS complex of a PVC originating in the LV will be mostly positive; a PVC from the RV will be mostly negative (see pp. 174–175)

b) Ventricular escape beats
☐ If impulses from higher centers (SA or AV junction) are not generated or do not reach the ventricles, the ventricles will initiate their own "escape" beat

☐ Three or more ventricular escape beats occurring in a row are termed *idioventricular rhythm*—the rate is usually 20 to 60 beats/min

☐ Ventricular rates of 60 to 100 beats/min are termed *accelerated idioventricular rhythm*

☐ QRS complex of these types of rhythms are wide and bizarre; their morphology may vary depending on the site of the focus

c) Ventricular tachycardia
☐ Three or more consecutive PVCs
☐ May occur or cease suddenly or may be sustained
☐ The RR interval is mostly regular; QRS complexes are usually wide and bizarre
☐ Ventricular rates may be 100 to 250 beats/min
☐ The SA node may continue to activate the atria in the normal fashion while the ventricular ectopic focus stimulates the ventricles. Therefore, P waves will be visible within the QRS complex but have no association to them. Occasionally they will capture part of the ventri-

cle, resulting in fusion beats, which is diagnostic
of ventricular tachycardia

☐ Supraventricular tachycardia (SVT) with aberration can easily simulate ventricular tachycardia, making the differential diagnosis very difficult

● Check the first beat of the tachycardia; if
there is a premature P wave present indicating a probable PAC, then the dysrhythmia
favors SVT with aberration. If the episode
starts with a PVC, then ventricular tachycardia is the diagnosis. If the first beat is not
observable, the differentiation between ventricular ectopy and SVT with aberration is
most difficult

● Any of the following three characteristics
favor ventricular tachycardia over SVT with
aberration

— Marked left-axis deviation ($> -30°$)
— Left peak of QRS complex is taller than
the right in lead V_1
— An rS configuration in lead V_6

d) Torsades de pointes (twist of points)

☐ A form of ventricular tachycardia

☐ Irregular and wide QRS complexes that undu-
late and seem to twist about an isoelectric axis

☐ Usually associated with a prolonged QT interval
(> 0.50 second) and prominent U waves

☐ Heart rates from 150 to 250 beats/min

☐ Can be seen in the setting of electrolyte imbalance especially with a decrease in potassium,
magnesium, or calcium) or in association with
drug therapy especially quinidine, procainamide, amiodarone, disopyramide, lidocaine, and
tricyclic antidepressants

☐ *Do not* treat this dysrhythmia with the usual
class 1 antidysrhythmics. Correct the causative
factor and defibrillate as needed. Often, temporary overdrive pacing may be needed until the
causative factor is removed

e) Ventricular fibrillation

☐ Uncoordinated, chaotic depolarization of the
ventricles produces erratic waveforms with no
discernible PQRST complexes

   ☐ The ECG shows an undulating irregular base-line (coarse or fine)

  f) Ventricular standstill (asystole)

   ☐ Complete cessation of ventricular activity

   ☐ P wave present if the underlying sinus rhythm is maintained

 (7) AV conduction defects

  a) First-degree AV block

   ☐ The impulse initiated at the SA node is delayed at the AV junction, producing a PR interval greater than 0.20 second

   ☐ Every sinus beat is conducted to the ventricles, producing a normal QRS complex; there is a P wave for every QRS complex

  b) Second-degree AV block—some of the sinus impulses are not conducted through the AV junctional tissue and bundle branches. Because of this, some P waves may not be followed by a QRS complex. There are two basic types

   ☐ Type I (also called Mobitz I or Wenckebach)—pathologic process located in the AV junction

    ● The delay of conduction through the AV junction progressively increases (gradually increasing the PR interval) until a sinus impulse fails to conduct through the AV junctional tissue; produces a dropped QRS at varying or constant intervals

    ● RR interval shortens as the PR interval increases

    ● PP interval remains constant

    ● P waves and QRS complex are normal

    ● Atrial impulses and associated ventricular response varies and often occurs in groups (e.g., 5:4, 4:3, 3:2 ratios), termed *grouped beating*

   ☐ Type II (also called Mobitz II)—less common than type I, involves the bundle branches, and carries a worse prognosis because it often leads to third-degree heart block

    ● SA node discharges regularly, producing a constant PP interval

    ● At times, one or more P waves do not conduct through to the ventricles, producing a 2:1, 3:1 type of conduction

- The pause due to the nonconducted P wave usually equals twice the normal RR interval
- PR intervals are constant in all conducted beats in contrast to type I
- RR interval will vary depending on the degree of block
- PP interval remains constant

c) Third-degree (complete) AV block (pathology can occur anywhere in the AV junctional area but usually involves the bundle of His or both the right and left bundle branches)

☐ There is no conduction of sinus impulses through the AV junctional tissue

☐ Two pacemakers become apparent; the SA node fires in its normal fashion, and since there is a complete block, the junctional or ventricular tissue will respond as an escape pacemaker producing two completely independent rhythms

☐ The P waves and QRS complexes are not associated with each other

☐ PP intervals are regular, and the rate is typical of sinus rhythm (60 to 100 beats/min)

☐ RR interval is also regular but the rate will depend on the inherent rate of the escape pacemaker; junctional (40 to 60 beats/min) or ventricular (< 40 beats/min)

(8) Intraventricular conduction defects

a) Left bundle branch block (LBBB)

☐ Due to a block in the left bundle branch, the right bundle branch is activated first. The impulse spreads to the right ventricle and then back to the septum and over to the left bundle distal to the blockage to then activate the left ventricle

☐ Prolonged activation time of the septum and the left ventricle produces a wide (> 0.12 second) QRS complex

☐ Best leads for diagnosis are V_1 and V_6

- V_1—a predominately negative complex of QS or rS pattern
- V_6—always positive with a broad, notched R wave
- Absence of the normal small q wave and S wave in leads I, aVL, V_5, and V_6

b) Right bundle branch block (RBBB)

☐ The left ventricle and septum are activated normally. The impulse then spreads to the RV from the LV with resultant activation
☐ The QRS complex is prolonged (> 0.12 second)
☐ There is a broad S wave in leads I, aVL, and V_6
☐ In lead V_1, the QRS complex is triphasic with an rSR′ configuration
☐ In lead V_6, the QRS complex is also triphasic with a qRS configuration

   c) Left anterior hemiblock
☐ Owing to a lesion in the anterior fascicle of the left bundle, the impulse travels through the posterior fascicle first, then through the anterior fascicle
☐ Produces left axis deviation of −45° or greater
☐ Small R and large S waves found in leads II, III, and aVF
☐ Small Q and large R waves in leads I and aVL
☐ QRS is at upper limits of normal duration

   d) Left posterior hemiblock
☐ Owing to a lesion in the posterior fascicle of the left bundle, the impulse travels through the anterior fascicle first and then to the posterior fascicle
☐ Produces right axis deviation of +120° or more
☐ Small Q and tall R waves in leads II, III, and aVF
☐ Small R waves and large S waves in leads I and aVR
☐ RV hypertrophy must be excluded clinically before diagnosis of left posterior hemiblock can be made

(9) Miscellaneous
   a) Wolff-Parkinson-White (W-P-W) syndrome
☐ An abnormal accessory pathway (bundle of Kent) exists between the atria and ventricles. The impulse conducts rapidly down this anomalous pathway to directly stimulate the ventricles bypassing the AV node (preexcitation)
☐ The impulse from the SA node also travels normally through the AV node to stimulate the ventricles. Hence, the ventricles are stimulated from two directions
☐ The QRS complex produced represents the de-

polarization of the ventricles as a fusion of two stimuli

☐ Since the initial impulse bypasses the AV node, there is no delay. This causes a shortened PR interval (less than 0.12 second) and a slurred upstroke to the R wave, known as a delta wave

☐ As the ventricles depolarize from the impulse coming through the AV node, the QRS complex produced is normal. The delta wave fuses with the RS part of the QRS complex. The total fused complex is usually greater than 0.12 second but may also be normal

☐ W-P-W syndrome is further divided into two types: type A has upright QRS deflections with inverted T waves and depressed ST segments in leads V_1–V_3; type B has negative QRS deflections and upright T waves and elevated ST segments in leads V_1–V_3

☐ W-P-W syndrome occurs most often in young adults; it may be constant or intermittent and is often associated with PSVT due to a circus movement or atrial fibrillation. W-P-W syndrome by itself is not significant, but the tachydysrhythmias associated with the syndrome may be severe enough that surgical ablation is required

(c) ECG interpretation of ischemia, injury, infarction (see pp. 225–226)

(d) ECG changes of pericarditis (see p. 248)

(e) ECG changes of myocardial trauma
  (1) Dysrhythmias
  (2) Pattern of pericarditis
  (3) Nonspecific ST and T wave changes
  (4) Infarction pattern
  (5) AV conduction defects

(f) ECG changes with potassium imbalances
  (1) Hypokalemia
    a) Prominent U wave
    b) T wave amplitude decreased
    c) ST segment depressed
    d) PR interval may be prolonged
    e) Prolonged QTc interval
  (2) Hyperkalemia
    a) The action potential curve decreases in height,

which has the effect of slowing conduction; may even lead to heart blocks

  b) The action potential duration is shortened, which causes a T wave symmetrically peaked, narrowed, and elevated at serum levels >5.5 mEq/L

  c) At higher levels (6.5 mEq/L and above) the PR interval increases, the P wave amplitude diminishes or may disappear, and the QRS complex widens

(g) ECG changes with calcium imbalances

  (1) Calcium imbalances affect phase 2 of the action potential curve by either shortening or lengthening this phase. The results with hypocalcemia are a prolonged QTc interval and a prolonged isoelectric ST segment. The results with hypercalcemia are a shortened QTc interval and a shortened or absent ST segment

g. Stress electrocardiography (exercise stress tests)

  i. Definition: an electrocardiogram performed during exercise

  ii. Indications for stress tests

  (a) Detects unknown and suspected coronary artery disease

  (b) In patients who have known coronary artery disease (such as post myocardial infarction, post angioplasty, or coronary artery bypass surgery), it is used to evaluate their response to exercise and is a functional assessment to stratify patients by risk

  (c) To evaluate the postsurgical or medical treatment for coronary artery disease

  (d) To monitor patient's progress while enrolled in a cardiac rehabilitation program

  (e) To evaluate dysrhythmias, especially exercise-induced ventricular tachycardia

  (f) To screen persons entering physical fitness programs and to screen high-risk professionals (e.g., airline pilots)

  iii. Contraindications to exercise stress tests may be

  (a) Impending, acute, or healing myocardial infarction

  (b) Unstable (preinfarction) angina

  (c) Uncompensated congestive heart failure

  (d) Severe aortic stenosis

  (e) Severe illnesses such as infections, asthma, and renal failure

  (f) Severe left main coronary artery disease

  (g) Uncontrolled, severe hypertension

  (h) Uncontrolled dysrhythmias; conduction defects greater than first-degree AV block

  (i) Acute pericarditis or myocarditis

iv. Types of stress protocols
  (a) Bruce protocol—intense exercise using a motor-driven treadmill over a short period of time with increasing increments in treadmill elevation and speed
  (b) Naughton protocol—uses gentle work loads but for longer durations in time; best suited for high-risk patients
v. Findings suggestive of ischemia and coronary artery disease
  (a) 1 mm or greater transient ST segment depression 80 msec after the J point (the point where the ST segment "takes off" from the QRS complex—the QRS complex–ST segment junction)
vi. Findings suggestive of severe coronary artery disease (disease of three or more vessels or the left main coronary artery)
  (a) Protracted ST segment depression, greater than 2 mm at 80 msec after the J point
  (b) Recovery time of ST segment changes or symptoms back to normal takes > 8 minutes
  (c) Exercise-induced hypotension
  (d) Exercise-induced ventricular tachycardia
h. Holter monitoring
  i. An ECG recorded over a 24-hour period
  ii. Used to document
    (a) Suspected dysrhythmias that a resting or stress ECG does not demonstrate because of their short time in use
    (b) Effects of surgical and medical treatment regimens for known dysrhythmias, heart blocks, preexcitation syndromes
    (c) Pacemaker function
    (d) Silent ischemia
  iii. Records on leads II and V_5
  iv. Patient keeps a diary in order to monitor periods of symptoms (chest pain, palpitations, syncope) and activities
  v. Tape is analyzed and compared with patient's diary to determine whether symptoms and ECG changes correlate so that therapy can be instituted

3. **Invasive methods of cardiac diagnosis**
  a. Cardiac catheterization
    i. Purpose—general
      (a) To define clinically suspected lesions (i.e., of arteries, valves, muscle tissue, anatomy)
      (b) To evaluate severity of lesions
      (c) To assess pathophysiology of cardiac disorders
      (d) To provide information on LV function
      (e) To allow for measurement of pressures in the heart
      (f) To measure cardiac output

(g) To measure blood gas content

ii. Technique

    (a) Catheterization of right side of heart performed via the right femoral or brachial vein and advanced into the RA

    (b) Catheter can be advanced through the tricuspid valve into the RV to the pulmonary artery to collect the necessary data

    (c) Catheterization of left side of heart performed retrogradely via the femoral or brachial artery or through a transseptal approach through the RA via the foramen ovale into the LA

    (d) Catheter is advanced into LA, LV, and aorta, measuring pressures in the chambers and vessels. The injection of contrast medium allows for evaluation of LV wall motion and integrity of the myocardium

    (e) Pressures are measured and blood samples from various parts of the heart are analyzed to determine oxygen saturations; to identify and assess the severity of shunts due to ventricular and atrial septal defects and patent ductus arteriosus; and to assess for valvular disease (Fig. 2–12)

iii. Cardiac output (CO)—determined during cardiac catheterization

    (a) Definition—the amount of blood ejected by the LV in 1 minute

    (b) Cardiac output is a product of stroke volume (SV) and heart rate (HR)

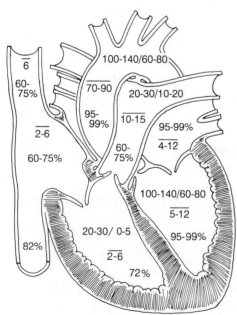

Figure 2–12. Normal oxygen saturations and normal systolic, diastolic (00/00), and mean pressure (0) ranges of the chambers and vessels of the heart.

$$CO = SV \times HR$$

(1) SV is the amount of blood ejected by the LV with each contraction. It is the difference between LV end-diastolic volume and LV end-systolic volume (SV = EDV − ESV; 60 to 130 ml)

(c) Normal CO = 4 to 8 L/min

(d) Most common methods to determine CO are Fick method, indicator-dilution technique, and the thermodilution technique

(e) Factors affecting CO

    (1) Changes in heart rate—excessively high heart rates decrease diastolic filling time, ultimately decreasing CO

    (2) Changes in contractility affecting stroke volume

        a) Increased sympathetic activity causes increased myocardial contractility (positive inotropy) and thus more blood is ejected (increased SV); this increases cardiac output

        b) Preload—when muscle fibers are stretched owing to increased preload, force of contraction increases; thus SV and CO increase

        c) Changes in resistance such as increased or decreased afterload will affect SV and CO (i.e., high afterloads decrease SV and CO)

    (3) Changes in venous return to heart affecting preload

        a) Reduction in total blood volume decreases venous return and preload. This causes a fall in cardiac filling, SV, and CO

        b) Venous constriction decreases venous pooling and increases venous return to the heart. This process increases preload, cardiac filling, SV, and CO

(f) CO decreased due to

    (1) Dysrhythmias

    (2) Hypovolemia

    (3) Mitral stenosis/mitral insufficiency

    (4) Cardiac tamponade

    (5) Constrictive pericarditis

    (6) Restrictive cardiomyopathies

    (7) Myocardial infarction with LV failure

    (8) Increased afterload (secondary to aortic stenosis, increased systemic vascular resistance)

    (9) Drugs with negative inotropic effects

    (10) Metabolic disorders

    (11) Hypothermia

        (g) CO increased due to

           (1) Sepsis

           (2) Hyperthyroid states

           (3) Hyperflow states with hepatic or mesenteric shunting

    iv. Complications of cardiac catheterization

        (a) Cardiac dysrhythmias

        (b) Conduction disturbances

        (c) Arterial thrombosis or embolus and dissection in limb (due to arterial injury, a clot forms and may dislodge, or a plaque may be dislodged)

        (d) Perforation of atria, arteries, or ventricle can lead to cardiac tamponade

        (e) Systemic emboli (may cause cerebrovascular accident, pulmonary embolism, myocardial infarction)

        (f) Renal shutdown or oliguria due to contrast media

        (g) Allergic reactions to contrast media

        (h) Sepsis

        (i) Hypovolemia (due to diuresis from contrast medium)

        (j) Hemorrhage or hematoma at insertion site

        (k) Death

    v. Cardiac index (CI)

        (a) CI is the CO corrected for differences in body size (a CO of 4 L/min may be adequate for a 100-lb woman but inadequate for a 200-lb man)

        (b) Based on body surface area (BSA) determined from a nomogram first described by Dubois

$$CI = CO/BSA$$

        (c) Normal CI is 2.5 to 4.0 L/min/m²

        (d) CI of 2 L/min/m² or less is incompatible with life

        (e) Increased CI due to

           (1) Exercise

           (2) Mild tachydysrhythmias (in a healthy heart)

        (f) Decreased CI due to

           (1) Decreased myocardial contractility (e.g., due to myocardial infarction, congestive heart failure, cardiomyopathy, electrolyte imbalances)

           (2) Increased afterload (e.g., due to valvular stenosis and pulmonary hypertension)

           (3) Changes in preload (e.g., due to hypovolemia or valvular incompetence or stenosis)

           (4) Tachydysrhythmias/irregular rhythms—decrease diastolic filling time and cause loss of atrial kick

  b. Ventriculography

    i. Definition: radiopaque contrast medium is injected into LV cavity, allowing the LV wall motion to be visualized on film (cineangiogram) or video

  ii. Purpose

    (a) To evaluate ventricular wall motion and contour

      (1) Akinetic areas—parts of ventricular wall with no motion (i.e., not contracting)

      (2) Hypokinetic areas—parts of ventricular wall with less than normal motion in systole

      (3) Dyskinetic areas—parts of ventricular wall with paradoxic motion

    (b) To detect ventricular aneurysms

    (c) To evaluate the mitral valve

    (d) To determine prognosis in patients selected for cardiac surgery

    (e) To determine LV function by measuring

      (1) End-diastolic volume

      (2) End-systolic volume

      (3) Stroke volume

      (4) Ejection fraction

    (f) RV can be similarly evaluated

    (g) To demonstrate shunts

c. Aortography

  i. Definition: radiopaque contrast medium is injected, allowing the aorta, the valve leaflets, and the major vessels of the aorta to be visualized and recorded on film

  ii. Purpose: to determine/diagnose the following

    (a) Aortic valve insufficiency

    (b) Aneurysms or dissections of ascending aorta

    (c) Coarctation of the aorta

    (d) Injuries to the aorta and/or major branches

d. Coronary arteriography

  i. Radiopaque contrast material is injected into the ostia of the right and left coronary arteries. This allows for visualization of the coronary arterial circulation and recording on film

  ii. Purpose

    (a) To study extent of coronary artery disease by noting areas and extent of lesions (for coronary arteries other than the left main, an obstruction of 75% or more is considered significant; for the left main, 50% or more is considered significant)

    (b) To evaluate ischemic heart disease

    (c) To evaluate atypical angina and coronary arterial spasm

    (d) To study patients with myocardial disease in order to rule out coronary artery disease

    (e) To perform intracoronary thrombolysis (see p. 227)

(f) To perform percutaneous transluminal coronary angioplasty (see PTCA, p. 211)

e. Electrophysiology studies (EPS)

　　i. Definition: series of programmed electrical stimuli are applied to the heart (using pacing electrodes guided under fluoroscopy) to induce dysrhythmias

　　ii. Purpose is to reproduce dysrhythmias under a controlled environment in order to determine the best mode of therapy for control (e.g., medications, pacemaker, ablation procedures)

　　iii. Patient selection

　　　　(a) Patients who have uncontrolled ventricular or supraventricular tachydysrhythmias with conventional medical therapy

　　　　(b) Patients identified at high risk for sudden cardiac death syndrome but who do not have reproducible ventricular dysrhythmias with the use of noninvasive techniques

　　　　(c) Patients with unexplained, recurrent syncopal episodes due to suspected cardiac etiology but not reproducible using noninvasive techniques

f. Bedside hemodynamic monitoring via flow-directed balloon-tipped catheter (see Figs. 2–12 and 2–13)

　　i. Allows for continuous bedside hemodynamic monitoring so that vascular tone, myocardial contractility, and fluid balance can be assessed and effectively managed

　　ii. Can measure right atrial pressure (RAP) through the proximal port of the catheter

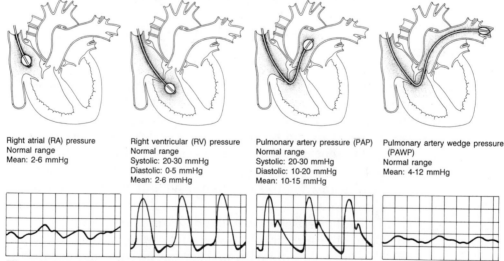

Right atrial (RA) pressure
Normal range
Mean: 2-6 mmHg

Right ventricular (RV) pressure
Normal range
Systolic: 20-30 mmHg
Diastolic: 0-5 mmHg
Mean: 2-6 mmHg

Pulmonary artery pressure (PAP)
Normal range
Systolic: 20-30 mmHg
Diastolic: 10-20 mmHg
Mean: 10-15 mmHg

Pulmonary artery wedge pressure
(PAWP)
Normal range
Mean: 4-12 mmHg

Figure 2–13. Flow-directed balloon-tipped catheter as it passes through the right side of the heart, wedging in a distal pulmonary artery with corresponding pressure waveforms and normal values.

(a) RAP is a determinant of RV end-diastolic pressure; reflects venous return to the right side of the heart
(b) Normal RAP = 2 to 6 mm Hg
(c) Elevated RA pressure may indicate
    (1) RV failure
    (2) Tricuspid valve dysfunction
    (3) Pulmonary hypertension
    (4) Chronic LV failure
    (5) Constrictive pericarditis
    (6) Cardiac tamponade
    (7) Ventricular septal defect with left-to-right shunt
    (8) Pulmonic stenosis
    (9) Chronic obstructive pulmonary disease
   (10) RV infarction
(d) Decreased RA pressure may indicate
    (1) Hypovolemia (e.g., due to diuretics, blood loss, burns, vomiting)
    (2) Venodilation (e.g., due to drugs [nitrates], hypersensitivity reactions)
(e) Central venous pressure (CVP)—reflects pressure in the great veins
    (1) Used to monitor blood volume, RV function, and central venous return
    (2) Previously used as a direct reflection of RAP but no longer
    (3) Can be measured in cm H_2O or mm Hg depending on the system being used
       a) To convert mm Hg to cm H_2O, multiply mm Hg × 1.36
       b) Examples

$$3 \text{ mm Hg} \times 1.36 = 4.1 \text{ cm } H_2O$$
$$9 \text{ mm Hg} \times 1.36 = 12.2 \text{ cm } H_2O$$
$$15 \text{ mm Hg} \times 1.36 = 20.4 \text{ cm } H_2O$$

    (4) Normal CVP—varies from patient to patient. One patient may be stable at a CVP of 5 cm H_2O and another may not. Therefore it is important to monitor the trends in the CVP readings and the clinical picture of the patient in relation to those readings (e.g., heart sounds, urine output changes, breath sounds). As a general rule, a CVP of 2 to 8 cm H_2O or 2 to 6 mm Hg is considered within normal limits.
    (5) CVP is decreased with negative-pressure breathing and shock and increased by positive-pressure breath-

ing, straining, increased blood volume, and heart failure

iii. Measures RV pressures

(a) Normal systolic RV pressure = 20 to 30 mm Hg; normal diastolic pressure = 0 to 5 mm Hg with an end-diastolic pressure of 2 to 6 mm Hg

(b) Elevated RV pressures seen in

(1) RV failure

(2) Constrictive pericarditis

(3) Cardiac tamponade

(4) Congestive heart failure

(5) Pulmonary hypertension

(6) Ventricular septal defect with left-to-right shunt

iv. Measures pulmonary artery (PA) pressure and pulmonary capillary wedge pressure (PCWP) through the distal port (see Fig. 2–13)

(a) Obtain readings according to prescribed routine, evaluating trends and reporting significant changes

(b) Pressure readings can be obtained with patient in any position provided that transducer is at same level as phlebostatic axis. Phlebostatic axis is an imaginary point defined by intersection of two imaginary lines. One line is drawn from fourth intercostal space from sternum to edge of chest and down to the side. Other line is drawn in middle of lateral chest wall from last rib to axilla. Point of intersection of these two lines is the phlebostatic axis

(c) PA pressure reflects left- and right-sided heart pressures

(d) PA systolic pressure represents pressure produced by RV (normal = 20 to 30 mm Hg)

(e) Elevation of PA pressure is associated with

(1) Atrial or ventricular septal defects causing increased pulmonary blood flow due to the left-to-right shunt

(2) Pulmonary hypertension (increases pulmonary vascular resistance)

(3) LV failure and mitral stenosis (increases pulmonary venous pressure)

(f) PA diastolic pressure reflects LVEDP and is used as a measure of LV function and diastolic filling pressures (normal < 10 to 20 mm Hg), hence preload

(g) PA diastolic pressure is elevated in

(1) LV failure

(2) Mitral stenosis

(3) Pulmonary hypertension

(4) Increased pulmonary blood flow due to left-to-right shunts (as in atrial and ventricular septal defects)

(h) PA diastolic pressure does not reflect LVEDP in heart rates greater than 125 beats/min, in chronic obstructive pulmonary disease, adult respiratory distress syndrome, mitral stenosis, or pulmonary embolism (in these instances, the PCWP must be used)

(i) PA mean ($\overline{PA}$)—normally less than 20 mm Hg (used primarily for hemodynamic calculations and not clinically important)

(j) PCWP (or pulmonary artery wedge pressure [PAWP]) is a reflection of LA pressure and is used to assess LV filling pressures (LVEDP)

(1) Balloon of catheter is inflated, wedging in a small branch of the PA (see Fig. 2–13)

(2) PCWP should be 2 to 5 mm Hg less than PA diastolic (4 to 12 mm Hg)

(3) PCWP is elevated in

   a) LV failure
   b) Constrictive pericarditis
   c) Mitral valve stenosis or insufficiency
   d) Fluid overload
   e) Ischemia

(4) PCWP is decreased in

   a) Hypovolemia
   b) Afterload reduction with use of vasodilating drugs

(5) Prevention of complications associated with the flow-directed balloon-tipped catheter

   a) Ensure that balloon is deflated after wedge pressure is obtained to prevent pulmonary infarctions
   b) Monitor waveform to ensure that the catheter is not wedged when balloon is deflated and that the catheter has not slipped back into the right ventricle (potential for ectopy is great)
   c) 0.8 to 1.5 ml of air is used to inflate the balloon. Use only the syringe that comes with the catheter to inflate the balloon. Other syringes may lead to accidental overinflation of the balloon and possible rupture, thus causing emboli or infarcts
   d) Ensure that the catheter is inserted under sterile technique (use of a catheter guard over the pulmonary artery catheter will ensure sterility and allow for adjustments); change dressings over insertion site per hospital policy; examine site for signs and symptoms of infection, phlebitis
   e) Ensure catheter introducer sheath is sutured to the skin to prevent migration of the catheter,

which can cause ventricular ectopy, possible perforation of RA, RV, or PA or pulmonary infarction due to wedging

    f) Maintain patency of the system with pressurized heparinized drip to prevent clot formation at end of catheter and possible embolization

    g) Check distal extremities for pulses, swelling, discoloration, and temperature changes suggestive of circulatory impairment

    h) Ensure that all electrical equipment in the area is operating correctly and grounded properly and that wiring is intact in order to prevent electrically induced ventricular fibrillation

(k) Mixed venous oxygen saturation (Sv_{O_2}) can be measured (using a special fiberoptic pulmonary artery catheter) by aspirating blood through the distal lumen. The data collected are recorded continuously, both digitally and printed in strip chart form

    (1) Sv_{O_2} rapidly reflects the extent to which the body's demand for oxygen is met by the amount of oxygen supplied

    (2) The oxygen supply to tissues depends on

        a) The content of oxygen in the arterial blood (both dissolved in the plasma and reflected by Pa_{O_2} and attached to hemoglobin as reflected by arterial oxygen saturation—Sa_{O_2})

        b) Efficiency of cardiac output—increased CO increases oxygen delivery to the tissues; decreased CO decreases availability of oxygen to the tissues

    (3) Critically ill patients have greatly increased demands for oxygen at the cellular level owing to a variety of conditions (e.g., fever, seizures, anxiety, pain)

    (4) The first compensatory mechanism of increasing CO to meet the demands may not be possible in severely compromised patients; hence, the body increases oxygen extraction from the blood to improve oxygenation of the tissues. This results in a fall in the Sv_{O_2} (significant if <60%), indicating changes in the patient's condition that produce an oxygen imbalance

    (5) Normal Sv_{O_2} = 60% to 80%

    (6) Increased Sv_{O_2} (80% to 95%) reflecting decreased oxygen demand may be due to

        a) Hypothermia

        b) Sepsis

(7) Decreased Sv_{O_2} (<60%) reflecting increased oxygen demand or decrease in oxygen delivery may be due to
    a) Dysrhythmias decreasing blood pressure
    b) Fever
    c) Pain
    d) Seizures
    e) Pump failure (e.g., due to shock, myocardial infarction, dysrhythmias)
    f) Hemorrhage
    g) Respiratory failure (adult respiratory distress syndrome, pulmonary edema)
    h) Hypoxia
(8) Sv_{O_2} monitoring is useful in monitoring the patient's response to nursing care and other medical regimens such as drug therapy; also decreases the need for frequent arterial blood gases and cardiac output determinations

(l) Left atrial pressure (LAP) measurements
  (1) Catheter inserted into the left atrium during cardiac surgery and brought out the chest wall to be connected to pressure monitoring devices providing continuous display of the LA pressure (versus obtaining the PCWP by inflating the balloon)
  (2) LAP is the most accurate measurement of LV preload and in the normal heart is the same as LVEDP
  (3) Normal LAP = 4 to 12 mm Hg
  (4) LAP waveform consists of an "a" wave, which represents LA contraction, and a "v" wave, representing filling of the LA while mitral valve is still closed
  (5) Increased LAP may be due to
    a) Decreased myocardial contractility (ventricles do not eject as much blood as normal hence the pressure is reflected back to the LA)
    b) Tachydysrhythmias (the ventricles are unable to empty as normal and the increased pressure is reflected back to the LA)
    c) Fluid overload
    d) Mitral stenosis
  (6) Decreased LAP may be due to hypovolemia as in hemorrhage postoperatively or systemic vascular dilatation during rewarming, etc.
  (7) Potential problems associated with LA catheters
    a) Air embolism—make sure all connections are secure; do not administer medications via this cath-

eter; use air filters between the tubing and the catheter; do not flush this line manually
   b) Clot formation—assure system is continually flushed with a pressurized heparin solution
   c) Infection
   d) Electrical hazards—assure proper grounding of all bedside apparatus
   e) Cardiac tamponade
(m) Coronary angioscopy
   (1) The endothelial surface of coronary arteries is examined using high-resolution flexible fiberoptic angioscopes
   (2) Clinical symptoms correlate highly with angioscopic findings
   (3) Chronic, stable angina is associated with a smooth-surfaced atheroma without hemorrhage or ulceration—termed *noncomplex atheroma*
   (4) Accelerated angina is associated with plaque ulceration, which is termed *complex* because the surface of the atheroma is ragged and intimal hemorrhage is present
   (5) Unstable angina at rest is associated with a partially occlusive thrombus
   (6) Since unstable coronary disease is associated with complex intimal abnormalities, it is conceivable that medical therapy can be instituted based on clinical symptomatology (i.e., anticoagulation, antiplatelet and thrombolytic therapy)

COMMONLY ENCOUNTERED NURSING DIAGNOSES

Potential for Anxiety, Depression, and Denial, related to threat of death, threat to or change of health status, threat to or change in body image, threat to or change in role functioning affecting socioeconomic status, or knowledge deficit

1. **Assessment for defining characteristics**
   a. Patient exhibits signs of anxiety (i.e., restlessness, insomnia, anorexia, palpitations, increased respirations, nausea, vomiting, dry mouth, increased muscular tension especially seen as facial tension, poor eye contact, acting out by exhibiting bouts of anger or withdrawing, increased heart rate, increased blood pressure, difficulty concentrating) or states inability to cope

b. Patient exhibits signs of depression (i.e., decreased energy drive, unresponsiveness, irritability, weeping or crying, feelings of helplessness) and verbalizes inability to cope and to make decisions

c. Patient exhibits signs of denial (i.e., does not follow the nursing/medical plan of care, will not talk about the present crisis, is inappropriately cheerful, makes statements that are unrealistic for the present time)

2. Expected outcomes

a. Uses effective coping mechanisms to manage the anxiety
b. States increased feelings of comfort
c. Appears less anxious and less depressed
d. Realistically appraises the crisis situation and its ramifications on self
e. Verbalizes feelings freely

3. Nursing interventions

a. Explain all procedures to the patient in a simple, concise, and reassuring manner. Repeat information as needed
b. Treat the patient as a person
c. Provide for a comfortable environment; decrease stimuli, and organize nursing tasks to allow for adequate rest periods
d. Give the patient as much control over the environment and other activities (such as self-care) as possible
e. Encourage the patient to discuss feelings and concerns
f. Teach patient relaxation techniques
g. Use therapeutic touch
h. If needed, provide sedatives or hypnotics as ordered
i. Provide for diversional activities
j. Accept patient's denial when it is beneficial to decrease the anxiety but do not reinforce it
k. Provide opportunities for family/significant others to be with patient, participate in the care, etc.
l. Initiate consultations with psychiatric liaison personnel as needed
m. Begin teaching when patient indicates readiness to learn

4. Evaluation of nursing care

a. Patient expresses fears, anxieties, needs; appears less tense; is able to maintain eye contact; is able to rest and sleep; exhibits decreased muscular tension; has normal heart rate; and communicates appropriately
b. Patient exhibits increased levels of energy and engages in conversation and less weeping
c. Patient makes appropriate decisions regarding self, cooperates with the plan of care, is able to talk about the crisis event and its ramifications on self and family, and is able to discuss future plans

Potential for Nosocomial Bacteremia, related to invasive lines/Foley catheter, and Nosocomial Pneumonia, related to required bed rest

1. **Assessment for defining characteristics**
   a. Temperature above patient's normal
   b. Redness, warmth, and drainage from insertion/incision sites
   c. Elevated leukocyte count
   d. Urine shows leukocytes
   e. Rales/rhonchi present on auscultation of lungs
   f. Egophony, bronchophony, or whispered pectoriloquy present
   g. Chest x-ray film shows consolidation
2. **Expected outcome:** patient is free of infection
3. **Nursing interventions**
   a. Inspect skin for redness, extreme warmth, or drainage from incisions, and peripheral, arterial, and venous lines
   b. Ensure aseptic handling of all intravenous lines
   c. Administer antibiotics as prescribed
   d. Report elevation in temperature and changes in laboratory data indicative of infectious process (i.e., increased leukocyte count with increased neutrophils)
   e. Change intravenous tubing as hospital policy dictates
   f. Change dressings every 24 hours or more often if needed
   g. Remove mucus secretions from respiratory tract via usual nursing techniques
   h. Encourage deep breathing and coughing and use of incentive spirometer
   i. Assess respiratory status and monitor for adventitious breath sounds (crackles, rhonchi, friction rubs)
   j. Assist patient to change position on a regular basis
      i. Provide air or egg crate mattresses, especially if patient is elderly
      ii. Give gentle massage to bony prominences
   k. Monitor hydration status and administer fluids as ordered
   l. Perform aseptic urinary catheter care per unit standards
   m. Monitor urine for color, odor, sediment, etc.
   n. Discontinue all catheters, intravenous lines, and drains as soon as possible
4. **Evaluation of nursing care**
   a. All invasive insertion sites are without signs of infection
   b. Patient is afebrile
   c. Patient's lungs are clear to auscultation without crackles or rhonchi
   d. Chest x-ray film is clear without atelectasis or pneumonia
   e. Laboratory data do not reflect infectious process
   f. Patient's skin remains intact with normal turgor

Potential for Confusion, related to sensory overload/ICU psychosis/sleep deprivation

1. **Assessment for defining characteristics**
   a. Patient is disoriented to person, time, and place
   b. Patient exhibits periods of agitation and irritability
   c. Patient experiences visual, auditory, and tactile hallucinations
   d. Patient does not follow simple commands or instructions
   e. Patient is unable to sleep normally
   f. Patient exhibits disordered thought patterns
2. **Expected outcomes**
   a. Remains oriented with no disorders in thought pattern
   b. Is able to follow instructions
   c. Has no indications of hallucinations
   d. Rests normally
3. **Nursing interventions**
   a. Try to provide restful environment by eliminating extraneous sounds as much as possible; organize nursing activities so as to provide periods of rest throughout the day and sleep during the night; dim lights; limit visiting
   b. Remove external tactile stimuli as soon as possible (e.g., tubes, drains, tape)
   c. Continuously orient patient; provide calender, clock, and newspaper; if there are windows, allow patient to see daylight and darkness
   d. If patient is confused, protect from self-injury; institute falls protocol, restrain per unit standards
   e. If in pain, administer medications as ordered
4. **Evaluation of nursing care**
   a. Patient is able to answer questions appropriately regarding person, time, and place
   b. Patient maintains normal rest/sleep patterns
   c. Patient remains free of self-injury

Potential for Impairment of Skin Integrity secondary to altered tissue perfusion, edema, immobility

1. **Assessment for defining characteristics**
   a. Edema present
   b. Patient immobile due to illness
   c. Nutritional status may be less than optimal
   d. Skin turgor altered
   e. Denuded skin over bony prominences
   f. Patient diaphoretic
   g. Altered sensorium (patient unaware of pain and pressure)
2. **Expected outcomes**
   a. Absence of reddened areas
   b. Skin remains intact

3. Nursing interventions

  a. Assess patient's skin, checking bony prominences and other pressure areas for redness, blistering of skin, or breaks in skin
  b. Palpate peripheral pulses to assess circulatory status
  c. Keep skin clean and dry. Clean any bodily excrement immediately since these are extremely irritating to the skin and promote bacterial growth and hence necrosis of skin
  d. If patient is able to cooperate, encourage to change positions
  e. Change patient's position at least every 2 hours, rotating from side to chest to side to back unless contraindicated
  f. Place patient on egg crate, sheepskin, or alternating-pressure mattress
  g. Massage skin, especially bony prominences, with lotion
  h. Position patient using pillows for support and to relieve pressure
  i. To reduce shearing forces, keep head of bed up less than 30°
  j. Keep bottom sheets dry and without wrinkles
  k. Provide active or passive range of motion exercises
  l. Monitor laboratory values that have an effect on skin (i.e., hematocrit, hemoglobin, blood urea nitrogen, albumin, bilirubin, electrolytes)
  m. Provide adequate nutrition

4. Evaluation of nursing care

  a. Skin is without reddened areas or breaks
  b. Patient voices no complaints of pain associated with pressure on skin

Potential for Knowledge Deficit

1. Assessment for defining characteristics

  a. Patient requests information
  b. Patient incorrectly relates instructions taught to him
  c. Patient incorrectly identifies medications, their uses, dosage, time schedule, and side effects

2. Expected outcomes

  a. Verbalizes understanding of the disease process, causes, treatment regimen, and life-style changes he must take to prevent/control complications or recurrence
  b. Verbalizes symptoms of recurrence and complications to be reported
  c. Verbalizes understanding of all medications, their uses, dosage, times of administration, and side effects
  d. Verbalizes understanding of diet regimen/restrictions

3. Nursing interventions

  a. Monitor readiness to learn and determine best methods for teaching/learning (i.e., structured, unstructured). Incorporate family/significant others (SO) when possible
  b. Plan periods of time for one-to-one interaction with patient

    c. Teach patient/SO about the disease process and all its ramifications

    d. Discuss procedures/factors that may place patient at risk for future similar events

    e. Provide printed instructions to take home regarding medications, signs and symptoms, activity regimens (including sexual activity), dietary restrictions, and what to do if questions, problems, and signs and symptoms arise

    f. Have patient demonstrate all psychomotor skills necessary for home care when appropriate

    g. Initiate community health and social service consultations as necessary for follow-up care

    h. Stress need for follow-up care

4. Evaluation of nursing care

    a. Patient/SO relate appropriate compliance factors to all nursing/medical regimen

    b. Patient/SO are able to return demonstrate correct procedures regarding home self-care measures

    c. Patient/SO relate symptoms requiring notification of physician

    d. Patient/SO relate factors that place patient at risk for recurrence

PATIENT HEALTH PROBLEMS

Coronary Artery Disease (CAD): Process in which the coronary artery vasculature is partially to totally occluded by the atherosclerotic process

1. Pathophysiology ("response to injury" theory)

    a. Endothelial cells in the intima of the artery are mechanically or chemically injured. This alters the structure of the cells, making them permeable to circulating liproproteins (the first phase of CAD formation)

    b. Platelets adhere and aggregate at the site of injury and macrophages migrate to the area as a result of the injury. Liproproteins enter the smooth muscle cells of the intimal layer, all of which promote the development of a "fatty streak" (the second phase of CAD formation)

    c. Repeated long-term injury to the endothelial cells eventually leads to the development of a "fibrofatty plaque" (the third phase of CAD formation). This is a pearly white accumulation in the intimal lining consisting mostly of smooth muscle cells but also collagen-producing fibroblasts and macrophages. It can be extensive enough such that the deposits begin to protrude into the lumen, obstructing blood flow (an atherosclerotic plaque)

    d. The process occurs repeatedly, progressively narrowing the vessel. Vessels in the area may hemorrhage, which further increases the size of the plaque. The fibrofatty plaque can actually rupture, forming a thrombus, which then may partially or totally obstruct the artery

   e. This process occurs mostly at bifurcations and at the proximal end of the artery, although distal lesions do occur
   f. The atherosclerotic process causes
      i. A decreased blood flow and oxygen supply to the myocardium
      ii. An imbalance between myocardial oxygen supply and demand, resulting in a state termed *coronary insufficiency*

2. **Etiology or precipitating factors**
   a. Heredity: tends to run in families
   b. Age: more prevalent in older age groups
   c. Gender: more prevalent in men then in women (prior to menopause)
   d. Hypertension: systolic blood pressure >160 and/or diastolic >95 mm Hg
   e. Diabetes mellitus: patients with diabetes mellitus are two times more likely to develop CAD than those without diabetes mellitus
   f. Cigarette smoking: smokers have a risk two to six times higher of death from CAD than nonsmokers
   g. Hyperlipidemia: high levels of triglycerides and low-density and very low-density lipoproteins are associated with an increased risk of CAD
   h. Obesity: obesity itself has been shown to be positively associated with an increase in CAD. In addition, it also contributes to the development of hypertension and diabetes
   i. Sedentary life style: controversial as to whether it is a risk factor by itself; however, studies do show a low positive relationship between inactivity and CAD.
   j. Stress: it was previously believed that the type A personality was twice as prone to CAD as compared with others. Current studies are now challenging this theory

3. **Nursing assessment data base.** CAD in itself will present no symptomatology. It is only when the patient suffers sequelae of CAD that CAD is diagnosed or if the patient has a stress test as part of a physical examination and does not pass. The possible sequelae of CAD are listed below, several of which will be covered in this chapter as separate entities. Each entity will include its own unique aspects for nursing history, nursing examination, diagnostic findings, and nursing diagnoses. The clinical presentation of CAD may be manifested by any of the following
   a. Angina pectoris
   b. Myocardial infarction
   c. Congestive heart failure
   d. Sudden cardiac death
   e. Dysrhythmias
   f. Cardiomegaly
   g. Mitral insufficiency
   h. Ventricular aneurysm/rupture

    i. Cardiogenic shock

    j. May exhibit no symptomatology

Angina Pectoris: A state of transient myocardial ischemia without cell death

1. Pathophysiology (see that for CAD, p. 205)

2. Etiology or precipitating factors

    a. Atherosclerotic heart disease

    b. Hypertension

    c. Aortic valve disease

    d. Anemia

    e. Dysrhythmias (especially tachydysrhythmias)

    f. Thyrotoxicosis

    g. Shock

    h. Congestive heart failure

    i. Aortitis

    j. Coronary artery spasm

    k. Precipitating factors include physical activity (not necessarily strenuous), ingestion of large meals, recumbent positions that may precipitate nocturnal angina, cold exposure, and anxiety

3. Nursing assessment data base

    a. Nursing history

        i. Subjective findings—consist of the patient's "chief complaint": the patient may describe symptoms of discomfort (rather than pain), such as burning, squeezing, aching, heaviness, pressure sensation, smothering, or indigestion-type symptoms

        ii. Objective findings

            (a) Etiologic or precipating factors—to elicit more objective data regarding the angina, have the patient describe it using the following PQRST system

                (1) *P* for provocative—have patient describe what activities bring on the angina (e.g., physical activity, resting, sleeping). Also ascertain what the patient does to relieve the pain (e.g., rests, takes nitroglycerin) and whether these measures are effective

                (2) *Q* for quality—how does the discomfort feel (see subjective findings). Also determine if it is accompanied by other symptoms such as sweating, nausea, palpitations, shortness of breath

                (3) *R* for region/radiation—where is the discomfort and does it radiate? Most often it radiates to arms, jaw (patient may complain of a toothache), and back between scapulae

                (4) *S* for severity—have patient rate the discomfort on a

scale of 1–10, with 1 being the least and 10 being the worst pain ever experienced by the patient

 (5) *T* for timing—ascertain when the discomfort began and how long it lasts. Was it sudden or gradual? It usually lasts only 1 to 4 minutes and subsides gradually when the precipitating factors are removed

  a) Forms of angina pectoris

   ☐ Stable angina—angina that has not increased in severity or frequency over a period of several months

   ☐ Unstable angina—new onset angina or angina in which the quality of pain has changed or increased in frequency, duration, and/or severity. It usually occurs with lessened exertion and/or rest

   ☐ Prinzmetal's (variant) angina—angina that may occur at rest, long after exercise, or while asleep. It is usually due to coronary vasospasm

 (b) Family history (see p. 152)

 (c) Social history (see p. 153)

 (d) Medication history (see p. 153)

 b. Nursing examination of the patient

  i. Inspection (see p. 153)

  ii. Palpation (see p. 154)

  iii. Percussion (see p. 156)

  iv. Auscultation (see p. 156)

 c. Diagnostic study findings (for review see p. 166)

  i. Stress electrocardiography: may or may not be positive (see p. 188)

  ii. Selective coronary arteriography: areas of lesions will be noted on the cineangiogram; also confirms valvular disease that may be causing the angina

  iii. Electrocardiogram may or may not show evidence of myocardial injury or damage (see p. 226)

  iv. Cardiac isoenzyme levels are not elevated with angina

  v. Echocardiogram (see p. 168) may show abnormal function of the valves, wall motion abnormalities, and hypertrophy

4. Nursing diagnoses

 a. See Commonly Encountered Nursing Diagnoses (pp. 200–205)

 b. Alteration in comfort (chest pain), related to myocardial ischemia due to atherosclerosis/coronary spasm

  i. Assessment for defining characteristics

   (a) Patient appears very anxious

   (b) Patient may clench fist over sternum

   (c) May see autonomic responses such as diaphoresis, blood

pressure and pulse rate change, and pupillary dilatation; respiratory rate may increase or decrease
- (d) Have patient describe the discomfort—see p. 207 to determine if it is characteristic of angina
- (e) On physical examination note any changes from the normal cardiac examination (e.g., S_3, S_4, distended neck veins)

ii. Expected outcomes
- (a) Patient verbalizes relief of pain
- (b) Patient able to tolerate increased activity without recurrence of pain

iii. Nursing interventions
- (a) Have patient stop any activity; place back into bed, preferably in semi-Fowler's position; rest
- (b) Administer oxygen therapy per unit standards
- (c) Take vital signs
- (d) Take 12-lead ECG
- (e) Administer nitroglycerin per unit standards
- (f) Maintain a quiet, calm environment
- (g) Ensure patient has a patent intravenous line
- (h) Administer and titrate drugs to reduce/eliminate angina. The goal is to decrease myocardial oxygen demand and improve oxygen supply.
  - (1) Nitroglycerin—administer intravenous form for unstable angina (p. 216); other forms with short-term or longer lasting effects (i.e., sublingual, oral, topical, inhalation)
  - (2) Beta-adrenergic blocking agents (see p. 220)
  - (3) Calcium-channel blocking agents (see Table 2–1 and p. 221)
- (i) May have to prepare the patient/SO for percutaneous

Table 2–1. COMPARISON OF CALCIUM CHANNEL BLOCKERS: THEIR EFFECTS ON THE HEART AND VASCULATURE

	Name of Drug*		
Effect	**Verapamil**	**Diltiazem**	**Nifedipine**
Heart rate	↓ ↓	↓ ↓	− or ↑
AV conduction	↓ ↓ ↓	↓ ↓	−
Systemic vasodilation	↑ ↑	↑	↑ ↑ ↑
Coronary vasodilation	↑ ↑	↑ ↑	↑ ↑ ↑
Myocardial contractility	↓ ↓	− or ↓	− or ↑

*The more arrows, the greater the degree of effect.
Adapted from Tillisch, J.: Information presented at the AACN National Teaching Institute, 1983.

transluminal coronary angioplasty (PTCA) (Fig. 2–14)—a nonoperative procedure to increase the inner diameter of coronary arteries that have been stenosed due to coronary artery disease. A successful procedure results in the improvement of blood flow to the myocardium distal to the blockage, thus decreasing or eliminating angina and preventing myocardial infarctions

(1) Indications for PTCA
    a) Unstable or chronic angina
    b) Post coronary artery bypass grafting with postoperative angina
    c) Acute and post acute myocardial infarction
(2) Patient selection—the ideal patient has
    a) Single- or double-vessel disease (excluding the left main) with at least 50% stenosis
    b) A lesion that is discrete, preferably proximal, noncalcific, concentric, and not located near any bifurcations
    c) The potential to survive emergency surgery if the procedure is complicated or fails
(3) More aggressive approaches are now undertaken in patients with multivessel disease, in patients with saphenous vein grafts (from previous coronary artery

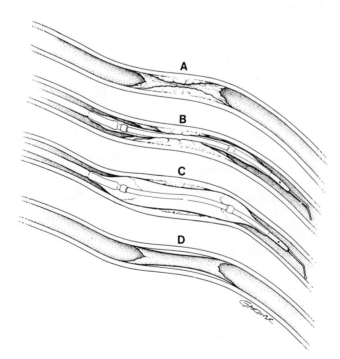

Figure 2–14. Percutaneous transluminal coronary angioplasty (PTCA). *A.* Catheter advancing toward the atherosclerotic plaque. *B.* Balloon placed into the plaque. *C.* Balloon inflated. *D.* Balloon removed leaving plaque depressed against the arterial wall.

bypass grafting) that have occluded over time and in totally occluded arteries

(4) Contraindicated in
   a) Left main CAD, especially when the patient is not considered a good surgical risk
   b) Variant angina
   c) In vessels stenosed at the orifice by the aortic wall
   d) In patients with critical valvular disease (not due to infarction)

(5) PTCA procedure
   a) Procedure is performed in the cardiac catheterization laboratory under fluoroscopy
   b) The balloon catheter is placed across the stenosis and inflated several times
   c) This procedure enlarges the diameter of the lumen by compressing the plaque against the walls of the artery and by splitting the intima of the artery stretching the overall vessel diameter. The effect of this is to increase the blood flow to the myocardium

(6) A postprocedure coronary arteriogram is recorded to document the results

(7) Potential complications of the procedure
   a) Dissection of the coronary artery (may require immediate coronary artery bypass grafting)
   b) Acute coronary occlusion due to dissection or spasm of the artery
   c) Myocardial infarction
   d) Pericardial tamponade (due to RV rupture from pacemaker lead)
   e) Hypotension may occur in reaction to contrast media injected to perform the angiogram
   f) Owing to cannulation of the femoral or brachial artery, and anticoagulation for the procedure, there may be bleeding, hematoma formation, retroperitoneal bleeding, and decreased or absent peripheral pulses distal to the insertion site
   g) Reperfusion dysrhythmias with resultant decrease in cardiac output and hypotension
   h) Vasovagal reaction as sheath is manipulated
   i) Restenosis of the artery within the first 6 months

(8) Implications for nursing
   a) Must prepare the patient/SO for the procedure—similar to that of usual cardiac catheterization procedure

      b) Potential for coronary artery bypass grafting must be discussed

      c) Supportive nursing techniques must be employed to decrease anxiety for patient/SO

      d) Discuss routines patient will experience post-PTCA procedure (see below)

      e) Nursing care post-PTCA procedure:
- ☐ Monitor for all potential complications discussed previously
- ☐ Bed rest for 8 hours with head of bed elevated no more than 30°
- ☐ The affected limb must be kept straight and relatively immobile. Use a sandbag over insertion site for 2 to 4 hours after procedure
- ☐ Serial ECGs and cardiac monitoring for 24 hours; observe for dysrhythmias
- ☐ Monitor hemodynamics and vital signs as ordered
- ☐ Monitor pulses, warmth, and sensation of affected limb; assess for bleeding and hematoma at insertion site
- ☐ Patient will be on heparin drip post PTCA; monitor blood tests (especially hematocrit, clotting studies); urine, emesis, stools for guaiac; central nervous system for cerebral hemorrhage; limit blood drawing to only as necessary or use arterial line if in place
- ☐ Monitor respiratory system for respiratory distress; encourage coughing and deep breathing—use incentive spirometry

      f) Teach patient about postdischarge anticoagulation medications and necessity for follow-up care, what to do if angina recurs, use of nitroglycerin, and reduction of risk factors

  (j) Patient/SO may have to be prepared for coronary artery reconstruction (endarterectomy or coronary artery bypass grafting using saphenous veins and internal mammary arteries)

    (1) Endarterectomy—distal, diffuse CAD is surgically removed rather than bypassed

      a) Arteriotomy—small areas of plaque may be excised through the arteriotomy or the artery may have to be split open and the plaque dissected from the vessel wall

      b) The coronary artery may have to be reconstructed

after removal of the plaque (which entails removing the intima) using a saphenous vein patch

(2) Coronary artery bypass grafting using saphenous vein grafts—the saphenous vein is used to create a conduit: one end of the graft is sewn onto the aorta; the other end is then sewn onto the affected coronary artery distal to the blockage. This reroutes coronary blood flow, bypassing the blockage and delivering oxygen to the deprived myocardium

(3) Coronary artery bypass grafting using internal mammary arteries

   a) These arteries are now used more often than systemic veins because their patency rate over time is greater

   b) Their use avoids the need for leg incisions to harvest the saphenous veins. This eliminates leg complications and discomfort for the patient.

   c) These arteries can be grafted much the same as systemic veins, but more often one end stays attached to the subclavian artery from which it originates and the other end is sewn onto the coronary artery distal to the blockage

(4) Patient selection criteria

   a) Angina unresponsive to medical therapy

   b) Blockage greater than 50% of the arterial diameter

   c) Critical left main coronary artery disease or three-vessel disease

   d) Emergent conditions such as preinfarction angina or acute myocardial infarction with unresponsive anginal pain and hemodynamic instability or as a result of a complication incurred during coronary angiography or PTCA

(5) Potential complications arising during surgery

   a) Intraoperative stroke or myocardial infarction

   b) Excessive bleeding

   c) Inability of the heart to resume pumping again once disconnected from the heart–lung machine; may need the intra-aortic balloon pump (see p. 231) or the ventricular assist device (VAD) (see p. 233) to support the heart

   d) Death

(6) Potential complications during the *immediate* postoperative period

   a) Low cardiac output (CO) syndrome/hypotension (may be due to inadequate volume replacement, fluid shifts [third spacing], hemorrhage; leads to decreased systemic perfusion which affects the kidneys, brain, heart, etc.)

b) Hemorrhage/bleeding disorders (more prone with the use of internal mammary arteries because the intercostal arteries are clipped from the internal mammary artery, hence more chance of hemorrhage; often longer pump times when internal mammary artery grafts are used, hence more chance of blood dyscrasias)

c) Hypertension (important to control—the increased afterload increases myocardial work and myocardial oxygen consumption, which may lead to failure or infarcts, and increases the potential for bleeding from anastomotic sites; grafts can actually disconnect)

d) Cardiac tamponade (noted by decreased CO, increased central venous pressure, pulsus paradoxus, widening cardiac silhouette on x-ray film, equaling of left- and right-sided heart pressures, decreased arterial pressure, marked decrease in chest tube output, distant heart sounds)

e) Dysrhythmias (usually due to electrolyte imbalances, acid–base imbalances, hypoxemia, drug toxicity, hypothermia, anesthetic agents)

f) Myocardial infarction

g) Respiratory failure (evidenced by acid–base imbalances, hypoxia, alveolar hypoventilation)

h) Renal failure (usually due to reduced CO and intravascular volume)

i) Electrolyte imbalances—common after coronary artery bypass grafting, especially hypokalemia

(7) Selected drugs used to maintain hemodynamic stability after coronary artery bypass grafting

a) Sodium nitroprusside

☐ Relaxes vascular smooth muscle, which causes vasodilation

☐ This decreases preload by reducing LV filling pressures

☐ Also reduces afterload by decreasing the systemic and pulmonary vascular resistance, which results in an increased CO

☐ Indicated when diminished CO is due at least in part to increased systemic vascular resis-

tance, such as after cardiac surgery, hypertensive crisis, or congestive heart failure
☐ Contraindicated in aortic stenosis or coarctation of the aorta
☐ Action is immediate and brief; effect will end 1 to 2 minutes after infusion is stopped
☐ Must be delivered by a volumetric infusion pump for safety
☐ Patient's blood pressure should be monitored via an arterial line and hemodynamics via a flow-directed balloon-tipped catheter
☐ Rate of infusion is determined by blood pressure and hemodynamic parameters (e.g., PCWP, CO)
☐ Calculated in micrograms per kilogram of body weight per minute (μg/kg/min)

b) Dopamine
☐ Has alpha- and beta-adrenergic effects as well as dopaminergic effects
☐ Its positive inotropic effects increase CO, blood pressure, and cerebral blood flow at moderate doses of 2 to 10 μg/kg/min
☐ Increases renal and mesenteric blood flow at low doses (1 to 2 μg/kg/min), thus increasing glomerular filtration rate and urinary output (dopaminergic effects)
☐ Doses > 10 μg/kg/min effect pure alpha stimulation, causing peripheral vasoconstriction (with resultant increased systemic vascular resistance and increased afterload) and loss of renal and mesenteric dilation
☐ Dopamine is indicated in low CO/hypotension, shock due to myocardial infarction, sepsis, and renal failure
☐ Dopamine is contraindicated in uncorrected tachydysrhythmias
☐ Alpha stimulation will cause peripheral vasoconstriction—check skin for color, temperature, capillary refill
☐ Should be infused via a central line or large vein. Extravasation causes tissue necrosis and sloughing. (If extravasation occurs, stop infusion; phentolamine [Regitine] is injected around the site to lessen the effects of the dopamine)
☐ Must be infused by volumetric infusion pump for accuracy and safety

☐ Should have an arterial line to monitor blood pressure

c) Dobutamine

☐ Stimulates beta receptors in the heart

☐ Is a direct-acting, positive-inotropic agent

☐ Increases stroke volume and CO by increasing contractility

☐ Systemic vascular resistance is usually decreased

☐ Less positive inotropic than dopamine

☐ Minimal vasoconstriction peripherally

☐ No renal effect as with dopamine, except when CO increases

☐ Is indicated in low CO, hypotensive states

☐ Is contraindicated in hypovolemia, hypertrophic cardiomyopathy (see p. 256), and severe aortic stenosis

☐ Infuse via a volumetric infusion pump

☐ Should have an arterial line to monitor blood pressure

☐ Monitor for tachydysrhythmias and ventricular ectopy

☐ May cause decreased blood pressure in low doses, especially if patient is volume depleted owing to initial diuresis. Rule out volume depletion before administering, so that a contracted vascular system does not further reduce tissue perfusion

d) Nitroglycerin

☐ Rapid acting

☐ Relaxes smooth muscle causing venous dilation. This causes systemic pooling of blood, decreased venous return, and decreased preload (this reduces myocardial oxygen demand and consumption)

☐ Vasodilates coronary arteries, improving blood flow and oxygenation to the myocardium

☐ Indicated for LV failure, post cardiac surgery, hypertension, angina pectoris, congestive heart failure

☐ Intravenous nitroglycerin if used early can help prevent or limit ischemia and may reduce infarct size. Should be given immediately with onset of chest pain for best results

□ Readily absorbed into plastic bags and tubing—use special nonabsorbable administration sets

□ Patient must have an arterial line to monitor blood pressure

□ Should infuse via a volumetric infusion pump for accuracy and safety

□ Patient's hemodynamics should be monitored with pulmonary artery catheter and arterial line

□ Intravenous nitroglycerin usually started at 5 μg/min and titrated to the lowest amount that produces the desired effect

□ Do not stop administering nitroglycerin abruptly; wean the patient by reducing the flow rate 5 to 10 μg every 15 minutes and observe for returning symptoms such as hypertension or ischemic symptoms

□ Side effects—hypotension, sweating, nausea, tachydysrhythmias and bradydysrhythmias, headache

  iv. Evaluation of nursing care

    (a) Patient will not experience anginal attacks or attacks will be less severe

    (b) Patient is without dysrhythmias, as evidenced by cardiac monitoring

    (c) Vital signs remain within normal limits for that patient

    (d) ECG shows stable, nonlethal rhythm

    (e) Laboratory data on arterial blood gases and electrolytes are within normal limits for patient

    (f) Patient appears calm

    (g) Patient/SO will identify risk factors associated with coronary artery disease and determine patient's own risk factors

    (h) Patient/SO will describe appropriate methods they will use in order to control risk factors

    (i) Patient/SO will identify precipitating factors of angina, will show evidence of understanding about each medication that patient is taking, and will describe signs and symptoms indicative of advancing disease

 c. Potential for decreased CO and tissue perfusion: related to dysrhythmias and conduction defects

  i. Assessment for defining characteristics

    (a) Hemodynamic readings vary from normal

    (b) Dysrhythmias noted on monitor/ECG

    (c) Decreased peripheral pulses

   (d) Cyanosis

   (e) Altered mental status

   (f) Oliguria, anuria

   (g) Decreased blood pressure

   (h) Cold, clammy skin

   (i) Sluggish capillary refill

   (j) Abnormal electrolyte and digoxin levels

   (k) Hypoxia

   (l) Dyspnea, shortness of breath

 ii. Expected outcomes

   (a) Patient is free of dysrhythmias

   (b) CO is adequate to maintain hemodynamic stability and to maintain cerebral, renal, myocardial, and peripheral perfusion. (Patient is without chest pain or dysrhythmias, has urine output more than 30 ml/hr, and is oriented to time, person, and place.)

   (c) Patient is calm

 iii. Nursing interventions (monitored patient)

   (a) Document rhythm strip per unit standards, and note what lead patient is monitored in

   (b) Obtain 12-lead ECG when a dysrhythmia is noted

   (c) Ascertain patient's response to the dysrhythmia, verbally and with vital signs

   (d) Notify physician especially for dysrhythmias that cause hemodynamic changes

   (e) Support myocardium by administering oxygen therapy

   (f) Monitor/evaluate all vital signs and hemodynamic parameters, noting trends of deviation from expected normals

   (g) Administer fluids as ordered to maintain adequate LVEDP

   (h) Monitor for heart failure (S_3, S_4) and presence of jugular venous distention, hepatojugular reflux, murmurs

   (i) Monitor intake and output closely (keep urine output at least 30 ml/hr)

   (j) Evaluate peripheral pulses for bilateral equality, pulse deficits

   (k) Observe for central nervous system disturbance (e.g., confusion, restlessness, agitation, dizziness)

   (l) Assess for other signs of decreased perfusion (e.g., cool skin, sluggish capillary refill)

   (m) Place patient in semi-Fowler's position

   (n) Monitor electrolytes, blood urea nitrogen, creatinine, acid–base balance

   (o) Weigh patient daily

   (p) Administer vasoactive drugs as ordered—assess patient's

response by monitoring hemodynamic parameters; titrate drugs to maintain blood pressure at prescribed parameters

(q) Observe patient for signs suggestive of inadequate myocardial perfusion (e.g., chest pain, congestive heart failure, pulmonary edema, shock state, dysrhythmias)

(r) Monitor oxygen status, via arterial blood gas analysis, Sv_{O_2}, pulse oximeter

(s) Auscultate lungs for rales, rhonchi

(t) Assist patient with planned, graduated levels of activity; allow patient to rest between nursing activities

(u) Provide environment conducive to rest

(v) Administer narcotics and analgesics as ordered

(w) Prevent complications associated with the use of the flow-directed balloon tipped catheter (see p. 197)

(x) Support myocardium through the administration of pharmacologic agents (see pp. 214–217) and antidysrhythmics per orders

(1) The grouping of drugs is based on the drug's electrophysiologic action on the heart and its autonomic effects

(2) The purpose of antidysrhythmic drug therapy is to depress pacemaker activity and to modify areas with impaired conduction. This is achieved by altering the sodium and calcium channels, prolonging the effective refractory period of the action potential (AP) curve, and blocking sympathetic effects on the heart

(3) Class I drugs—depress the maximum rate of depolarization by depressing the fast sodium channels during phase 0 of the AP curve. They also depress the conduction of the cardiac impulse and decrease the excitability of the heart. Class I drugs are subdivided into three groups based on the intensity of their action

(4) Class I-A

a) Moderately depress the rate of depolarization and prolong repolarization by lengthening phase 3 of the AP curve; are negative inotropic agents and decrease automaticity, excitability, and conduction velocity

b) Useful in controlling the reentry type of dysrhythmias originating in the atria, AV junction, or ventricles

c) Examples—quinidine, procainamide, disopyramide phosphate

(5) Class I-B drugs

a) Suppress ventricular automaticity by decreasing

slope of phase 4 of AP curve and increasing the threshold potential of the ventricles. Some act on the Purkinje fibers themselves; others decrease automaticity throughout the heart. They shorten phase 3 of AP curve

b) Act selectively on ischemic or diseased tissue; block conduction and interrupt reentry circuits; are indicated in the treatment of symptomatic ventricular dysrhythmias

c) Examples—lidocaine, phenytoin, tocainide, mexiletine

(6) Class I-C drugs

a) Greatly prolong cardiac conduction (more than class I-A and I-B drugs) and markedly depress His-Purkinje and intraventricular conduction

b) Are very effective for use on drug-resistant ventricular dysrhythmias, particularly ventricular tachycardiaa

c) Examples—flecainide, encainide

(7) Class II drugs—beta-adrenergic blockers. As a group, these drugs block the effects of beta₁ stimulation on the heart. As a result, myocardial contractility is depressed, AV conduction time is prolonged, the heart rate is slowed (preserving oxygen consumption), and blood pressure decreases. Because the heart rate is slowed, diastolic filling time is increased—this improves coronary perfusion and myocardial oxygen supply

a) This is accomplished by

☐ Depressing SA node automaticity

☐ Increasing refractory period of atrial and AV junctional tissue

☐ Shortening the AP duration and the refractory period of the Purkinje fibers

b) Useful in controlling ventricular response to supraventricular tachycardia secondary to reentry mechanism, atrial dysrhythmias, angina, and hypertension

c) Are indicated in treatment of hypertension, angina pectoris, obstructive hypertrophic cardiomyopathies, and tachydysrhythmias of reentrant origin

d) Are contraindicated in cardiac failure, cardiogenic shock, bronchial asthma, sinus bradycardia, insulin-dependent diabetes, and greater than first-degree AV block *e)* Side effects—excessive slowing of heart rate, hypotension, fatigue, insomnia, depression, gastrointestinal upset, impotence

f) Examples—propranolol, metoprolol, nadolol, timolol, atenolol

(8) Class III drugs—prolong the effective refractory period, with little effect on conduction throughout the heart

    a) Amiodarone suppresses SA and AV node automaticity and increases the effective refractory period thus prolonging repolarization and refractoriness of all cardiac tissue. Used for both supraventricular and ventricular tachydysrhythmias

    b) Bretylium increases the threshold potential and prolongs the effective refractory period of ventricular and Purkinje fibers. Is used mainly for the treatment of ventricular tachycardia and ventricular fibrillation in patients not responding to other agents (e.g., lidocaine and procainamide)

(9) Class IV drugs—calcium-channel blockers (see Table 2–1)

    a) Alter the electrochemical properties of myocardial cells, causing them to react more slowly to electrical impulses. Depresses automaticity in the SA and AV nodes.

    b) Block the slow calcium current in the AV junctional tissue. This prolongs the conduction time in the AV junction and increases its refractory period

    c) Decrease the movement of calcium into the smooth muscle (decreasing afterload by decreasing systemic vascular resistance and improving coronary blood flow and oxygen supply) and myocardial cells (producing a negative inotropic effect)

    d) Some decrease the rate of discharge from SA node and inhibit conduction through the AV junction—negative chronotropic and dromotropic effects. This helps reduce myocardial oxygen demand and increase myocardial oxygen supply (by increasing diastolic filling time when heart rate slows)

    e) Verapamil is a calcium-channel blocker with the stated effects above. (Nifedipine and diltiazem predominantly affect the vascular smooth muscle tone by decreasing the actin–myosin ability to bind calcium. This results in dilatation of the coronary arteries. Hence, these are drugs commonly used to control angina.)

    f) Are indicated in the treatment of supraventricular tachydysrhythmias due to AV junctional reentry and reentry involving accessory AV pathways; since they directly vasodilate the coronaries, they are effective to prevent coronary vasospasm of Prinzmetal's angina and chronic and unstable angina

    g) Are contraindicated in hypotensive states, LV dysfunction, and AV blocks

    h) Side effects—dizziness, flushing, headache, gastrointestinal upset, nervousness, bradycardia, hypotension, conduction disturbances

    i) May be given in combination with beta blockers and nitrates

(10) Digitalis glycosides—these are not classed as antidysrhythmics. However, they have effects on the heart and the electroconductive system and hence are used to treat certain supraventricular tachycardias (i.e., they slow down the rates of atrial fibrillation, atrial flutter, and paroxysmal atrial tachycardia) and are used to treat congestive heart failure

    a) Decrease automaticity in the SA node and increase automaticity in atrial and ventricular muscle

    b) Slow conduction velocity through the AV junctional tissue and Purkinje fibers; thus ventricular response is slowed

    c) Increase the effective refractory period on the AV junctional tissue and Purkinje fibers

    d) Have negative chronotropic and positive inotropic effects

    e) Also help improve stroke volume and CO; relieve congestion; as a result, blood flow to kidneys is improved and urine output increases

    f) Therapeutic serum level of digoxin is 0.8 to 2.4 ng/ml

    g) Patients become more toxic in the presence of decreased renal and liver function, hypokalemia, hypomagnesemia, hypocalcemia, alkalosis, and hypoxia

    h) Signs of toxicity are any dysrhythmias or conduction defects, gastrointestinal upset, visual disturbances, headache, fatigue, and restlessness

iv. Evaluation of nursing care
    (a) Hemodynamic readings within normal limits
    (b) Without dysrhythmias
    (c) Peripheral pulses present and equal bilaterally
    (d) Vital signs within normal limits
    (e) Skin warm and dry; mucosa pink
    (f) Capillary refill brisk
    (g) Urine output > 30 ml/hr
    (h) Sv_{O_2} >60% to 80%; arterial blood gases within normal limits; lungs clear to auscultation
    (i) Without S_3, S_4, positive hepatojugular reflux and jugular venous distention
    (j) Electrolytes, blood urea nitrogen, and creatinine values within normal limits
    (k) Patient oriented to person, time, and place,
    (l) Patient remains calm
    (m) Patient is pain free

Myocardial Infarction (MI): Necrosis of myocardial tissue due to relative or absolute lack of blood supply to the myocardium
1. Pathophysiology (see that for coronary artery disease, p. 205)
2. Etiology or precipitating factors
    a. Atherosclerotic heart disease (CAD; see p. 205)
    b. Coronary artery spasm
    c. Coronary artery embolism
3. Nursing assessment data base
    a. Nursing history
       i. Subjective findings—see angina, p. 207
      ii. Objective findings
         (a) See angina, p. 207
         (b) Also observe for complications associated with MI
            (1) Dysrhythmias and conduction defects of all types
            (2) Congestive heart failure, pulmonary edema (see p. 242)
            (3) Cardiogenic shock (see p. 299)
            (4) Systemic or pulmonary thromboembolism
            (5) Papillary muscle rupture, mitral insufficiency (see p. 261)
            (6) Dressler's syndrome (pericarditis occurring 2 to 4 weeks after MI; probably due to an autoimmune antibody response from released antigens of necrotic myocardial tissue)
            (7) Ventricular aneurysm/rupture
            (8) Ventricular septal defect (see p. 275)
    b. Nursing examination of the patient (review pp. 152–166)

i. Inspection
(a) Patient very anxious, fearful, weak
(b) Complains of constant chest pressure or discomfort that may be described as severe; it generally lasts longer than 30 minutes or more and is unrelieved with rest or nitrates. Patient may describe radiation of the discomfort to the neck, jaw, or either arm (most often left) or may describe this as the only discomfort he experiences
(c) Patient may experience nausea and/or vomiting
(d) May be cyanotic
(e) Dysrhythmias noted on ECG
(f) Shortness of breath
ii. Palpation
(a) Skin diaphoretic, cold, and clammy
(b) Thrills, heaves, abnormal PMI; irregular, slow, fast, or thready pulses
iii. Percussion: noncontributory
iv. Auscultation
(a) Ventricular (diastolic) gallop S_3 or presystolic (atrial) gallop S_4
(b) Pericardial friction rub
(c) Murmurs
(d) Rales
c. Diagnostic study findings
i. Laboratory findings
(a) Increased leukocyte count, sedimentation rate, and serum enzyme levels
(b) Creatinine phosphokinase (CPK)—normally elevated within 4 to 6 hours, peaks 12 to 24 hours, and lasts for 2 to 3 days. Elevation of CPK alone is not solely indicative of MI because it may be elevated for a variety of reasons, such as surgical procedures or trauma
(c) Lactate dehydrogenase (LDH)—normally elevated within 8 to 12 hours, peaks in 2 to 4 days, and lasts for 10 to 14 days. This enzyme also is not specific to myocardial tissue and its level may be elevated for other reasons as well
(d) Serum glutamic oxaloacetic transaminase (SGOT) is not often used as an indicator of an infarct
(e) Isoenzymes are more specific for cardiac muscle damage
(1) CPK-MB—very specific for myocardial infarction; will not rise in patients with transient cardiac chest pain or in association with surgical procedures as CPK-MM and BB isoenzymes do. Should be 4% greater than total CPK for definitive diagnosis of MI

(2) LDH$_1$ is specific for MI over LDH$_{2-5}$. If the total LDH is elevated and LDH$_1$ is the predominant isoenzyme, then the diagnosis of MI can be confirmed

Enzyme	Onset	Peak	Return to Normal
CPK-MB	4–6 hours	12–24 hours	72–96 hours
LDH$_1$	6–24 hours	24–48 hours	72–96 hours

  ii. Radiopharmaceutical studies (see p. 167) will show areas of infarcts, defects in RV and LV wall motion, and abnormal ejection fraction
 iii. MUGA is used to evaluate the RV and LV wall motion (see p. 167)
  iv. Echocardiogram—two-dimensional echocardiogram is more useful in the diagnosis of RV infarcts than the traditional M-mode echocardiogram. It documents increased RV cavity size, RV performance, and segmental wall motion abnormalities
   v. PET scans (see p. 168)
  vi. Pathologic changes found on ECG (for correlation of clinical manifestations with CAD locations, see Table 2–2)

Table 2–2. CORRELATION OF CORONARY DISEASE LOCATIONS WITH CLINICAL MANIFESTATIONS

Location of Occluding Lesion	Clinical Manifestations
Left main coronary artery	Massive left ventricular infarction
Left anterior descending coronary artery	Anterior infarction with Q waves in the precordial (V) leads Septal infarction with Q waves in leads V$_1$–V$_3$ Apical infarction Right bundle branch block with left anterior hemiblock Mobitz type II heart block and complete heart block
Left circumflex coronary artery	Lateral or inferolateral infarction True posterior infarction
Right coronary artery	Inferior infarction with Q waves in leads II, III, and aVF AV conduction disturbances (first-degree AV block, Mobitz type I or Wenckebach second-degree AV block) Cardiovascular reflexes (bradycardia, hypotension) Right ventricular infarction evidenced by: Elevated systemic venous pressure Decreased cardiac output Minimal to absent pulmonary congestion

Adapted from Conner, R. P.: Coronary artery anatomy: The electrocardiograph—clinical correlation. Crit. Care Nurse 3:72, 1983.

(a) Ischemia
   (1) ST segment depression
   (2) T-wave inversion
   (3) Both changes above may be seen in all leads
(b) Injury—a stage beyond ischemia, but still reversible
   (1) Subendocardial injury—ST segment depression greater than 1 mm; usually transient and returns to normal when the pain subsides
   (2) Subepicardial injury—ST segment and T wave elevation. Usually seen in patients with Prinzmetal's angina and often precedes MI
(c) MI—in general
   (1) Q waves—pathologic, must be at least 0.04 second (1 mm) wide and one fourth of the height of the QRS complex in leads facing the infarction
   (2) ST segment changes
      a) Elevated in leads over or facing infarcted area
      b) Reciprocal changes (ST segment depression) will be found in leads 180° from area of infarction
   (3) T wave changes
      a) May occur hours or weeks after the infarct
      b) Within the early hours of infarction, peaked upright T waves may be seen in leads over the infarct
      c) In leads with ST segment elevation, T wave is often inverted
      d) After several hours or days, the ST segment becomes isoelectric and the T wave may remain inverted
      e) T wave changes may last for weeks and return to normal or remain inverted for the rest of the patient's life
   (4) Changes must be seen in at least two leads. In addition, Q wave changes are normally seen in the lateral precordial leads, representing septal depolarization
(d) ECG changes associated with various sites of acute LV infarcts. Indicative changes—Q wave, ST segment elevation, T wave inversion
   (1) Acute anterior infarction
      a) Indicative changes in leads V_{1-4}
      b) Reciprocal changes in leads II, III, and aVF
   (2) Anterolateral infarction
      a) Q wave and inverted T wave in leads I, aVL, and V_{4-6}
      b) Changes in leads V_{1-6} will be found with extensive anterolateral infarction

       (3) Anteroseptal infarction

          a) Indicative changes found in one or more of leads V_{1-4}

       (4) Inferior (diaphragmatic) infarction

          a) Indicative changes in leads II, III, aVF, and occasionally the lateral precordial leads

          b) Reciprocal changes in leads I, aVL, and precordial leads of anterior chest

       (5) Lateral wall infarction

          a) Indicative changes seen in leads I, aVL, and V_{5-6}

          b) Reciprocal changes in leads II, III, and aVF

       (6) Posterior wall infarction

          a) No leads truly reflect posterior surface of the heart

          b) Diagnosis of infarct is inferred from reciprocal changes seen in anterior chest leads V_{1-3}

          c) Abnormally tall R waves seen in V_1 and V_2

          d) ST segment depression in leads V_{1-3}

          e) Tall T waves in leads V_{1-3}

       (7) Subendocardial infarction (non–Q wave MI)—infarcts of endocardial surface do not produce abnormal Q waves in facing leads because part of myocardium is still electroactive

          a) No abnormal Q waves seen

          b) ST segment depression and T wave inversion in leads facing epicardial surface overlying infarct

    (e) ECG changes associated with RV infarction (using right precordial chest leads)

       (1) Suspect RV infarction in the setting of inferior wall infarction

       (2) In RV infarction, ST elevation will be seen in leads V_{4-6}

4. Nursing diagnoses

   a. See Commonly Encountered Nursing Diagnoses, pp. 200–205

   b. Alteration in comfort (chest pain), related to decreased coronary blood flow inducing myocardial ischemia or infarct. The patient may be a candidate for intracoronary (performed during coronary arteriography) or intravenous thrombolysis (Table 2–3). The patient/SO will have to be prepared for this procedure using the usual teaching methods. The major goal is to decrease the mortality rate during the acute period and increase myocardial salvage. Thrombolysis accomplishes this by lysing the fibrin clot

     i. Assessment for defining characteristics

       (a) Patient must be symptomatic for less than 4 hours

       (b) Angina for at least 30 minutes' duration not relieved with nitroglycerin

Table 2–3. THROMBOLYTIC AGENTS

Thrombolytic Agent	Source	Mode of Action	Agent Characteristics	Route Administered	Dosage	Resultant Effects/ Complications
Streptokinase	Enzyme derived from beta-hemolytic *Streptococcus* bacteria	A catalyst in converting plasminogen to plasmin, which then dissolves the clot	Pharmacologic half-life is 18 minutes; has systemic lytic effects (because of circulating plasmin); lasting 24–36 hours	Intravenous	750,000–1.5 million IU (total dose) (Brewer & Marks, 1986); up to 2 million IU (total dose) (Quaal, 1986)	Potential for hemorrhage, allergic reactions, reperfusion dysrhythmias
Streptokinase	Same	Same	Same	Intracoronary	130,000–400,000 IU (total dose) (Brewer & Marks, 1986); 130,000–295,000 IU (total dose) (Quaal, 1986); 100,000–400,000 IU (total dose) (Tilkian & Daily, 1986)	Same
Urokinase	Enzyme produced by human renal parenchymal cells; it is secreted by the kidney and obtained from urine	Acts directly on plasminogen forming plasmin, which dissolves the clot	Nonantigenic; much fewer systemic lytic effects than streptokinase; half-life is 20 minutes; thrombolytic effects last 12–24 hours	Intracoronary Intravenous	2,000–24,000 U/min (Rentrop, 1985); 250,000–2 million IU (total dose) (Tilkian & Daily, 1986) 4,000–8,000 U/min (Topol, 1987); 2–3 million U (total dose) (Topol, 1987)	No allergic responses; decreased potential for hemorrhage
Tissue plasminogen activator	Serine protease produced naturally by the body found in tissues including endothelium and organs	Converts to plasmin only when it comes in contact with the fibrin clot surface; it is the body's own natural fibrinolytic system	Nonantigenic; systemic lytic effects; very short half-life (2 minutes); thrombolytic effects last only 25–50 minutes	Intravenous	0.5–1.0 mg/kg over 60–90 minutes (Quaal, 1986); usual total dose is 100 mg	No allergic responses; no systemic lytic effects

(c) Ensuing MI with persistent ST segment elevation even with nitroglycerin (in two leads or more)

(d) Coronary artery thrombus secondary to angiographic studies or PTCA

(e) Potential contraindications for thrombolytic therapy

   (1) Recent surgical procedures (within 2 weeks)

   (2) Pregnancy or recent delivery

   (3) History of cerebrovascular disease (less than 3 months)

   (4) Uncontrolled hypertension

   (5) Recent major trauma (less than 6 months)

   (6) Bleeding disorders or recent history of a hemorrhagic event

   (7) Recent organ biopsy

(8) Prolonged cardiopulmonary resuscitation

(9) Severe, advanced illnesses

(10) Severe renal or hepatic disease

ii. Expected outcomes

(a) The coronary artery usually reopens within 30 to 90 minutes. Coronary perfusion increases, which improves myocardial oxygenation with relief of symptoms

(b) The zones of myocardial ischemia and the size of infarcted area are limited

(c) Ventricular function is improved, maintaining an adequate SV and CO

(d) Dysrhythmias are reduced

(e) ECG shows ST segment returns to baseline levels

(f) CPK and CPK-MB will peak and return to normal more rapidly than the usual time frames

iii. Nursing interventions

(a) Be aware of the various thrombolytic agents used (see Table 2–3)

(b) Observe for reperfusion dysrhythmias as blood flow is reestablished; ventricular dysrhythmias are common—monitor ECG; watch for hypotension and bradycardia; administer antidysrhythmics as ordered (usually lidocaine)

(c) Streptokinase, urokinase, and tissue plasminogen activator (t-PA) may cause bleeding into peripheral areas such as the site of the invasive procedure, gums, retroperitoneal cavity, and gastrointestinal tract owing to their nonspecific systemic effects

(1) Monitor patient's coagulation studies

(2) Observe for ecchymotic areas especially at the flank; complaints of back pain

(3) Immobilize the affected limb

(4) Avoid intramuscular injections and arterial needle-sticks for at least 24 hours after the therapy; do not remove central lines while the patient is still thrombolytic

(5) Test stools, emesis, and urine for occult blood

(6) Observe for hypotension

(7) Monitor for neurologic changes

(d) The thrombolytic agent (especially streptokinase) may cause an allergic reaction. Monitor for urticaria, fever, bronchospasm, dyspnea, dysrhythmias, and flushing

(e) Reocclusion may occur—monitor ECG for ST segment changes and dysrhythmias, especially bradycardia; hypotension may occur and the patient may complain of chest pain; the patient is kept on heparin following the thrombolytic therapy—keep PTT at twice that of control

iv. Evaluation of nursing care

(a) ECG shows normal sinus rhythm

(b) Vital signs within normal limits

(c) Patient without signs and symptoms of bleeding (i.e., stools, nasogastric aspirate, and urine are guaiac negative)

(d) Coagulation studies within normal limits

(e) Patient remains neurologically intact—alert, oriented

(f) No complaints of chest pain; ECG is without signs of ischemia or infarct

c. Potential for decreased CO and tissue perfusion, related to dysrhythmias and conduction defects and to depressed ventricular function

i. Assessment for defining characteristics (see p. 217)

ii. Expected outcomes

(a) See p. 218

(b) Patient will have normal ventricular function/hemodynamics providing normal tissue perfusion throughout the body

iii. Nursing interventions—in general, interventions are aimed at decreasing the work load on the heart in order to decrease the myocardial oxygen demand and increasing the myocardial oxygen supply to the heart thus minimizing the size of the infarct. This includes the administration of pharmacologic agents and mechanical device support, all of which has the best success rate within the first 6 hours from the onset of chest pain. Studies show that attempts at limiting size of the infarct after this 6-hour period are much less successful; therapy is then aimed at recognizing and treating complications from the MI

(a) See pp. 218–222

(b) In setting of inferior wall MI, assess for RV infarction

(1) Take 12-lead ECG on left and right chest (see pp. 225–227 for changes associated with LV and RV infarcts)

(2) Monitor hemodynamics and note parameters indicative of LV and RV infarcts

Parameter	Normal	RV Infarct	LV Infarct
RA pressure (CVP)	2–6 mm Hg	↑	Normal
PA systolic (RVP)	20–30 mm Hg	↓	Normal or ↑
PA diastolic	10–20 mm Hg	↓	↑
PCWP	4–12 mm Hg	↓	↑
LVEDP	5–12 mm Hg	↓	↑
CO	4–8 L/min	↓	↓
CI	2.5–4.0 L/min/m²	↓	↓
SVR	900–1400/sec/cm⁻⁵	↑	↑

(3) Note for other signs of pending ventricular failure (see congestive heart failure, p. 243)

(4) Administer medications to control afterload, preload, myocardial contractility, and dysrhythmias (nitroglycerin, nitroprusside, dopamine, dobutamine, digoxin, antidysrhythmics to allow the ventricle to work more effectively without increasing stroke work

(c) If the patient fails to progress with traditional therapies, placement of the intra-aortic balloon pump (IABP) is warranted. Patient/SO will have to be prepared for the procedure

(1) Purpose—to decrease myocardial oxygen demand by decreasing myocardial work load, to increase coronary perfusion, and to decrease afterload. This helps limit infarct size if initiated early enough, prevent cardiogenic shock, and improve CO and thus tissue perfusion

(2) Uses—in cardiogenic shock post acute MI, for circulatory support post cardiac surgery if the ventricle fails, in patients with refractory angina when traditional therapy fails, in septic shock, in patients who are poor cardiac risks but need some general surgical procedure, and during cardiac catheterization in high-risk cardiac patients

(3) A balloon catheter is placed via femoral artery into the descending thoracic aorta

(4) The inflation and deflation of the balloon is synchronized with the patient's ECG

   a) The balloon is inflated during diastole—this augments diastolic pressure, which increases coronary blood flow and myocardial oxygen supply. This will improve myocardial contractility

   b) The balloon is deflated just before systole creating a vacuum effect. This helps the ventricle to empty its contents more fully, reducing the LVEDP. In addition, deflation in systole reduces the afterload for the LV (impedance to forward blood flow), decreasing its myocardial oxygen requirements

(5) Contraindications—in patients with aortic insufficiency or severe peripheral vascular disease; if patient has had a past aortofemoral/aortoiliac bypass graft this would prohibit a femoral insertion

(6) Potential complications associated with the use of IABP

   a) Ischemia of the limb distal to insertion site

   b) Dissection of the aorta

        c) Thrombocytopenia

        d) Septicemia

        e) Infection at insertion site

(7) Nursing care associated with the use of the IABP

        a) Monitor vital signs, especially heart rate (IABP timing is based on the heart rate—when rate changes, adjustments in timing of the balloon may have to be made)

        b) Monitor mean arterial pressure—to assess volume status; it should improve with the use of IABP

        c) PCWP—will provide data regarding volume status

        d) Monitor for and treat dysrhythmias early. Irregular dysrhythmias will decrease the effectiveness of the IABP

        e) Assess for effective cardiac output—mentation, urine output, color of skin/mucous membranes, capillary refill; all should be adequate, indicating good response to the treatment

        f) Assess the peripheral pulses, and document their presence and any change from baseline assessment; assess for color, temperature, and sensation changes as compared with other limb. Notify physician of any changes

        g) Monitor insertion site for hemorrhage/hematoma secondary to poor insertion technique and/or anticoagulation

        h) To prevent aortic/femoral injury, elevate head of bed no greater than 30°; patient must not flex leg (log roll patient when turning)

        i) Monitor for migration of catheter up aorta by assessing the pulses in the left arm. If pulses are decreased or absent, then migration has occurred (indicating occlusion of subclavian artery)

        j) Monitor for side effects of anticoagulation: abnormal PT, PTT, platelet count; send all stools, and nasogastric aspirations for guaiac test; check urine for hematuria; note petechiae and oozing of blood from any insertion sites

        k) Monitor for IABP malfunction—must be well versed with this machine and be able to troubleshoot or perfusion technician should be available at all times to intervene

        l) Monitor for signs of local and systemic infection; change dressings per unit standards

        m) Prevent complications related to immobility such

as skin breakdown and respiratory compromise via the usual nursing measures

(d) If the patient does not respond to IABP, the ventricular assist device (VAD) is another option.

    (1) VAD may be used on the left ventricle (LVAD), right ventricle (RVAD), or both (BIVAD)

    (2) In contrast to the IABP, which only augments CO by up to 15%, the VAD provides total support to the heart and circulation. This allows the heart to recover from any type of insult

    (3) The goals of VADs are to provide a CO (CI) sufficient enough to support the tissues and organs with perfusion while allowing the heart to rest and recover from the insult

    (4) Indicated in patients who develop cardiogenic shock post MI or postcardiotomy ventricular failure, in patients awaiting cardiac transplantation whose hearts are no longer able to maintain life, and in patients who cannot be weaned from cardiopulmonary bypass during cardiac surgery

    (5) Contraindicated in patients who

        a) Have sustained prolonged cardiac arrest with central nervous system damage

        b) Are considered to have irreversible myocardial muscle damage and probably unable to be weaned from the VAD

        c) Have chronic liver disease

        d) Are septic

        e) Have severe renal failure

    (6) VADs are often used in conjunction with the IABP in patients with multisystem organ failure

    (7) VADs are most often used in conjunction with the IABP

    (8) VADs are more easily connected to the patient when the chest is open as during surgery. With LVADs, blood is diverted from the LA, bypassing the LV, routed to the pump, and returned to the patient via cannulation of the ascending or transverse aorta. With RVADs, blood is shunted from the RA, bypassing the RV, routed to the pump, and returned to the patient via cannulation of the pulmonary artery

    (9) The cannulae can exit from either the sternal incision or separate parasternal incisions. The chest is then closed. (The chest may remain open in certain instances.)

(10) Nursing implications with VADs

 a) Must work closely with the perfusionist, who usually is responsible for the pump's functioning

 b) Continually assess patient for signs that VAD is working and providing adequate CO—hence, adequate perfusion (monitor intake and output; check capillary refill and temperature and color of skin; assess central nervous system state, i.e., mentation; assess peripheral pulses, vital signs, and hemodynamic parameters. *NOTE:* cardiac output is accurate only with LVADs, not RVADs)

 c) Provide pharmacologic support and adjust to maintain the required parameters as ordered (inotropics to maintain blood pressure and CO, nitroprusside to adjust the SVR, and prophylactic antibiotics)

 d) Monitor for dysrhythmias and intervene per unit standards

 e) Monitor for complications associated with the use of the VAD (thromboembolism, hemolysis) and other signs of complications, such as bleeding (patient is anticoagulated); renal, respiratory, and ventricular failure; infection (both systemic and local); air emboli; and thrombi

 f) While patient is bedridden, provide measures to prevent the hazards of immobility

 g) Must use strict aseptic technique

(11) Weaning begins when the patient's ventricle shows ability to provide support to the total CO. If the patient can maintain a MAP greater than 60 mm Hg, RA and LA pressures less than 20 to 25 mm Hg, and a CI greater than 1.8 L/min, the VAD flow rate is decreased. This makes the patient's ventricle assume more of a role in maintaining total blood flow. The CO, MAP, and mixed venous blood gases are evaluated at this time to assess the functioning of the ventricle. The process continues until the patient is able to provide sole support of blood flow

(e) If the patient is unable to maintain a normal sinus rhythm and/or has conduction defects (all of which may adversely affect CO and functioning of the IABP/VAD), then temporary/permanent cardiac pacing may be warranted

(1) Purpose of cardiac pacing is to provide an extrinsic electrical impulse to the heart so that it depolarizes and ultimately contracts

(2) Indications for pacing

a) Sick sinus syndrome (may require permanent pacing)

b) Symptomatic bradydysrhythmias

c) Second-degree AV block—type I (Wenckebach) may require temporary pacing. However, type I is usually a side effect from drug therapy and reversible with cessation of the drug

d) Second-degree AV block—type II (Mobitz) will probably require a permanent pacemaker

e) Third-degree AV block—when there is total cessation of conduction through the AV junction, the rate of the ventricular escape rhythm that results would not be sufficient enough in most patients to maintain an adequate CO (usually at rates below 40 beats/min). A pacemaker will be required, especially if there is associated symptomatic bradycardia, resultant congestive heart failure, or asystolic periods greater than 3 seconds

f) May be used to override a tachydysrhythmia that resists conversion by drug or electrical cardioversion

g) Very sensitive carotid sinus syndrome causing severe sinus bradycardia and/or AV blocks will probably require a permanent pacemaker

h) Post cardiac surgery

(3) Equipment

a) Leads—made up of a wire and an electrode at the distal end that is in contact with the endocardium. It may be a unipolar or bipolar electrode. The proximal end attaches to a pulse generator (pacemaker)

b) Pulse generator (pacemaker)—power provided by lithium electrochemical cells
   □ Produces the electrical stimulus to initiate depolarization of the myocardium
   □ Manifestation of pacemaker on ECG (Fig. 2–15)—when pacemaker is in control, it produces a pacing artifact (spike) on the ECG prior to the depolarization waveform, indicating capture

c) Temporary pacemakers—used for short-term pacing. Routes of pacing
   □ Transthoracic epicardial pacing—electrodes may be attached to the epicardium (atrium, ventricle, or both) during cardiac surgery (in anticipation of dysrhythmias and conduction

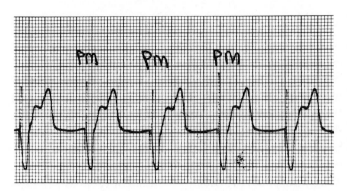

Figure 2–15. Electrocardiographic rhythm strip showing appropriate pacemaker capture *(PM)*. A pacemaker spike immediately precedes each ventricular complex. (From Sanderson, R. G., and Kurth, C. L.: The Cardiac Patient: A Comprehensive Approach, 2nd ed. W. B. Saunders Co., Philadelphia, 1983, p. 233.)

defects postoperatively); proximal end then exits through the chest wall and attaches to the generator
- ☐ Transvenous endocardial pacing—the pacing catheter is placed via a percutaneous route into the RV or RA appendage for pacing. The proximal end is then attached to the generator
- ☐ External transcutaneous pacemaker—used during cardiac arrests while awaiting the placement of a transvenous catheter. Skin electrodes (conducting pads) are placed over the base and apex of the heart. They are connected to an external synchronous or asynchronous pacemaker that can deliver 50 to 200 mV

d) Permanent pacemakers—the leads are placed into the endocardium with the help of fluoroscopy usually through the transvenous approach. The generator is then implanted into the patient (usually over the pectoralis major muscle or over the abdomen). These pacemakers are often programmable, that is, as the patient's requirements for pacing change, so can the settings of the pacemaker usually without any invasive procedures

e) Modes of pacing
- ☐ Asynchronous (fixed-rate) pacemakers. These discharge impulses to either the atrium, ventricle, or both at a pre-set rate regardless of any intrinsic electrical activity. This mode is reserved for those instances when no electrical activity is present in the atrium or ventricle to avoid any competition between the pacemaker and the heart's own impulses and thus avoid the possibility of lethal ventricular dysrhythmias

☐ Synchronous (demand) pacemakers are most often used today. These are able to sense the patient's own inherent impulses. An optimal heart rate is determined for the patient. If the patient's rate falls below that set rate, the pacemaker will sense this and discharge an impulse to the appropriate chamber(s), causing the rate to remain at the prescribed level. Dual-chamber synchronous pacing is optimal to use since it is the closest to the physiologic normal; it maintains normal AV sequence of electrical depolarization and therefore facilitates atrial kick. CO is greatly enhanced. In addition, some AV sequential pacemakers are rate responsive. They discharge impulses based on the patient's physiologic need. AV sequential pacemakers also eliminate competition and the resultant complications (Fig. 2–16).

☐ Pacemakers can be set to pace either chamber or both, sense either chamber or both, sense one and pace the other, etc. Some are programmable, and some can detect tachycardias and terminate the dysrhythmia automatically or be activated by the patient when they perceive a fast rate. There are many combinations. The Inter-Society Commission for Heart Disease (ISCHD) has developed a coding system that explains functioning of the pacemaker (Table 2–4)

f) Complications associated with the insertion of pacemakers

☐ Infection either systemic or local

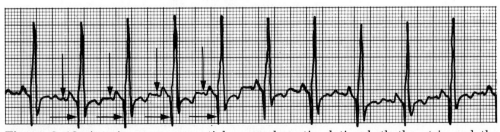

Figure 2–16. Arteriovenous sequential pacemaker stimulating both the atria and the ventricles. Vertical arrows indicate atrial pacing spikes; horizontal arrows indicate ventricular pacing spikes. (From Hudak, C. M., et al.: Critical Care Nursing. J. B. Lippincott Co., Philadelphia, 1986, p. 148.)

Table 2–4. PACEMAKER CODE (1987)

Code Positions				
I *Chamber* *Paced*	*II* *Chamber* *Sensed*	*III* *Response to* *Sensing*	*IV* *Programmable* *Functions*	*V* *Antitachyarrhythmia* *Functions*
V, ventricle	V, ventricle	T, triggers pacing	P, programmable rate and/or output	P, overdrive pacing
A, atrium	A, atrium	I, inhibits pacing	M, multiprogrammability of rate, output, sensitivity, etc.	S, shock D, dual (P&S)
D, double	D, double	D, triggers and inhibits pacing	C, communicating functions (telemetry)	O, none
O, none	O, none	O, none	R, rate modulation O, none	

(From Phillips, R. E., and Feeney, M. K.: The Cardiac Rhythms: A Systematic Approach to Interpretation, 3rd ed. Philadelphia, W. B. Saunders, 1990; modified from Bernstein, A. D., Camm, A. J., Fletcher, R. D., et al.: The NASPE/BPEG generic pacemaker code for antibradyarrhythmia and adoptive-rate pacing and antitachyarrhythmia devices. PACE 10:794–799, 1987.)

□ Pneumothorax especially when the subclavian vein is used for insertion

□ Myocardial perforation

□ Hematoma

□ Dysrhythmias

□ Accidental electrocution

g) Complications associated with the components of the pacemaker system itself

□ Component failure to discharge (pace)—can be due to

● Battery failure

● Lead dislodgement

● Fracture of the lead wire inside the catheter

● Disconnections between catheter and the generator

● Sensing malfunction—these problems will be manifested on the ECG by a loss of the pacemaker spike (Fig. 2–17)

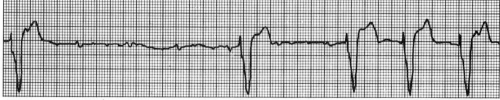

Figure 2–17. VVI pacemaker. Failure to discharge (pace) is indicated by lack of pacemaker spike at appropriate intervals. (From Hudak, C. M., et al.: Critical Care Nursing. J. B. Lippincott Co., Philadelphia, 1986, p. 151.)

Figure 2–18. Failure of pulse generator to capture. (From Phillips, R. E., and Feeney, M. K.: The Cardiac Rhythms, 2nd ed. W. B. Saunders Co., Philadelphia, 1980, p. 347.)

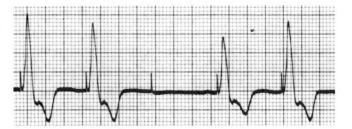

☐ Failure to capture (Fig. 2–18) due to
  ● Low voltage
  ● Battery failure
  ● Faulty connections between the pulse generator and catheter
  ● Improper position of catheter
  ● Catheter wire fracture
  ● Fibrosis at catheter tip
  ● Fracture of catheter
☐ Failure to sense (Fig. 2–19)—the pulse generator fails to sense the patient's own rhythm because of
  ● Improper position of catheter tip/lead dislodgement
  ● Battery failure
  ● Sensitivity is set too low
  ● Fractured wire in catheter—pacemaker spikes occur on the ECG without regard for the patient's inherent rhythm (stimulus may fall during vulnerable period of T wave and induce ventricular tachycardia)—known as pacemaker competition

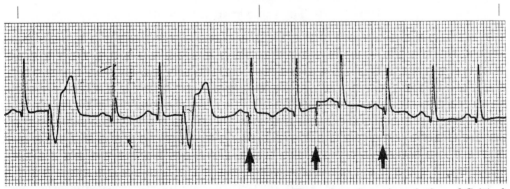

Figure 2–19. Failure of pulse generator to sense. (From American Association of Critical Care Nurses: Methods in Critical Care. The AACN Manual. W. B. Saunders Co., Philadelphia, 1980, p. 145.)

h) Nursing implications for patients with temporary pacemakers

☐ Teach patient/SO regarding need for the pacemaker and about the procedure for placement

☐ Older models whose terminals and connections to temporary unit are exposed must be shielded (use a rubber glove) to prevent contact with sources of 60-cycle currents in order to prevent ventricular fibrillation and getting wet from fluids causing electrical hazard

☐ Ensure all equipment in room is grounded. Avoid simultaneous contact with electrical equipment and patient at the same time

☐ Wear rubber gloves when adjusting electrodes

☐ Cover dials of pacemaker with plastic shield to prevent accidental changes in settings

☐ Limit motion of the extremity at the insertion site. Stabilize arm, catheter, and pacemaker to armboard and avoid movement of arm above shoulder level. Do not lift patient from under the arm. If leg is insertion site, likewise limit its motion especially hip flexion and outward rotation

☐ Ensure that no AC radio, TV, electric shaver, or electric bed are used by the patient

☐ Observe catheter site daily for signs and symptoms of infection

☐ Monitor ECG, obtain rhythm strips per unit standards to document functioning of pacemaker and to detect complications

☐ Monitor vital signs

☐ In the event of cardiac arrest

● Turn pacer on if it is off

● Ensure that the pacing threshold is high enough for pacer to capture by increasing the output (milliamperage)

● Ensure that rate is at least 60 beats/min

● Some pacemakers require them to be disconnected or turned off if patient requires defibrillation; know which type the patient has

i) Nursing implications for patients with permanent pacemakers

☐ Teach patient/SO about the need for and the procedure to implant the pacemaker

☐ Teach patient/SO to check pacemaker function—count pulse daily for a full minute at same time every day; if rate slows five or more beats, check again and, if still slow, call physician

☐ Teach patient/SO to report signs and symptoms, including dizziness; fainting spells; prolonged weakness or fatigue; palpitations; prolonged hiccoughing; swelling of legs, ankles, arms, or wrists; chest pain; difficulty breathing; fever; and redness, swelling, or drainage at surgical site

☐ Stress importance to patient of carrying an identification card at all times, showing patient's name; physician's name, address, and phone number; and type of pacemaker. The wearing of a medical alert bracelet is advisable

☐ Discuss prescribed medications that patient is taking to include name, purpose, dosages, times to be taken, and side effects

☐ Traveling or relocating
  ● Patient should inform physician before traveling; carry list of physicians or hospitals in localities with prepared medical summary to give them
  ● In event of a move, patient should immediately find a new physician for follow-up care

☐ Return to work
  ● Physician will recommend appropriate time to return to work
  ● If job is strenuous, plan modifications or alternatives

☐ Driving a car usually resumes after a month

☐ Exercise
  ● Physician will advise time to begin exercise
  ● Regular, moderate exercise is recommended
  ● Contact sports should be avoided

☐ Sexual relations
  ● Patient can return to degree of activity desired and tolerable
  ● A woman with a pacemaker can tolerate pregnancy

iv. Evaluation of nursing care
    (a) See pp. 222–223
    (b) If patient has an IABP or a VAD
       (1) Patient will exhibit signs of improved CO and tissue perfusion

(2) Peripheral pulses in upper and lower extremities are present and equal bilaterally

(3) Skin warm to touch bilaterally

(4) Patient without signs of bleeding (guaiac tests negative, no hematuria, etc.), no hematoma at insertion site; PT and PTT at recommended levels

(5) Without signs of infection, either local or systemic

(c) If patient has a pacemaker

(1) Patient/SO will verbalize an understanding of the need for and the procedure to place the pacemaker

(2) Pacemaker shows appropriate capture on ECG; without signs of failure to pace, sense, and capture

(3) Patient exhibits no signs of local/systemic infection

(4) Patient/SO relate

  a) Appropriate measures to take when traveling
  b) How to monitor the pacemaker for proper function
  c) Measures to take if pacemaker shows signs of failure

Congestive Heart Failure/Pulmonary Edema: A state in which there is impaired cardiac function such that the ventricle is unable to maintain a CO sufficient to meet the metabolic needs of the body. The LV, RV, or both may fail.

1. Pathophysiology

a. Left-sided heart failure—the diseased LV cannot pump blood returning from the lungs into systemic circulation (decreased contractility) adequately, decreasing CO and elevating LV pressures and volume

b. The LA is then unable to empty its contents into the LV. This raises the pressures within the LA

c. Increased LA pressure is reflected back to the lungs, producing pulmonary congestion

  i. If pressure exceeds pulmonary capillary oncotic pressure (30 mm Hg), fluid will leak into pulmonary interstitial space, resulting in pulmonary edema

  ii. There is decreased oxygenation of blood as oxygen/carbon dioxide exchange is impeded

d. As pressure continues to increase in lungs, pressure in right side of heart increases owing to increased pressure in pulmonary vasculature

e. Right side of heart cannot pump its blood into pulmonary system owing to this increase in pressure

f. Venous return is impeded as the right side of the heart now fails

g. Pressure continues to build, and eventually body organs become congested with venous blood

h. Right-sided heart failure may occur first in the setting of RV infarct

2. **Etiology or precipitating factors**

Left-sided Heart Failure	Right-sided Heart Failure
Atherosclerotic heart disease	Left-sided heart failure
Acute LV MI	Atherosclerotic heart disease
Tachy/bradycardia	Acute RV MI
Cardiomyopathy	Tachy/bradycardia
Increased circulating volume	Pulmonary embolism
Aortic stenosis, aortic insufficiency	Fluid overload, excess sodium intake
Ventricular septal defect	Mitral stenosis
Cardiac tamponade	Atrial or ventricular septal defect
Constrictive pericarditis	Pulmonary outflow stenosis
Mitral stenosis, mitral insufficiency	Chronic obstructive pulmonary disease—pulmonary hypertension (cor pulmonale)

3. **Nursing assessment data base**
   a. Nursing history
      i. Subjective findings: patient may complain of chest discomfort, shortness of breath, orthopnea, paroxysmal nocturnal dyspnea, weight gain, decreased urination, swelling of extremities, etc.
      ii. Objective findings

Left-sided Heart Failure	Right-sided Heart Failure
Anxiety	Hepatomegaly
Orthopnea	Splenomegaly
Dyspnea, dyspnea on exertion, nocturnal dyspnea	Dependent pitting edema
Cough with frothy sputum	Venous distention, hepatojugular reflux
Tachypnea	Bounding pulses
Diaphoresis	Oliguria
Basilar rales, rhonchi	Dysrhythmias
Cyanosis	Elevated CVP, RA, and RV pressures
Hypoxia, respiratory acidosis	Kussmaul's sign
Elevated PA diastolic, PCWP	Murmur of tricuspid insufficiency
Nocturia	S_3, S_4 heart sounds
Mental confusion	Fatigue, weakness
S_3, S_4 heart sounds	Abdominal pain
Fatigue, weakness, lethargy	Anorexia
Murmur of mitral insufficiency	Chest x-ray film shows enlarged RA and RV
Chest x-ray film shows enlarged LV and LA, pulmonary effusion	Weight gain
Pulsus alternans	

(a) In the setting of MI with LV failure, the patient may be classified into one of four classes based on objective findings (devised by Killip). Prompt aggressive therapy is the key to reducing the mortality rate
   (1) Class I—no failure
      a) No clinical or x-ray signs of failure
      b) Excellent short- and long-term prognosis

    (2) Class II—early, mild to moderate failure. Character-
ized by

    a) S_3

    b) Dysrhythmias

    c) Crackles in lower bases

    d) Pulmonary congestion on x-ray film

    e) Condition worsens on exertion

    f) Low CO

    g) Short-term mortality is three to five times greater
than patients in class I

    (3) Class III—acute pulmonary edema

    a) Extreme dyspnea

    b) Anxiety

    c) Orthopnea

    d) Diffuse pulmonary congestion with interstitial and
alveolar edema

    e) S_3

    f) Mortality is five times greater than patients in
class I

    (4) Class IV—cardiogenic shock. For signs and symptoms,
see pp. 304–305

  b. Nursing examination of the patient (see objective findings in section
just presented)

  c. Diagnostic study findings: based mainly on the pathophysiologic
findings stated in previous section (mostly found on physical examination)

4. **Nursing diagnoses**

  a. See Commonly Encountered Nursing Diagnoses, pp. 200–205

  b. Decreased CO and tissue perfusion related to damaged myocardium,
decreased contractile state, dysrhythmias, and conduction defects

  c. Potential for excess fluid volume due to ineffective pumping of the
heart

    i. Assessment for defining characteristics (see p. 243)

    ii. Expected outcomes

    (a) Volume status is stabilized as evidenced by normal respi-
ratory examination, lungs clear on x-ray film, normal
cardiac examination, decrease in edema, decrease in
weight, balanced intake and output

    iii. Nursing interventions

    (a) Monitor ECG and institute appropriate therapy if dys-
rhythmias occur

    (b) Provide for bed rest—semi-Fowler's position for ease of
breathing

    (c) Administer oxygen therapy

    (d) Monitor intake and output closely

   (e) Follow fluid and sodium restrictions closely

   (f) Observe for signs and symptoms of decreased perfusion to brain—if patient is disoriented, protect from injury

   (g) Weigh patient daily

   (h) Assess patient for signs and symptoms indicating excessive systemic fluid volume (i.e., distended neck veins, peripheral edema, hepatic/visceral congestion)

   (i) Monitor laboratory data, especially arterial blood gases, electrolytes, especially potassium (patient may be receiving cardiac glycosides, potential for toxicity is greater with hypokalemia, and patient may become hypokalemic on diuretics)

   (j) Maintain relaxed, quiet environment to provide rest

   (k) Organize nursing care to allow for rest periods

   (l) Monitor hemodynamic parameters closely, especially when using vasoactive drugs

   (m) Note any changes in patient from initial physical examination to detect worsening of congestive heart failure

   (n) If patient is on bed rest for prolonged period, institute measures to prevent hazards of immobility

   (o) Administer diuretics as ordered

      (1) Some diuretics inhibit the distal renal tubular reabsorption of sodium and some inhibit chloride transport in the ascending loop of Henle

      (2) Effects (regardless of their site of action) are to promote excretion of water from the body

      (3) Complications

         a) Electrolyte imbalances, particularly decrease in sodium and potassium levels

         b) Fatigue

         c) Hypovolemia

         d) Nausea, vomiting

         e) Headache

         f) Dry mouth

         g) Muscle cramps

         h) Dizziness

   (p) Assess cardiac and respiratory system for signs of failure

   (q) In extreme cases may have to assist in phlebotomy or use rotating tourniquets (usually when pulmonary edema is present)

   (r) Administer positive inotropic drugs as ordered

      (1) Cardiac glycosides

      (2) Amrinone

         a) Directly increases myocardial contractility without

increasing the heart rate by increasing cellular levels of cyclic adenosine monophosphate (AMP)

   b) Directly relaxes vascular smooth muscle producing peripheral vasodilation (decreases afterload and preload)
   c) Used when patient does not respond to glycosides, diuretics, and vasodilators
   d) Initial bolus of 0.75 to 1.5 µg/kg over 2 to 3 minutes followed by an infusion of 5 to 10 µg/kg/min. Total dose not to exceed 18 mg/kg in 24 hours
   e) Side effects include thrombocytopenia, hypotension, dysrhythmias, and hypersensitivity reactions
   f) Nursing implications
      ☐ Monitor blood pressure closely and if it falls, then stop infusion
      ☐ Contraindicated in patients with severe pulmonic or aortic valvular disease
      ☐ Monitor platelet count
   (s) Administer morphine as ordered
      (1) Induces vasodilation; decreases venous return to heart
      (2) Reduces pain
      (3) Decreases anxiety
      (4) Decreases myocardial oxygen consumption
      (5) Side effects include decreases in respiration (apnea, hypoventilation), bradydysrhythmias, and hypotension
   (t) Administer vasodilators as ordered—improve LV function by lowering systemic vascular resistance (and thus decreasing afterload); increase venous capacitance; decrease preload
      (1) Nitroglycerin
      (2) Sodium nitroprusside
   (u) Provide explanations; begin teaching patient/SO in preparation for discharge
iv. Evaluation of nursing care
   (a) See pp. 222–223
   (b) For evaluation for discharge, patient/SO
      (1) Will relate foods high in sodium and will plan appropriate meals, which will be low in sodium
      (2) Will list at least four foods rich in potassium
      (3) Will demonstrate proper method to monitor pulse
      (4) Will list three symptoms that indicate worsening of condition, whether from congestive heart failure or side effects from drugs

(5) Will relate name, purpose, dose, frequency, and side effects of medications being taken

Pericarditis: An inflammation of the pericardial sac
1. **Pathophysiology**
   a. The inflammation is usually a manifestation of a more generalized disease process
   b. Fibrin may deposit on the serous pericardium, causing constrictive pericarditis
   c. Effusions into pericardial sac may occur, causing restrictive pericarditis (cardiac tamponade/effusion)
   d. The fibrin process or the effusion will interfere with the heart's ability to fill adequately
   e. Eventually, the systemic and pulmonary venous pressures increase, systemic blood pressure decreases, and CO falls
2. **Etiology or precipitating factors**
   a. Idiopathic or nonspecific
   b. Acute myocardial infarction (Dressler's syndrome)
   c. Postcardiotomy syndrome or post thoracotomy
   d. Connective tissue diseases such as lupus erythematosus, polyarteritis nodosa, and scleroderma
   e. Infections
      i. Bacterial
      ii. Viral
      iii. Fungal
      iv. Protozoal
      v. Tuberculosis
   f. Trauma (pentrating or nonpenetrating, including surgical procedures such as pacemaker insertion)
   g. Neoplasms (especially metastatic tumors from the lung and breast, melanomas, lymphomas)
   h. Dissecting aortic aneurysms
   i. Radiation therapy to thorax
   j. Uremia
   k. Drug induced
      i. Procainamide
      ii. Hydralazine
      iii. Phenytoin
      iv. Daunorubicin
      v. Penicillin
      vi. Phenylbutazone
      vii. Minoxidil
3. **Nursing assessment data base**
   a. Nursing history
      i. Subjective findings

        (a) Patient complains of sharp or stabbing precordial pain increased with inspiration, lying down, or turning of thorax; may be relieved by leaning forward

        (b) Patient may relate more nonspecific complaints such as fever, joint discomfort, fatigue, weight loss (suggest a systemic disease causing pericarditis)

    ii. Objective findings

        (a) Patient has a history of any of the etiologic findings discussed previously

        (b) Patient has recent history of taking immunosuppressive drugs (i.e., corticosteroids)

b. Nursing examination of the patient (depending on the severity of the pericarditis, may see any or all of the following on physical examination)

    i. Inspection

        (a) Dyspnea/orthopnea

        (b) Cough, hemoptysis

        (c) Mental confusion, restlessness

        (d) Cyanosis

        (e) Pallor

        (f) Jugular venous distention

        (g) Kussmaul's sign (rise in CVP on inspiration) seen in patients with constrictive pericarditis

        (h) Pulsus paradoxus

    ii. Palpation

        (a) Tachycardia

        (b) Fever

        (c) Hepatojugular reflux

        (d) Decreased or absent peripheral pulses

    iii. Percussion: noncontributory

    iv. Auscultation

        (a) Pericardial friction rub

        (b) Heart sounds are usually normal except muffled/distant with effusions

        (c) May hear S_2 and S_3 if failure is present

        (d) If valvular dysfunction, then murmurs may be heard

        (e) Narrowed pulse pressure

c. Diagnostic findings

    i. ECG changes with acute pericarditis

        (a) ST segment elevation in two or three limb leads

        (b) ST segment elevation in precordial leads

        (c) ST segment depression in V_1 and aVR

        (d) T wave inverted after ST segment is isoelectric again

    ii. Laboratory studies

        (a) Complete blood cell count may show leukocytosis

(b) Cardiac isoenzymes may be elevated if associated with myocardial infarction

(c) Blood cultures to identify causative organisms and their sensitivity to antibiotics

(d) Antinuclear antibody (ANA) will be positive in connective tissue diseases

(e) Blood urea nitrogen used to evaluate renal status especially when CO is affected

(f) Increased sedimentation rate

iii. Radiologic examination: may be normal or may show cardiac enlargement owing to pericardial effusion, infiltrates of lungs

iv. Echocardiography: may show pericardial effusion, vegetation of valves, and RA and RV chamber dilatation

v. Cardiac catheterization used to

(a) Evaluate severity of constriction

(b) Check need for pericardiotomy

(c) Differentiate diagnosis of pericarditis from restrictive cardiomyopathy

(d) If constriction or tamponade is present, then RV and LV filling pressures increase; CO falls with resultant decrease in blood pressure, narrowed pulse pressures, and equalization of left- and right-sided heart filling pressures

4. Nursing diagnoses

a. See Commonly Encountered Nursing Diagnoses, pp. 200–205

b. Alteration in tissue perfusion related to decreased contractile state from the inflammatory process: see pp. 217–223

c. Alteration in comfort/pain due to the pericarditis

i. Assessment for defining characteristics

(a) Patient verbalizes sharp, stabbing type of pain

(b) Patient displays guarding behavior, impaired thought process, altered time perception, facial expressions of pain

(c) Patient appears anxious

ii. Expected outcomes

(a) Absence of pain

(b) Laboratory values return to normal

iii. Nursing interventions

(a) Assess patient for pain and observe for nonverbal cues of pain

(b) If pain is present, then ascertain its description using PQRST method (see pp. 207–208)

(c) Position patient for comfort—often sitting up and leaning forward will help to increase comfort

(d) Administer medications to relieve pain as ordered (analgesics, narcotics, anti-inflammatory agents)

       (e) Administer antimicrobials if they are not the cause of pericarditis

       (f) If pericarditis is due to uremia, then prepare for dialysis

  iv. Evaluation of nursing care

       (a) Patient states pain is less/or alleviated

       (b) Patient appears more calm, less anxious

       (c) Thought processes within normal limits

       (d) Patient laboratory values show antimicrobial therapy is working (i.e., leukocyte count, complete blood cell count returning to normal or within normal limits, blood cultures negative, etc.)

d. Potential for complications such as tamponade (secondary to effusions), dysrhythmias, congestive heart failure, and death

  i. Assessment for defining characteristics

       (a) See p. 249

       (b) Dysrhythmias seen on ECG

       (c) See p. 243, objective findings of left- and right-sided heart failure

  ii. Expected outcomes

       (a) Patient without tamponade

       (b) Hemodynamics and vital signs within normal limits

       (c) Patient without dysrhythmias

       (d) Patient without signs and symptoms of congestive heart failure

  iii. Nursing interventions

       (a) Monitor patient closely for signs of hemodynamic changes indicative of tamponade; record and report appropriately

       (b) Continuously monitor patient for dysrhythmias and treat according to unit standards

       (c) Monitor for signs and symptoms listed in nursing examination of the patient, p. 248

       (d) Prepare patient for any tests needed to further evaluate status of patient (i.e., x-ray studies, echocardiography, contrast studies, etc.)

       (e) Monitor patient for signs of congestive heart failure

       (f) Keep patient on bed rest

       (g) Continually assess patient's level of anxiety; provide quiet, relaxed environment to reduce stress/anxiety and promote rest

       (h) If tamponade occurs

          (1) Place patient in Fowler's position

          (2) Administer oxygen therapy as ordered

          (3) Prepare patient for pericardiocentesis

          (4) Have emergency equipment readily available

          (5) Monitor peripheral pulses for perfusion

        (i) Ensure a patent intravenous line

  iv. Evaluation of nursing care

     (a) Patient without signs or symptoms of tamponade

     (b) Hemodynamic pressures, vital signs within normal limits without pulsus paradoxus

     (c) Patient is calm

     (d) Patient without signs and symptoms of congestive heart failure

     (e) Cardiac rate and rhythm are normal, without dysrhythmias

Infective Endocarditis: An infection of the heart's endocardial surface and/or the valves

1. Pathophysiology

  a. Direct trauma due to high-velocity turbulent blood flow from valvular insufficiency, septal defects, or local trauma (indwelling catheters, artificial valves) can predispose the endothelial surface to injury. As a response, there is the deposition of platelets and fibrin forming microscopic platelet–fibrin thrombi. This stage is known as nonbacterial thrombotic endocarditis (NBTE).

  b. The heart (particularly the valves) is now set up for colonization by bacteria. Bacteria from other infections in the body (skin, genitourinary tract, lungs, mouth) attach to the valves

  c. As the bacteria or other organisms grow, they cause the deposition of platelets and fibrin (valves on the left side of the heart are more often affected than valves on the right side of the heart), forming vegetations. Eventually valvular tissue is deformed or destroyed by the vegetations and the valves become incompetent

  d. Chronic antigenemia and antibodies cause increased levels of immune complexes in the blood. These cause hypersensitivity reactions (allergic vasculitis) in peripheral parts of the body involving arterioles, vessel walls, and tissue surrounding the vessels

  e. Embolization of the infective material may occur and spread through the body

2. Etiology or precipitating factors

  a. Organisms involved: just about any organism can cause endocarditis. Common organisms involved are

     i. *Streptococcus viridans*—most prevalent causative organism

    ii. *Staphylococcus aureus*

    iii. Enterococci

    iv. *Staphylococcus epidermidis*

     v. *Streptococcus pneumoniae*

    vi. *Pseudomonas aeruginosa*

   vii. *Candida albicans*

  viii. *Aspergillus fumigatus*

b. Rheumatic heart disease predisposes the valves to an infectious endocarditis process
c. Open-heart surgical procedures (especially with prosthetic valve replacements)
d. Congenital heart defects (e.g., ventricular septal defects)
e. Genitourinary surgery
f. Gynecologic/obstetric surgery
g. Dental procedures (extractions)
h. Abscesses on skin
i. Invasive tests, monitoring
j. Intravenous drug abuse
k. Immunosuppressive therapy

3. **Nursing assessment data base**
   a. Nursing history
      i. Subjective findings
         (a) Ascertain patient's chief complaint and history of present illness
         (b) Patient may complain of fever, chills, fatigue, anorexia, nausea, vomiting, arthralgias, myalgias (all due to the bacteremia), back pain (cause unknown), decreased or loss of visual fields (due to embolization), and dyspnea
      ii. Objective findings: patient relates history of any of the etiologic factors listed previously
   b. Nursing examination of the patient
      i. Inspection
         (a) Clubbing of fingers
         (b) May show signs and symptoms of heart failure
         (c) Splinter hemorrhages of nails (due to emboli or allergic vasculitis)
         (d) Petechiae (due to emboli or allergic vasculitis) may be seen on the conjunctiva, chest, abdomen, and mucosa of mouth
         (e) Roth spots (round or oval white spots seen on the retina) (due to emboli or allergic vasculitis)
         (f) Purpuritic pustular skin lesions (due to emboli)
         (g) Janeway lesions (due to allergic vasculitis) are painless lesions on palms and soles
         (h) Osler's nodes (due to emboli or allergic vasculitis) are painful nodules on fingers and toes
         (i) If patient is monitored with ECG, may see conduction disturbances or dysrhythmias if conductive system is affected
         (j) If embolization to brain, may see central nervous system disturbances (e.g., hemiplegia, confusion, headache, tran-

sient ischemic attacks, aphasia, ataxia, changes in level of consciousness)

  (k) Hematuria and oliguria if kidney is infarcted from emboli; glomerulonephritis due to allergic, immunologic reactions

  (l) Tachypnea, dyspnea, hemoptysis, sudden pain in chest or shoulder, cyanosis, and restlessness if lung infarcted

  (m) ECG may show signs of infarction if emboli to heart are present

  ii. Palpation

    (a) Abdominal pain (due to mesenteric emboli)

    (b) Decreased or no pulses in cold limbs, (due to emboli)

    (c) Splenomegaly or pain due to splenic infarction

    (d) May palpate thrills if murmurs are present

    (e) If congestive heart failure is present, then hepatojugular reflux, jugular venous distention, peripheral edema, etc. (see p. 243)

  iii. Percussion

    (a) If there is associated pericardial effusion, may be able to percuss dullness in lower half of sternum

  iv. Auscultation

    (a) Murmurs of insufficiency and stenosis of all valves is possible (due to vegetations on the valve leaflets)

    (b) Decreased or absent breath sounds or adventitious breath sounds if lungs infarcted

    (c) Rales heard if LV fails

 c. Diagnostic findings

  i. Laboratory data

    (a) Leukocytosis

    (b) Anemia

    (c) Elevated sedimentation rate

    (d) Positive blood cultures

    (e) Elevated rheumatoid factor may be present along with elevated circulating immune complex levels

    (f) Abnormal laboratory values associated with affected organs (e.g., kidneys, lungs, heart)

  ii. Echocardiography: may show presence of vegetations on the valves and degree of valvular dysfunction

4. Nursing diagnoses

 a. See Commonly Encountered Nursing Diagnoses, pp. 200–205

 b. Potential for alteration in tissue perfusion due to altered cardiac output related to valvular dysfunction, congestive heart failure, and fluid volume excess

  i. Assessment for defining characteristics

    (a) See pp. 217–218

  ii. Expected outcomes

      (a) CO will be sufficient to maintain adequate tissue perfusion to all parts of body

      (b) Patient will be free of signs and symptoms of congestive heart failure

   iii. Nursing interventions

      (a) Monitor all vital signs and hemodynamic pressures and report changes

      (b) Monitor ECG; watch for dysrhythmias, conduction defects, signs of infarction; and intervene per unit standards

      (c) Assess patient for signs and symptoms of congestive heart failure (see p. 243)

      (d) Monitor for cardiac murmurs

      (e) Additional interventions, see pp. 244–246

   iv. Evaluation of nursing care

      (a) See pp. 222–223

      (b) Patient remains in normal sinus rhythm

      (c) Normal heart sounds without murmurs

c. Ineffective thermoregulation secondary to the infection

   i. Assessment for defining characteristics

      (a) Fluctuations in body temperature between above normal and normal

      (b) If hyperthermic, may see flushed skin; patient feels warm to touch and may be tachypneic and/or tachycardic; extreme hyperthermia may induce seizures; mental status changes may be noted

   ii. Expected outcomes

      (a) Patient will be afebrile

      (b) Patient will have negative blood cultures

      (c) Patient will not be dehydrated, as evidenced by normal turgor, balanced intake and output, normal temperature, and moist mucosa

   iii. Nursing interventions

      (a) Monitor vital signs per unit standards

      (b) Provide measures to reduce the hyperthermia (i.e., administer antimicrobials as ordered, antipyretics, and cooling measures if too hyperthermic; encourage fluid intake [if no evidence of congestive heart failure])

      (c) Assess patient for dehydration

      (d) Monitor intake and output, and weigh patient daily

      (e) Draw blood cultures per unit standards if temperature spikes

   iv. Evaluation of nursing care

      (a) Patient's temperature returns to normal

      (b) Blood cultures negative

      (c) Skin with normal turgor and moist mucous membranes

(d) Intake equals output
d. Potential for embolic episodes secondary to vegetations on the valves
   i. Assessment for defining characteristics
      (a) Patient complains of abdominal pain
      (b) Hematuria
      (c) Central nervous system dysfunction (i.e., altered level of consciousness, strokelike symptoms, seizures)
      (d) Patient complains of chest pain
      (e) Patient exhibits signs of cutaneous embolization (see pp. 252–253)
      (f) Patient's vital signs abnormal
   ii. Expected outcomes
      (a) Patient will be free of/or resolution of systemic embolization
      (b) Affected organs will show normal function as evidenced by normal results of diagnostic tests
      (c) Extremities will have adequate circulation
   iii. Nursing interventions: *NOTE:* This type of embolization is not treated as thrombic embolization (i.e., with anticoagulants); instead treatment is aimed at the infection and treated with antimicrobials
      (a) Continually assess patient for signs and symptoms of systemic embolization
      (b) Observe extremities for positive Homans' sign, swelling, erythema, decreased or absent pulses, coolness, and decreased capillary refill
      (c) Assess patient for signs and symptoms of myocardial infarction; monitor ECG
      (d) Prepare patient for any diagnostic testing
      (e) Send all stools for guaiac test; hematest urine and nasogastric aspirations, etc.
      (f) Monitor all laboratory data for abnormalities suggestive of organ failure
      (g) If pulmonary, myocardial, or cerebral embolism occurs, administer oxygen therapy, position patient for comfort and ease of breathing, and administer pain medication as ordered
      (h) If embolization occurs more than once, patient may have to be prepared for valve replacement
      (i) Patient may need valve repair; prepare patient accordingly
   iv. Evaluation of nursing care
      (a) Patient is free of systemic embolization
      (b) If embolization has occurred, then patient is free of sequelae (without hematuria, with intact central nervous system, without respiratory distress, and with normal ECG,

laboratory values within normal limits, no abdominal pain, negative guaiac tests, etc.)

Cardiomyopathy: A chronic or subacute disorder of heart muscle with obscure or often unknown causes. It often involves the endocardial and sometimes the pericardial layers of the heart. It is most commonly grouped into three classifications: dilated (congestive), hypertrophic (both obstructive and nonobstructive), or restrictive

1. Pathophysiology
   a. Dilated (most common)
       i. Myocardial fibers (fibrils) degenerate
       ii. Fibrotic tissue increases
       iii. Myocardial metabolism is disrupted
       iv. Severe dilatation of the heart occurs often affecting all four chambers
       v. Myocardial contractility decreases, resulting in decreased stroke volume, ejection fraction, and low CO
       vi. There is papillary muscle dysfunction secondary to LV dilatation, resulting in mitral insufficiency
       vii. Congestive heart failure develops, often becoming refractory to treatment, with resultant death
   b. Hypertrophic
       i. Hypertrophy of heart muscle includes the ventricular septum and the free wall of the ventricle
       ii. There may or may not be an LV outflow tract obstruction (previously called idiopathic hypertrophic subaortic stenosis [IHSS], now more commonly referred to as hypertrophic obstructive cardiomyopathy [HOCM])
       iii. Ventricles become rigid
       iv. Left ventricular compliance is decreased
       v. CO may be normal, low, or high
       vi. The process may continue for years with no obvious problems or with slow onset of symptoms or may end with sudden cardiac death as a first sign of the disease process
   c. Restrictive (least common)
       i. Fibroelastic tissue and cellular or molecular material infiltrates the myocardium, endocardium, and subendocardium
       ii. The heart becomes very noncompliant and cannot distend and contract well in diastole or systole
       iii. LVEDP increases: end result is low CO with resultant congestive failure and death
2. Etiology or precipitating factors (It is difficult to say what the causative agent(s) may be, but the following are often associated with the disease process.)
   a. Dilated

      i. Idiopathic
     ii. Infection: viral, bacterial, parasitic, fungal, protozoal
   iii. Metabolic: hypokalemia, chronic hypophosphatemia, thiamine deficiency, protein deficiency, hypocalcemia
   iv. Toxins: alcohol, lead, arsenic, uremia, certain chemotherapeutic drugs
    v. Peripartum or postpartum (common in women with multiple pregnancy older than age 30)
   vi. Neuromuscular disorders: muscular dystrophy, myotonic dystrophy
  vii. Connective tissue disorders: lupus erythematosus, rheumatoid disease, polyarteritis, scleroderma
 viii. Beriberi
   ix. Infiltrative disorders: sarcoid, amyloid

  b. Hypertrophic
      i. Idiopathic
     ii. Strong familial component
   iii. Neuromuscular disorders: Friedreich's ataxia
   iv. Metabolic: hypoparathyroidism

  c. Restrictive
      i. Idiopathic
     ii. Infiltrative: sarcoid, amyloid, hemochromatosis, neoplasms
   iii. Endomyocardial fibrosis
   iv. Glycogen and mucopolysaccharide deposition
    v. Radiation
   vi. Scleroderma

3. Nursing assessment data base
  a. Nursing history
      i. Subjective findings
        (a) Ascertain patient's chief complaint and history of present illness. Patient may complain of aches, fever, syncope, palpitations, dyspnea, orthopnea, fatigue, and other congestive heart failure/pulmonary congestion type symptoms
     ii. Objective findings
        (a) Collect data to rule out other disease processes, such as hypertension, pericarditis, and toxemia
        (b) Collect data to decipher potential etiologic factors such as recent infections, drinking history, current use of medications, pregnancy, and any endocrine disorders
        (c) Patient gives family history of cardiomyopathy or sudden death in young adults
  b. Nursing examination of the patient (Table 2–5)
  c. Diagnostic study findings
      i. Chest x-ray film

Table 2–5. PHYSICAL FINDINGS ASSOCIATED WITH DILATED, HYPERTROPHIC, AND RESTRICTIVE CARDIOMYOPATHY

Cardiomyopathy	Patient Complaint	Inspection	Palpation	Percussion	Auscultation
Dilated	Dyspnea on exertion, orthopnea, fatigue, palpitations	Clinical manifestations of CHF, dysrhythmias on monitor, conduction defects	Narrow pulse pressure, pulsus alternans, cool skin, +PMI laterally displaced, left ventricular heave, peripheral edema, hepatomegaly	Cardiac enlargement, dullness in bases of lungs	Irregular heart beat, third and fourth heart sounds, mitral and tricuspid insufficiency, pulmonary rales
Hypertrophic	Dyspnea on exertion, orthopnea, PND, angina, syncope, palpitations	Dyspnea, orthopnea	Forceful and laterally displaced apical impulse, systolic thrill		Fourth heart sound, may hear a third heart sound, split second heart sound, systolic ejection murmur
Restrictive	Fatigue, weakness, dyspnea on exertion, anorexia, poor exercise tolerance	Dysrhythmias, distended neck veins, Kussmaul's sign	Edema, ascites, +HJR, right upper quadrant pain	Cardiac enlargement, pulmonary congestion	Third and fourth heart sounds, mitral and tricuspid insufficiency

(a) Dilated—in advanced stages, generalized cardiomegaly is seen; pulmonary congestion, pleural effusions, etc., may be seen in congestive heart failure

(b) Hypertrophic—may be normal, but LV hypertrophy and LA enlargement may be seen

(c) Restrictive—often normal; may show mild cardiomegaly with LA and LV enlargement

ii. ECG

(a) Dysrhythmias or conduction defects (i.e., sinus tachycardia, atrial fibrillation, ventricular ectopy, bundle branch blocks)

(b) LA and LV enlargement

(c) Infarction type of changes

iii. Cardiac catheterization

(a) Dilated—in LV failure, the LVEDP, PCWP, and PAP will be elevated, decreasing CO. If RV failure occurs, then the RVEDP, RA, and CVP pressures also rise

(b) Hypertrophic—elevated LVEDP

(c) Restrictive—elevated RVEDP and LVEDP and elevated RA and LA pressures

iv. Echocardiography (both M-mode and two-dimensional)

(a) Dilated—LV dilatation, decreased contractility of LV and RV, elevated end-systolic and end-diastolic volumes, reduced ejection fraction; may show thrombi in LV; demon-

strates functioning of the valves and progressive changes over time
   (b) Hypertrophic—LV hypertrophy, asymmetric septal hypertrophy
   (c) Restrictive—LA enlargement, LV wall thickening; LV wall movement may be reduced
v. Radionuclide tests: may see increased ventricular volumes, decreased ejection fraction, increased uptake in patients with amyloid, defects in cardiac wall in patients with neoplasms, sarcoid

4. Nursing diagnoses
   a. See Commonly Encountered Nursing Diagnoses, pp. 200–205
   b. Decreased CO and tissue perfusion related to depressed ventricular function, dysrhythmias, and conduction defects
   c. Decreased CO and tissue perfusion related to hypertrophic cardiomyopathy and dilated cardiomyopathy
      i. Assessment for defining characteristics
         (a) See Table 2–5
         (b) Signs of congestive failure (see p. 243)
         (c) Dysrhythmias, particularly atrial and ventricular on ECG
         (d) Hemodynamic readings abnormal
      ii. Expected outcomes
         (a) Patient will have an adequate CO to maintain tissue perfusion
         (b) Patient/SO will be aware of activities that aggravate the symptoms of hypertrophic cardiomyopathy
      iii. Nursing interventions
         (a) Hypertrophic
            (1) Administer medications to reduce outflow tract obstruction and improve LV outflow gradient and relieve syncope, angina, dyspnea, and dysrhythmias (i.e., propranolol, verapamil, nifedipine)
            (2) Avoid administering isoproterenol, dopamine, digitalis preparations (in the early stages prior to congestive heart failure) since they increase contractility and hence the obstruction
            (3) Administer anticoagulants when patient is in atrial fibrillation
            (4) See pp. 218–219 for other related nursing interventions
            (5) Instruct patients to avoid activities that may increase the obstruction such as strenuous exercise, Valsalva maneuvers, and sitting or standing suddenly
            (6) Since stress aggravates the outflow obstruction, help

patient identify stressors and teach methods of stress reduction

    (7) Since patient is at risk for endocarditis, instruct patient to notify his dentist prior to any dental/surgical procedures (for prophylactic antibiotics)

  (b) Dilated

    (1) Administer inotropics such as digitalis preparations, amrinone, and dobutamine to improve myocardial contractility and decrease the failure

    (2) Administer diuretics to relieve the congestion

    (3) Administer afterload- and preload-reducing agents such as nitroprusside and nitroglycerin to decrease myocardial work load, improve CO, and decrease pulmonary venous pressure

  (c) In end-stage disease, patient may be candidate for cardiac transplant

  iv. Evaluation of nursing care

    (a) See pp. 222–223

    (b) Patient/SO relates measures to prevent increase in obstruction

    (c) Patient/SO demonstrates effective methods of stress reduction

d. Potential for impaired gas exchange secondary to pulmonary vascular congestion or pulmonary embolism

  i. Assessment for defining characteristics

    (a) Patients at risk are those in older age groups, immobile patients on bed rest, and patients in congestive heart failure, in atrial fibrillation, or who have a dilated myocardium

    (b) Central nervous system symptoms: confusion, somnolence

    (c) Restlessness

    (d) Irritability

    (e) Hypercapnia

    (f) Hypoxia

    (g) Inability to remove secretions

    (h) Tachycardia

    (i) Tachypnea

    (j) Hemoptysis

    (k) Chest discomfort/pain

    (l) Anxiety

    (m) Elevated pulmonary artery pressures

    (n) S_3

    (o) Rales

  ii. Expected outcomes

    (a) Absence or resolution of pulmonary congestion

(b) Absence or resolution of pulmonary emboli

(c) Absence of respiratory distress

iii. Nursing interventions

(a) Employ preventive measures especially for high-risk patients

(1) Assist with passive/active exercises while patient is confined to bed

(2) Apply antithrombic stockings

(3) Encourage patient not to cross legs or feet; avoid using knee joint on Gatch bed

(4) Teach patient to avoid activities that cause straining (Valsalva maneuver)

(5) Administer anticoagulants as ordered (monitor PT and PTT; observe for bleeding)

(6) Position patient so that angulation at groin and knees is avoided; elevate legs when out of bed

(b) Prepare patient for any tests (e.g., lung scans) in the usual manner

(c) Monitor vital signs, hemodynamic parameters, and laboratory values as appropriate

(d) Observe for signs and symptoms listed in assessment for defining characteristics on p. 260

(e) Administer medications as ordered (e.g., digoxin, diuretics, potassium replacements)

(f) Administer supportive measures as situation dictates (e.g., oxygen therapy, pain medication, sedatives, emotional support)

iv. Evaluation of nursing care

(a) Patient is hemodynamically stable; vital signs within normal limits

(b) Patient is without embolic episodes or pulmonary congestion

(c) Lungs are clear to auscultation

(d) Patient is alert and oriented to time, person, and place

(e) All laboratory values, including arterial blood gases are within normal limits

(f) Patient is calm and relaxed

Mitral Insufficiency: The regurgitation of blood from the LV to the LA during ventricular systole owing to an incompetent mitral valve due to an acute or chronic condition

1. Pathophysiology

a. The mitral valve fails to close properly during ventricular systole

b. The LV ejects blood into the aorta and back into the LA as well.

More than 50% of stroke volume may be ejected from the LV into the LA

   c. Acute onset

      i. The LA pressures dramatically increase owing to volume overload. LA size initially remains small

      ii. Pulmonary edema rapidly ensues

      iii. LV function quickly deteriorates; LVEDP rises

      iv. The LV dilates and fails; CO decreases

      v. Pulmonary hypertension may develop owing to compression on pulmonary vascular bed

      vi. Death may ensue if disorder is not promptly treated

   d. Chronic onset

      i. The LA is very compliant and dilates; there is a slow increase in LA pressures but pulmonary artery pressures remain relatively normal (PA pressures may initially be elevated in the early course of the process)

      ii. Due to chronic volume overload on the LV (which occurs with insufficiency), the LV compensates with LV dilatation and eventually hypertrophy

      iii. Pulmonary venous pressures become elevated; pulmonary hypertension ensues, and PCWP rises

      iv. The dilated LV and LA also cause dysrhythmias, notably ventricular and atrial fibrillation

      v. Right-sided heart failure may occur

2. Etiology or precipitating factors

   a. Acute causes

      i. Trauma

      ii. Rheumatic valvular disease or endocarditis may cause rupture of the chordae tendineae

      iii. Papillary muscle dysfunction secondary to myocardial infarction

   b. Chronic causes

      i. Rheumatic heart disease

      ii. Congenital malformations of the mitral valve, chordae tendineae, or mitral ring

      iii. In association with other anomalies (e.g., AV canal, atrial septal defect, hypertrophic cardiomyopathy [obstructive type])

      iv. Prolapsed mitral valve

      v. LV dilatation from other causes

      vi. Marfan's syndrome

      vii. Endocarditis

      viii. Calcification

3. Nursing assessment data base

   a. Nursing history

      i. Subjective findings

      (a) Patient complains of
        (1) Dyspnea
        (2) Orthopnea
        (3) Paroxysmal nocturnal dyspnea
        (4) Weakness/fatigue
        (5) Palpitations
        (6) Symptoms of RV failure
   ii. Objective findings
      (a) Patient relates history of past rheumatic fever, streptococcal infection, endocarditis, ischemia, trauma, mitral valve prolapse

b. Nursing examination of the patient
   i. Inspection: if in failure, may see
      (a) Dyspnea
      (b) Anxiety
      (c) Diaphoresis
      (d) Cyanosis
      (e) Confusion
   ii. Palpation
      (a) PMI is laterally displaced, diffuse, and hyperdynamic
      (b) May feel a systolic thrill
      (c) Pulse may be irregular if in atrial fibrillation
      (d) Hepatomegaly (late sign)
   iii. Percussion
      (a) If heart is dilated, cardiac border will be more lateral
   iv. Auscultation
      (a) May hear rales when pulmonary congestion/edema is present
      (b) High-pitched blowing holosystolic murmur heard best at the apex with radiation to the axilla
      (c) S_2 is widely split
      (d) S_3; may hear an S_4

c. Diagnostic findings
   i. Radiologic
      (a) Chest x-ray film shows LA and LV enlargement in chronic forms; LA will not be enlarged with acute onset
      (b) May see calcification of mitral annulus
   ii. ECG
      (a) LV and LA enlargement
      (b) Dysrhythmias such as atrial fibrillation
   iii. Echocardiography: helps determine the etiology
      (a) LA and LV enlargement with increased wall motion in chronic mitral insufficiency
      (b) Prolapse of mitral valve, mitral annular calcification, flail leaflet, vegetations

(c) Abnormal regional wall motion if papillary muscle dysfunction is cause

   iv. Cardiac catheterization

      (a) Increased LVEDP and LAP

      (b) Increased PAP in chronic cases

      (c) Contrast medium flows from LV into LA during systole

      (d) Calculates regurgitant fraction

4. Nursing diagnoses

  a. See Commonly Encountered Nursing Diagnoses, pp. 200–205

  b. Alteration in CO and tissue perfusion related to valve dysfunction

    i. Assessment for defining characteristics

      (a) See pp. 217–218

    ii. Expected outcomes

      (a) CO will be sufficient enough to maintain adequate tissue perfusion to all parts of body

      (b) Patient will be free of signs and symptoms of congestive heart failure

   iii. Nursing interventions

      (a) Monitor all vital signs and hemodynamic pressures and report changes

      (b) Monitor ECG; watch for dysrhythmias especially ventricular and atrial fibrillation. Intervene per unit standards

      (c) Assess patient for signs and symptoms of congestive heart failure

      (d) Additional interventions, see pp. 244–246

      (e) If the valve is to be surgically repaired, then patient/SO must be prepared for the surgery. Provide explanation of the disease process, preoperative routines, the surgical procedure, including the types of valves used (i.e., Starr-Edwards, Bjork-Shiley, St. Jude Medical, Carpentier-Edwards, Ionescu-Shiley), and what is to be expected during the immediate postoperative period

     (f) Postoperative general care for valve repair is similar to postoperative care for most cardiac surgical operations, (e.g., coronary artery bypass grafting) in which a median sternotomy approach is used; assessing for and preventing the potential complications is of utmost importance (see pp. 213–217 for postoperative care)

     (g) Discharge instructions include the usual postoperative instructions for any heart surgery. If valve was replaced, then the importance of prophylactic antibiotic therapy must be stressed if patient undergoes any surgical/dental interventions in the future

   iv. Evaluation of nursing care

      (a) Hemodynamic stability is evidenced by normal vital signs, lack of dysrhythmias, or dysrhythmias under control without producing hemodynamic changes

(b) Patient does not exhibit an inappropriate amount of anxiety

(c) Patient verbalizes an understanding of the preoperative teachings discussed

(d) Postoperatively, patient is hemodynamically stable; vital signs within normal limits; PAP, PCWP, and CVP all within normal limits; patient is free of other potential complications as outlined on pp. 213–214

(e) On discharge, patient/SO relate an understanding of all postoperative care measures and particularly the need for antibiotic prophylaxis when undergoing future surgical/dental procedures and anticoagulant therapy

Mitral Stenosis: An obstruction of the mitral orifice that impedes the flow of blood from the LA to the LV during ventricular diastole

1. **Pathophysiology**

   a. There is progressive fibrosis, scarring, and calcification of the valve leaflets

   b. The commissures may fuse

   c. The mitral valve orifice is narrowed (in normal adult it is 3 to 5 cm^2)

   d. LA pressures increase as a compensatory mechanism to maintain normal LV filling. As the valve continues to narrow, the LA eventually dilates, often causing atrial fibrillation

   e. If the process continues and the valve orifice narrows to smaller than 1 cm^2, the patient becomes symptomatic with minimal exertion or at rest and usually severe pulmonary hypertension develops (patient becomes symptomatic with extreme exertion with valve stenosis to 2.1 to 2.5 cm^2; at 1.6 to 2.0 cm^2, the patient is symptomatic with moderate exertion)

   f. As the pulmonary capillary hydrostatic pressure rises over the plasma oncotic pressure, fluid escapes into the pulmonary interstitium and alveoli

   g. Pulmonary arteriolar vasoconstriction occurs, and, over time, RV pressures increase with eventual hypertrophy and dilatation. RV failure is inevitable

   h. The stenosis impedes forward blood flow and alone is often enough to decrease stroke volume and CO. In addition, there is the loss of atrial kick (due to the atrial fibrillation) and tachycardia results (compensatory mechanism to maintain some type of CO), all of which decrease LV filling time, further decreasing CO

   i. Atrial clots form, and systemic or cerebral emboli may ensue

2. **Etiology or precipitating factors**

    a. Rheumatic heart disease

    b. Congenital mitral stenosis

    c. Tumors of the LA

    d. Calcification of the mitral annulus

3. Nursing assessment data base

    a. Nursing history

       i. Subjective findings

          (a) Patient will note a gradual decline in physical activity over the years

          (b) Patient gives a history of

             (1) Dyspnea on exertion

             (2) Progressive fatigue

             (3) Cough, hemoptysis

             (4) Orthopnea

             (5) Fatigue

             (6) Signs and symptoms of right-sided congestive heart failure are late signs of mitral stenosis

             (7) Dysphagia (due to enlarged atrium)

       ii. Objective findings

          (a) History of rheumatic heart disease

          (b) History of congenital heart disease

          (c) History of repeated respiratory tract infections

          (d) Patient is often female and in her early 30s

    b. Nursing examination of the patient: findings depend on the degree of failure present

       i. Inspection

          (a) Any of the signs and symptoms of congestive heart failure

          (b) Cheeks may be ruddy (mitral facies)

          (c) Patient may look thin

       ii. Palpation

          (a) May feel RV lift if pulmonary hypertension is present; LV impulse is normal

          (b) Thrill present over apical area depending on the intensity of the murmur

      iii. Percussion: noncontributory

      iv. Auscultation

          (a) See p. 165 for characteristics of mitral stenosis

          (b) May have associated murmur of tricuspid insufficiency if RV failure exists and of pulmonary insufficiency if pulmonary hypertension exists

    c. Diagnostic findings

       i. Radiologic: chest x-ray film reveals

          (a) LA and RV hypertrophy

          (b) Calcification of mitral valve

(c) Interstitial edema, pulmonary vascular redistribution (due to high PCWP)

 ii. Cardiac catheterization

  (a) Calcification of mitral valve

  (b) Elevated LA pressures

  (c) Elevated RV and RA pressures when RV failure is present

  (d) Elevated pulmonary artery pressures, PCWP

 iii. Echocardiography

  (a) Thickened anterior and posterior mitral valve leaflets

  (b) Abnormal movement of leaflets

  (c) Enlarged LA with thrombus may be seen

  (d) Enlarged RV

 iv. ECG

  (a) RV hypertrophy pattern when pulmonary hypertension exists

  (b) Atrial fibrillation

  (c) LA enlargement noted by P mitrale

4. Nursing diagnoses

 a. See pp. 264–265

 b. Potential for systemic/pulmonary emboli related to clots in atrium

  i. Assessment for defining characteristics

   (a) Echocardiography suggests thrombi in LA

   (b) Extremities—patient complains of pain in calf and cold extremities or unequal temperature of extremities; extremities may exhibit pallor, rubor, or cyanosis; diminished or absent peripheral pulses (if arterial emboli); capillary refill sluggish and swelling in affected extremity

   (c) Pulmonary embolism—tachycardia, tachypnea, hypoxia, dyspnea, cough, hemoptysis, elevated PAP, hypotension, pain in chest, abnormal arterial blood gas values, cyanosis, lung scan positive for emboli

   (d) Central nervous system embolism—symptoms of stroke (i.e., paralysis, weakness, dysphasia, confusion, seizures)

   (e) Renal—hematuria, oliguria, back pain, rising blood urea nitrogen value

   (f) Splenic—pain in left upper quadrant with radiation to left shoulder

   (g) Mesenteric—pain in lower abdomen, bloody diarrhea, elevated leukocyte count, and erythrocyte sedimentation rate

   (h) Doppler ultrasound detects diminished/absent arterial/venous blood flow

   (i) Oscillometry used to detect arterial occlusions by measuring pulse volume

(j) Patient is at high risk when on bed rest, in atrial fibrillation, and/or in congestive heart failure

ii. Expected outcomes

(a) Absence or resolution of systemic/pulmonary emboli

(b) Patient is hemodynamically stable

iii. Nursing interventions

(a) Assess for signs and symptoms of peripheral systemic emboli (see assessment for defining characteristics, p. 267)

(b) Elevate extremities that have thromboemboli

(c) See pp. 244–246 for other nursing measures

Aortic Insufficiency: Because of an incompetent valve there is regurgitation of blood from the aorta to LV during ventricular diastole

1. **Pathophysiology**

a. Valve cusps may rupture; vegetations may develop; perforation of the cusps may occur with scarring, degeneration, or prolapse; valves may fibrose and shorten. All of these conditions (due to various causes) prevent the valve from closing properly

b. It can develop acutely. The increased blood flow to the LV produces volume overload, severely increasing the LVEDP

c. It can be a chronic process in which the LV compensates by increasing its forward stroke output to maintain adequate systemic flow (increasing myocardial oxygen demands). Eventually the LV dilates and hypertrophies; LVEDP rises as LV fails and decompensates; stroke volume decreases

d. In addition, there are low aortic diastolic pressures, which decreases blood flow to coronary arteries during diastole

2. **Etiology or precipitating factors**

a. Rheumatic endocarditis

b. Idiopathic calcification of the valve

c. Congenital malformations (ventricular septal defect, bicuspid aortic valve)

d. Bacterial endocarditis

e. Syphilis

f. Rheumatic spondylitis

g. Marfan's syndrome

h. Hypertension

i. Ehler-Danlos syndrome

j. Lupus erythematosus

k. Aortic dissection

l. Rupture of a sinus of Valsalva aneurysm

3. **Nursing assessment data base**

a. History

i. Subjective findings: patient complains of

(a) Easy fatigability

        (b) Dyspnea, paroxysmal nocturnal dyspnea

        (c) Orthopnea

        (d) Increased force of heartbeat, palpitations

        (e) Exertional chest pain (angina)

        (f) Exertional syncope

    ii. Objective findings

        (a) Patient has a positive history of any of the etiologic factors listed above

  b. Nursing examination of the patient

    i. Inspection

        (a) Signs and symptoms of left-sided heart failure

        (b) deMusset's sign (nodding of head)

        (c) Flushed appearance

    ii. Palpation

        (a) Forceful diffuse apical impulse, displaced laterally and downward (in chronic forms); no change in apical impulse with acute onset

        (b) Widened pulse pressure (increased systolic blood pressure, decreased diastolic blood pressure)

        (c) Abrupt rise and fall of carotids and other peripheral pulses; bounding (water-hammer) pulse

        (d) Positive Quinke's sign—visible capillary pulsation of nail beds when fingertip is pressed

        (e) Positive Hill's sign—the popliteal blood pressure is higher than brachial blood pressure by about 40 mm Hg (seen in severe aortic insufficiency)

    iii. Percussion

        (a) Cardiac border may be displaced laterally when cardiomegaly is present

    iv. Auscultation

        (a) High-pitched, blowing, decrescendo, systolic murmur

        (b) Grade I–II/IV in intensity

        (c) Best heard in aortic area and Erb's point

        (d) Often hear S_3 and/or S_4

  c. Diagnostic findings (depend on etiology)

    i. Radiologic: chest x-ray film reveals

        (a) LV enlargement

        (b) Calcified aortic valve

        (c) Pulmonary vascular redistribution; interstitial pulmonary edema may be present

    ii. ECG

        (a) LA and LV hypertrophy

        (b) Sinus tachycardia

    iii. Echocardiography

(a) Dilation of LV cavity with hyperdynamic wall motion in chronic cases

(b) Demonstrates abnormalities of the aortic valve; vegetations

iv. Radionuclide studies: help quantify the degree of regurgitation

v. Cardiac catheterization

(a) Increased LVEDP, LAP

(b) Increased PCWP

(c) Increased right-sided heart pressures in late stages

(d) Low systemic diastolic pressures

(e) Quantification of the insufficiency

4. Nursing diagnoses

a. See Commonly Encountered Nursing Diagnoses, pp. 200–205

b. Alteration in cardiac output and tissue perfusion related to valve dysfunction

i. Assessment for defining characteristics—see pp. 217–218

ii. Expected outcomes—see p. 264

iii. Nursing interventions

(a) See p. 264

(b) Administer the various medications prescribed for the patient (antibiotics, digitalis, diuretics, vasodilators, anticoagulants, oxygen) as ordered

(c) Teach patient/SO about need for a sodium-restricted diet, medications

(d) Encourage activity limitations

iv. Evaluation

(a) See pp. 264–265

(b) Patient/SO describe a diet low in sodium

Aortic Stenosis: Obstruction to the ejection of blood from the LV during systole. Stenosis may be supravalvular, subvalvular, or valvular

1. Pathophysiology

a. Afterload is increased (which the LV must overcome), regardless of the cause of obstruction to LV outflow

b. The LV hypertrophies over time in order to maintain stroke volume and adequate CO

c. This process decreases LV compliance, increasing the LVEDP. Eventually, the LV becomes stiff, fatigues, and dilates. This decreases stroke volume

d. The LA has to work harder to pump blood into the ventricle

e. LA pressures increase, which increase the pulmonary vascular pressure. This leads to pulmonary congestion and eventually increases the pressures in the right side of the heart

f. RV failure ensues

    g. The left side of the heart has to pump against an increased afterload. This increases myocardial oxygen demand

    h. LV hypertrophy and increased LVEDP cause decreased subendocardial coronary perfusion and subendocardial ischemia

2. Etiology or precipitating factors

    a. Rheumatic (the commissures fuse and the valve leaflets thicken and fibrose—symptoms usually seen in patients in their 50s and 60s)

    b. Senile calcific or degenerative aortic stenosis (deposits of calcium are found in the cusps of the valve itself—symptoms usually seen in patients in their 60s and 70s)

    c. Congenital biscuspid valve (symptoms usually seen in patients in their 40s and 50s)

3. Nursing assessment data base

    a. History

       i. Subjective findings: patient complains of

          (a) Syncope

          (b) Fatigue/weakness

          (c) Palpitations

          (d) Angina

          (e) If in left ventricular failure, the patient will have complaints as listed on p. 243

       ii. Objective findings

          (a) Patient has a history of any of the etiologic factors listed above

    b. Nursing examination of the patient: findings will vary widely depending on how the disease process has progressed (e.g., if left-sided failure is present) (see p. 243)

       i. Inspection

          (a) Patient may appear anxious

          (b) Respirations may be labored

          (c) Color of skin may reflect poor oxygenation due to decreased tissue perfusion; may also see shiny skin over shins and absence of hair

          (d) Mental status may be compromised

       ii. Palpation

          (a) Forceful, sustained apical impulse

          (b) May feel a systolic thrill in aortic area

          (c) Delayed carotid upstroke

          (d) Narrowed pulse pressure

      iii. Percussion: noncontributory

      iv. Auscultation

          (a) May hear a paradoxically split S_2

          (b) An S_3 or an S_4 may be present

          (c) A harsh, systolic ejection, crescendo-decrescendo murmur heard best in aortic area, radiating up the neck

   c. Diagnostic findings

      i. Radiologic

        (a) Chest x-ray film shows cardiac enlargement in late stages

        (b) Pulmonary vascular redistribution

        (c) A calcific aortic valve may be seen

     ii. ECG

        (a) With severe atrial stenosis, LA enlargement and LV hypertrophy and strain pattern exist

        (b) Left axis deviation

        (c) May note conduction defects such as left bundle branch block

        (d) Atrial fibrillation in late stages

    iii. Echocardiography

        (a) Decreased or no visible movement of the aortic valve

        (b) LA enlargement

        (c) LV hypertrophy

        (d) Abnormal valve orifice

    iv. Radionuclide studies determine LV function and ejection fraction

     v. Cardiac catheterization

        (a) Elevated LV systolic pressure and LVEDP

        (b) Elevated LAP

        (c) Pressure gradient between the LV and the aorta greater than 50 mm Hg

        (d) Aortic valve area is compromised (normal area is 3.0 to 3.5 cm^2, mild atrial stenosis = 1.0 to 1.2 cm^2, moderate = 0.7–1.0 cm^2, severe = <0.5 cm^2)

4. Nursing diagnoses: see p. 270

Atrial Septal Defect (ASD): A communicating defect of the septum between the two atria

1. Pathophysiology

   a. During fetal development, the formation of the atrium and atrial septum is interrupted

   b. Three common sites of defects (Fig. 2–20)

      i. Sinus venosus: located high in the septum at the junction of the RA and superior vena cava—least common

     ii. Ostium secundum: located in the middle of the septum to the right of the foramen ovale—most common

    iii. Ostium primum: located at the lower end of the septum

   c. Left side of heart has high pressure as compared with right side

   d. Blood flow is shunted during diastole from left to right initially, increasing pulmonary flow and producing volume overload of RA and RV

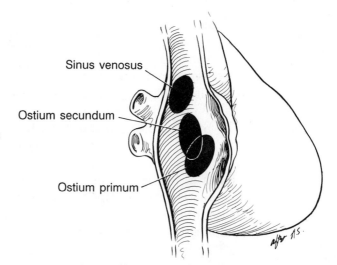

Figure 2–20. The three types of atrial septal defects.

Sinus venosus

Ostium secundum

Ostium primum

    e. Intimal proliferation and medial hypertrophy of pulmonary artery may develop over time and result in pulmonary hypertension

    f. The pulmonary hypertension may cause shunt to reverse right to left

2. Etiology or precipitating factors:

    a. Exact cause is unknown

    b. May be due to

       i. Maternal and fetal infections during first trimester of pregnancy (e.g., rubella)

       ii. Effects of drugs/medications

      iii. Dietary deficiencies during fetal development

      iv. Genetic factors

3. Nursing assessment data base

    a. Nursing history

       i. Subjective findings: complaints of

         (a) Fatigue

         (b) Dyspnea

         (c) Palpitations

       ii. Objective findings

         (a) Most common in women

         (b) History of increased incidence of pulmonary infections during childhood

    b. Nursing examination of the patient (Signs will vary depending on the direction of the shunt. When the shunt reverses to right to left, signs and symptoms of severe heart failure will be present.)

       i. Inspection

         (a) Patient is generally normal in appearance

         (b) Is acyanotic in the absence of right-to-left shunt

         (c) Signs of heart failure in older patients

    ii. Palpation

        (a) Systolic lift along left sternal border due to enlarged right ventricle

   iii. Percussion: noncontributory

   iv. Auscultation

        (a) Widely fixed split of S_2

        (b) Systolic ejection murmur; heard best in second left intercostal space; due to increased flow through the pulmonic valve

        (c) A diastolic murmur may be heard due to increased flow of blood through the tricuspid valve

  c. Diagnostic findings

     i. Radiologic: chest x-ray film reveals

        (a) Enlarged RA and RV

        (b) Increased pulmonary vascular markings

    ii. ECG

        (a) Atrial fibrillation and/or atrial flutter seen in older age groups

        (b) Right bundle branch block

        (c) Right axis deviation in secundum and sinus venosus defects

        (d) Left axis deviation in primum defects

   iii. Echocardiography

        (a) RV enlargement (M-mode)

        (b) The actual defect will be seen with two-dimensional echocardiography

   iv. Cardiac catheterization

        (a) Characteristic finding is an increase (step-up) in oxygen concentration in the RA

        (b) Increased pulmonary artery pressures may be noted

        (c) Determines severity of the shunt

4. Nursing diagnoses

  a. See Commonly Encountered Nursing Diagnoses, pp. 200–205

  b. Alteration in CO and tissue perfusion related to the septal defect

     i. Assessment for defining characteristics: see pp. 217–218

    ii. Expected outcomes: see pp. 264–265

   iii. Nursing interventions

        (a) Monitor all vital signs and hemodynamic pressures and report changes

        (b) Monitor ECG; watch for dysrhythmias, especially blocks

        (c) Assess patient for signs and symptoms of congestive heart failure

        (d) Additional interventions, see pp. 244–246

        (e) Administer prophylactic antibiotics to prevent endocarditis

(f) If the defect is to be surgically repaired, then patient/SO must be prepared for the surgery, including explanation of the disease process, preoperative routines, the surgical procedure, and what is to be expected during the immediate postoperative period

(g) Postoperative general care for septal repairs is similar to postoperative care for most cardiac surgical operations (e.g., coronary artery bypass grafting) in which a median sternotomy approach is used; assessing for and preventing the potential complications is of utmost importance (see pp. 213–217 for postoperative care)

iv. Evaluation of nursing care: see pp. 222–223

c. Potential for infectious process (infective endocarditis) secondary to this congenital heart defect: see pp. 251–252

d. Note additional information

i. Repair of the defect is recommended to prevent the complications of pulmonary hypertension and heart failure

ii. Repair of defect in children may be deferred to age 3 or 4 if symptoms are not severe

iii. In older children and young adults, the repair should be performed before pulmonary hypertension exists; otherwise pathophysiologic changes may be irreversible with ensuing death

iv. A median sternotomy or a right thoracotomy approach is used with cardiopulmonary bypass

v. The defect may be patched with pericardium or closed with suture

vi. Heart block is the most common complication following closure of ostium primum type defect because of injury to AV bundle. Temporary pacing may be required

Ventricular Septal Defect (VSD): A communicating defect of the septum between the two ventricles. It may occur in the muscular or membranous portion of the septum

1. Pathophysiology

a. Four common sites of defects based on their location in the interventricular septum (Fig. 2–21)

i. Supracristal defect: located between the crista supraventricularis and the pulmonic valve—least common

ii. Membranous defect: caudal to the crista supraventricularis—often spontaneously closes

iii. AV canal type defects: beneath the septal leaflet of the tricuspid valve where the AV conduction bundle is particularly susceptible to injury. Defects are usually large and involve the mitral and tricuspid valves

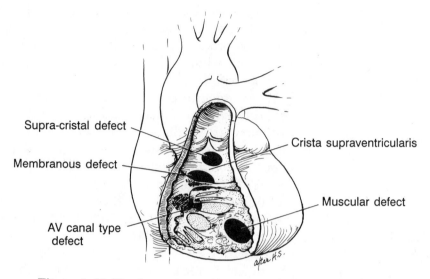

Supra-cristal defect

Membranous defect

AV canal type
defect

Crista supraventricularis

Muscular defect

Figure 2–21. The four common types of ventricular septal defects.

    iv. Muscular defect: in the muscular septum near the apex of the right ventricle—also often closes spontaneously
  b. Blood is shunted from the LV into the RV through the defect owing to the higher pressures in the LV
  c. The increase of blood shunted to the RV increases RV pressures and the pulmonary blood flow
  d. Increased pulmonary blood flow results in increased pulmonary venous return to the LA, thus overloading the left side of the heart and inducing failure
  e. In time, the increased pulmonary blood flow results in increased pulmonary vascular resistance, which increases the pulmonary resistance above systemic resistance
  f. This damages the vascular bed, and over time the injury becomes irreversible. The shunt then becomes reversed—right to left (Eisenmenger's syndrome)

2. Etiology or precipitating factors
  a. Exact cause is unknown
  b. May be due to
    i. Maternal and fetal infections during first trimester of pregnancy (e.g., rubella)
    ii. Effects of drugs/medications
    iii. Dietary deficiencies during fetal development
    iv. Effects of smoking, alcohol
    v. Genetic
    vi. Myocardial infarction
  c. During fetal development, the normal fusion between the aortopul-

monary septum and the primordial ventricular septum does not occur, resulting in supracristal and membranous type defects

d. AV canal type defect is caused by faulty fusion between endocardial cushions and primordial ventricular septum

e. Muscular defect is due to malformations of the primordial ventricular septum

3. Nursing assessment data base

a. Nursing history

    i. Subjective findings: complaints of

        (a) Fatigue

        (b) Dyspnea

    ii. Objective findings

        (a) Most common in males

        (b) Family history of heart defects

        (c) Mother was exposed to infectious process in first trimester; poor nutrition, smoked, intake of alcohol, drugs/medications

        (d) History of slow weight gain

        (e) Child may have difficulty feeding

b. Nursing examination of the patient (signs will vary depending on the size and direction of the shunt). Patients are often asymptomatic with small defects. Large defects will become evident at very early ages. When the shunt reverses to right to left, signs and symptoms of severe heart failure and cyanosis will be present

    i. Inspection

        (a) Pale

        (b) Frail looking, thin

        (c) Tachypnea

    ii. Percussion: noncontributory

    iii. Palpation

        (a) Systolic thrill over upper left sternal border

        (b) In later stages, PMI displaced laterally

    iv. Auscultation

        (a) Harsh holosystolic murmur, best heard at left of sternum, fourth intercostal space (the louder the murmur, the smaller the defect)

        (b) Murmurs of tricuspid, pulmonic, mitral, or aortic incompetence may be heard depending on the type of defect and the overall sequelae due to the defect

c. Diagnostic findings

    i. Radiologic (large defects)

        (a) Enlargement of LA and LV

        (b) Enlargement of RA and RV in presence of pulmonary artery hypertension

        (c) Increased pulmonary vascular markings

(d) Dilated pulmonary artery
ii. ECG
(a) LA and LV hypertrophy patterns
(b) RV hypertrophy
iii. Echocardiography
(a) The actual defect may be seen with two-dimensional echo-cardiography
(b) Chamber enlargement will be noted
iv. Cardiac catheterization: confirms size of defect
(a) Increased oxygen saturation in RV indicates left-to-right shunt
(b) Increased pressure in RV and pulmonary artery
(c) If right-to-left shunt, then oxygen saturation in arterial peripheral blood is reduced
(d) Ventriculography demonstrates the shunt
v. Radionuclide studies (technetium-99): shows the degree of left-to-right shunt

4. Nursing diagnoses
a. See Commonly Encountered Nursing Diagnoses, pp. 200–205
b. Alteration in CO and tissue perfusion related to septal defect
i. Assessment for defining characteristics: see pp. 217–218
ii. Expected outcomes: see p. 264
iii. Nursing interventions
(a) See p. 270
(b) Note additional information
(1) Asymptomatic patients who have no pathologic changes do not require surgery
(2) Patients require surgery when shunt is greater than 1.5:1 and symptoms arise; if there is failure to thrive; if there are repeated respiratory infections; if pulmonary pressures increase (but no reversal of the shunt yet); or if there is a large left-to-right shunt (greater than 1.5:1)
(3) Prefer to delay surgery to ages older than 1 year because of the slightly higher mortality rate in ages younger than 1 year
(4) Surgical repair is contraindicated when pulmonary pressure is equal to or greater than systemic pressure and there is a right-to-left shunt
(5) Surgical repair is accomplished via a median sternotomy approach using cardiopulmonary bypass
(6) Defects may be closed by primary suture, with a Dacron or pericardial patch
(7) Additional postoperative complications to be aware of are

> *a)* Pulmonary edema—due to high pulmonary vascular resistance
>
> *b)* Heart blocks due to injury to the conduction bundle (AV to bundle of His)

iv. Evaluation of nursing care: see p. 270

Patent Ductus Arteriosus (PDA): A persistent communication between the aorta and the pulmonary artery that fails to close after birth

1. Pathophysiology

a. Higher pressure in the aorta causes blood flow through the patent ductus into the pulmonary artery as a left-to-right shunt, recirculating oxygenated blood (Fig. 2–22)

b. The increased volume of blood may

  i. Dilate the pulmonary artery, possibly causing an aneurysm of the ductus

  ii. Increase pulmonary pressures and increase return of blood to LA and LV, overloading the left side of the heart with resultant LV hypertrophy and symptoms of left-sided heart failure; pulmonary congestion ensues over time

  iii. Increase pulmonary congestion; increased pressures also lead to increased work for the RV (which will enlarge over time)

c. If obstructive pulmonary vascular lesions develop, the pressure in the pulmonary artery will rise above the aortic pressure, causing the shunt to reverse to right-to-left (Eisenmenger's syndrome)

  i. Cyanosis and right-sided heart failure ensue

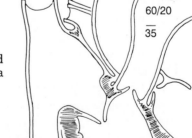

Figure 2–22. The anatomical defect and associated cardiac catheterization data of a patent ductus arteriosus.

ii. Deoxygenated blood is distributed to lower parts of the body below the ductus (causing cyanosis and clubbing of toes), while upper parts of the body receive oxygenated blood with no abnormalities

iii. All patients are candidates for infective endocarditis; vegetations may embolize to lungs, leading to infarctions and death

2. Etiology or precipitating factors

a. During fetal circulation, blood from the pulmonary artery flows through the ductus into the descending aorta in order to bypass the collapsed lungs. Normally, the ductus closes within 24 to 72 hours after birth, so that the blood goes to the lungs before reaching the systemic circulation. Closure of the duct is accomplished by the contraction of smooth muscles in the wall of the duct resulting from the increased oxygen tension. When the smooth muscles do not contract, as may happen when hypoxia occurs at birth, the ductus remains open

b. May be associated with other anomalies (e.g., atrial and ventricular septal defects)

c. Very common in association with congenital rubella, prematurity

d. Common in infants with lung disease and those born at high altitudes (chronic hypoxia)

3. Nursing assessment data base

a. Nursing history

  i. Subjective findings

    (a) Parent states child fatigues easily and feeds poorly

    (b) Increased number of respiratory tract infections

  ii. Objective findings

    (a) History of rubella during first trimester

    (b) History of hypoxia at birth

b. Nursing examination of patient

  i. Inspection

    (a) Signs of congestive heart failure depend on the size of the defect

    (b) May see cyanosis in lower parts of body and clubbing of toes while upper part of body is pink

  ii. Palpation

    (a) Bounding pulses with large PDAs

    (b) Hyperdynamic precordium

    (c) Prominent apical impulse

    (d) Systolic thrill in second left intercostal space

  iii. Percussion—noncontributory

  iv. Auscultation

    (a) Presence of a loud, continuous (in both systole and diastole) "machinery-like" murmur is indicative of PDA (due to the

pressure gradient between the aorta and the pulmonary artery); heard best at left upper sternal border
    (b) Widened pulse pressure
  c. Diagnostic findings
    i. Radiologic: chest x-ray film
      (a) LA and LV enlargement
      (b) Enlarged aorta (with large shunts) and pulmonary artery
      (c) Increased pulmonary vascular markings
    ii. ECG: LA and LV enlargement patterns with large shunts
    iii. Echocardiography: detects the PDA and reveals the enlarged chambers
    iv. Cardiac catheterization
      (a) Establishes the aortopulmonary communication and the size and direction of the shunt
      (b) Assesses pulmonary pressures and resistance; large shunts produce increases in pulmonary artery pressure
      (c) Step-up and increased pressures will be evident in pulmonary artery with right-to-left shunts; increased pressures in LA (see Fig. 2–22)

4. Nursing diagnoses
  a. See Commonly Encountered Nursing Diagnoses, pp. 200–205
  b. Alteration in CO and tissue perfusion related to the pathophysiologic changes of the PDA
    i. Assessment for defining characteristics: see pp. 217–218
    ii. Expected outcomes: see p. 218
    iii. Nursing interventions
      (a) See pp. 274–275
      (b) Postoperative nursing care involves the basic care for thoracotomy
      (c) Observe for postoperative complications—uncommon but include recurrent nerve injury, infections, bleeding, and possibility of a hemothorax or chylothorax
    iv. Evaluation of nursing care: see pp. 222–223
  c. Potential for infectious process (infective endocarditis) secondary to this congenital heart defect
  d. Note additional information
    i. Medical management of the PDA may be tried first by closing the PDA with prostaglandins, controlling the congestive heart failure with medications, decreasing the work load of the heart by decreasing energy expenditure, and providing adequate oxygenation
    ii. Surgery is contraindicated in cases of right-to-left shunts
    iii. Surgery is performed through a left thoracotomy incision
    iv. Once the duct is reached, it is ligated

Coarctation of the Aorta (COA): A narrowing of the aorta most commonly found distal to the left subclavian artery (Fig. 2–23)

1. Pathophysiology

 a. Smooth muscle of the ductus arteriosus extends into the aorta, and when the tissue contracts to close the duct after birth, narrowing of the aorta occurs

 b. Sometimes, the aortic medial tissue thickens and forms a ridge projecting into the lumen of the aorta. This also obstructs outflow from the LV

 c. Fetal development of the aortic arch may be abnormal

 d. Pressures proximal to the COA are increased, while pressures distal to the COA are decreased, forming a pressure gradient

 e. LV pressures increase, as do pressures in all vessels of the aortic arch. Over time, the LV hypertrophies, dilates, and can fail owing to this increase in afterload

 f. Upper parts of the body develop systemic hypertension, which also increases the afterload

 g. Collateral circulation develops (arising from the subclavian arteries), which feeds the lower parts of the body (compensating for the decrease in blood flow through the normal route). The collaterals involved are the internal mammary, epigastric, intercostal, lumbar, and thyrocervical arteries

 h. If left untreated, the person will die due to sequelae from the

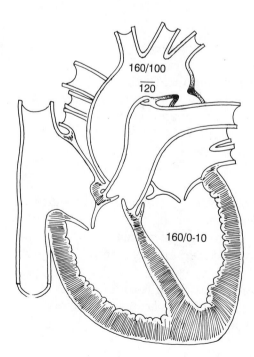

Figure 2–23. The anatomical defect and associated cardiac catheterization data of a coarctation of the aorta.

prolonged hypertension (i.e., strokes, coronary artery disease, congestive heart failure, aortic rupture or dissection)

    i. COA is classified as

        i. Preductal: located proximal to the ductus arteriosus

        ii. Postductal: located distal to the ductus arteriosus

2. Etiology or precipitating factors: see pathophysiology

3. Nursing assessment data base (Clinical manifestations will vary depending on the age of the person; most often persons are asymptomatic and the COA is discovered on routine examinations.)

  a. Nursing history

    i. Subjective: patient may complain of headaches, epistaxis, leg cramps

    ii. Objective: unremarkable in the asymptomatic patient

  b. Nursing examination of the patient

    i. Inspection

      (a) Upper body more developed than lower body, which may be underdeveloped

      (b) May see a heave over LV area due to LV hypertrophy

    ii. Palpation

      (a) Heave over LV

      (b) Forceful upper extremity pulses; typically weak and delayed or absent lower extremity pulses

      (c) Blood pressure in lower extremities is less than that in the upper extremities (just opposite of normal)

      (d) Collateral arteries may be palpated over the precordium, between ribs

    iii. Percussion: noncontributory

    iv. Auscultation

      (a) Systolic murmur heard best at left sternal border radiating to the neck or back between the scapulae

      (b) S_2 and S_3 may be heard owing to the failure or to the hypertension

  c. Diagnostic findings

    i. Radiologic: chest x-ray film

      (a) Enlarged left ventricle

      (b) The "3" sign: dilated ascending aorta followed by the constricted area followed by the poststenotic dilatation

      (c) Rib-notching of fourth through eighth ribs due to the collateral circulation of the intercostal arteries

    ii. ECG: LV and/or RV hypertrophy pattern

    iii. Cardiac catheterization (see Fig. 2–23): used to rule out other defects, measure the pressures in the aorta and the LV and RV, and assess the adequacy of collateral circulation. Aortogram is diagnostic of coarctation

4. Nursing diagnoses

a. See Commonly Encountered Nursing Diagnoses, pp. 200–205
b. Alteration in cardiac output and tissue perfusion related to the pathophysiologic changes of the coarctation
   i. Assessment for defining characteristics: see pp. 217–218
   ii. Expected outcomes: see p. 264
   iii. Nursing interventions: see p. 281
   iv. Evaluation of nursing care: see pp. 222–223
c. Potential for infectious process (infective endocarditis) secondary to this congenital heart defect
d. Note additional information
   i. The presence of heart failure and coarctation in infants signifies the presence of other anomalies
   ii. If coarctation is not associated with heart failure or hypertension, then surgery can be delayed to ages 3 to 5 but should be performed as soon as possible to avoid residual hypertension
   iii. Adults with coarctation can undergo surgery as long as an associated disease does not contraindicate the surgical procedure. The surgical correction will often decrease the hypertension and improve the failure
   iv. The operative procedure is performed through a left thoracotomy incision
   v. The coarctation is excised and either an end-to-end anastomosis is performed or a tubular prosthetic graft is inserted
   vi. The postoperative nursing care involves the basic care for thoracotomy
   vii. Postoperative complications to watch for are hemothorax, chylothorax, mesenteric vasculitis, and paradoxic hypertension

Hypertensive Crisis: An acute, life-threatening rise in blood pressure with severe end-organ damage and even death if left untreated
1. Pathophysiology
   a. Essential hypertension (elevated blood pressure of unknown cause) or secondary hypertension (elevated blood pressure due to a known cause, i.e., renal vascular disease, pheochromocytoma, coarctation of aorta, pregnancy) over time will produce changes in arterioles (necrosis and inflammation), which eventually cause a decrease in blood flow to end organs. Permanent damage may result (Table 2–6). Uncontrolled hypertension may then induce a sudden rise in blood pressure, which may lead to
   b. Accelerated hypertension: diastolic blood pressure of > 120 mm Hg associated with rapid vascular changes and retinal exudates and hemorrhages. If no treatment is instituted, this will progress to
   c. Malignant hypertension: associated with a diastolic blood pressure > 140 mm Hg, retinal exudates and hemorrhages, and also papilledema around the optic disc

Table 2–6. THE SEQUELAE OF HYPERTENSION: ITS EFFECTS ON END-ORGANS THAT MAY LEAD TO HYPERTENSIVE CRISIS

Hypertension		
Enhanced sympathetic stimulation Effects of renin–angiotension system (increased fluid retention, increased systemic vasoconstriction) Necrosis of arterioles Decreased blood flow to end-organs		
Heart	**Brain**	**Kidney**
Tachycardia	Loss of autoregulatory mechanisms	↓ Renal perfusion
↑ Cardiac output	Arterial spasm and ischemia lead to TIAs	↓ Ability to concentrate urine
↓ Perfusion → angina → MI	Weakened vessels → aneurysms → hemorrhage → CVA	↑ BUN, creatinine
CAD LV hypertrophy CHF Angina		↑ Proteinuria Kidney failure Uremia

  i. Large amounts of renin and angiotensin cause arterial dilatation and contraction. This produces turbulent blood flow, which causes microangiopathic hemolytic anemia and intravascular coagulation

  ii. The arterial walls swell with fluid, causing fibrinoid necrosis

 d. Hypertensive encephalopathy ensues: excessive elevation of blood pressure (>250/150) → dysfunction of cerebral autoregulation → vasospasms → ischemia → increased capillary pressure and permeability → cerebral edema and hemorrhage

2. Etiology or precipitating factors

 a. Untreated or inadequately treated essential or secondary hypertension

 b. Poor compliance with antihypertensive medication treatment plan

 c. Renal disease (acute glomerulonephritis, chronic pyelonephritis, renal vascular disease, renal secreting tumors, chronic renal failure)

 d. Toxemia of pregnancy

 e. Pheochromocytoma

 f. Pituitary tumors

 g. Coarctation of the aorta

 h. Concurrrent use of catecholamine precursors and monoamine oxidase (MAO) inhibitor drugs

 i. Adrenocortical hyperfunction

 j. Cushing's syndrome

 k. Polycythemia

 l. Atherosclerosis

3. Nursing assessment data base

   a. Nursing history: patient may or may not be able to respond to questioning; question significant others

      i. Subjective findings: complaints of severe headache, epistaxis

     ii. Objective findings

        (a) History of hypertension

        (b) Positive family history of hypertension

        (c) Higher incidence of essential hypertension in black females

        (d) Medication history positive for MAO inhibitors, oral contraceptives, anti-inflammatory agents, appetite suppressants

        (e) Diet history: high intake of sodium

        (f) History of any of the etiologic factors listed previously

        (g) Evidence of complications of hypertension (coronary artery disease, renal dysfunction)

        (h) History of other risk factors (diabetes, obesity, smoking, hyperlipidemia, stress)

   b. Nursing examination of the patient

      i. Clinical presentation: accelerated hypertension

        (a) Diastolic pressure > 120 mm Hg

        (b) Retinopathy with exudates

        (c) Retinal hemorrhages

        (d) Headache

        (e) Restlessness

        (f) Epistaxis

        (g) Tachycardia

        (h) Rales

        (i) S_3, S_4

        (j) Bruit over femoral area, anteriorly over renal vasculature, carotids, abdominal aorta

     ii. Clinical presentation: malignant hypertension

        (a) Diastolic pressure > 140 mm Hg

        (b) Papilledema of optic disc

        (c) Retinopathy

        (d) Headache

        (e) Blurred vision

        (f) Dyspnea

        (g) Chest pain

        (h) Others as in accelerated hypertension

    iii. Clinical presentation: hypertensive encephalopathy

        (a) Blood pressure > 250/150 mm Hg

        (b) Retinopathy

        (c) Papilledema of optic disc

        (d) Severe headache

        (e) Vomiting

(f) Mental status changes

(g) Transitory focal neurologic signs (e.g., nystagmus)

(h) Localized weakness

(i) Seizures

(j) Diuresis

(k) Coma

c. Diagnostic findings

i. Laboratory: must find the cause of the hypertension if possible and its effects on end organs

(a) Complete blood cell count—hematocrit is decreased in renal failure and polycythemia associated with renal disease

(b) Serum blood urea nitrogen and creatinine clearance values will be elevated if renal disease is present

(c) Serum glucose level elevated in Cushing's syndrome, pheochromocytoma, and diabetes—all possible causes of hypertension

(d) Urinalysis—routine; especially important is the presence of proteinuria (indicates renal disease) and hematuria (malignant nephrosclerosis)

(e) Urinary vanillylmandelic acid (VMA)—catecholamines are elevated in pheochromocytoma (an etiologic factor in hypertension)

(f) Serum uric acid—hyperuricemia is associated with renal failure

(g) Serum potassium—used to rule out primary aldosteronism, which causes hypokalemia and hypertension

ii. Radiologic findings

(a) Renal arteriography—used to show renal artery stenosis, atherosclerosis, lesions, and dysplasias as cause of hypertension

(b) Intravenous pyelography—may indicate presence of kidney disease; cannot differentiate what type

(c) Chest x-ray film may reveal cardiomegaly

iii. ECG: may reveal signs of LV hypertrophy, ischemia

iv. CT scan: will show diffuse brain edema in patients with encephalopathy and will also demonstrate hemorrhage

4. **Nursing diagnoses:** hypertensive crisis is a life-threatening event. Rapid stabilization of blood pressure is the prime goal!

a. Elevated blood pressure secondary to accelerated/malignant hypertension

i. Assessment for defining characteristics

(a) Patient exhibits signs and symptoms as described above

ii. Expected outcomes

(a) Blood pressure will return to normal limits

iii. Nursing interventions
   (a) Continually reassure patient and family/SO
   (b) Maintain a calm, quiet environment
   (c) Assist in the insertion of hemodynamic monitoring lines to monitor patient's response to therapy
   (d) Administer drugs as ordered (Table 2–7)
   (e) Administer diuretics (furosemide, ethacrynic acid) as ordered
   (f) Monitor patient's response to drugs and titrate to maintain desired blood pressure level

Table 2–7. DRUGS USED IN THE MANAGEMENT OF HYPERTENSIVE CRISIS

Drug	Dose	Comments	Side Effects
Vasodilators			
Sodium nitroprusside (Nipride)	0.5–10 µg/kg/min continuous IV	Instant onset of action; must monitor patient closely and infuse with central line	Nausea and vomiting, HTN, restlessness, agitation, tachycardia
Diazoxide (Hyperstat)	50–100 mg IV bolus q 5–10 minutes until BP is lowered; total dose up to 300 mg	Rapid onset of action (3–5 minutes); sustained effect 4–12 hours; contraindicated in aortic dissection	Nausea and vomiting, tachycardia, headache, hyperglycemia, flushing, angina, hypotension
Hydralazine (Apresoline)	10–20 mg (mixed in at least 20 ml) IV bolus or 10–50 mg IM; both until desired BP obtained	Rapid onset (20–30 minutes); duration of action 3–6 hours; contraindicated in aortic dissection	Headache, tachycardia, palpitations, angina, flushing, vomiting
Nitroglycerin	5 µg/min continuous IV titrated to desired effect	Instant onset of action; 2–3 minutes duration of action	Palpitations, headache, tachycardia, restlessness, hypotension, abdominal pain
Sympathetic Blocking Agents			
Trimethaphan camsylate (Arfonad)	40–90 µg/kg/min continuous infusion or 1000 mg/L	Rapid onset of action (5–10 minutes); duration of action 5–10 minutes	Urinary retention, dry mouth, paralysis of pupillary reflex, paralytic ileus
Methyldopa (Aldomet)	250–600 mg diluted in 100 ml given over 30–60 minutes IV	Onset in 2–3 hours; sustained effect 4–8 hours; contraindicated in hypertensive encephalopathy	Drowsiness
Phentolamine (Regitine)	5–10 mg IM or 5–10 mg rapid bolus or 200 mg/L continuous IV infusion	Instant onset with duration of 5–20 minutes	Tachycardia, flushing, headache, palpitations

    (g) Monitor patient for side effects of the administered drugs (see Table 2–7)

    (h) Monitor intake and output closely

    (i) Monitor ECG for dysrhythmias

    (j) Monitor patient for any complaints of sudden chest pain (dissecting aortic aneurysm), changes in level of consciousness, nausea, vomiting, headache, visual changes—all of which indicate an increase in intracranial pressure

  iv. Evaluation of nursing care

    (a) Patient's blood pressure within prescribed limits

    (b) Without signs and symptoms of accelerated or malignant hypertension or hypertensive encephalopathy

    (c) Without side effects from the drug therapy

    (d) ECG—normal sinus rhythm

b. Potential for hypotension secondary to diuretic and antihypertensive drug therapy

  i. Assessment for defining characteristics

    (a) Blood pressure below prescribed limits

    (b) Urine output below prescribed limits

    (c) Altered serum electrolytes

    (d) May exhibit hypovolemic shock-type symptoms

  ii. Expected outcomes

    (a) Blood pressure within normal limits

    (b) ECG—normal sinus rhythm

    (c) Normovolemia

  iii. Nursing interventions

    (a) Monitor hemodynamic pressures closely

    (b) Monitor patient's response to the drug therapy, and report values that reflect hypotension

    (c) Titrate/stop antihypertensive drugs

    (d) Administer fluids to restore volume

    (e) Monitor electrolytes for abnormalities

    (f) Monitor ECG continuously

  iv. Evaluation of nursing care

    (a) Blood pressure is within prescribed limits

    (b) Hemodynamics reflect adequate filling pressures, CO, etc.

    (c) Electrolytes within normal limits

    (d) ECG—normal sinus rhythm

c. Potential for knowledge deficit related to denial, lack of knowledge, and anxiety (see pp. 200–205)

Peripheral Vascular Disease: Vascular disorders of arteries and veins (usually degenerative) that supply the extremities

1. Pathophysiology (arterial only)

  a. Atherosclerotic process

     i. Affects mostly the intima of the artery, but the underlying media is secondarily affected by the degenerative process, severely weakening the wall of the artery

     ii. The systemic blood pressure increases the tension and focal weakness. It may result in an aneurysm over time

     iii. Mural thrombi line the surface of the aneurysm, decreasing the lumen's diameter and setting up for potential emboli

     iv. If no intervention, the aneurysm may rupture and death can ensue. Sometimes the ruptured vessel may be tamponaded by surrounding structures allowing time for surgical intervention

  b. Degenerative structural changes in the media of the artery combined with loss of smooth muscle cells lead to dissection. Pressure during systole causes intimal tear, and blood enters the media. Over time the blood continues to tear the media over a varying length of the artery. This thin-walled channel can easily rupture

  c. Invasion of the wall of the artery by microorganisms leads to medial weakening and proliferation of fibrous tissue

  d. Most common sequelae of peripheral atherosclerosis

     i. Aneurysms (see Fig. 2–24)

       (a) Abdominal aortic aneurysm (AAA) (usually involves aorta between the renal and iliac arteries)

       (b) Thoracic aortic aneurysm (TAA)

         (1) Usually of ascending, transverse, or descending parts of aorta

         (2) Most frequent in men in their 60s and 70s

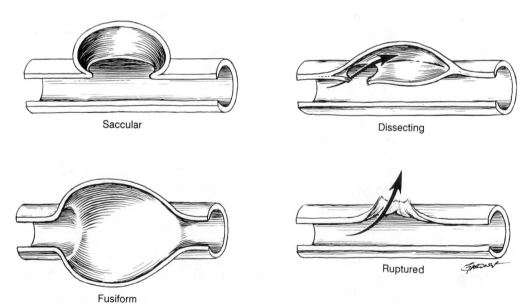

Saccular

Dissecting

Fusiform

Ruptured

Figure 2–24. Types of aortic aneurysms. *A.* Sacculated. *B.* Fusiform. *C.* Dissecting. *D.* Ruptured.

(c) Ruptured aneurysms

(d) Aneurysm of iliac, femoral, and popliteal arteries

(e) Aortic dissection (not a true aneurysm)—classified according to the anatomy of the aorta involved

    (1) Type I tear—just above aortic valve and extends distally to abdominal aorta

    (2) Type II tear—localized from ascending aorta to aortic arch

    (3) Type III tear—begins distal to left subclavian and extends distally

  ii. Occlusive disease of aortoiliacs, carotid, vertebral, subclavian

  iii. Mural thrombi and embolization to lower extremities

2. Etiologic or precipitating factors

a. Atherosclerosis

b. Syphilitic aortitis: commonly involves the ascending aorta and aortic arch during the tertiary stage.

c. Cystic medial necrosis: noninflammatory focal accumulation of mucoid material in the media causes the structural changes in the arterial wall. Cause is not known but it is associated with Marfan's syndrome

d. Marfan's syndrome: increased elasticity of the walls of the aorta due to deficiency of collagen and connective tissue

e. Severe hypertension will compound the effects of medial deterioration

f. Pregnancy: hormonal changes associated with pregnancy affect the smooth muscle and the media of the aorta

g. Trauma: especially rapid deceleration; blunt type of trauma can tear the intima of the thoracic aorta and form a dissecting aneurysm

h. Congenital abnormalities

i. Infectious arteritis other than syphilis

3. Nursing assessment data base

a. Nursing history

  i. Subjective: patient complains of

    (a) Abdominal aortic aneurysm (AAA)

      (1) Feeling pulsations in abdominal area

      (2) Dull abdominal or low back (impending rupture) ache/pain

      (3) Nausea and vomiting (pressure against the duodenum)

      (4) Ruptured: severe, sudden, continuous abdominal pain, radiating to the back, hips, scrotum; nausea and vomiting; syncope

    (b) Thoracic aortic aneurysm (TAA)

      (1) Sudden, tearing pain in chest radiating to shoulders, neck, and back

    (2) Cough, hoarseness, weak voice due to pressure against recurrent laryngeal nerve

    (3) Dysphagia due to pressure on the esophagus

    (4) Dyspnea due to pressure on the trachea

   (c) Aortic dissection

    (1) Sudden, sharp, tearing pain in chest radiating to shoulders, neck, back, and abdomen

   (d) Occlusive disease

    (1) Intermittent claudication of hip, buttocks, thigh, calf, foot; severe pain in toes; ulcers that do not heal

    (2) Impotence

    (3) Severe extremity pain, pallor, loss of pulses, paresthesias; paralysis is associated with acute thrombosis of AAA

    (4) Carotids—transient ischemic attacks, monocular visual disturbances, sensory or motor deficits, expressive or receptive dysphasia

  ii. Objective findings

   (a) Positive history of arteriosclerosis (e.g., coronary artery disease, cerebrovascular accident)

   (b) Positive risk factors for atherosclerosis

   (c) Family history of atherosclerosis

   (d) Recent history of deceleration-type trauma (pertaining to aneurysm only)

 b. Nursing examination of the patient

  i. Aneurysms

   (a) Inspection

    (1) Precordial pulsations

   (b) Palpation

    (1) Pulsating abdominal mass

    (2) Bounding pulses (abdominal aortic aneurysm)

   (c) Percussion—noncontributory

   (d) Auscultation

    (1) Bruits—abdominal aorta, femoral, renal, popliteal

    (2) Murmur of aortic insufficiency when aneurysm involves the aortic ring

  ii. Arterial occlusions

   (a) Inspection

    (1) Ulcers/gangrene in extremities

    (2) Pale, mottled, extremities on elevation; rubor on dependency of extremities

    (3) Extremities may be asymmetric; difference noted in calf circumference

    (4) Tropic changes of skin on extremities due to impaired circulation

(5) Retinal arterial emboli with carotid disease
- (b) Palpation
  - (1) Weak, nonexistent or unequal peripheral pulses
  - (2) Cool skin
  - (3) Sluggish capillary refill
  - (4) Pulsatile mass in popliteal fossa indicative of popliteal aneurysm
- (c) Auscultation—bruits. Check over all arteries and heart (to rule out radiation sound from a murmur)

c. Diagnostic study findings
  - i. ECG: noncontributory
  - ii. Chest x-ray film: increased aortic diameter, right deviation of trachea; pleural effusions
  - iii. Anteroposterior and lateral films of the abdomen will demonstrate the aneurysm
  - iv. Aortography
    - (a) Determines the origin and extent of the dissection and shows a double lumen
  - v. Computed tomography demonstrates the lumen diameter, wall thickness, and length of the aneurysm and amount of mural thrombi that may be present
  - vi. Arteriography
    - (a) Assesses peripheral vascular disease by providing morphologic visualization of the arterial lumen
    - (b) Provides information to decide if artery is a candidate for reconstruction by assessing extent of disease and evaluating extent of collateral circulation available
    - (c) Also used to assess aneurysms or arteriovenous fistulas
  - vii. Laboratory values
    - (a) Complete blood cell count—decreased hemoglobin and hematocrit; increased leukocyte count
    - (b) Increased blood urea nitrogen and creatinine values; proteinuria and hematuria indicate compromise of kidneys
  - viii. Doppler ultrasound
    - (a) Assesses peripheral arterial and cerebrovascular blood flow/velocity
    - (b) Picks up sound generated by moving blood through vessels. Totally occluded vessels do not transmit sound
  - ix. Ultrasonic scanning: two-dimensional echos of soft tissue provide images of arterial walls
  - x. Plethysmography: assesses peripheral arterial and cerebrovascular disease by analyzing pulse waves, limb blood flow, limb blood content, and limb blood pressure

4. **Nursing diagnoses**

a. Potential for alteration in tissue perfusion related to arterial occlusive disease, aneurysm, dissection, or perioperative complications
   i. Assessment for defining characteristics: see nursing assessment data base
   ii. Expected outcomes
      (a) Absence of pain
      (b) Patient remains or attains hemodynamic stability
      (c) Without postoperative complications; graft remains patent, no emboli, no infection, adequate perfusion to extremities, palpable pulses, warm extremities
      (d) Patient/SO are less anxious and able to rest
      (e) Patient/SO understand discharge instructions (follow-up appointments, activity regimen, medication regimen, signs/symptoms requiring medical attention)
   iii. Nursing interventions
      (a) Assess patient for signs and symptoms discussed under assessment, above
      (b) Prepare patient for preoperative evaluation studies; discuss the disease process, rationale for the tests and what patient will experience
      (c) Encourage verbalization of fears/anxiety; support patient/SO
      (d) Prepare patient/SO for operative procedure, need for surgery, and expected outcomes
         (1) Repair of thoracic and abdominal aortic aneurysms and dissections
            a) The aneurysm is repaired generally when it reaches 6 cm in diameter or more. The danger of rupture increases dramatically at larger diameters. The goal is to prevent complications (i.e., rupture, stroke, organ ischemia)
            b) For thoracic aneurysms, especially those of the ascending aorta (Fig. 2–25), a median sternotomy approach is used. The aorta may have to be cross clamped, and extracorporeal circulation may be required to bypass the aorta. The aneurysm is endarterectomized; a Dacron graft is then inserted to establish continuity of flow. If the aortic valve is incompetent, then repair of the valve is warranted at the same time
            c) Thoracoabdominal aortic aneurysms are more complicated because of the various arteries that arise from this section of the aorta feeding visceral organs (Fig. 2–26)
               ☐ Two approaches are used—an anterolateral tho-

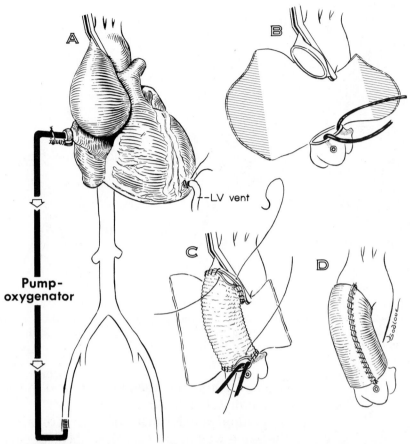

Figure 2–25. Repair of ascending aortic aneurysm. *A.* Extracorporeal circulation is used. Aorta is cross-clamped distal to aneurysm, and left ventricular vent is inserted. *B.* After opening of aneurysm, coronary cannulae are inserted. *C.* Insertion of woven Dacron graft. *D.* Aneurysmal wall is closed over prosthesis. (From Fairbairn, J. F., et al., eds.: Allen-Barker-Hines Peripheral Vascular Diseases, 4th ed. W. B. Saunders Co., Philadelphia, 1972, p. 297.)

racotomy and a xiphopubic midline abdominal incision

☐ A Dacron graft is anastomosed end-to-side of the aorta above the aneurysm, tunneled through the diaphragm, and anastomosed end-to-side of the aorta below the aneurysm

☐ Flow is established through the graft by occluding the thoracic aorta distal to the upper anastomosis

☐ Small Dacron grafts are then anastomosed to the larger bypass graft—the opposite ends are then anastomosed to the celiac, mesenteric, and renal arteries, and blood flow is established

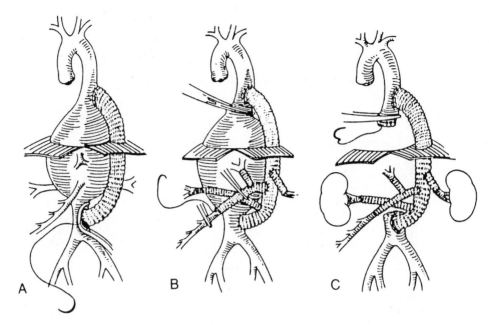

Figure 2–26. Technique for bypassing and resecting a thoracoabdominal aneurysm, involving celiac, mesenteric, and renal arteries. (From Gay, W. A., ed. Cardiovascular Surgery. Harper & Row Publishers, Philadelphia, 1984, chap. 3, p. 17.)

    ☐ The aneurysm is then excised, and the proximal and distal ends are oversewn

    d) Abdominal aortic aneurysms are repaired much the same way as already described. Depending on the length of the aneurysm, the Dacron graft may be tubular or bifurcated

(2) Repair of occlusive disease of lower extremities

    a) Indicated when patient experiences ischemic pain at rest, disabling claudication, ulcers that do not heal, and gangrene

    b) For aortoiliac or aortofemoral disease (Fig. 2–27) the artery may be endartarectomized and reconstructed or a bypass graft may be placed

    c) For femoropopliteal disease, the saphenous vein is most often used for grafting much the same way coronary artery bypass grafting is performed (Fig. 2–28)

(e) Immediate postoperative care

(1) Monitor vital signs and hemodynamic parameters closely—keep systolic blood pressure below 120 mm Hg with administration of drugs as ordered (antihypertensives, analgesics). (Hypertension may induce

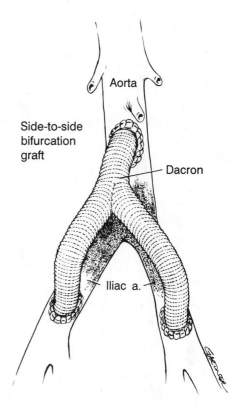

Aorta

Side-to-side
bifurcation
graft

Dacron

Iliac a.

Figure 2–27. Side-to-side bypass graft for aortoiliac disease.

bleeding postoperatively due to the pressure on the suture lines.)

(2) Check peripheral pulses (may need Doppler) for temperature, color, capillary refill, and petechiae, and report changes from baseline status every hour for 24 hours

(3) Monitor for central nervous system dysfunction (due to repairs of ascending and thoracic aortic aneurysms) (e.g., confusion, restlessness, headache)

(4) Monitor abdominal girth or limb girth (whichever applies) as ordered to assess for hemorrhage

(5) Monitor for hemorrhage/hypovolemia—hypotension, tachycardia, weak pulses, altered sensorium, decreased hemodynamic values

(6) Monitor ECG for signs of ischemia, injury, and dysrhythmias

(7) Monitor renal status closely—urine output; amount; specific gravity; and presence of hematuria. (Certain surgical procedures may impair blood flow to the kidneys.)

(8) Patient may have been hypothermic during surgery—

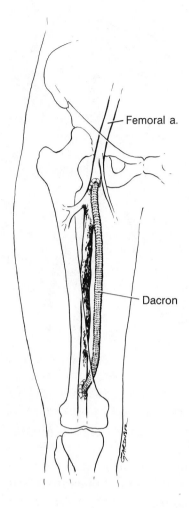

Femoral a.

Dacron

Figure 2–28. Bypass graft for femoropopliteal disease with use of saphenous vein.

rewarm slowly and prevent overshoot into hyperthermic stage

(9) Assess respiratory status—patient will have difficulty deep breathing and coughing. Encourage deep breathing and coughing and use of incentive spirometer; use humidified oxygen

(10) Maintain a quiet, calm atmosphere; explain all procedures to patient to help reduce anxiety

(11) Provide adequate oxygenation; monitor arterial blood gases

(12) Monitor other laboratory values for abnormalities (e.g., electrolytes, blood urea nitrogen, creatinine, PT, PTT)

(13) For aortic repairs, keep head of bed elevated no more than 45° for first 3 days

(14) Patient must not flex or cross leg after revascularization of femoral artery

(15) Expect an ileus with thoracoabdominal repairs—keep bowel decompressed with nasogastric tube; monitor output

(16) Monitor for watery, bloody diarrhea—indicates ischemic bowel (due to reduced perfusion during surgery)

(17) Monitor for peripheral signs and symptoms of spinal cord ischemia such as paralysis of lower extremities and bowel and bladder paralysis

   iv. Evaluation of nursing care

     (a) Hemodynamic parameters, vital signs all within normal limits

     (b) Patient calm, no complaints of pain

     (c) Palpable pulses of affected extremities, limbs warm; capillary refill brisk; color pink

     (d) No evidence of hemorrhage

     (e) Patient alert and oriented to time, person, and place

     (f) Urine output >30 ml/hr, hematest negative, specific gravity within normal limits

     (g) ECG—normal sinus rhythm, without blocks or evidence of myocardial infarction

     (h) Lungs clear to auscultation

  b. See Commonly Encountered Nursing Diagnoses, pp. 200–205

Shock: A syndrome due to a variety of pathophysiologic alterations of the cardiovascular and pulmonary systems that have a net result of decreased cellular perfusion and oxygen transport to all parts of the body

1. Pathophysiology

  a. Compensatory mechanisms of shock. These mechanisms attempt to prevent deterioration of circulation during shock by attempting to return CO and arterial pressure to normal limits, thus improving tissue perfusion and preventing organ necrosis

    i. Baroreceptor reflex—a drop in mean arterial pressure or pulse pressure results in decreased stretching of arterial baroreceptors and loss of their inhibitory effect on the vasomotor center. This sympathetic vasomotor stimulation causes secretion of norepinephrine at endings of vasoconstrictor nerves and stimulation of vasoconstrictors throughout the body and heart, resulting in

     (a) Arteriolar constriction

     (b) Venous constriction

     (c) Increased force and rate of cardiac contraction

    ii. Norepinephrine-epinephrine vasoconstrictor mechanism: stimulation of vasomotor center also stimulates adrenal medulla to secrete norepinephrine and epinephrine, further assisting vaso-constriction throughout the body

iii. Central nervous system ischemic response: when mean arterial pressure drops below 50 mm Hg, ischemia and resultant elevated carbon dioxide levels in vasomotor center cause extremely powerful sympathetic stimulation. Degree of vasoconstriction caused by this response is so severe that peripheral vessels may become totally occluded

iv. Widespread reflex venoconstriction—intense vasoconstriction in splanchnic area of subcutaneous and pulmonary veins helps maintain filling pressure of heart

v. Constriction of afferent and efferent arterioles of kidneys: reduced renal artery pressure results in renal arteriolar constriction, causing decreased glomerular filtration and renal plasma flow and resulting in decrease in urine output and increase in sodium retention

vi. Activation of renin-angiotensin system: reduced renal afferent arteriolar pressure stimulates baroreceptors in juxtaglomerular cells and activates the renin-angiotensin system, assisting in elevation of arterial pressure, causing

(a) Vasoconstriction of arterioles and, to a lesser extent, veins

(b) Increased renal tubular reabsorption of sodium and water

(c) Stimulation of adrenal cortex to increase production of aldosterone, which causes retention of renal sodium, thus expanding extracellular fluid volume

vii. Shifting of tissue fluid into capillaries: because of decrease in capillary hydrostatic pressure from arteriolar constriction and decreased venous pressure, fluid moves into capillaries from interstitial and intracellular spaces

b. Regardless of the cause of shock, once the compensatory mechanisms fail, the pathophysiologic process that follows is the same for all forms. *NOTE:* prompt intervention can alter the process and prevent the development of the irreversible stage and death

i. Cellular hypoxia induces anaerobic metabolism and lactic acid production occurs, decreasing the pH at the capillary level

ii. As a result

(a) Myocardial contractility is decreased (directly decreasing CO)

(b) The peripheral vascular bed dilates, increasing the vascular space. This results in reduction of effective circulating volume without actual blood loss

(c) Also, permeability of capillary bed is increased, leading to shift of fluid into third space and further decreasing circulating volume

iii. Postcapillary vasoconstriction in the peripheral vascular bed results in pooling and stasis of blood. The blood coagulates, occluding the capillaries. Tissues supplied by the capillaries die. The body's own fibrinolytic activity lyses the clotted blood, which all leads to disseminated intravascular coagulation (DIC)

iv. Both decreased myocardial contractility and dilated peripheral vascular bed decrease venous return to the heart (decrease preload); CO falls and blood pressure drops, reducing delivery of oxygen to the tissues and resulting in organ failure

   (a) Myocardial depression—when arterial pressure falls below level required to maintain coronary blood flow, myocardial ischemia and depression occur, further decreasing cardiac output and blood flow. Myocardial depressant factor (MDF) released by the pancreas contributes to the myocardial failure. MDF and lysosomal enzymes together progress shock to the irreversible stage

v. Vasomotor center depression: severe cerebral ischemia leads to depression of vasomotor center and elimination of sympathetic stimulation, resulting in pooling of blood in periphery and further reducing venous return and CO

vi. Vascular failure: arterial and venous dilation can occur from decrease in nutrients to vessels during shock, causing decrease in blood flow to vital organs and pooling of blood in the venous bed

vii. Thrombosis of small vessels: plugs in small vessels may form because of continued tissue metabolism in presence of sluggish blood flow. Agglutination of erythrocytes, leukocytes, and platelets may be precipitated by

   (a) Platelet aggregation by catecholamines

   (b) Damage to endothelial lining of small vessels, with subsequent deposition of fibrin and accumulation of microthrombi

   (c) Hypoxia increasing the rigidity of erythrocytes

   (d) Release of vasoactive peptides and anaphylatoxins as a result of complement activation

viii. Release of toxins of ischemic tissues

   (a) Myocardial toxic factor (MTF) is released late in septic shock and depresses myocardial contractility by interfering with function of calcium ions in excitation–contraction coupling process. It is believed that pancreatic ischemia causes release of proteolytic enzymes, which either stimulate release of MTF or alter plasma proteins to form new toxic substance

   (b) Endotoxin is released from bodies of dead gram-negative bacteria in intestines. Diminished blood flow and depression of normal antibacterial defense mechanism of reticuloendothelial system enhance its absorption. Endotoxin causes vascular dilation and cardiac depression

  ix. Cellular deterioration

    (a) Active transport of sodium and potassium through cell membrane is reduced

    (b) Mitochondrial activity is depressed

    (c) Loss of integrity of lysosomal membranes causes release of acid hydrolases that degrade protein, carbohydrates, and fats

    (d) Cellular metabolism of nutrients is depressed

  x. Acidosis: inadequate tissue perfusion leads to increased anaerobic glycolysis and production of lactic acid. Resulting lactic acidosis depresses myocardium and decreases peripheral vascular responsiveness to catecholamines

  xi. Tissue necrosis: prolonged diversion of blood from kidneys, liver, gastrointestinal tract, etc., contributes to increasing anaerobic metabolism in these areas, resulting in cell death and tissue necrosis

  xii. Deterioration of microcirculation: spasm of precapillary sphincters and venules is a compensatory mechanism of shock, but when vasoconstriction is prolonged, continued ischemia and local acidosis cause dilation of precapillary sphincters, while more resistant venules remain constricted. Blood enters capillaries but pools and stagnates. This continual increase in capillary hydrostatic pressure causes fluid to leave vascular system in increasing amounts. Capillary walls eventually lose their integrity and slough

  xiii. If there is no or inadequate intervention, cells continue to die owing to the inadequate microcirculation. Necrosis of various organs occurs and death ensues

2. **Etiology or precipitating factors**

  a. Cardiogenic shock: inadequate pumping of the heart, resulting in decreased systemic blood flow and inadequate tissue perfusion. Causes include

    i. Myocardial infarction (patient must lose 40% to 45% of LV myocardium)

    ii. Acute dysrhythmias

    iii. Severe congestive heart failure

    iv. Pulmonary embolism

    v. Cardiac tamponade

    vi. Cardiomyopathy

    vii. Surgical or spontaneous damage to valves

    viii. Any form of severe myocardial injury

  b. Hypovolemic shock: loss of blood, plasma, or water to exterior or into tissues, leading to decreased circulating blood volume and venous return, reduced CO, and inadequate tissue perfusion. Causes include

    i. External loss of blood, plasma, and body fluids due to hemorrhage from trauma, surgical procedures, burns, and dehydration (from diarrhea, vomiting, diabetic ketosis, diabetes insipidus)

    ii. Internal loss of blood, plasma, or fluids due to third spacing into peritoneal cavity (ascites from cirrhosis), leakage of fluid into intestines, intestinal obstruction and hemorrhage from ruptured spleen, pancreatitis, hemothorax, etc.

c. Septic shock: massive infection causing vasodilation and inadequate tissue perfusion, usually following endotoxemia or bacteremia due to gram-negative bacilli or gram-positive cocci. Causes include

    i. Septicemia

    ii. Localized infection gaining entry into systemic circulation (especially from urinary tract procedures, indwelling catheters, invasive monitoring, etc.)

    iii. Postabortion and postpartum infection

    iv. Immunosuppressant therapy (chemotherapy, corticosteroids)

    v. Alcoholism

    vi. Bone marrow suppression

    vii. Burns

    viii. Hyperalimentation, IV therapy

d. Anaphylactic shock: histamine is released into the bloodstream following an allergic, antigen–antibody reaction. There is a subsequent increase in capillary permeability and widespread dilation of arterioles and capillary beds, all of which reduce venous return to the heart. Causes include

    i. Diagnostic tests: contrast media

    ii. Drug therapy (penicillin)

    iii. Food intolerances

    iv. Bite or sting from animals and insects

    v. Blood transfusion incompatibilities

e. Neurogenic shock: generalized vasodilation because of decreased neurogenic tone to vessels. Blood volume is within normal limits, but capacity of blood vessels is increased; consequently, peripheral pooling occurs, resulting in diminished venous return and reduced CO. Causes include

    i. General anesthesia

    ii. Spinal anesthesia

    iii. Epidural block

    iv. Spinal cord injury

    v. Ganglion-blocking or other antihypertensive drugs

    vi. Ingestion of barbituates or phenothiazines

    vii. Vasovagal syncope

    viii. Direct damage to vasomotor center of medulla

ix. Altered function of vasomotor center in response to low blood glucose (insulin shock)

3. **Nursing assessment data base**: clinical manifestations may vary depending on the type of shock

a. Nursing history

    i. Subjective findings: patient/SO gives a history of any of the etiologic factors presented above

    ii. Objective findings: same

b. Nursing examination of patient

    i. Common clinical presentations

      (a) Inspection

        (1) Irritability and anxiety may occur in early shock because of increased secretion of epinephrine from sympathetic stimulation or from hypoxia

        (2) Apathy, lethargy, confusion, and coma occur as shock progresses to later stages, because of acidosis and decreased cerebral blood flow

        (3) Cyanosis occurs due to reduced hemoglobin in blood

        (4) Initially, tachypnea is the result of chemoreceptor stimulation from reduced arterial pressure, but, as shock progresses, it is a result of medullary respiratory stimulation from metabolic acidosis

      (b) Palpation

        (1) Hypotension usually results from a decrease in stroke volume and cardiac output (blood pressure initially may be normal or high because of sympathetic stimulation)

        (2) Tachycardia with weak, thready pulse is a result of sympathetic vasoconstriction

        (3) Decreased pulse pressure results from decrease in stroke volume

        (4) Cool, pale, clammy skin is result of peripheral vasoconstriction from sympathetic stimulation (except in early stages of septic shock)

        (5) Hypothermia (except in septic shock) is result of decreased metabolism

      (c) Percussion—noncontributory

      (d) Auscultation—noncontributory

    ii. Clinical presentation specific to cardiogenic shock

      (a) Elevated CVP with distended neck veins

      (b) Decreased CO

      (c) Decreased CI (<2.0 L/min/m^2)

      (d) Hypotension (systolic blood pressure <80 mm Hg)

      (e) Elevated PCWP (>18 mm Hg)

      (f) Elevated systemic vascular resistance

        (g) Pulmonary congestion
        (h) Peripheral edema
- iii. Clinical presentation specific to hypovolemic shock
        (a) Decreased CVP
        (b) Decreased CO
        (c) Decreased PAP
        (d) Decreased PCWP
        (e) Flat neck veins
- iv. Clinical presentation specific to septic shock
        (a) Hyperdynamic (warm) septic shock. After the patient develops septicemia and the body's defenses become compromised, the hyperdynamic phase ensues
            (1) Systemic vascular resistance decreases (due to massive peripheral vasodilation)
            (2) CO tends to increase initially (but may remain normal) due to the decreased systemic vascular resistance
            (3) Blood pressure falls (mean arterial pressure <60 mm Hg) even though CO is increased, decreasing tissue perfusion (especially to major organs)
            (4) The patient presents with tachycardia, tachypnea, decreased urine output, hyperthermia, chills, warm flushed skin, and sensorial changes such as confusion, restlessness, and disorientation. Pulmonary interstitial edema and atelectasis may develop with resultant adventitious breath sounds. Hypoxemia and abnormal arterial blood gas values reflect a compromised respiratory system; eventually the patient progresses to adult respiratory distress syndrome
        (b) Hypodynamic (cold) phase. This phase follows the hyperdynamic phase if intervention is not successful. It is characterized by
            (1) Low CO and low CI
            (2) Elevated systemic vascular resistance but profound hypotension
            (3) Decreased tissue perfusion
            (4) Severe tachycardia
            (5) Peripheral pulses are weak and thready or absent
            (6) Skin is cold, clammy, and pale
            (7) Hypothermia
            (8) Eventually there is multiple organ failure; patient becomes comatose and dies
- v. Clinical presentation specific to anaphylaxis
        (a) Urticaria
        (b) Laryngeal edema with bronchospasm producing stridor, wheezing, severe respiratory distress

(c) Hypotension

(d) Dysrhythmias

(e) ECG changes suggestive of ischemia

(f) Seizure activity

(g) Nausea and vomiting

(h) Abdominal pain

(i) Diarrhea

(j) Anxiety

(k) Confusion

(l) Warm moist skin

vi. Clinical presentation specific to neurogenic shock (due to the profound vasodilation, there is pooling of blood in the arterioles and veins, resulting in hypvolemic type symptoms)

(a) Decreased systemic vascular resistance

(b) Decreased CO and CI

(c) Profound hypotension

(d) Bradycardia

(e) Signs and symptoms of decreased tissue perfusion to major organs—decreased urinary output, tachypnea, nausea, vomiting, restlessness, confusion

c. Diagnostic findings

i. Common findings for all forms of shock

(a) Arterial blood gases—respiratory alkalosis progressing to metabolic acidosis. This occurs initially as compensatory mechanism to blow off carbon dioxide because of increasing lactic acidosis. As shock progresses, metabolic acidosis develops as respiratory compensation fails

(b) In presence of volume depletion, hematocrit is elevated (hemoconcentration) but drops (hemodilution) as volume deficit is replaced

(c) Decreased serum bicarbonate

(d) Elevated serum lactate

(e) Elevated blood urea nitrogen

(f) Elevated creatinine

(g) Hyperkalemia due to oliguria and inadequate tissue perfusion

(h) Elevated urine specific gravity

(i) Elevated urine osmolarity

(j) Decreased urine creatinine clearance

(k) Altered hematologic studies suggestive of disseminated intravascular coagulation (DIC)

(l) Elevated serum enzymes suggestive of cardiac and liver impairment

ii. Diagnostic findings specific to septic shock

(a) Leukocytosis usually occurs with a shift to left (refers to increased production of neutrophils, an indicator of acute infection)

(b) Thrombocytopenia (secondary to DIC)

(c) Abnormal PT and PTT, reflecting deficiency in clotting factors (secondary to DIC)

(d) Blood cultures identifying causative pathogen (cultures may be negative because bacteremia can be intermittent or patient may already have received antibiotic therapy, thus masking diagnosis)

4. **Nursing diagnoses common to all forms of shock**

   a. Decreased CO and hence tissue perfusion related to decreased circulating blood volume

      i. Assessment for defining characteristics: see pp. 217–218

      ii. Expected outcomes: see p. 218

      iii. Nursing interventions

         (a) See pp. 218–222

         (b) Expand blood volume by administration of blood, plasma expanders, albumin, and electrolyte solutions as ordered

         (c) Management specific to cardiogenic shock

            (1) Administer vasopressors—beta-adrenergic stimulators (dopamine, dobutamine) and alpha-adrenergic stimulator (norepinephrine)

            (2) Afterload increases and deleteriously affects cardiac function—administer vasodilators as ordered (sodium nitroprusside, intravenous nitroglycerin)

            (3) Patient may be placed on the intra-aortic balloon pump

            (4) Other measures aimed at improving cardiac function (i.e., improving oxygenation, decreasing work load on the heart, improving LV function, decreasing patient stress). These concepts have been stressed throughout this chapter, and all can be applied to this aspect of shock

         (d) Management specific to hypovolemic shock

            (1) In the acute phase of hemorrhage, a pneumatic anti-shock garment may be used to increase blood pressure and tamponade the hemorrhage

            (2) Vasopressors generally are contraindicated because normal sympathetic response is capable of producing maximal tolerable vasoconstriction

            (3) Replace volume as indicated above

         (e) Management specific to septic shock

            (1) Administer prescribed antibiotics

            (2) Administer beta-receptor stimulants, which have a positive inotropic effect on the heart and vasodilate microcirculation

(3) Vasopressors that stimulate alpha-adrenergic receptors are contraindicated

(4) Administer corticosteroids during early phase of shock—major benefit is stabilization of lysosomal membrane

(5) Monitor all insertion/invasive sites per unit standards for signs of infection and change sites per unit standards

(6) Monitor all drainage from wounds, lungs, and urinary tract for signs indicating infection; culture all drainage

(f) Management specific to anaphylactic shock

(1) Immediately discontinue the infusion of the antigen

(2) Administer sympathomimetic (epinephrine), which will

    a) Stimulate alpha-receptors, causing vasoconstriction of peripheral blood vessels

    b) Stimulate beta$_1$-receptors, producing positive inotropic and positive chronotropic effects

    c) Stimulate beta$_2$-receptors, which induces bronchodilation

    d) Prevent further histamine release

    e) Counteract circulatory failure and bronchospasm

(3) Administer antihistamines (diphenhydramine) to block histamine receptors and counteract urticaria, itching, and swelling

(4) Administer adrenocortical corticosteroids to stabilize damaged capillary walls and counteract the flow of fluid and proteins into the extravascular spaces

iv. Evaluation of nursing care: see pp. 222–223

b. Potential for impaired gas exchange related to fluid accumulation within the interstitium decreasing diffusion of oxygen

i. Assessment for defining characteristics

(a) Tachypnea, dyspnea

(b) Arterial blood gases—respiratory alkalosis

(c) Bilateral rales

(d) Mental status changes—confusion, restlessness, irritability

(e) Chest x-ray film shows increased pulmonary infiltrates, pulmonary edema

(f) Increased PAP, PCWP, PVR

ii. Expected outcomes

(a) Patient breathes easier, with normal rate and depth of respirations

(b) Arterial blood gases within normal limits

      (c) Lungs clear to auscultation, without adventitious lung sounds

      (d) Patient is oriented to time, person, and place

      (e) Patient is calm

      (f) Chest x-ray film is clear

      (g) Hemodynamic parameters within normal limits

  iii. Nursing interventions

      (a) Assess patient's level of consciousness

      (b) Maintain patent airway—if ventilated then suction per standards

      (c) Monitor patient's respiratory status by assessing lungs for signs of infiltrates and observing patient's color and respiratory rate and character

      (d) Institute nursing actions to mobilize secretions—incentive spirometry, changing positions, chest wall percussion, and postural drainage; deliver humidified oxygen

      (e) Observe for onset of adult respiratory distress syndrome

      (f) Correct acid–base disturbances as ordered (shock produces complex abnormalities due to hypoxia, tachypnea, hypocapnia, lactic acidosis). This will entail fluid replacement, improvement of perfusion, maintenance of airway, possibly mechanical ventilation, and treatment with sedatives and paralyzing agents)

  iv. Evaluation of nursing care: see expected outcomes

  c. Potential for bleeding: related to decreased amount of coagulation factors (DIC): see Chapter 3

  d. See Commonly Encountered Nursing Diagnoses, pp. 200–205

References

Abela, G. S., et al.: Laser recanalization of occluded atherosclerotic arteries in vivo and in vitro. Circulation 71:403–411, 1985.

Ahnve, S.: Correction of QT interval for heart rate: Review of different formulas and the use of Bazett's formula in myocardial infarction. Am. Heart J. 109:568–573, 1985.

American Association of Critical Care Nurses: Methods in Critical Care. The AACN Manual. W. B. Saunders Co., Philadelphia, 1980, p. 145.

Andreoli, K. G., et al.: Comprehensive Cardiac Care, 6th ed. C. V. Mosby Co., St. Louis, 1987.

Appleton, D. L., and Quaglia, J. D.: Vascular disease and postoperative nursing management. Crit. Care Nurse 5(5):34–42, 1985.

Balk, R. N., and Bone, R. C. (eds.): Critical Care Clinics—Septic Shock. W. B. Saunders Co., Philadelphia, 1989.

Bass, J. L., et al.: Flow in the aorta and patent ductus arteriosus in infants with aortic atresia or aortic stenosis: A pulsed Doppler ultrasound study. Circulation 74:315–322, 1986.

Bentley, L. J.: Radionuclide imaging techniques in the diagnosis and treatment of coronary artery disease. Focus Crit. Care 14(6):27–36, 1987.

Berne, R. M., and Levy, M. N.: Cardiovascular Physiology, 5th ed. C. V. Mosby Co., St. Louis, 1986.

Berron, K.: Role of ventricular assist device in acute myocardial infarction. Crit. Care Nurs. Q. 12(2):25–37, 1989.

Blumlein, S., et al.: Quantitation of mitral regurgitation by Doppler echocardiography. Circulation 74:306–314, 1986.

Braunwald, E.: Heart Disease: A Textbook of Cardiovascular Medicine. W. B. Saunders Co., Philadelphia, 1984.

Brewer, C. C., and Marks, J. E.: Streptokinase and tissue plasminogen activator in acute myocardial infarction. Heart Lung 15:552–558, 1986.

Bullas, J. B., and Pfister, S. M.: Variant angina. Crit. Care Nurse 7(4):9–12, 1987.

Bumann, R., and Speltz, M.: Decreased cardiac output: A nursing diagnosis. Dimens. Crit. Care Nurs. 8(1):6–15, 1989.

Cameron, A., et al.: Bypass surgery with the internal mammary artery graft: 15-year follow-up. Circulation 74(suppl III):1130–1136, 1986.

Carlson, S.: IV Nitroglycerine: Reducing complications at high dosages. Dimens. Crit. Care Nurs. 7(2):83–89, 1988.

Carpentino, L. J.: Nursing Diagnosis Application to Clinical Practice. J. B. Lippincott Co., Philadelphia, 1987.

Conner, R. P.: The electrocardiographic diagnosis of posterior myocardial infarction. Crit. Care Nurse 5(2):20–24, 1985.

Conover, M. B.: Pocket Nurse Guide to Electrocardiography. C. V. Mosby Co., St. Louis, 1986.

Cooper, J., and Marriott, H. J.: Why are so many critical care nurses unable to recognize ventricular tachycardia in the 12-lead electrocardiogram? Heart Lung 18(3):243–247, 1989.

Correia, J. A., and Alpert, N. M.: Positron-emission tomography in cardiology. Radiol. Clin. North Am. 23:783–793, 1985.

Curran, C. C., and Mathewson, M.: Use of cardiac glycosides in the critically ill. Crit. Care Nurse 7(6):31–43, 1987.

Daily, E. K., and Schroeder, J. S.: Techniques in Bedside Hemodynamic Monitoring, 3rd ed. C. V. Mosby Co., St. Louis, 1984.

Davidson, L. J., and Brown, S.: Continuous SvO_2 monitoring: A tool for analyzing hemodynamic status. Heart Lung 15(3):287–292, 1986.

DeAngelis, R.: Amiodarone. Crit. Care Nurse 6(6):12–16, 1986.

Dixon, M. B.: Acute aortic dissection. J. Cardiovasc. Nurs. 1(2):24–35, 1987.

Dixon, M. B., and Nunnelee, J.: Arterial reconstruction for atherosclerotic occlusive disease. J. Cardiovasc. Nurs. 1(2):36–49, 1987.

Dreifus, L. S. (ed.): Cardiovascular Clinics—Pacemaker Therapy. F. A. Davis Co., Philadelphia, 1983, p. 137.

Eberts, M. A.: Advances in the pharmacologic management of angina pectoris. J. Cardiovasc. Nurs. 1:15–29, 1986.

Erickson, S.: Wolff-Parkinson-White syndrome: A review and an update. Crit. Care Nurse 9(5):28–35, 1989.

Fairbairn, J. F., et al.: Allen-Barker-Hines Peripheral Vascular Diseases, 4th ed. W. B. Saunders Co., Philadelphia, 1972.

Finkelmeier, B. A., and Salinger, M. H.: Dual-chamber cardiac pacing: An overview. Crit. Care Nurse 6(5):12–28, 1986.

Fisher, J., et al.: The management of cardiogenic shock. Clin. Cardiol. Pract. 1(1):23–42, 1984.

Fontaine, G., et al.: Torsade de pointes: Definition and management. Mod. Concepts Cardiovasc. Dis. 51:103–108, 1982.

Fox, K., and Ilsey, C. D.: The Essentials of Exercise Electrocardiography. Current Medical Literature, Ltd., London, 1984.

Gay, W. A. (ed.): Cardiovascular Surgery. Harper & Row, Philadelphia, 1984.

Genton, R.: Management of congestive heart failure in patients with acute myocardial infarction. JAMA 256:2556–2560, 1986.

Girlando, R. M., et al.: Coarctation of the aorta. Crit. Care Nurse 8(1):38–50, 1988.

Goldbaum, T. S., et al.: Cardiac tamponade following percutaneous transluminal coronary angioplasty: Four case reports. Cathet. Cardiovasc. Diagn. 11:413–416, 1985.

Grimes, J., and Burns, E.: Health Assessment in Nursing Practice, 2nd ed. Jones and Bartlett, Boston, 1987.

Guyton, A. C.: Textbook of Medical Physiology, 7th ed. W. B. Saunders Co., Philadelphia, 1986.

Hardy, G. R.: SvO_2 Continuous monitoring techniques. Dimens. Crit. Care Nurs. 7(1):8–17, 1988.

Heger, J. W., et al.: Cardiology for the House Officer. Williams & Wilkins Co., Baltimore, 1983, pp. 38–205.

Henry, S.: Anti-arrhythmic drug therapy. Calif. Nurs. Rev. 8(6):38–40, 1986.

Hotter, A. N.: Preventing cardiovascular complications following AAA surgery. Dimens. Crit. Care Nurs. 6(1):10–18, 1987.

Hudak, C. M., et al.: Critical Care Nursing: A Holistic Approach, 4th ed. J. B. Lippincott Co., Philadelphia, 1986.

Jansen, K. J., and McFadden, P. M.: Postoperative nursing management in patients undergoing myocardial revascularization with the internal mammary artery bypass. Heart Lung 15:48–54, 1986.

Jaquith, S. M.: Continuous measurement of SvO_2 clinical applications and advantages for critical care nursing. Crit. Care Nurse 5(2):40–44, 1985.

Johanson, B. C., et al.: Standards for Critical Care. C. V. Mosby Co., St. Louis, 1985.

Johnson, C. T., and Conan, M.: Relationship between the prolonged QTc interval and ventricular fibrillation. Heart Lung 15(2):141–150, 1986.

Johnson, R., and Swartz, M. H.: A Simplified Approach to Electrocardiography. W. B. Saunders Co., Philadelphia, 1986.

Kanter, K. R., et al.: Bridging to cardiac transplantation with pulsatile ventricular assist devices. Ann. Thorac. Surg. 46(2):134–140, 1988.

Katz, A. M.: Mechanisms of action and differences in calcium channel blockers. Am. J. Cardiol. 58:20D–22D, 1986.

Katz, A. M., et al.: Cellular actions and pharmacology of the calcium channel blocking drugs. Am. J. Med. 77(suppl 2B):2–10, 1984.

Kim, M. J., et al.: Pocket Guide to Nursing Diagnoses, 3rd ed. C. V. Mosby Co., St. Louis, 1989.

King, S. B., and Douglas, J. S.: Coronary Arteriography and Angioplasty. McGraw-Hill Book Co., New York, 1985.

Kinney, M. R., Packa, D. R., and Dunbar, S. B.: AACN's Clinical Reference for Critical-Care Nursing, 2nd ed. McGraw-Hill Book Co., New York, 1989.

Kleven, M. R.: Comparison of thrombolytic agents: Mechanism of action, efficacy and safety. Heart Lung 17(6):750–755, 1988.

Kloner, R. A. (ed.): Guide to Cardiology. John Wiley & Sons, New York, 1984.

Korsmeyer, C., et al.: The nurse's role in thrombolytic therapy for acute MI. Crit. Care Nurse 7(6):22–30, 1987.

Kutcher, K. L.: Cardiac electrophysiologic mapping techniques. Focus Crit. Care 12(4):26–30, 1985.

Lanoue, A. S., et al.: Percutaneous transluminal coronary angioplasty: Nonoperative treatment of coronary artery disease. J. Cardiovasc. Nurs. 1:30–44, 1986.

Lazarus, M., et al.: Cardiac arrhythmias: Diagnosis and treatment. Crit Care Nurse 8(7):57–65, 1988.

Loan, T.: Nursing interaction with patients undergoing coronary angioplasty. Heart Lung 15(4):368–375, 1986.

Loop, F. D., et al.: Influence of the internal mammary artery graft on 10-year survival and other cardiac events. N. Engl. J. Med. 314:1–6, 1986.

Mandel, W. J.: Cardiac Arrhythmias, Their Mechanisms, Diagnosis and Management. J. B. Lippincott Co., Philadelphia, 1980.

Marrie, T. J.: Infective endocarditis: A serious and changing disease. Crit. Care Nurse 7:31–46, 1987.

Marriott, H. J., and Conover, M. B.: Advanced Concepts in Arrhythmias. C. V. Mosby Co., St. Louis, 1983.

Martchetta, S., and Stennis, E.: Ventricular assist devices: Applications for critical care. J. Cardiovasc. Nurs. 2(2):39–55, 1988.

Metcalfe, K.: Understanding Cardiac Pacing: A Guide for Nurses. Appleton-Century-Crofts, Norwalk, Conn., 1986.

Millar, S. (ed.): AACN Procedure Manual for Critical Care. W. B. Saunders Co., Philadelphia, 1985.

Miller, C. L.: Medication in angina. Focus Crit. Care 15(4):23–29, 1988.

Miller, D. H., and Boer, J. S.: The cardiomyopathies, a pathophysiologic approach to therapeutic management. Arch. Intern. Med. 143:2157–2162, 1983.

Milligan, K. S.: Tissue-type plasminogen activator: A new fibrinolytic agent. Heart Lung 16:69–74, 1987.

Misinski, M.: Pathophysiology of acute myocardial infarction: A rationale for thrombolytic therapy. Heart Lung 17(suppl):743–750, 1988.

Morganroth, J.: A review of the uses and limitations of tocainide-A class 1B antiarrhythmic agent. Am. Heart J. 110:856–863, 1985.

Mulford, E.: Nursing perspectives for the patient receiving postoperative ventricular assistance in the critical care unit. Heart Lung 16:246–255, 1987.

Nappi, J. M., and Anderson, J. L.: Flecainide: A new prototype antiarrhythmic agent. Pharmacotherapy 5:209–221, 1985.

Niemyski, P., and Hallstedt, L. F.: Patient selection and management in thrombolytic therapy: Nursing implications. Crit. Care Nurs. Q. 12(2):8–24, 1989.

Olearchyk, A. S., and Magovern, G. J.: Internal mammary artery grafting. J. Thorac. Cardiovasc. Surg. 92:1082–1087, 1986.

Osbakken, M., and Yuschok, T.: Evaluation of ventricular function with gated cardiac magnetic resonance imaging. Cathet. Cardiovasc. Diagn. 12:156–160, 1986.

Perry, A. G., and Potter, P. A. (eds.): Shock—Comprehensive Nursing Management. C. V. Mosby Co., St. Louis, 1983.

Phillips, R. E., and Feeney, M. K.: The Cardiac Rhythms, 2nd ed. W. B. Saunders Co., Philadelphia, 1980.

Quaal, S. J.: Thrombolytic therapy: An overview. J. Cardiovasc. Nurs. 1:45–56, 1986.

Rakel, R. E. (ed.): Conn's Current Therapy. W. B. Saunders Co., Philadelphia, 1988.

Rentrop, K. P.: Thrombolytic therapy in patients with acute myocardial infarction. Circulation 71:627–631, 1985.

Rice, V.: Shock management: II. Pharmacologic intervention. Crit. Care Nurse 5(1):42–57, 1985.

Rice, V.: Shock, a clinical syndrome: IV: Nursing intervention. Crit. Care Nurse 4(5):34–43, 1984.

Roberts, S. L.: Cardiogenic shock: Decreased coronary artery tissue perfusion. Dimens. Crit. Care Nurs. 7(4):196–208, 1988.

Robinson, J. S.: Acute right ventricular infarction: Recognition, evaluation and treatment. Crit. Care Nurse 7(4):42–53, 1987.

Rodriguez, S. W., and Reed, R. L.: Thrombolytic therapy for MI. Am. J. Nurs. 87:631–640, 1987.

Rossignol, M., et al.: Treatment of right ventricular infarction. Focus Crit. Care 12(6):20–25, 1985.

Rushmer, R. F.: Cardiovascular Dynamics, 3rd ed. W. B. Saunders Co., Philadelphia, 1970.

Ruzevich, S. A. et al.: Nursing care of the patient with a pneumatic ventricular assist device. Heart Lung 17:399–497, 1988.

Sanderson, R. G., and Kurth, C. L.: The Cardiac Patient: A Comprehensive Approach, 2nd ed. W. B. Saunders Co., Philadelphia, 1983.

Schakenbach, L. H.: Physiologic dynamics of acquired valvular heart disease. J. Cardiovasc. Nurs. 1(2):1–17, 1987.

Schelbert, H. R.: Positron-emission tomography: Assessment of myocardial blood flow and metabolism. Circulation 72(suppl IV):122–133, 1985.

Schroeder, S. A., et al. (eds.): Current Medical Diagnoses and Treatment. Appleton and Lange, Norwalk, Conn., 1988.

Schwartz, G. R., et al. (eds.): Principles and Practice of Emergency Medicine, 2nd ed., vol. 2. W. B. Saunders Co., Philadelphia, 1986.

Scrima, D. A.: Infective endocarditis: Nursing considerations. Crit. Care Nurse 7:47–56, 1987.

Selwyn, A. P., and Smith, T. W.: Current and future directions for clinical investigation of the heart with positron-emission tomography. Circulation 72(suppl IV):31–38, 1985.

Shepard, N., et al.: A guide to arrhythmia interpretation and management. Crit. Care Nurse 2(5):59–85, 1982.

Sherman, C. T., et al.: Coronary angioscopy in patients with unstable angina pectoris. N. Engl. J. Med. 315:913–919, 1986.

Shoemaker, W. C., et al.: Textbook of Critical Care, 2nd ed. W. B. Saunders Co., Philadelphia, 1988.

Sipperly, M. E.: Thrombolytic therapy update. Crit. Care Nurse 5:30–33, 1985.

Somberg, J. C., and Tepper, D.: Flecainide: A new antiarrhythmic agent. Am. Heart J. 112:808–813, 1986.

Sommers, M. S. (ed.): Difficult Diagnoses in Critical Care Nursing. Aspen Publishers, Rockville, Md., 1989.

Steger, K. E., et al.: Drug-induced torsade des pointes: Case report and implications for the critical care staff. Heart Lung 15:200–202, 1986.

Stein, E.: Clinical Electrocardiography: A Self Study Course. Lea & Febiger, Philadelphia, 1987.

Stone, K. S., and Scordo, K. A.: Understanding the calcium channel blockers. Heart Lung 13:563–571, 1984.

Sullam, P. M., et al.: Pathogenesis of endocarditis. Am. J. Med. 78(suppl 6B):110–115, 1985.

Summers, C., and O'Mara, S. R.: Assessment and treatment of life-threatening ventricular arrhythmias: The role of programmed electrical stimulation, intraoperative mapping and endocardial resection. Heart Lung 14(2):130–141, 1985.

Taylor, G. J., et al.: Intravenous versus intracoronary streptokinase therapy for acute myocardial infarction in community hospitals. Am. J. Cardiol. 54:256–260, 1984.

Taylor, T.: Monitoring left atrial pressures in the open-heart surgical patient. Crit. Care Nurse 6(2):62–68, 1986.

Tector, A. J., et al.: Expanding the use of the internal mammary artery to improve patency of coronary artery bypass grafting. J. Thorac. Cardiovasc. Surg. 91:9–16, 1986.

Tilkian, A. G., and Daily, E. K. (eds.): Cardiovascular Procedures: Diagnostic Techniques and Therapeutic Procedures. C. V. Mosby Co., St. Louis, 1986.

TIMI Study Group.: The thrombolysis in myocardial infarction (TIMI) trial, phase 1 findings. N. Engl. J. Med. 312:932–936, 1985.

Tinkler, J., and Rapin, M.: Care of the Critically Ill Patient. Springer-Verlag, New York, 1983.

Topol, E. J.: Clinical use of streptokinase and urokinase therapy for acute myocardial infarct. Heart Lung 16(6):760–774, 1987.

Touloukian, J. E.: Calcium channel blocking agents: Physiologic basis of nursing intervention. Heart Lung 14:342–348, 1985.

Valentine, R. P., et al.: Intravenous versus intracoronary streptokinase in acute myocardial infarction. Am. J. Cardiol. 55:309–315, 1985.

Walsh, D. G., et al.: Use of tissue plasminogen activator in emergency department for acute myocardial infarction. Ann. Emerg. Med. 16:243–247, 1987.

Weinberger, M. H.: Antihypertensive therapy and lipids. Am. J. Med. 80(suppl 2A):64–70, 1986.

Wescott, B. L.: Tissue plasminogen activator: A new advancement in fibrinolytic therapy. Focus Crit. Care 13(6):22–26, 1986.

White, K. M.: Completing the hemodynamic picture: SvO_2. Heart Lung 14:272–279, 1985.

Williams, E. M.: A classification of antiarrhythmic action reassessed after a decade of new drugs. J. Clin Pharmacol. 24:129–147, 1984.

Wilson, D. B., and Vacek, J. L.: Angina and coronary artery disease. Postgrad. Med. 84:77–84, 1988.

Wyngaarden, J. B., and Smith, L. H. (eds.): Cecil Textbook of Medicine, 18th ed., vol. 1. W. B. Saunders Co., Philadelphia, 1988.

Yabek, S. M., et al.: Effects of flecainide on the cellular electrophysiology of neonatal and adult fibers. Am. Heart J. 113:70–76, 1987.

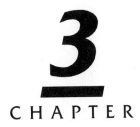

CHAPTER

The Neurologic System

Diana L. Nikas, R.N., M.N., CCRN, CNRN, FCCM

PHYSIOLOGIC ANATOMY

Brain

1. **Coverings**
   a. Scalp
      i. Galea aponeurotica: freely movable, dense, fibrous tissue that covers the skull and absorbs the force of external trauma
      ii. Fatty and vascular layer: subcutaneous layer between the skin and galea containing blood vessels that contract poorly when injured
      iii. Subaponeurotic space: space beneath the galea that contains diploic and emissary veins
   b. Skull
      i. Bones: frontal, parietal, temporal, and occipital
      ii. Rigid cavity: houses and protects brain and has volume of 1400 to 1500 ml (Fig. 3–1)
      iii. Composition: an inner table and an outer table, separated by diploic space (cancellous bone). This arrangement provides maximal strength with an economy of weight
      iv. Fossae: three depressions in base of skull—anterior, middle, and posterior (Fig. 3–2)
   c. Meninges (Fig. 3–3)
      i. Dura mater
         (a) Outermost covering of brain consisting of two layers of tough fibrous tissue
         (1) Outer layer is periosteum of bone

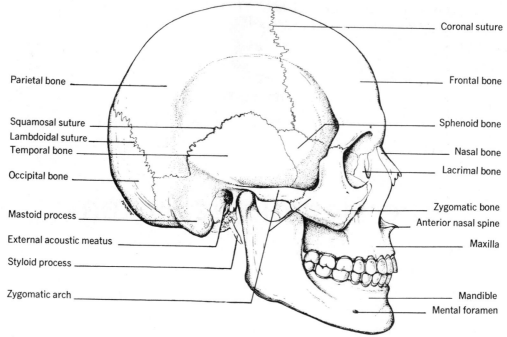

Parietal bone

Squamosal suture
Lambdoidal suture
Temporal bone

Occipital bone

Mastoid process

External acoustic meatus

Styloid process

Zygomatic arch

Coronal suture

Frontal bone

Sphenoid bone

Nasal bone

Lacrimal bone

Zygomatic bone
Anterior nasal spine

Maxilla

Mandible
Mental foramen

Figure 3–1. Bones of the skull. (From Chaffee, E. E., and Greisheimer, E. M.: Basic Physiology and Anatomy, 3rd ed. J. B. Lippincott Co., Philadelphia, 1974, p. 62.)

    (2) Inner layer forms falx cerebri and tentorium cerebelli
  (b) Meningeal arteries and venous sinuses lie within clefts formed by separation of inner and outer layers of dura
 ii. Arachnoid mater
  (a) Fine, fibrous, elastic layer that lies between dura mater and pia mater
  (b) Subarachnoid space
    (1) Lies between arachnoid mater and pia mater
    (2) Separates widely at base of brain to form subarachnoid cisterna
    (3) Contains larger blood vessels of brain
    (4) Contains cerebrospinal fluid (CSF), which completely surrounds brain and spinal cord and acts as shock absorber
  (c) Arachnoid villi—projections of arachnoid mater that serve as channels for absorption of CSF into venous system (pacchionian bodies are large arachnoid villi distributed along superior sagittal sinus)
 iii. Pia mater
  (a) Delicate layer that adheres to surface of brain and spinal cord
  (b) Follows sulci and gyri of brain and carries branches of cerebral arteries with it

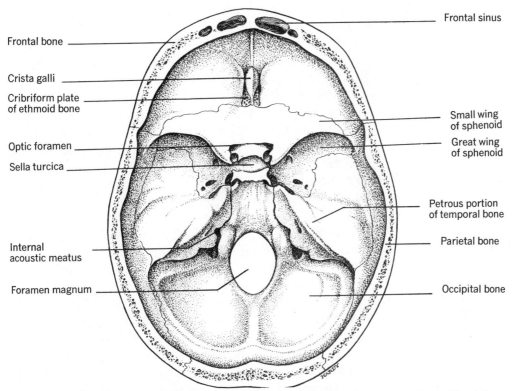

Frontal sinus

Frontal bone

Crista galli

Cribriform plate
of ethmoid bone

Small wing
of sphenoid

Great wing
of sphenoid

Optic foramen

Sella turcica

Petrous portion
of temporal bone

Parietal bone

Internal
acoustic meatus

Foramen magnum

Occipital bone

Figure 3–2. Base of skull. (From Chaffee, E. E., and Greisheimer, E. M.: Basic Physiology and Anatomy, 3rd ed. J. B. Lippincott Co., Philadelphia, 1974, p. 63.)

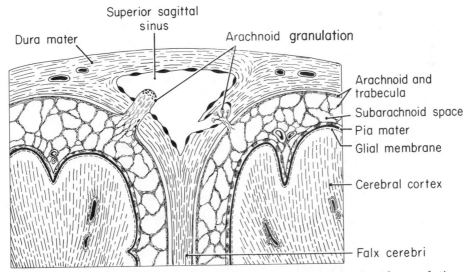

Superior sagittal
sinus

Dura mater

Arachnoid granulation

Arachnoid and
trabecula

Subarachnoid space

Pia mater

Glial membrane

Cerebral cortex

Falx cerebri

Figure 3–3. Diagram of meningeal-cortical relationships. Arachnoid granulations may penetrate dural sinus or terminate in a lateral lacuna of the sinus. The pia is firmly anchored to cortex by the glial membrane. (From Carpenter, M. B.: Core Text of Neuroanatomy, 2nd ed. © 1978, the Williams & Wilkins Company, Baltimore.)

       (c) Blood vessels of pia form choroid plexus

2. Divisions of the brain

  a. Cerebrum: consists of

    i. Telencephalon: two cerebral hemispheres separated by longitudinal fissure and joined by corpus callosum

      (a) Functional localization in cortex

        (1) Frontal lobe—responsible for voluntary motor function (origin of pyramidal motor system) and higher mental functions such as judgment and foresight, affect, and personality

        (2) Temporal lobes—responsible for hearing, speech in dominant hemisphere, vestibular sense, behavior, and emotion

        (3) Parietal lobe—responsible for sensory function, sensory association areas, and higher level processing of general sensory modalities (e.g., stereognosis)

        (4) Occipital lobe—responsible for vision

        (5) Corpus callosum—commissural fibers that transfer learned discriminations, sensory experience, and memory from one cerebral hemisphere to the other

        (6) Cerebral dominance—in right-handed and some left-handed persons, left cerebral hemisphere is dominant for verbal, linguistic, arithmetical, calculating, and analytic functions. Nondominant hemisphere is generally believed to be concerned with geometric, spatial, visual, pattern, and musical functions

      (b) Basal ganglia (also called basal nuclei) (Fig. 3–4)

        (1) Include caudate nucleus, putamen, globus pallidus, claustrum, subthalamic nucleus, and substantia nigra

        (2) Exert regulating and controlling influences on motor integration; suppress muscle tone; influence postural reflexes—a major center of the extrapyramidal motor system

    ii. Diencephalon: consists of

      (a) Thalamus—anatomically forms lateral walls of third ventricle; subdivided into several nuclei on basis of fiber connections and phylogenetic connections

        (1) Certain nuclei receive specific sensory input from general senses, taste, vision, and hearing and relay it to cerebral cortex

        (2) Other nuclei participate in affective aspects of brain function, are functionally related to association areas of cortex, or have a role in motor function and ascending reticular activating system

      (b) Hypothalamus—forms ventral part of diencephalon, facing

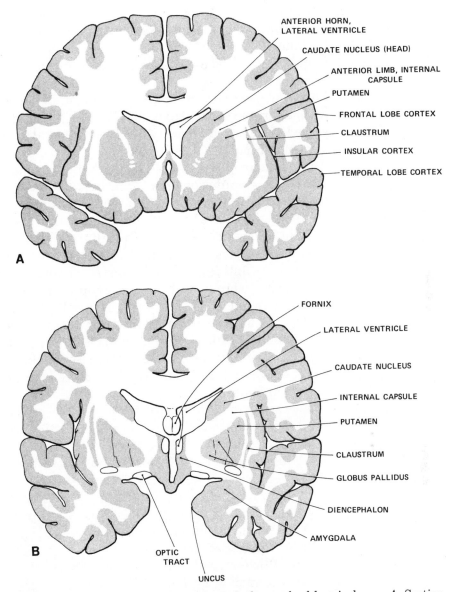

Figure 3–4. Two coronal sections through the cerebral hemispheres. *A.* Section through the rostral part of the frontal lobe to show the relationship of the basal ganglia to the surrounding telencephalic structures. *B.* Section through the caudal part of the frontal lobe, showing the location of the basal ganglia lateral to the diencephalon. (From Gilman, S., and Winans, S. S.: Manter and Gatz's Essentials of Clinical Neuroanatomy and Neurophysiology, 6th ed. F. A. Davis Company, Philadelphia, 1982.)

third ventricle medially. Hypothalamic nuclei intercon-
nect with each other and with limbic system, midbrain,
thalamus, and pituitary gland. Functions include

(1) Temperature regulation (anterior and posterior hypothalamus)

(2) Regulation of food and water intake (ventromedial and
lateral regions)

(3) Behavior—as part of limbic system, it is concerned
with aggressive and sexual behavior. It may be involved with sleep along with other central nervous
system (CNS) structures

(4) Autonomic responses—parasympathetic responses are
elicited by stimulation of anterior hypothalamus; sympathetic responses may be elicited by stimulation of
posterior and lateral hypothalamic nuclei

(5) Control hormonal secretion of pituitary gland

   a) Posterior pituitary (neurohypophysis)—stores and
releases antidiuretic hormone (ADH) and oxytocin,
which are produced by the supraoptic and paraventricular nuclei, respectively, of hypothalamus

     ☐ Increased serum osmolarity or decreased extra-
cellular fluid volume stimulates ADH synthesis
and release. ADH causes increased reabsorption
of water from distal tubule and collecting duct
of nephron

     ☐ Oxytocin stimulates contraction of uterus under
appropriate circumstances and ejection of milk
from lactating breast

   b) Anterior pituitary (adenohypophysis)—hormonal
secretion from anterior pituitary is under control
of pituitary releasing/inhibiting factors produced
in hypothalamus and transported to anterior pituitary via a pituitary portal system. Hormones
thus influenced are

     ☐ Follicle-stimulating hormone (FSH)

     ☐ Luteinizing hormone (LH)

     ☐ Prolactin

     ☐ Thyroid-stimulating hormone (TSH)

     ☐ Adrenocorticotropic hormone (ACTH)

     ☐ Somatotropic hormone (STH) or growth hor-
mone (GH)

iii. Limbic system (Fig. 3–5)

  (a) Composed of cingulate and parahippocampal gyri, hippo-
campal formation, part of amygdaloid nucleus, hypothalamus, and anterior nucleus of thalamus

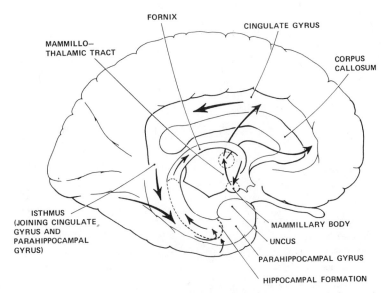

Figure 3–5. The Papez circuit *(arrows)* diagrammed on a schematic view of the limbic system on the medial surface of the cerebral hemisphere. (From Gilman, S., and Winans, S. S.: Manter and Gatz's Essentials of Clinical Neuroanatomy and Neurophysiology, 6th ed. F. A. Davis Company, Philadelphia, 1982.)

(b) Responsible for affective aspect of emotional behavior as well as visceral responses accompanying them; also involved in some aspects of memory

b. Brain stem (Fig. 3–6)

   i. Midbrain (mesencephalon): located between pons and diencephalon

      (a) Contains nuclei of third (oculomotor) and fourth (trochlear) cranial nerves

      (b) Contains motor and sensory pathways

      (c) Tectal region (inferior and superior colliculi) is concerned with auditory and visual systems

      (d) Connected to cerebellum via superior cerebellar peduncles

   ii. Pons: located between midbrain and medulla; on ventral surface appears to form a bridge connecting right and left cerebellar hemispheres

      (a) Contains nuclei of fifth (trigeminal), sixth (abducens), and seventh (facial) cranial nerves. Some nuclei of acoustic (eighth cranial nerve) are found in pons

      (b) On basal portion of pons middle cerebellar peduncles provide extensive connections between cerebral cortex and cerebellum, thus ensuring maximal motor efficiency

      (c) Contains motor and sensory pathways

   iii. Medulla: located between pons and spinal cord

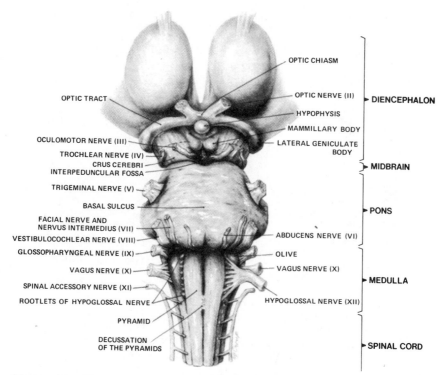

Figure 3–6. The ventral surface of the human brain stem and diencephalon. (From Gilman, S., and Winans, S. S.: Manter and Gatz's Essentials of Clinical Neuroanatomy and Neurophysiology, 6th ed. F. A. Davis Company, Philadelphia, 1982.)

      (a) Contains nuclei of the eighth (acoustic), ninth (glossopharyngeal), tenth (vagus), eleventh (spinal accessory), and twelfth (hypoglossal) cranial nerves

      (b) Motor and sensory tracts of spinal cord continue into medulla

      (c) Attached to cerebellum via inferior cerebellar peduncles

    iv. Reticular formation: diffuse cellular network of brain stem with axons projecting to thalamus, cortex, spinal cord, and cerebellum

      (a) Ascending reticular activating system is essential for arousal from sleep, alert wakefulness, focusing of attention, and perceptual association. Destructive lesions of upper pons and midbrain produce coma

      (b) Descending reticular system may inhibit or facilitate activity of motor neurons controlling skeletal musculature

    v. Respiratory and cardiovascular centers have been identified within the brain stem

  c. Cerebellum: lies in posterior fossa posterior to brain stem. It is separated from the cerebrum by the tentorium cerebelli

i. Influences muscle tone in relation to equilibrium, locomotion, posture, and nonstereotyped movements
ii. Especially important in synchronization of muscle action
iii. Input is from spinal, brain stem, and cerebral centers; output is via descending pathways (e.g., corticospinal, vestibulospinal, and reticulospinal tracts)

3. Cerebral blood supply (Fig. 3–7)
  a. Arterial: supplied by two paired systems of vessels—the internal carotid and vertebral artery systems
    i. Internal carotid system: internal carotid arteries arise from common carotid arteries. Branches of this system include
      (a) Anterior cerebral arteries—supply medial aspect of frontal and parietal lobes and corpus callosum
      (b) Anterior communicating artery—connects right and left anterior cerebral arteries
      (c) Middle cerebral arteries—supply most of lateral surfaces of frontal, temporal, and parietal lobe; it is the largest, most important branch of the internal carotid system
      (d) Posterior communicating arteries—connect posterior cerebral arteries with internal carotid arteries
    ii. Vertebral system: vertebral arteries arise from subclavian arteries and join at lower border of pons to form basilar artery. Branches of this system include
      (a) Posterior inferior cerebellar arteries (PICA)—branches of

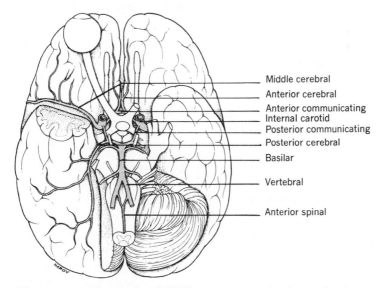

Middle cerebral
Anterior cerebral
Anterior communicating
Internal carotid
Posterior communicating
Posterior cerebral
Basilar
Vertebral
Anterior spinal

Figure 3–7. The circle of Willis as seen at the base of a brain that has been removed from the skull. (From Chaffee, E. E., and Greisheimer, E. M.: Basic Physiology and Anatomy, 3rd ed. J. B. Lippincott Co., Philadelphia, 1974, p. 301.)

vertebral arteries that supply posterior and inferior portions of cerebellum

(b) Anterior spinal artery—supplies anterior half to three fourths of the spinal cord and medial aspect of the brain stem

(c) Posterior cerebral arteries—branches of basilar artery that supply posterior parietal lobe and inferior portion of temporal and occipital lobes

(d) Superior cerebellar and anterior inferior cerebellar arteries—branches of basilar artery that supply brain stem and cerebellum

iii. Circle of Willis—anastomosis of arteries at base of brain formed by short segment of internal carotid and anterior and posterior cerebral arteries that are connected by an anterior communicating artery and two posterior communicating arteries. This anastomosis permits collateral circulation if one of the carotid or vertebral arteries becomes occluded. Effectiveness of this mechanism is affected by patency of the vessels and anomalous vessels

iv. Meningeal arteries: branches of external carotid arteries that supply dura mater

(a) Anterior meningeal artery—supplies anterior portion of dura, over frontal tips

(b) Middle meningeal artery—supplies most of dura (i.e., posterior portion of frontal area, all of temporal and parietal, and part of occipital area)

(c) Posterior meningeal artery—supplies occipital area of dura

(d) Pia and arachnoid derive their blood supply from internal carotid and vertebral arteries

v. Cerebral blood flow (CBF)

(a) CBF varies with changes in cerebral perfusion pressure (CPP) and diameter of cerebrovascular bed

(1) CPP is difference between mean arterial pressure (MAP) and intracranial pressure (ICP). CPP = MAP − ICP. Normal CPP is above 60 mm Hg.

(2) Diameter of cerebrovascular bed influenced by

a) Autoregulation—an alteration in diameter of resistance vessels (arterioles) that maintains constant blood flow over a range of perfusion pressures. The limits of autoregulation are mean arterial pressures between 50 and 150 mm Hg

b) Hypercapnia (Pa_{CO_2} > 45 mm Hg) and to a lesser extent hypoxemia (Pa_{O_2} < 60 mm Hg) lead to vasodilation and increased CBF

b. Venous: cerebrum has external veins that lie in subarachnoid space on surfaces of hemispheres and internal veins that drain the central core of cerebrum and lie beneath the corpus callosum (Fig. 3–8)

    i. Both external and internal venous systems empty into venous sinuses that lie between dural layers

        (a) Superior sagittal sinus—lies in attached border of falx cerebri. Superior cerebral veins empty into it

        (b) Inferior sagittal sinus—lies along free border of falx cerebri and receives blood from medial aspects of hemispheres

        (c) Straight sinus—lies in attachment of falx cerebri to tentorium and drains system of internal cerebral veins

        (d) Transverse sinus—lies in bony groove along fixed edge of tentorium cerebelli and is usually continuous with straight sinus

        (e) Other sinuses include cavernous, circular, superior pe-

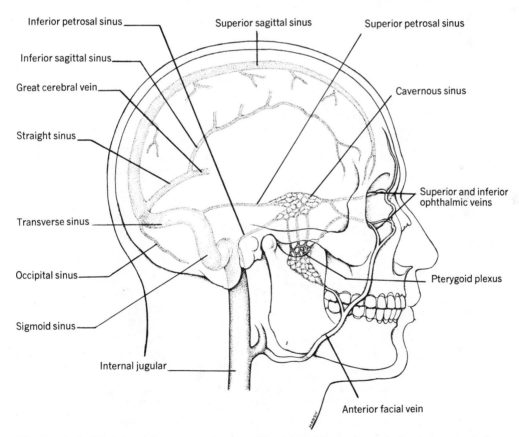

Figure 3–8. The cranial venous sinuses. The sigmoid portion of the transverse sinus continues as the internal jugular vein. (From Chaffee, E. E., and Greisheimer, E. M.: Basic Physiology and Anatomy, 3rd ed. J. B. Lippincott, Philadelphia, 1974, p. 309.)

trosal, inferior petrosal, basilar, sphenoparietal, and occipital

    (f) Emissary veins—connect dural sinuses with veins outside cranial cavity

  ii. Internal jugular veins: collect blood from dural venous sinuses

4. Ventricular system and cerebrospinal fluid (CSF)

  a. Communicating system within brain: composed of four cavities containing CSF (Fig. 3–9)

    i. Lateral ventricles: the largest of the ventricles; one lies in each cerebral hemisphere. Anterior horn of lateral ventricles lies in frontal lobe; body extends back through parietal lobe to posterior horn, which extends into occipital lobe. Inferior horn lies in temporal lobe

    ii. Third ventricle: lies in midline between two lateral ventricles. Lateral walls are formed by the two thalami, which are connected by band of gray matter called massa intermedia

    iii. Fourth ventricle: lies in posterior fossa and is continuous with aqueduct of Sylvius superiorly and central canal inferiorly

  b. Function

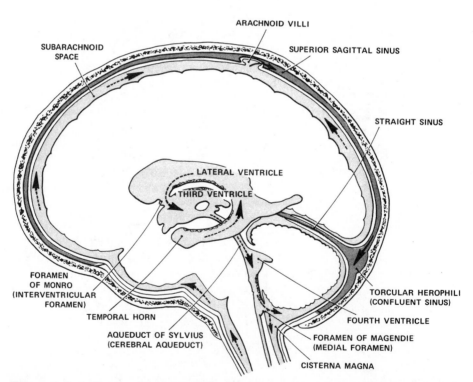

Figure 3–9. A diagram illustrating the circulation of the cerebrospinal fluid. (From Gilman, S., and Winans, S. S.: Manter and Gatz's Essentials of Clinical Neuroanatomy and Neurophysiology, 6th ed. F. A. Davis Company, Philadelphia, 1982.)

     i. CSF cushions brain and spinal cord and decreases their effective weight

    ii. Displacement of CSF out of cranial cavity (and, to an extent, increased reabsorption of CSF) compensates for changes in intracranial volume

   iii. Role in metabolism is uncertain

c. Properties

     i. Clear, colorless, odorless

    ii. Specific gravity: 1.007

   iii. pH: 7.35

   iv. Chloride: 120 to 130 mEq/L

    v. Sodium: 140 to 142 mEq/L

   vi. Glucose: 60% of serum glucose level

  vii. Protein

     (a) Lumbar—15 to 45 mg/dl

     (b) Cisternal—10 to 25 mg/dl

     (c) Ventricular—5 to 15 mg/dl

 viii. Cells

     (a) Leukocytes—0 to 5/mm^3

     (b) Erythrocytes—0/mm^3

   ix. Ventricular system and subarachnoid space contain 125 to 150 ml of CSF; rate of synthesis is estimated to be 500 ml/day. CSF is distributed as follows

     (a) 90 ml in lumbar subarachnoid space

     (b) 25 ml in ventricles

     (c) 35 ml in rest of subarachnoid space

    x. Pressure: 80 to 180 mm H_2O, measured at lumbar level, with patient in side-lying position

d. Formation

     i. Choroid plexus: tuft of capillaries covered by epithelial cells. It is the principal source of CSF and is found within all ventricles

    ii. Majority (95%) of CSF is produced in lateral ventricles. Remainder is formed in third and fourth ventricles

   iii. Small amounts may be produced by blood vessels of brain and meningeal linings

   iv. Process of osmosis across walls of choroid plexus is believed to be responsible for most CSF produced, although the composition differs from a simple ultrafiltrate of plasma. Active transport of sodium, potassium, and chloride creates an osmotic gradient favoring movement of water across epithelial cells of choroid plexus into the ventricles

e. Circulation

     i. CSF circulates from lateral ventricles through interventricular foramen (foramen of Monro) to third ventricle and, via aqueduct of Sylvius, to fourth ventricle

      ii. From fourth ventricle, CSF circulates to cisterna and subarachnoid space via foramina of Luschka and Magendie

  f. Absorption

      i. Arachnoid granulations consist of numerous arachnoid villi located along superior sagittal sinus

      ii. Most CSF is absorbed via arachnoid villi that project from subarachnoid space into dural sinuses

      iii. Hydrostatic pressure gradient between CSF and venous sinus is one factor that determines CSF absorption

5. Cells of nervous system (Fig. 3–10)

  a. Neurons: transmitters of nerve impulses (information)

      i. 10 billion in CNS

      ii. Functions include

        (a) Receiving input from other neurons, primarily via dendrites and cell body

        (b) Summation of inhibitory or excitatory postsynaptic potentials, eventually leading to an action potential

        (c) Conducting action potentials along axon-to-axon terminal

        (d) Transferring information by synaptic transmission to other neurons, muscle cells, or gland cells

      iii. Components of each cell

        (a) Cell body (soma or perikaryon)—carries out metabolic functions of cell; contains nucleus and cytoplasmic organelles (i.e., neurofibrils, neurofilaments, microtubules, Nissl material, mitochondria, Golgi apparatus)

        (b) Dendrites—extensions of cell body that conduct impulses toward cell body. Dendritic zone—receptive area of neuron. Each neuron may have numerous dendrites

        (c) Axon hillock—thickened area of cell body from which axon originates

        (d) Axon—conducts impulses away from cell body. It is usually myelinated. Outside the brain, axons are also covered with neurilemma. Each neuron possesses one axon

        (e) Myelin sheath—a white protein–lipid complex that surrounds some axons; laid down by Schwann cells in peripheral nervous system and by oligodendrocytes in CNS

        (f) Nodes of Ranvier—periodic constrictions along axon where it is not covered by myelin. Impulse is conducted from node to node (saltatory conduction) and thus is speeded up

        (g) Synaptic knobs (terminal buttons or axon telodendria)—contain vesicles in which neurotransmitter substances are stored

  b. Neuroglial cells: form supporting structure for nervous system

      i. About ten times as numerous as neurons

      ii. Four types

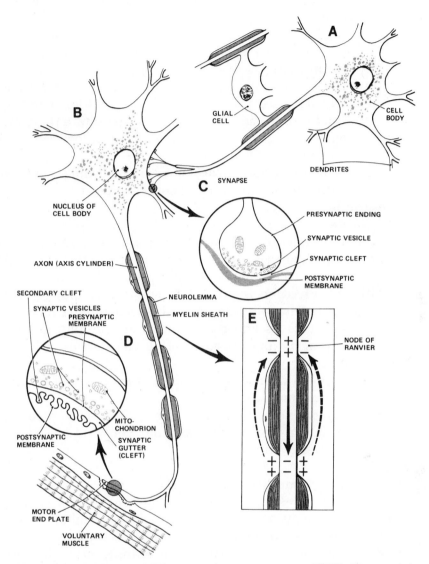

Figure 3–10. Neurons of the central nervous system (CNS). Neuron *A* is confined to the CNS and terminates on neuron *B* at a typical chemical synapse *(C)*. Neuron *B* is a ventral horn cell; its axon extends into a peripheral nerve and innervates a striated (voluntary) muscle at the myoneural junction (motor end plate, *D*). In *E* the action potential is moving in the direction of the solid arrow inside the axon; the dashed arrows indicate the direction of flow of the action current. (From Gilman, S., and Winans, S. S.: Manter and Gatz's Essentials of Clinical Neuroanatomy and Neurophysiology, 6th ed. F. A. Davis Company, Philadelphia, 1982.)

(a) Microglia—no special function known under normal conditions, but they phagocytize tissue debris when nervous tissue is damaged

(b) Oligodendroglia—responsible for myelin formation. They seem to have symbiotic relationship with nerve cells within CNS

(c) Astrocytes—function uncertain. They send many end-feet to blood vessels, may provide nutrients for neurons, contribute to basic structure of blood–brain barrier, and constitute structural and supporting framework for nerve cells and capillaries

(d) Ependyma—specialized glial tissue lining ventricles of brain and central canal of spinal cord

6. Brain metabolism

a. Carbohydrate

   i. Brain has high metabolic energy requirements and uses glucose as its principal source of energy in production of adenosine triphosphate (ATP) necessary in cellular processes

   ii. Although glycogen is present in small amounts, glycolysis is not sufficient to maintain adequate production of ATP

   iii. Glucose serves as major contributor in building amino acids and fatty acids and is source of carbon dioxide, which helps regulate pH

   iv. Hypoglycemia depresses cerebral metabolism and may lead to convulsions, coma, and death

   v. Hyperglycemia has no known direct effect on nervous system function but may cause intracellular dehydration, with resultant cerebral dysfunction

b. Oxygen

   i. Oxygen consumption averages about 49 ml/min, or about 20% of total-body resting oxygen consumption

   ii. Constant supply of oxygen is essential to normal brain function; cytotoxic cerebral edema results within seconds of anoxia

   iii. Energy for metabolic activities of brain is normally produced by oxidative metabolism of glucose, but rate increases markedly during hypoxia

c. Blood–brain barrier: special permeability characteristics of brain capillaries and choroid plexus act to limit transfer of certain substances into extracellular fluid (ECF) or CSF of brain. It is believed to be due to unique membranous ultrastructure of endothelial cells of vessels in the brain with "tight" junctions and the end-feet projections of the astrocytes

   i. Water, carbon dioxide, oxygen, and glucose cross cerebral capillaries with ease. Uptake of other substances, such as ions, is much slower in comparison to uptake by other organs. These substances may be transported by stereospecific transport systems

    ii. Functions to maintain homeostatic environment of neurons in CNS by determining level of metabolism and ionic composition of tissue fluids

   iii. Of clinical significance in treating and diagnosing disease of CNS. Blood–brain barrier is often disrupted in injured tissue, leading to increased permeability

   iv. Blood–CSF barrier permits selective transport from blood to ventricular system. Substances placed into CSF diffuse readily into interstitial fluid of brain

d. Vitamins: several vitamins are essential for normal CNS functioning. Because these vitamins function as coenzymes for enzyme systems, deficiencies cause neurologic symptoms, probably by reducing activity of one or more enzyme systems

    i. Thiamine (vitamin B_1): important in formation of compounds of Krebs' cycle. Deficiencies cause necrosis of cell bodies of cranial nerve nuclei in brain stem and may also affect areas of diencephalon

    ii. Vitamin B_{12}: deficiencies lead to combined subacute degeneration of spinal cord and peripheral nerves, although exact mechanism is not clearly established

   iii. Pyridoxine (vitamin B_6): a coenzyme for a variety of enzymatic reactions. Seizures appear to be principal reaction to deficiencies

   iv. Nicotinic acid: required for enzymatic synthesis of coenzymes. Deficiencies cause pellagra, characterized by dermatitis and disturbances in mentation

e. Cerebral neurotransmitters: chemical mediators of nerve impulse transmission

    i. Acetylcholine (ACh): found in cholinergic fibers of autonomic nervous system (ANS) and nerves to skeletal muscles. ACh may also be involved in drinking behavior

    ii. Norepinephrine (NE): found in adrenergic fibers of ANS. Produced in locus ceruleus nucleus of brain stem, it is implicated in feeding behavior, temperature control, and sleep, particularly paradoxic (rapid eye movement [REM]) sleep

   iii. Dopamine (DA): found in substantia nigra and corpus striatum. It acts as an inhibitory transmitter (e.g., inhibits release of prolactin). It is found in decreased amounts in Parkinson's disease and is also associated with eating and drinking behavior and possibly with sexual behavior

   iv. Gamma-aminobutyric acid (GABA): found at some synaptic junctions and in substantia nigra. It acts as an inhibitory transmitter. It is found in decreased amounts in Huntington's chorea

    v. Serotonin (5-HT): produced in raphe nuclei of brain stem. It is also found in high concentrations in hypothalamus, midbrain, and caudate nucleus and is implicated in sleep behavior, particularly slow wave and possibly REM sleep

7. Synaptic transmission of impulses

  a. Nerve impulse: nerve cells that are excited by electrical, chemical, or mechanical stimuli produce an impulse that is transmitted (or conducted) along the nerve fibers in an active, self-propagating process requiring expenditure of energy. This mechanism allows one part of the body to "communicate" with other parts of the body

  b. Synapse: a junction between one neuron and the next that permits unidirectional conduction of an impulse from presynaptic to postsynaptic neurons

  c. Excitatory neurotransmitter: a substance secreted by presynaptic knobs or vesicles (usually located at axon terminal) that excite a postsynaptic neuron. Released when cell membrane is polarized by nerve impulse

  d. Depolarization: causes increase in permeability of cell membrane resulting in intracellular flow of sodium ions

    i. Increased levels of intracellular Na^+ cause decrease in resting membrane potential (RMP)

    ii. RMP is voltage difference across a cell membrane, with inside negative to outside

    iii. Change in RMP is called the excitatory postsynaptic potential (EPSP)

  e. Action potential: if transient voltage change that occurs with depolarization is of sufficient magnitude (i.e., threshold level), an action potential occurs. Once initiated, it is self-propagated and spreads like a wave over membrane

  f. Summation: simultaneous excitation of successively greater numbers of excitatory presynaptic terminals (or rapidly successive discharges from same presynaptic terminal) that cause progressive increase in postsynaptic potential

    i. Facilitation: if summated postsynaptic potential is less than its threshold for excitation, neuron is said to be facilitated but not excited. No action potential occurs

    ii. Rate of discharge of neuron is dependent on summated postsynaptic potential in relation to threshold for excitation

      (a) Complete refraction (neuron is incapable of producing an action potential) limits the frequency of impulses a cell can generate

      (b) Relative refraction means that neuron can be excited again, but only with summation above threshold

  g. Repolarization

        i. At peak of action potential, cell membrane again becomes impermeable to sodium and RMP returns toward normal

        ii. Cell also becomes more permeable to potassium, and RMP returns to normal with aid of sodium–potassium pump, which pumps sodium out of cell and potassium into cell

  h. Inhibition

        i. Inhibitory postsynaptic potential (IPSP)

          (a) Hyperpolarization of cell membrane is caused by secretion of an inhibitory transmitter (perhaps GABA) by presynaptic terminals of inhibitory neurons

          (b) Results in increase in negativity of RMP caused by increased permeability of cells to potassium and chloride

          (c) This causes decreased excitability and inhibition of impulse transmission

        ii. Presynaptic inhibition: causes inhibition by reducing amount of neurotransmitter substance released from excitatory presynaptic endings and thus reducing to subthreshold levels the magnitude of EPSP they produce

Spine and Spinal Cord

1. **Vertebral column**

  a. Composed of 33 vertebrae

        i. Cervical

          (a) Seven vertebrae that support muscles of head and neck

          (b) Smallest of all vertebrae

          (c) Atlas (first cervical vertebra)—articulates with occipital bone superiorly and with axis inferiorly

          (d) Axis (second cervical vertebra)

            (1) Articulates with atlas and allows for rotation of head

            (2) Odontoid process (dens)—a projection of axis that articulates with atlas

        ii. Thoracic

          (a) Twelve vertebrae

          (b) Articulate with ribs and support muscles of chest

        iii. Lumbar

          (a) Five vertebrae that support back muscles

          (b) Largest and strongest of vertebrae

          (c) Site of most herniated intervertebral discs

        iv. Sacral: five vertebrae fused to form a large triangular bone called the sacrum

        v. Coccygeal: four rudimentary vertebrae with rudimentary bodies, articulating facets, and transverse processes

  b. Typical vertebra

        i. Body: solid portion of vertebra, lying anteriorly

   ii. Arch: made up of
    (a) Spinous process
    (b) Transverse processes, one on either side of spinous process
    (c) Lamina that connects spinous process to transverse process
   iii. Articular processes: portions of vertebra that come into contact with vertebrae above and below
   iv. Intervertebral foramina: openings through which spinal nerves pass
   v. Spinal foramina: openings through which spinal cord passes
   vi. Intervertebral disc
    (a) Layer of fibrocartilage found between bodies of adjoining vertebrae
    (b) Acts as shock absorber
    (c) Composed of anulus fibrosus (tough outer layer) and nucleus pulposus (gelatinous inner layer)

 2. Spinal cord (Fig. 3–11)
  a. Location: extends from superior border of atlas (first cervical vertebra) to upper border of second lumbar vertebra
   i. Continuous with medulla oblongata
   ii. Conus medullaris: caudal end of spinal cord
   iii. Central canal: opening in center of spinal cord that contains CSF and is continuous with fourth ventricle
   iv. Filum terminale: non-neural filament that extends from conus medullaris to its attachment to first coccygeal segment; has no known functional significance
  b. Meninges: continuous with those covering the brain
   i. Pia mater: vascular; attached to spinal cord, spinal roots, and filum terminale
   ii. Arachnoid mater: extends to second sacral level where it merges with filum terminale
    (a) Subarachnoid space—contains CSF; surrounds spinal cord
    (b) Lumbar cistern—subarachnoid space between conus medullaris and second sacral level
   iii. Dura mater: surrounds arachnoid and merges with filum terminale. Ends as blind sac at second sacral vertebra
  c. Gray matter (Fig. 3–12)
   i. H-shaped, internal mass of gray substance surrounded by white matter
   ii. Anterior gray column (anterior horn): contains cell bodies of efferent or motor fibers
   iii. Lateral column: contains preganglionic fibers of autonomic nervous system and is prominent in upper cervical, thoracic, and midsacral regions
   iv. Posterior gray column (posterior horn): contains cell bodies of afferent or sensory fibers

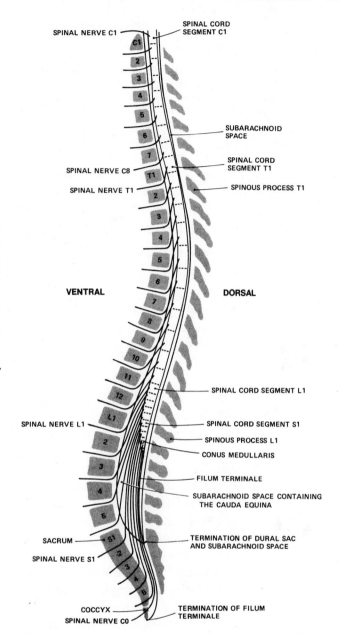

Figure 3–11. Diagram of the relationship of the spinal cord segments and spinal nerve roots to the dural sac and vertebrae of the spinal column. The bodies of the individual vertebrae on the ventral side of the spinal cord are numbered. The spinous processes of the vertebrae are dorsal to the cord. (From Gilman, S., and Winans, S. S.: Manter and Gatz's Essentials of Clinical Neuroanatomy and Neurophysiology, 6th ed. F. A. Davis Company, Philadelphia, 1982.)

d. White matter (see Fig. 3–12)
  i. Composed of three longitudinal columns (funiculi): anterior, lateral, posterior columns
  ii. Contains mostly myelinated axons
  iii. Funiculi contain tracts (fasciculi) that are functionally distinct (i.e., have same or similar origin, course, and termination) and are classified as
    (a) Ascending or sensory tracts—pathways to brain for impulses entering cord via dorsal root of spinal nerves

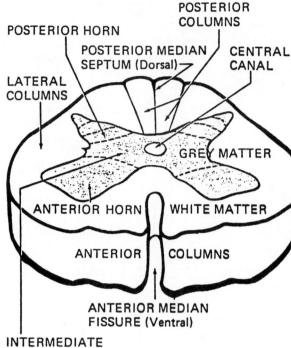

Figure 3–12. Parts of the spinal cord. (From Snyder, M., and Jackle, M.: Neurologic Problems— A Critical Care Nursing Focus. Robert J. Brady Company, Bowie, Md., 1981.)

    (b) Descending or motor tracts—transmit impulses from brain to motor neurons of spinal cord and exit via ventral root of spinal nerves

    (c) Short ascending and descending fibers that begin in one area of spinal cord and terminate in another

  iv. Each tract is named to indicate

    (a) Column in which it travels

    (b) Location of its cells of origin

    (c) Location of axon termination

  v. Ascending tracts of clinical significance (Fig. 3–13)

    (a) Fasciculus gracilis and fasciculus cuneatus—posterior white columns

      (1) Fibers enter the dorsal root of the spinal nerve and ascend in posterior funiculus

      (2) Convey position and vibratory sense, joint and two-point discrimination, tactile localization

    (b) Lateral spinothalamic tract

      (1) Originates in posterior horn; crosses over via anterior white commissure to contralateral funiculus before ascending to thalamus

      (2) Conveys pain and temperature sensation

    (c) Anterior spinothalamic tract

      (1) Originates in posterior horn; crosses over to opposite

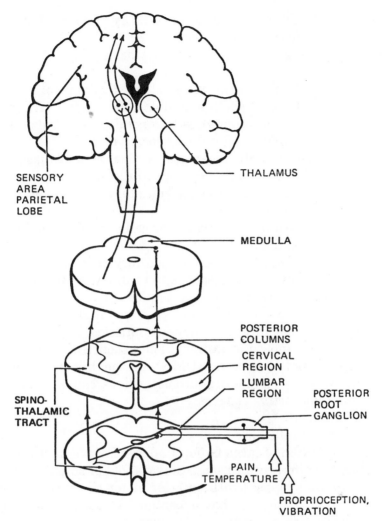

Figure 3–13. Sensory tracts. (From Snyder, M., and Jackle, M.: Neurologic Problems—A Critical Care Nursing Focus. Robert J. Brady Company, Bowie, Md., 1981.)

          side of cord via anterior white commissure and ascends to thalamus in anterolateral funiculus

    (2) Conveys light touch, pressure, and pain and temperature sensation

  (d) Dorsal and ventral spinocerebellar tracts

    (1) Originate in posterior horn; ascend to cerebellum via lateral funiculus. Dorsal is uncrossed tract; ventral is crossed tract

    (2) Convey proprioceptive data influencing muscle tone and synergy

  (e) Spinotectal tract

    (1) Originates in cells of posterior horn

(2) Transmits general sensory information to tectum (roof) of midbrain

vi. Descending tracts of clinical significance (Fig. 3–14)
   (a) Rubrospinal tract
      (1) Originates in red nucleus of midbrain; receives fibers from cerebellum and descends in lateral funiculus
      (2) Conveys impulses to control muscle tone and synergy
   (b) Ventral and lateral corticospinal tracts
      (1) Originate in cerebral cortical motor areas and descend in lateral and anterior funiculi
      (2) Carry impulses for voluntary movement
   (c) Tectospinal tract
      (1) Originates in superior colliculus; descends in anterior funiculus
      (2) Mediates optic and auditory reflexes (e.g., reflex head turning in response to visual or auditory stimuli)
e. Upper and lower motor neurons (Fig. 3–15)
   i. Lower motor neurons (LMN) are spinal and cranial motor neurons that directly innervate muscles. Lesions cause flaccid paralysis, muscular atrophy, and absence of reflex responses
   ii. Upper motor neurons (UMN) in the brain and spinal cord activate lower motor neurons. Lesions cause spastic paralysis and hyperactive reflexes

3. **Reflexes** (Fig. 3–16)
   a. Monosynaptic reflex arc
      i. Stimulation of large Group I afferent nerve fibers sends impulses to spinal cord through dorsal roots of spinal nerve
      ii. Impulse synapses with anterior motor neurons, sending out an efferent discharge that is confined to axons supplying muscle from which afferent impulse originated
   b. Polysynaptic reflex arc
      i. Stimulation of small afferent axons of muscle nerves causes synapses with interneurons, leading to asynchronous discharge of motor neurons
      ii. Polysynaptic discharge is distributed in motor axons supplying ipsilateral flexor muscles and contralateral extensor muscles
   c. Law of reciprocal innervation: impulses that excite motor neurons supplying a particular muscle also inhibit motor neurons of antagonistic muscles

Peripheral Nervous System

1. **Spinal nerves**
   a. Thirty-one symmetrically arranged pairs: a sensory (dorsal) root and a motor (ventral) root—8 cervical pairs, 12 thoracic pairs, 5 lumbar pairs, 5 sacral pairs, 1 coccygeal pair

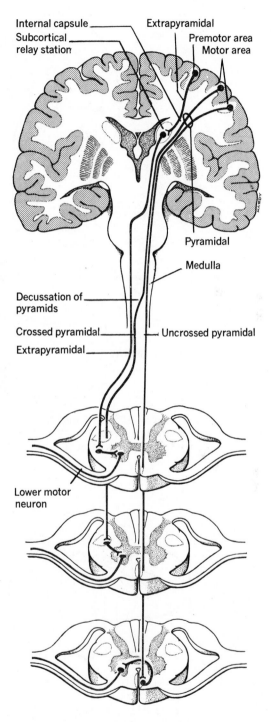

Figure 3–14. Diagram of motor pathways between the cerebral cortex, one of the subcortical relay stations, and lower motor neurons in the spinal cord. Decussation (crossing) of fibers means that each side of the brain controls skeletal muscles on the opposite side of the body. (From Chaffee, E. E., and Greisheimer, E. M.: Basic Physiology and Anatomy, 3rd ed. J. B. Lippincott Co., Philadelphia, 1974, p. 202.)

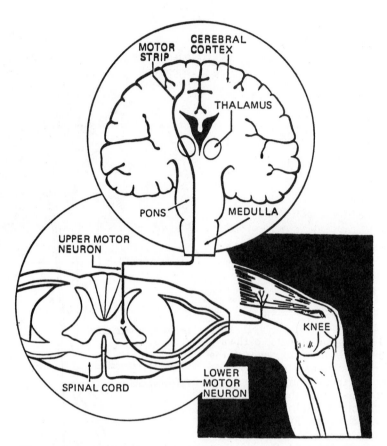

Figure 3–15. UMN and LMN. (From Snyder, M., and Jackle, M.: Neurologic Problems—A Critical Care Nursing Focus. Robert J. Brady Company, Bowie, Md., 1981.)

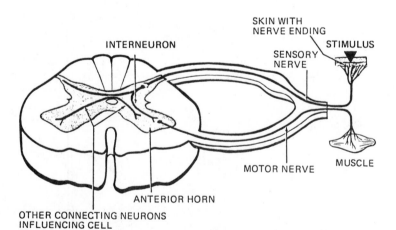

Figure 3–16. A reflex is a basic stimulus-response pattern that operates without voluntary or conscious control. (From Snyder, M., and Jackle, M.: Neurologic Problems—A Critical Care Nursing Focus. Robert J. Brady Company, Bowie, Md., 1981.)

b. Fibers of spinal nerve
   i. Meningeal branches: carry sensory and vasomotor innervation to spinal meninges
   ii. Motor fibers: originate in anterior gray column of spinal cord, form ventral root of spinal nerve, and pass to skeletal muscles
   iii. Sensory fibers: originate in spinal ganglia of dorsal roots; peripheral branches distribute to visceral and somatic structures as mediators of sensory impulses to CNS
   iv. Autonomic fibers
      (a) Sympathetic
         (1) Originate from cells that lie between posterior and anterior gray columns from T1 to L2 cord segment
         (2) Innervate viscera, blood vessels, glands, and smooth muscle
      (b) Parasympathetic
         (1) Arise from neurons of the third, seventh, ninth, and tenth cranial nerves and cord segments S2–4
         (2) Pass to pelvic and lower abdominal viscera and smooth muscles and glands of head
c. Cauda equina: spinal nerves arising from lumbosacral portion of spinal cord contained within lumbar cistern
d. Dermatomes: area of skin supplied by dorsal roots (sensory innervation) of a single spinal nerve
e. Plexuses: network of spinal nerve roots
   i. Cervical
      (a) Composed of anterior rami of C1–4
      (b) Has cutaneous, motor, and phrenic branches
   ii. Brachial
      (a) Composed of anterior rami of C5–8 and T1
      (b) Nerves arising from here include circumflex, musculocutaneous, ulnar, median, and radial
   iii. Lumbar
      (a) Composed of anterior rami of L1–4
      (b) Branches are lateral femoral cutaneous, femoral, and genitofemoral
   iv. Sacral
      (a) Composed of anterior rami of L4 and L5 and S1–4
      (b) Branches include sciatic and pudendal
2. **Neuromuscular transmission** (Fig. 3–17)
   a. Physiologic anatomy
      i. Motor end plate (neuromuscular junction): a specialized region where motor axon loses its myelin sheath and splays out in a flattened plate close to muscle fiber membrane
      ii. Synaptic cleft: space between nerve terminal and muscle fiber membrane

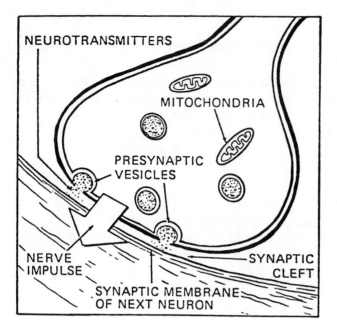

Figure 3–17. Impulse transmission across the synapse. The synaptic knob is at the end of the axon. The presynaptic vesicles contain precursors of chemical substances that are neurotransmitters. When the neurotransmitters are secreted, they diffuse across the synaptic cleft and cause the synaptic membrane of the next neuron to depolarize. The impulse wave then starts down the next neuron. (From Snyder, M., and Jackle, M.: Neurologic Problems—A Critical Care Nursing Focus. Robert J. Brady Company, Bowie, Md., 1981.)

     iii. Synaptic gutter: area of muscle fiber membrane characterized by numerous folds, which increase surface area available for neurotransmitter substance to act

     iv. Vesicles: structures of nerve terminal that store and release neurotransmitter substance acetylcholine

  b. Release of acetylcholine: when action potential reaches neuromuscular junction, vesicles release acetylcholine into synaptic cleft. Amount released depends on magnitude of action potential and presence of calcium. Acetylcholine attaches to receptor sites on postjunctional muscle membrane and increases its permeability to sodium and potassium

  c. End-plate potential: motor-nerve action potential caused by depolarization owing to sodium influx and potassium efflux. Differs from action potential in that it is local (i.e., nonpropagated) and is graded, rather than all or nothing

  d. Muscle contraction: action potentials are subsequently formed on either side of an end plate and conducted in both directions along the muscle fiber, initiating a series of events that result in muscle contraction

  e. Acetylcholinesterase: catalyzes hydrolysis of acetylcholine to choline and acetic acid and thus limits duration of acetylcholine action on the end plate and ensures production of only one action potential. Acetylcholine is then resynthesized in the presence of choline acetylase and coenzyme A acetate

3. Cranial nerves (Fig. 3–18)

  a. Olfactory (I)

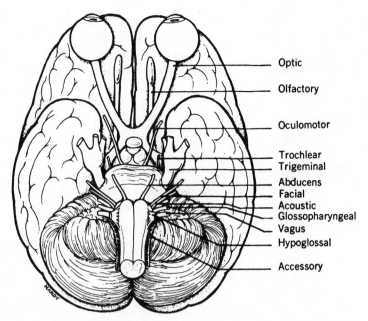

Figure 3–18. Base of brain showing entrance or exit of cranial nerves. The eyeballs are shown schematically in relation to the optic nerves. (From Chaffee, E. E., and Greisheimer, E. M.: Basic Physiology and Anatomy, 3rd ed. J. B. Lippincott, Philadelphia, 1974, p. 212.)

    i. Receptors are located in nasal mucosa. Fibers pass through cribriform plate to olfactory bulb, which, in turn, forms olfactory tract. Peripheral and central connections of this nerve are numerous and complex

    ii. A sensory nerve responsible for smell

b. Optic (II)

    i. Fibers originate from ganglion cells of retina. At optic chiasm, fibers from nasal half of retina cross; those from temporal half do not. Fibers continue as optic tracts to lateral geniculate bodies and then to occipital cortex

    ii. A sensory nerve concerned with vision

c. Oculomotor (III)

    i. Nuclei are located in midbrain. Preganglionic parasympathetic fibers originate in Edinger-Westphal nucleus and accompany other oculomotor fibers into orbit, where they terminate in ciliary ganglion. Postganglionic fibers pass to constrictor pupillae and ciliary muscles of eye to cause pupillary constriction in response to light

    ii. Motor fibers supply extraocular muscles: inferior rectus (depresses and adducts eye), medial rectus (adducts eye), superior rectus (elevates and adducts eye), inferior oblique (elevates and abducts eye), levator palpebrae (raises upper eyelid)

    d. Trochlear (IV)
        i. Originates caudal to oculomotor nucleus in midbrain. It is the only cranial nerve to originate from dorsal aspect of brain stem
       ii. Supplies superior oblique muscle, which abducts and depresses eye

    e. Trigeminal (V)
        i. Sensory fibers arise from cells in semilunar or gasserian ganglion. Nerve is attached to lateral aspect of pons. Motor fibers leave pons ventromedial to sensory roots
       ii. Three sensory divisions
          (a) Ophthalmic branch provides sensation to forehead, eyes, nose, temples, paranasal sinuses, and part of nasal mucosa
          (b) Maxillary branch provides sensation to upper jaw, teeth, lip, cheeks, hard palate, maxillary sinuses, and nasal mucosa
          (c) Mandibular branch provides sensation to lower jaw, teeth, lip, buccal mucosa, tongue, and part of external ear, auditory meatus, and meninges
      iii. Motor fibers innervate muscles of mastication: temporalis and masseter muscles

    f. Abducens (VI)
        i. Emerges at caudal border of pons near midline and enters orbit with oculomotor and trochlear nerves
       ii. Supplies lateral rectus muscle, which abducts eye

    g. Facial (VII)
        i. Fibers originate in caudal portion of pons at junction of pons and medulla, lateral to abducens nerve
       ii. Motor portions of nerve innervate all muscles of facial expression, plus salivary and lacrimal glands. Sensory portion of nerve conveys taste from anterior two thirds of tongue

    h. Acoustic (VIII) (vestibulocochlear nerve)
        i. Emerges from brain stem at pontomedullary junction and has two divisions
          (a) Cochlear nerve—fibers from cells in spiral ganglion end either in organ of Corti (peripheral fibers) or ventral and dorsal cochlear nuclei in medulla (central fibers). Fibers from these nuclei proceed to inferior colliculi and then to medial geniculate nuclei of thalamus, before ending on auditory cortex of temporal lobe
          (b) Vestibular nerve—fibers from cells in vestibular ganglion pass to semicircular canals and maculas and to vestibular nuclei in brain stem
       ii. Cochlear nerve is responsible for hearing; vestibular nerve aids in maintaining equilibrium and coordinating head and eye movements

i. Glossopharyngeal (IX)

    i. Sensory fibers arise from cells at back of tongue, pharynx, and palate and enter medulla behind facial nerve. Motor fibers originate from nucleus in medulla to innervate stylopharyngeus muscle

    ii. Sensory fibers provide sensation to pharynx, soft palate, and posterior third of tongue. They also supply special receptors in carotid body and carotid sinus concerned with reflex control of respiration, blood pressure, and heart rate

    iii. Motor fibers participate with those of vagus nerve in swallowing mechanism

j. Vagus (X)

    i. Sensory fibers originate in cells in ganglia just below jugular foramen and enter medulla just behind glossopharyngeal nerve. Motor fibers leave medulla and join sensory part of nerve. Parasympathetic fibers are distributed to abdominal and thoracic viscera

    ii. Sensory fibers provide sensation to palate and pharynx (along with glossopharyngeal nerve), and to larynx (vagus nerve alone)

    iii. Motor fibers innervate palatal muscles, pharyngeal muscles (along with glossopharyngeal nerve), and laryngeal muscles

    iv. Postganglionic parasympathetic fibers inhibit heart rate and adrenal secretion; they stimulate gastrointestinal peristalsis and gastric, hepatic, and pancreatic glandular secretion

k. Spinal accessory (XI)

    i. Motor fibers arise from lateral surface of medulla and upper cervical spinal cord

    ii. Supplies trapezius (elevates shoulders) and sternocleidomastoid muscles (tilts, turns, and thrusts head forward)

l. Hypoglossal (XII)

    i. Motor fibers originate in ventromedial sulcus of medulla

    ii. Innervates muscles of tongue

4. **Autonomic nervous system (ANS)** (Fig. 3–19)

a. Structure

    i. Composed of two neuron chains

    ii. Preganglionic cell bodies are located within lateral gray column of spinal cord or homologous motor nuclei of cranial nerves

    iii. Most preganglionic axons are myelinated and synapse on cell bodies of postganglionic neurons located outside CNS

    iv. Axons of postganglionic neurons terminate on visceral effectors

b. Divisions

    i. Sympathetic (thoracolumbar)

        (a) Preganglionic axons leave spinal cord in ventral roots of T1 to L2 and pass to

            (1) Paravertebral sympathetic ganglion chain via white

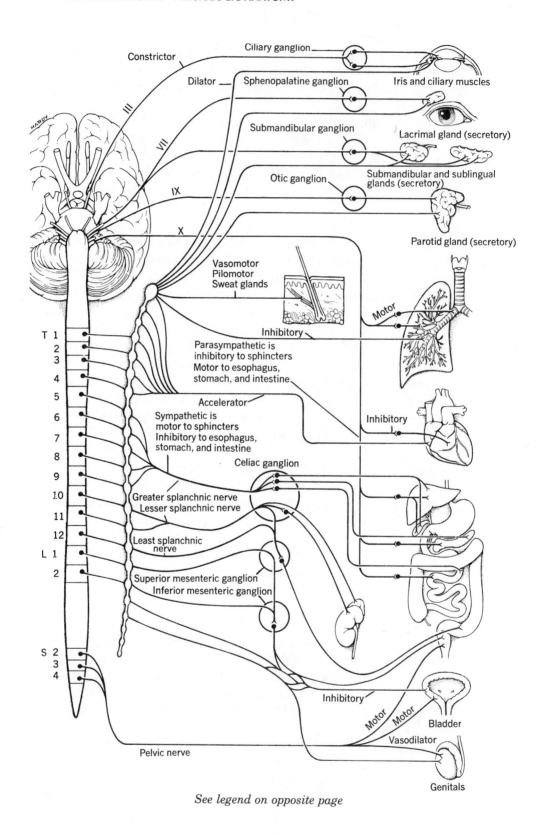

Constrictor

Ciliary ganglion

Dilator

Sphenopalatine ganglion

Iris and ciliary muscles

III

Submandibular ganglion

VII

Lacrimal gland (secretory)

Otic ganglion

IX

Submandibular and sublingual glands (secretory)

X

Parotid gland (secretory)

Vasomotor
Pilomotor
Sweat glands

Motor

Inhibitory

T 1
2
3
4
5
6
7
8
9
10
11
12
L 1
2

Parasympathetic is inhibitory to sphincters Motor to esophagus, stomach, and intestine

Accelerator

Sympathetic is motor to sphincters Inhibitory to esophagus, stomach, and intestine

Inhibitory

Celiac ganglion

Greater splanchnic nerve
Lesser splanchnic nerve

Least splanchnic nerve

Superior mesenteric ganglion
Inferior mesenteric ganglion

S 2
3
4

Inhibitory

Motor

Motor

Bladder

Vasodilator

Pelvic nerve

Genitals

See legend on opposite page

rami communicantes, ending on cell bodies of postganglionic neurons

    (2) Collateral ganglia, ending on postganglionic neurons close to viscera

  (b) Postganglionic axons pass to

    (1) Viscera via sympathetic nerves

    (2) Gray rami communicantes; they are then distributed to autonomic effectors in areas supplied by these spinal nerves

  (c) Segmental distribution of sympathetic fibers

    (1) T1—up sympathetic chain to head

    (2) T2—into neck

    (3) T3–6—thorax

    (4) T7–11—abdomen

    (5) T12, L1, L2—legs

  (d) Functions

    (1) Generally antagonistic to parasympathetic activity

    (2) Can synapse with many postganglionic fibers

    (3) Sympathetic stimulation dilates pupils and bronchioles, relaxes smooth muscles of gastrointestinal tract, increases blood pressure by constricting blood vessels, increases heart rate, increases secretion of adrenal medulla

    (4) Brought into widespread activity under emergency conditions, and gives rise to mass responses of body systems

ii. Parasympathetic (craniosacral)

  (a) Preganglionic cell bodies are in gray matter of brain stem and middle three segments of sacral cord

  (b) Preganglionic fibers end on short postganglionic neurons located on or near visceral structures

  (c) Supplies visceral structures in head via oculomotor, facial, and glossopharyngeal nerves and those in thorax and upper abdomen via vagus nerve

  (d) Sacral outflow supplies pelvic viscera via pelvic branches of S2–4

  (e) Gives rise to localized reactions, rather than mass action of sympathetic stimulation

  (f) Parasympathetic stimulation constricts pupils; contracts

---

Figure 3–19. Diagram of the automatic nervous system, including parasympathetic or craniosacral fibers and sympathetic or thoracolumbar fibers. Note that most organs have a double nerve supply. (From Chaffee, E. E., and Greisheimer, E. M.: Basic Physiology and Anatomy, 3rd ed. J. B. Lippincott, Philadelphia, 1974, p. 222.)

smooth muscle of stomach, intestine, and bladder; slows heart rate; stimulates secretion of most glands
 c. Chemical mediation: ANS is divided into cholinergic and adrenergic divisions based on chemical mediator (i.e., neurotransmitter substance liberated)
   i. Cholinergic neurons release acetylcholine and include
     (a) All preganglionic neurons except sympathetic preganglionic neurons to adrenal medulla
     (b) Parasympathetic postganglionic neurons
     (c) Sympathetic postganglionic neurons to sweat glands and skeletal muscle blood vessels (vasodilator)
   ii. Adrenergic neurons release norepinephrine and include
     (a) Sympathetic postganglionic endings, except as noted above
     (b) Sympathetic preganglionic neurons to adrenal medulla
     (c) Constrictor fibers of skeletal muscle blood vessels

NURSING ASSESSMENT DATA BASE

Nursing History

1. **Patient health history**
   a. Current and significant past medical history of all major systems, including traumatic injury
   b. Chronologic sequence of onset and development of each neurologic symptom
   c. Factors that relieve or exacerbate symptoms
   d. Difficulties with activities of daily living
   e. Childhood diseases
2. **Family history**
   a. Diabetes mellitus
   b. Cardiac disease
   c. Hypertension
   d. Cancer
   e. Neurologic disorders
3. **Social history and habits**
   a. Smoking: past, present, amount, duration of use
   b. Illicit drug use or abuse
   c. Alcohol intake: past, present, amount, duration of use
   d. Type of work
   e. Hobbies, recreation
4. **Medication history**
   a. Anticonvulsants
   b. Tranquilizers, sedatives
   c. Anticoagulants

d. Aspirin
e. Cardiac, including antihypertensives
f. Other

Nursing Examination of Patient

1. Inspection

a. General cerebral functions: mental status examination
   i. General behavior and appearance: dress, grooming, demeanor
   ii. Sensorium: level of consciousness or awareness, attention span, memory, insight, orientation, calculation
   iii. Intellectual capacity: bright, average, dull, demented, retarded
   iv. Emotional state: mood, affective responses
   v. Thought content, judgment: illusions, hallucinations, delusions
   vi. Conversation: stream of talk, sentence structure

b. Speech: evaluate for
   i. Dysphonia: difficulty producing the voice sound (vagus nerve dysfunction)
   ii. Dysarthria: difficulty with articulation (upper motor neuron, lower motor neuron, or muscular lesion)
   iii. Dysprosody: difficulty with stress of syllables, inflections, pitch of voice, rhythm
   iv. Dysphasia: difficulty in expression or understanding of words (dominant hemisphere, usually the left)

c. Head and face
   i. Facial gestalt, mobility, emotional expression
   ii. Eyes for ptosis, symmetry of width of palpebral fissures
   iii. Contour of nose, mouth, chin, ears
   iv. Hair of scalp, eyebrows, beard
   v. Head for abnormalities in shape or symmetry

d. Cranial nerves
   i. Olfactory (I): testing each nostril separately, ask patient to identify familiar nonirritating odors such as cloves, coffee, or perfume. Loss of sense of smell is called anosmia
   ii. Optic (II)
      (a) Visual acuity may be tested with a Snellen chart or grossly with newsprint
      (b) Inspect optic fundi ophthalmoscopically
      (c) Determine visual fields by confrontation. Ask patient to fixate on an object in the distance and bring finger from periphery into patient's field of vision. By positioning yourself directly in front of patient you can compare his visual fields with yours. Test each eye individually
      (d) Lesions of retina, optic nerve, optic tract, lateral geniculate

body, geniculocalcarine tract, or occipital lobe will result in loss of sight in all or part of visual field

(1) Unilateral blindness (Fig. 3–20A) is caused by lesions of eye, retina, or optic nerve

(2) Bitemporal hemianopsia (Fig. 3–20B) is caused by lesions affecting the optic chiasm

(3) Left (or right) homonymous hemianopsia (Fig. 3–20C) is caused by lesions of the right (or left) optic tract

(4) Left (or right) homonymous hemianopsia with macular sparing (Fig. 3–20D) is caused by lesions of geniculocalcarine tract

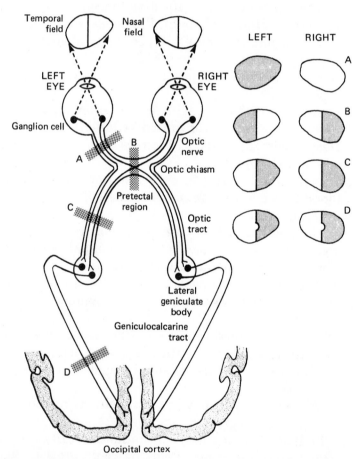

Figure 3–20. Visual pathways. Lesions at the points marked by the letters cause the visual field defects shown in the diagrams on the right. Occipital lesions may spare the fibers from the macula (as in D) because of the separation in the brain of these fibers from the others subserving vision. (Reproduced, with permission, from Ganong, W. F.: Review of Medical Physiology, 14th ed. Copyright Appleton & Lange Publications, 1989.)

iii. Oculomotor (III), trochlear (IV), and abducens (VI)
   (a) Examine size and shape of pupils and pupillary light reflexes—direct, consensual, and accommodation
      (1) Direct light reflex—constriction of pupil when stimulated by light. This tests the afferent limb of the optic nerve and the efferent limb of the oculomotor nerve
      (2) Consensual light reflex—constriction of opposite pupil when light stimulates only one eye. This differentiates lesions of the optic nerve from lesions of the oculomotor nerve
      (3) Accommodation reflex: convergence of eyes, constriction of pupils, and thickening of lens. Occurs when person looks at a close object
   (b) Check range of ocular movements by having patient's eyes following your finger through all fields of gaze. Observe for nystagmus at rest and during ocular movements
iv. Trigeminal (V)
   (a) Sensory
      (1) Test forehead, cheeks, and jaw on each side of face. Use wisp of cotton for light touch, pin for pinprick, and test tubes of hot and cold water for temperature
      (2) Corneal reflex—touch cornea with wisp of cotton. Observe for reflex blinking. This tests the afferent limb of the trigeminal nerve and the efferent limb of the facial nerve of the reflex arc
   (b) Motor—ask patient to clench his teeth and palpate masseter and temporal muscles. Assess ability to chew
v. Facial (VII)
   (a) Ask patient to raise his eyebrows, frown, smile, and open eyes against resistance. Note strength and symmetry of facial muscles
   (b) Test taste on anterior two thirds of tongue by applying salt and sugar to both sides of tongue. Ask patient to identify the taste prior to closing mouth
vi. Acoustic (VIII)
   (a) Cochlear (hearing)
      (1) Hearing acuity—cover one ear and test the other with watch or whisper. If deficit is suggested, proceed to (2) and (3) following
      (2) Weber's test—place stem of tuning fork on midline vertex of skull. Normally there is no lateralization of sound. When sound is referred to better-hearing ear, decreased hearing is because of impaired function of cochlear nerve
      (3) Rinne's test—place tuning fork on mastoid bone; when

sound is no longer heard, place in front of ear. Since air conduction is normally greater than bone conduction, middle-ear disease is suspected in patients who can hear the tuning fork better when placed on mastoid bone

(b) Vestibular

(1) Patient complaints of vertigo, nausea, anxiety, signs of nystagmus, postural deviation, pallor, sweating, hypotension, and vomiting—all may indicate vestibular nerve dysfunction

(2) Caloric irrigation test—position patient 30° from supine to bring semicircular canals to a vertical plane. After checking to ensure an unoccluded ear canal and an intact tympanic membrane, irrigate canal with cold water. When the pathway from the vestibular portion of the acoustic nerve to the oculomotor and abducens nerves is intact, the response in an awake patient will consist of vertigo, nausea, and horizontal nystagmus (fast component) toward unirrigated side, postural deviation, and past-pointing to irrigated side. In a patient with impaired vestibular function, some or all of these responses may be abnormal

vii. Glossopharyngeal (IX) and vagus (X)

(a) Ask patient to open his mouth and say "Ah"; observe for symmetric elevation of palatal arch

(b) Gag reflex—stroke palatal arch with a tongue blade. Palate should elevate, and the patient should have a gag response. This tests the afferent limb of the glossopharyngeal nerve and the efferent limb of the vagus nerve

(c) Speech—appraise articulation. If defect is suspected, have patient say "Kuh, Kuh, Kuh," "La, La, La," and "Mi, Mi, Mi." This tests competency of soft palate, tongue, and lips, respectively

(d) Swallowing—if patient is dysarthric or dysphagic, assess ability to swallow water. If patient is unable to follow commands, observe ability to handle secretions

(e) Carotid sinus reflex—pressure over carotid sinus normally produces slowing of heart rate and fall in blood pressure

(f) Hoarseness—may indicate damage to vagal nerve. Laryngoscopic examination may be indicated

viii. Spinal accessory (XI)

(a) Inspect sternocleidomastoid and trapezius muscles for size and symmetry

(b) See p. 360–361 for other tests of spinal accessory nerve (XI) function

ix. Hypoglossal (XII) (see p. 361)

    (a) Inspect tongue for atrophy while at rest

    (b) Check alignment of tongue when protruded by comparing median raphe with notch between medial incisors

e. Motor system

    i. Observe size and contour of muscles: note atrophy, hypertrophy, asymmetry, joint malalignments, or involuntary movements, such as fasciculations, tics, tremors, or abnormal positions

    ii. Strength testing (see p. 361)

    iii. Muscle tone (see Palpation, p. 360)

    iv. Muscle stretch reflexes (deep tendon reflexes) (see Percussion, p. 361)

    v. Superficial reflexes: tested by stroking skin with moderately sharp object

        (a) Upper abdominal (T7–9) and lower abdominal (T11–12)—umbilicus normally deviates toward quadrant tested; this response is absent with upper motor neuron lesions

        (b) Cremasteric (L1–2)—stroking thigh causes elevation of ipsilateral testicle; this response is absent with upper motor neuron lesions

        (c) Plantar (S1–2)

            (1) Stroking lateral aspect of sole of foot causes flexion of great toe

            (2) An abnormal response, seen with upper motor neuron lesions, is extension of great toe—Babinski sign

            (3) There are other methods to elicit extensor-plantar response, but all indicate same pathologic process

        (d) Other abnormal reflexes that indicate diffuse cerebral dysfunction

            (1) Grasp reflex: patient grasps when something is placed in his hand and does not release on command

            (2) Snout reflex: pursing of lips when side of mouth is touched

            (3) Glabellar reflex: repeated blinking in response to tapping on forehead

f. Cerebellar function

    i. Testing depends on ability of patient to perform volitional movements; that is, the motor system related to area being tested must be intact (e.g., hemiplegic or comatose patient cannot perform cerebellar function tests because of inability to perform voluntary movements, not because of cerebellar dysfunction)

    ii. Four major clinical signs of dysfunction and tests used to detect them are

(a) Dystaxia (intention tremor or incoordination of volitional movements)
  (1) Observe for swaying when patient stands with feet together, first with eyes open, then closed (Romberg test)
  (2) Gait dystaxia—detected by observing patient for a wide-based gait while walking and assessing ability to perform tandem (heel-to-toe) walking
  (3) Arm dystaxia—detected by finger-to-nose test (asking patient to touch his nose, then the examiner's finger) and rapid-alternating movement test (asking patient to slap his thigh first with palm and then with back of his hand in quick alternating movements)
  (4) Leg dystaxia—detected by heel-to-shin test (patient is asked to run heel from opposite knee down shin)
(b) Hypotonia (lack of muscle tone)
  (1) Inspect patient for rag-doll postures and gait
  (2) Observe for lack of muscular resistance when passively moving patient's extremity
  (3) In patients with cerebellar dysfunction, leg continues to swing like a pendulum after tendon reflex is elicited
  (4) Postural dysequilibrium may be elicited by rebound tests—wrist-slapping and arm-pulling
(c) Nystagmus (jerky, oscillatory eye movements)
  (1) Inspect and have patient follow your finger through fields of gaze
  (2) Nystagmus results from lesions of eye, cerebellum, vestibular system, or their brain stem pathways and has different clinical characteristics. Interpretation of findings thus may require consultation
(d) Dysarthria (inability to articulate speech sounds)—see test for glossopharyngeal and vagus nerves. May result from dysfunction of acoustic (VIII), glossopharyngeal (IX), vagus (X), or hypoglossal (XII) nerves or cerebellar dysfunction that interferes with coordination of the muscles innervated by these nerves

g. Sensory system
  i. Tested with patient's eyes closed: one side of body is compared with the other
  ii. Determine whether the distribution of sensory loss is dermatomal, related to peripheral nerve(s) or central pathway, or nonorganic
  iii. Broad dermatomal areas are
    (a) C3–4—"cape" area of shoulders
    (b) C5–T1—surface of arms

        (c) T2 abuts on C4 over "cape" area of shoulders

        (d) T4—nipple line

        (e) T10—umbilicus

        (f) L5—great toe

        (g) S1—small toe

        (h) S4–5—perianal area

   iv. Superficial sensory modalities

        (a) Light touch—touch hands, trunk, and feet with wisp of cotton

        (b) Pain—using a pin, gently touch hands, trunk, and feet. Ask patient to identify when being touched by sharp and dull ends of pin

        (c) Temperature—ask patient to discriminate between hot and cold test tubes of water touched to hands, trunk, and feet

   v. Deep sensory modalities

        (a) Vibration—apply vibrating tuning fork to bony prominences and soft tissue and ask patient to report when he feels vibration. Apply fork to a toe or finger and place your finger under the digit. Patient should report feeling vibration of tuning fork longer than you can

        (b) Proprioception (position sense)—ask patient to close his eyes and report whether his finger or toe is being moved up or down

   vi. Cortical/discriminatory sensation—receptors, sensory pathways, and primary receptive cortical area must be intact for accurate interpretation of following tests. Ability to perform tests accurately thus assesses association portions (parietal lobe) of cortex

        (a) Stereognosis—ask patient, without aid of vision, to identify familiar objects placed in his hand

        (b) Topognosia—ask patient to identify which finger the examiner is touching, and whether it is on right or left side

        (c) Graphognosia—ask patient to identify numbers or letters traced on skin of palm or fingers

        (d) Tactile inattention—determine whether patient can identify that he has been touched on both sides of his body simultaneously

h. Assessment of patient with altered state of consciousness

   i. Consciousness is an awareness of self and environment. Disturbances in consciousness can result from extensive bilateral cerebral lesions, from injury to diencephalon or pontomesencephalic (pons/midbrain) reticular formation, or from metabolic abnormalities. Unilateral lesions of cerebrum and lesions of medulla or spinal cord do not cause coma

 ii. Level of consciousness
  (a) Determine stimuli necessary to arouse patient. Does he respond when his name is called? Does he have to be touched or shaken? Are painful stimuli necessary? Does he have no response at all?
  (b) Describe patient's behavior once aroused. Is he oriented or confused as to person, place, time, environment? Is he restless, irritable, combative? Does he follow verbal commands?
  (c) Describe patient's verbal response. Is his speech clear, garbled, or confused? Does he use inappropriate words? Does he make incomprehensible sounds? Does he have any verbal response?
  (d) Determine patient's best motor response. Does he obey verbal commands? Does he localize or withdraw from noxious stimuli? Does he exhibit abnormal flexor or extensor posturing? Is there no response at all to stimuli (i.e., is he flaccid)?
  (e) Responses to the above assessment parameters should be charted in detail to provide a clear picture of the patient's level of consciousness. Terms such as stuporous, obtunded, semi-comatose, and comatose should be avoided because patients do not fit neatly into one defined area
 iii. Glasgow Coma Score (GCS): This standardized tool assesses many of the same areas of level of consciousness as described above. The patient's responses are graded, and the scores for the three categories are summed. The GCS ranges from 3 to 15, with 15 being normal
  (a) Eye opening—assesses arousal state
   (1) "Spontaneously" (GCS = 4)—patient opens eyes without stimulation
   (2) "To voice" (GCS = 3)—opens eyes when spoken to
   (3) "To pain" (GCS = 2)—opens eyes when noxious stimuli applied
   (4) "None" (GCS = 1)—does not open eyes to any stimulus
  (b) Best motor response—record best motor response of arms
   (1) Assesses both arousal and content of consciousness
   (2) "Obeys" (GCS = 6)—follows simple commands
   (3) "Localizes" (GCS = 5)—patient attempts to remove noxious stimuli. Assessed by applying pressure to supraorbital ridge or trapezius muscle
   (4) "Withdraws" (GCS = 4)—arm or leg is pulled away from painful stimuli of examiner who applies pressure to nail beds
   (5) "Abnormal flexion" (GCS = 3)—adduction, internal ro-

tation, and rigid flexion of hand and arm with the hand clenched and thumb grasped in hand (decorticate posturing)

(6) "Abnormal extension" (GCS = 2)—adduction, internal rotation, and rigid extension, the thumb is grasped in a clenched fist (decerebrate posturing)

(7) "Flaccid" (GCS = 1)—no motor movements of any kind

(c) Best verbal response—assessment of content of consciousness both in terms of ability to produce speech as a function of consciousness and quality of speech

    (1) "Oriented" (GCS = 5)—can state his name, where he is, and date

    (2) "Confused" (GCS = 4)—cannot state either who he is, where he is, or date

    (3) "Inappropriate words" (GCS = 3)—words spoken with no specific intent at communicating

    (4) "Incomprehensible sounds" (GCS = 2)—grunts, groans, other sounds

    (5) "None" (GCS = 1)—no attempt at vocalizing. Assessment of speech is impaired in patients who are intubated, who speak only a foreign language, who are very young, or who have global aphasia. This does not indicate total loss of brain function

iv. Pupillary responses

(a) Describe shape of pupil. Irregularly shaped pupils can be caused by direct trauma, cataracts, or other ocular dysfunction. An oval pupil has been noted to accompany tentorial herniation and increased intracranial pressure

(b) Describe size of pupils in millimeters or in comparison to one another (e.g., right pupil larger or smaller than left). Pupil size represents balance between parasympathetic and sympathetic innervation. Unequal pupils (anisocoria) results from

    (1) Disruption of parasympathetic fibers of oculomotor nerve and/or compression of nucleus by mass lesions or tentorial herniation, causing the ipsilateral pupil to dilate

    (2) Disruption of sympathetic pathways (e.g., cervical spinal cord injury), resulting in a constricted pupil on the ipsilateral side (Horner's syndrome)

(c) Pupillary light reflexes test the integrity of the optic (afferent limb) and oculomotor (efferent limb) nerves

    (1) Describe direct light reflex as brisk, sluggish, or nonreactive. Lost with oculomotor (parasympathetic) or

optic nerve injury but retained with sympathetic disruption

(2) Describe consensual light reflex as present or absent. Remains intact when oculomotor nerve and midbrain connections are intact. A blind eye, therefore, will lose direct light reflex but retain consensual reflex. Cortical blindness does not affect either direct or consensual reflexes

(d) Describe ciliospinal reflex (ipsilateral pupillary dilatation in response to pinching the trapezius muscle) as present or absent. Lost with interruption of sympathetic fibers of oculomotor nerve

v. Motor ability

(a) If patient is able to follow verbal commands, assess strength and tone of extremities as described previously

(b) If patient is unable to follow verbal commands, assess motor ability by observing which extremities he moves spontaneously or in response to noxious stimuli

(c) Hemiparesis or hemiplegia may also be detected by lifting both arms off bed and releasing them simultaneously. Hemiparetic side will fall faster and more limply than normal side. Repeat maneuver with legs

(d) Paratonia is increased muscular resistance of any part of body to passive movement. It usually accompanies diffuse forebrain dysfunction but when seen unilaterally is associated with lesions of frontal lobe and increased intracranial pressure

(e) Flexor posturing (decorticate rigidity) consists of flexion and adduction of upper extremity with extension, internal rotation, and plantar flexion in lower extremity. Associated with lesions of internal capsule (a compact band of afferent and efferent fibers near upper part of brain stem) or cerebral hemispheres

(f) Extensor posturing (decerebrate rigidity) is characterized by extension, adduction, and hyperpronation of upper extremities and plantar flexion of lower extremities. Results from lesions at the pontomesencephalic level

(g) Unilateral, bilateral, or mixed responses may occur

(h) Deep tendon reflexes—may be diminished initially after acute intracranial injury due to cerebral shock. Hyperreflexia and appearance of Babinski reflexes are indicative of upper motor neuron lesions. Clonus may also be present

vi. Cranial nerves

(a) Optic (II) is indirectly tested by pupillary light reflexes, since optic nerve (II) is afferent limb of this reflex arc. Oculomotor (III) is efferent limb of reflex arc

(b) Trigeminal (V)—see p. 351 for testing. An alternate method for testing the trigeminal-facial nerve (V-VII) arc is to apply pressure to the supraorbital ridge and observe facial grimacing, which will be decreased or absent on same side as hemiplegia

(c) Vestibular portion of the acoustic nerve (VIII) and its connections with the oculomotor (III) and abducens (VI) nerves provide information regarding integrity of brain stem. Can be tested by

(1) Caloric irrigation test (oculovestibular reflex)—see p. 352. A normal coma response (i.e., one showing the connections between acoustic (VIII), oculomotor (III), and abducens (VI) nerves to be intact) consists of nystagmus and deviation of the eyes toward irrigated ear

(2) Doll's eye test (oculocephalic reflex). In a comatose patient who has intact connections between acoustic (VIII), oculomotor (III), and abducens (VI) nerves, brisk turning of patient's head will cause the eyes to move in opposite direction. This is described as doll's eyes present. Absent doll's eyes result in the eyes remaining in a fixed position. *CAUTION:* before doing this maneuver, be sure that a cervical spine injury has been ruled out

(d) Glossopharyngeal (IX) and vagus (X) nerves are tested by the gag reflex

vii. Vital signs

(a) Temperature

(1) Hyperthermia increases metabolic needs of an already compromised CNS. Usually indicates infection, extreme restlessness, or seizure activity

(2) Hypothermia, if extreme, can lead to cardiac dysrhythmias and has not been consistently proven to be of therapeutic value in preventing or treating secondary effects of cerebral insult

(b) Respirations

(1) Hypercapnia or hypoxia leads to vasodilatation, increased cerebral blood volume (CBV), and, in patient with compromised intracranial dynamics, increased intracranial pressure

(2) Respiratory dysrhythmias often correlate with lesions at various levels, although effects are variable and influenced by other factors

        a) Post-hyperventilation apnea—patient with metabolic or structural forebrain disease will have a period of apnea after taking deep breaths sufficient to lower Pa_{CO_2} to below normal. This response is abolished in sleep or obtundation

        b) Cheyne-Stokes respiration—a pattern that alternately crescendos to hyperpnea and decrescendos to apnea. Associated with bilateral lesions of cerebral hemispheres, basal ganglia, or metabolic lesions

        c) Central neurogenic hyperventilation—sustained, regular, rapid, and deep hyperpnea. Seen in patients with lesions of midbrain, often secondary to transtentorial herniation and midpontine lesions

        d) Apneustic breathing—an end-inspiratory pause, often followed with expiratory pauses. Indicates injury to respiratory mechanisms at mid or caudal pontine level

        e) Ataxic breathing (Biot's)—completely irregular pattern with both deep and shallow breaths occurring randomly. Represents disruption of medullary inspiratory and expiratory neurons and thus occurs with lesions of posterior fossa

        f) Cluster breathing—disorganized sequence of breaths with irregular periods of apnea. Seen in patients with lesions of caudal pons or rostral medulla

    (c) Pulse and blood pressure

       (1) Although of vital importance in overall assessment and care of critically ill patients, pulse and blood pressure are notoriously unreliable parameters in CNS disease. When changes do occur, they are seen late in course of increasing intracranial pressure and thus are of little clinical use in determining increased intracranial pressure

       (2) Cushing's reflex is an increase in systolic pressure greater than the increase in diastolic pressure. This reflex leads to widening pulse pressure and occasionally to reflex slowing of pulse. It is a late sign of intracranial hypertension

2. Palpation

  a. Skull for lumps, depressions, tenderness

  b. Carotid and temporal arteries

  c. Spinal accessory (CN XI)—see p. 352

    i. Ask patient to turn head and not allow you to force it back toward midline. Palpate opposite sternocleidomastoid muscle

    ii. Ask patient to shrug shoulders upward against resistance of your downward pressure on his shoulders. Note strength and contraction of trapezius muscles

    iii. Ask patient to push head forward against your hand. Assess strength of both sternocleidomastoid muscles

  d. Hypoglossal (CN XII)—see p. 353

    i. Have patient protrude tongue and push it to right and left. Have patient press tongue against inside of cheek while you assess its strength

  e. Motor system

    i. Palpate muscles if tenderness or spasm is suspected, or if muscles seem atrophic or hypertrophic

    ii. Strength testing

      (a) Shoulder girdle—press down on patient's arms after he abducts them to shoulder height. Check for scapular winging

      (b) Upper extremities—test biceps, triceps, wrist dorsiflexion, hand grasps, strength of finger abduction and extension

      (c) Lower extremities—test hip flexors, abductors and adductors, knee flexors and extensors (deep knee bend), foot dorsiflexors, invertors, evertors

      (d) Abdominal muscles—observe for umbilical migration as patient does a sit-up

      (e) Note whether weakness follows a distributional pattern such as proximal-distal, right-left, or upper-lower extremity. Grade strength as normal, minimal, moderate, or severe weakness or paralysis

  f. Muscle tone—note whether rigidity (increased muscular resistance throughout range of motion of joint), spasticity (increased muscular resistance to brisk movement of joint), or clonus (oscillation between flexion and extension of the foot when brisk pressure is applied to sole) is elicited by passive motion

3. Percussion

  a. Sinuses and mastoid processes for tenderness if patient complains of headaches

  b. Muscle stretch reflexes—elicited by percussing a tendon with a reflex hammer, which causes stretch of muscle spindles and subsequent contraction of muscle fibers. Compare response on one side with the other

    i. Hyperreflexia may indicate interruption of upper motor neuron pathways between cerebrum and lower motor neurons

    ii. Areflexia is most commonly caused by lesions of lower motor neurons

      iii. Jaw reflex (trigeminal nerve, CN V)
      iv. Biceps reflex (C5–6)
      v. Brachioradialis (C5–6)
      vi. Triceps (C7–8)
      vii. Finger flexion (C7–T1)
      viii. Quadriceps (patellar) (L2–4)
      ix. Achilles (ankle jerk) (L5–S1–3)

4. Auscultation

   a. Auscultate great vessels, eyes, temples, and mastoid processes for bruits

Diagnostic Studies

1. Laboratory findings

   a. Blood
      i. Complete blood cell count, differential, sedimentation rate
      ii. Chemistries
      iii. Electrolytes
      iv. Clotting profile
      v. Arterial blood gases
      vi. Toxicology: alcohol, drugs
   b. Urinalysis
   c. CSF: See p. 327 for normal values
      i. Gross description of appearance
      ii. Cell count
      iii. Protein: identify site specimen drawn
      iv. Wassermann test
      v. Culture and sensitivity
      vi. Glucose level: compare with serum levels
      vii. Specific gravity
      viii. pH

2. Radiologic findings

   a. Skull series: used to diagnose skull fractures and illustrate status of cranial sutures. May also aid in diagnosis of other abnormalities such as tumors, degenerative processes, and increased intracranial pressure by presence of calcifications, erosion, or exostosis of bone
   b. Spine series: used to diagnose fractures, dislocations, or degenerative processes of vertebrae
   c. Computed tomography (CT scan)
      i. Principle: x-ray beam is projected through narrow section of brain, and detectors at opposite side record transmission readings from tissues. Readings are fed into computer that derives absorption (or attenuation) of x-ray by tissues in path of beam. Computer prints out digital picture that may be converted to black and white image and displayed on oscilloscope or x-ray

film. Denser tissue (e.g., bone) absorbs more x-ray and appears whiter on final image. Scan may be repeated after the patient has received intravenous contrast agent that enhances some abnormal tissue

ii. Clinical use: valuable in diagnosis of almost all intracranial pathologic processes and of particular value in head trauma. Used alone or in conjunction with magnetic resonance imaging (MRI) in detecting tumors, hydrocephalus, cerebral edema, and infectious processes. Of more limited value in diagnosing vascular lesions such as aneurysms or arteriovenous malformations

iii. Pre- and post-procedure care: no specific pre-procedure care is necessary. If contrast enhancement is used, quantity and specific gravity of urine will be increased for approximately 8 hours post scan

d. Cerebral angiography

i. Principle: a contrast material is injected into one or more arteries in order to obtain radiographic visualization of intracranial or extracranial circulation

ii. Clinical use: particularly useful in diagnosis of vascular abnormalities such as aneurysms, arteriovenous malformations, vasospasm, or vascular tumors. Also aids in diagnosis of other intracranial abnormalities that cause stretching/displacement of vessels or change in their diameter

iii. Pre- and post-procedure care: patient may be premedicated, and a consent form should be signed. Post procedure, check injection site for bleeding or hematoma formation. Pressure dressings/ice may be applied. A major complication is stroke caused by dislodging of an atherosclerotic plaque from the wall of an artery or of a clot that had been formed at end of catheter or needle

e. Radioisotope brain scanning

i. Principle: a radioactive substance is introduced into the blood, and the brain is scanned to determine areas that have accumulated the substance. In some disorders, radioisotope accumulates in abnormal areas of brain in sufficient quantities to allow detection, probably owing to a breakdown in the blood–brain barrier or increased vascularity of lesion

ii. Clinical use: screening patients for presence of brain tumors and evaluating cerebrovascular disease and some infectious processes. Often used in conjunction with other diagnostic procedures

iii. Pre- and post-procedure care: radioisotope is injected at varying time intervals prior to scanning. No specific post-procedure care or complications

f. Myelography

     i. Principle: x-ray examination of spinal canal after injection of a radiopaque substance into subarachnoid space, usually in lumbar area

     ii. Clinical use: diagnosis of intervertebral disc disease, spinal cord tumors, and other diseases of or injuries to spinal cord

     iii. Pre- and post-procedure care: written consent should be obtained. Patient may complain of headache post procedure and usually is required to lie flat for 4 to 24 hours

3. **Other diagnostic findings**

  a. Electroencephalography (EEG)

     i. Principle: recording of electrical activity of brain by electrodes attached to scalp. Voltage fluctuations have rhythmicity depending on area of cerebrum being recorded and age and level of alertness of patient

     ii. Clinical use: most helpful in diagnosing epilepsy, space-occupying lesions, and (on occasion) coma. Used in many institutions to aid in diagnosis of cerebral death

     iii. Pre- and post-procedure care: pre-procedure care varies depending on institution and type of EEG (e.g., sleep EEG). Post-procedure care includes washing conductive paste from hair. No risks in this procedure

  b. Cerebral blood flow: xenon (^{133}Xe) inhalation

     i. Principle: there are a number of invasive and noninvasive methods of measuring cerebral blood flow. One noninvasive method that can be done at the bedside is the xenon isotope inhalation technique. The technique employs externally placed scintillation detectors to measure radioactive xenon inhaled by the patient. Flow is calculated regionally by the rate of decline in radioactivity

     ii. Clinical use: of primary use and importance in patients with cerebrovascular disorders such as stroke, arteriovenous malformations, or vasospasm from a subarachnoid hemorrhage

     iii. Pre- and post-procedure care: no specific care. The scintillation detectors are large, and their appearance may frighten the patient. The inhalation of a radioactive substance may also cause anxiety, and the safety of this gas should be emphasized to the patient. No risks involved in procedure

  c. Electromyography (EMG)

     i. Principle: needle electrodes are used to record electrical potentials from contracting muscle fibers. These are displayed on an oscilloscope

     ii. Clinical use: aid in diagnosis of lower motor neuron disease or muscle disorders due to denervation or myopathy

     iii. Pre- and post-procedure care: no risk to patient, although needle electrodes are uncomfortable

d. Nerve conduction velocity
    i. Principle: a large motor nerve trunk is stimulated with electrode, and a response is recorded in one of its muscles. Velocity of impulse conduction can be calculated from distance and time elapsed between stimulus and response
    ii. Clinical use: diagnosis of peripheral neuropathies and nerve compression. In myasthenia gravis, repetitive stimulation gives objective evidence of decreasing muscular strength
    iii. Pre- and post-procedure care: no risk to patient, although needle electrodes are uncomfortable
e. Lumbar puncture, cisternal puncture
    i. Principle: a needle is placed into subarachnoid space, usually at L4–5 interspace (or cisterna magna with a cisternal puncture)
    ii. Clinical use: to obtain CSF for laboratory examination, measure/reduce CSF pressure, as a route for administration of medications, or in preparation for other diagnostic studies (e.g., myelography)
    iii. Pre- and post-procedure care: for lumbar puncture: written consent may be obtained. Contraindicated in patient with increased intracranial pressure since it may lead to herniation of brain stem. Infection, headache, or backache may occur as complications. Patient is usually required to lie flat for a few hours post procedure. For cisternal puncture: written consent may be obtained. Injury to brain stem could occur and lead to changes in vital signs or to shock. Hemorrhage or infection may also occur. Patient is usually kept flat for 4 to 6 hours
f. Evoked potentials (EPs)
    i. Principle: electrodes are placed on the scalp appropriate to the type of evoked response tested (e.g., brain-stem auditory evoked response [BAER], visual evoked response [VER], or somatosensory evoked response [SER]). As stimulus is applied (i.e., clicking noise for BAER, strobe light or pattern-shift for VER, and electrical stimulation of peripheral nerve for SER), evoked response (potential) is amplified, averaged by computer, displayed on oscilloscope, and recorded on paper. Evoked potential wave latencies and amplitudes are compared with normal responses and right and left responses in subject
    ii. Clinical use: BAERs are useful in determining brain stem function. VERs are useful index of hemispheric function and in diagnosis of multiple sclerosis. SERs may demonstrate lesions of peripheral pathways, spinal cord, or brain stem. Multimodal evoked potentials (MEPs) (two or all three methods) may be done to confirm or refute clinical diagnosis. Evoked potentials are useful in determining prognosis in severe head injury

iii. Pre- and post-procedure care: no specific pre- or post-procedure care. Patients must have temperature above 97°F (36.1°C) prior to BAERs. No specific post-procedure care or complications

g. Magnetic resonance imaging (MRI)

i. Technique: when hydrogen protons are placed in a magnetic field, they will precess (or wobble) like a spinning top. When a strong magnetic field is applied, hydrogen protons align. A radiofrequency (RF) is then applied at right angles to main field. After the RF is turned off, hydrogen protons emit an absorbed RF signal as they return to original orientation. These signals are picked up by receiving coils and used to generate an MR image. A magnetic enhancing agent, gadolinium, is used to enhance some lesions for better interpretation

ii. Clinical use: because MRI focuses on the hydrogen ion (i.e., water), brain edema and infarcted tissue are readily detected. Rapidly moving protons in blood emit little signal, and altered flow patterns can be detected by measuring intensity variations. Soft tissue resolution is greater than that of CT scan. Because MRI is a reflection of hydrogen proton concentration, this technique has the potential for providing information about the chemical environment of tissues. Future MRI scanning techniques may use phosphate or carbon protons, which will delineate the chemical environment more clearly

iii. Pre- and post-procedure care: all metal objects must be removed from patient prior to scanning. Patients should be told of the need to lie very still and that they will be in a small confined space. No specific post-procedure care or complications

COMMONLY ENCOUNTERED NURSING DIAGNOSES

Alteration in Cerebral Tissue Perfusion related to increased intracranial pressure (ICP) (see Increased Intracranial Pressure)

1. **Assessment for defining characteristics**
   a. Altered level of consciousness
   b. Change in pupillary size and reactivity
   c. Change in motor ability
   d. Decrease in cerebral perfusion pressure (CPP) below 60 mm Hg
   e. Increase in ICP above 20 mm Hg
2. **Expected outcomes**
   a. Maintains CPP above 60 mm Hg
   b. Maintains ICP below 20 mm Hg
3. **Nursing interventions**

a. Assess neurologic status frequently
b. Calculate CPP if ICP monitoring device is in place
c. Maintain ICP monitoring device
d. Limiting suctioning to 15 seconds; hyperventilate and/or hyperoxygenate before and after suctioning to minimize ICP rises
e. Facilitate venous return: elevate head of bed 30° to 40°; maintain head and neck in anatomic alignment
f. Monitor ICP during care activities; space nursing care as necessary to keep ICP at baseline or below 20 mm Hg
g. Report changes in ICP to physician, including trend toward a climbing ICP even if it remains below 20 mm Hg
h. Maintain CSF drainage system at level ordered to prevent inadvertent loss of CSF. Drain CSF as ordered to maintain ICP at desired level (e.g., below 20 mm Hg)
i. Prevent Valsalva's maneuver by instructing patient to exhale when bearing down or moving in bed
j. Administer diuretics or other drugs to reduce ICP as ordered. Monitor and record response

4. **Evaluation of nursing care**
   a. CPP remains above 60 mm Hg
   b. ICP remains below 20 mm Hg

Impaired Gas Exchange related to altered oxygen supply or oxygen-carrying capacity

1. **Assessment for defining characteristics**
   a. Pa_{O_2} less than 80 mm Hg
   b. Restlessness, irritability
   c. Tachypnea
   d. Increased work of breathing
   e. Changes in pulse rate and blood pressure
   f. Decreased level of responsiveness
   g. Decreased hematocrit and hemoglobin levels
2. **Expected outcomes**
   a. Maintains Pa_{O_2} above 80 mm Hg
   b. Maintains hemoglobin and hematocrit above 10 g/dl and 30%, respectively
   c. Maintains or improves neurologic function
3. **Nursing interventions**
   a. Administer oxygen therapy as ordered
   b. Maintain positive end-expiratory pressure (PEEP) or continuous positive airway pressure (CPAP) as ordered
   c. Maintain adequate amount of circulating erythrocytes by administering blood and blood products as ordered
   d. Monitor arterial oxygen tension and saturation

  e. Assess pulmonary status per unit standards and as patient's condition requires

  f. Position to facilitate chest expansion

  g. Suction as necessary to keep airway clear

4. Evaluation of nursing care

  a. Pa_{O_2} is maintained about 80 mm Hg

  b. Hematocrit remains above 30%; hemoglobin remains above 10 g/dl

  c. Neurologic functioning remains stable or improves

***Ineffective Breathing Pattern** related to depressed level of consciousness, intracranial pathologic process, and metabolic imbalance*

1. Assessment for defining characteristics

  a. Tachypnea

  b. Shallow, rapid respirations

  c. Deep, labored respirations

  d. Pa_{CO_2} greater than 45 mm Hg or less than 30 mm Hg

  e. Altered level of responsiveness

  f. ICP greater than 20 mm Hg

  g. Nasal flaring

  h. Change in alveolar minute ventilation

  i. Laboratory evidence of acidosis (e.g., pH less than 7.35)

2. Expected outcomes

  a. Maintains Pa_{CO_2} below 45 mm Hg and at ordered level

  b. Maintains ICP below 20 mm Hg

  c. Maintains metabolic balance

3. Nursing interventions

  a. Monitor pulmonary status as patient's condition indicates

  b. Maintain mechanical ventilation as ordered

  c. Suction as necessary to keep airway patent

  d. Maintain Pa_{CO_2} within ordered range

  e. Monitor ICP; maintain below 20 mm Hg

  f. Administer sedation as ordered to maintain adequate ventilation

  g. Monitor neurologic status

  h. Monitor pH and lactate levels

4. Evaluation of nursing care

  a. Pa_{CO_2} is maintained below 45 mm Hg and as ordered

  b. ICP remains below 20 mm Hg

  c. Metabolic acidosis will not occur

***Ineffective Airway Clearance** related to increased secretions and depressed level of consciousness*

1. Assessment for defining characteristics

  a. Inability to cough effectively to clear airway

  b. Changes in rate, depth, or pattern of respiration

    c. Tachypnea

    d. Noisy respirations

    e. Decreased level of responsiveness

    f. Alteration in arterial blood gas values

    g. Adventitious breath sounds

    h. Dyspnea

    i. Fever

2. Expected outcomes

    a. Maintains patent airway

    b. Maintains arterial blood gases within ordered range

    c. Maintains ICP below 20 mm Hg

    d. Has no adventitious sounds

3. Nursing interventions

    a. Assess respiratory status and adventitious sounds as patient's condition indicates

    b. Turn patient every 2 hours; position to maintain mobility of secretions while keeping head of bed at 30°

    c. Suction as necessary to maintain patent airway; monitor ICP during suctioning, limit suctioning to 15 seconds, hyperventilate, and hyperoxygenate prior to and after suctioning

    d. Provide adequate humidification to airway as per standards

    e. Maintain adequate hydration as ordered

4. Evaluation of nursing care

    a. Patent airway maintained

    b. Arterial blood gases remain within ordered parameters

    c. ICP remains below 20 mm Hg

    d. Adventitious sounds absent

Potential Fluid Volume Deficit related to excessive loss and decreased intake

1. Assessment for defining characteristics

    a. Oliguria

    b. Weight loss

    c. Altered electrolytes (e.g., sodium > 150 mEq/L)

    d. Serum osmolality > 305 mOsm/L

    e. Urine specific gravity increased

    f. Low blood pressure

    g. Rapid, thready pulse

    h. Increased temperature

    i. History of osmotic or loop diuretic therapy, fluid restriction, or hemorrhage

    j. Low central venous or pulmonary capillary wedge pressures

    k. Altered coagulation studies

    l. Decreased level of responsiveness

    m. Urine output > 200 ml/hr; specific gravity < 1.005, as seen in diabetes insipidus

2. Expected outcomes

    a. Maintains stable vital signs and neurologic status

    b. Produces adequate urine output (i.e., between 30 and 100 ml/hr) with specific gravity 1.005 to 1.020

    c. Demonstrates electrolyte, osmolality, and clotting profile within normal limits

3. Nursing interventions

    a. Monitor vital signs and neurologic status every hour until stable

    b. Measure, record, and report intake and output

    c. Measure specific gravity every 2 to 4 hours

    d. Administer fluid and blood products as ordered. Record effectiveness

    e. Monitor central venous and pulmonary capillary wedge pressures. Report deviations from normal

    f. Monitor electrolyte values, serum osmolality, and clotting profile

    g. Weigh daily

    h. Administer exogenous pitressin as ordered; monitor response

4. Evaluation of nursing care

    a. Vital signs and neurologic status are maintained within expected range

    b. Urine output is maintained above 30 ml/hr

    c. Electrolytes, serum osmolality, and clotting profile are maintained in normal range

Fluid Volume Excess related to syndrome of inappropriate ADH or to excessive intake

1. Assessment for defining characteristics

    a. Decreased level of responsiveness

    b. Serum osmolality < 275 mOsm/L

    c. Serum sodium < 135 mEq/L

    d. Urine osmolality less than serum osmolality

    e. Increased blood pressure

    f. Seizures

    g. Edema

    h. ICP greater than 20 mm Hg

2. Expected outcomes

    a. Maintains sodium and serum osmolality within normal limits

    b. Maintains level of responsiveness

    c. Maintains ICP less than 20 mm Hg

3. Nursing interventions

    a. Monitor vital signs and neurologic status

    b. Monitor electrolytes and serum osmolality as ordered

    c. Observe for seizure activity

    d. Monitor ICP; report rises above 20 mm Hg

    e. Measure and record intake and output

    f. Restrict fluids as ordered; administer hypertonic saline as ordered

    g. Assess for edema

4. **Evaluation of nursing care**

    a. Serum sodium level and serum osmolality remain within normal limits

    b. Neurologic status remains stable

    c. ICP remains below 20 mm Hg

Potential for Infection related to invasive lines, monitoring and therapeutic devices, and traumatic and surgical wounds

1. **Assessment for defining characteristics**

    a. Presence of invasive monitoring lines (e.g., ICP, arterial line, central venous pressure, pulmonary artery catheter, intravenous lines)

    b. Presence of traumatic wounds

    c. Presence of surgical incision

    d. CSF otorrhea or rhinorrhea

    e. Leaking of CSF around ICP device

    f. Wet dressings

    g. Drainage devices

    h. Presence of tracheal intubation and humidified ventilation

2. **Expected outcomes**

    a. Wound and drainage cultures free of pathogens

    b. Clear and odorless respiratory secretions

    c. Wounds/incisions are clean, pink, and free of purulent drainage

    d. Intravenous lines show no signs of inflammation

3. **Nursing interventions**

    a. Minimize risk of infection by using good handwashing technique and wearing gloves to maintain asepsis

    b. Use aseptic technique when handling invasive lines

    c. Use aseptic technique when setting up monitoring systems

    d. Culture drainage and secretions per order or unit protocol

    e. Remove invasive line as soon as clinically possible per physician's order

    f. Change lines and tubings every 72 hours or per hospital protocol

    g. Rotate IV and ICP sites per hospital protocol

4. **Evaluation of nursing care**

    a. Cultures of drainage and secretions are sterile

    b. Wounds are healing without signs of infection

    c. Insertion sites are free of signs of infection

Impaired Verbal Communication related to expressive/receptive dysphasia

1. **Assessment for defining characteristics**

    a. Inability to speak
    b. Inability to name objects
    c. Perseveration
    d. Inability to speak sentences
    e. Unable to understand spoken or written language
    f. Use of inappropriate words
    g. Speech unrelated to environmental stimuli
    h. Incessant verbalization
    i. Disorientation
    j. Unable to follow commands

2. **Expected outcomes**
    a. Needs are met
    b. Effective methods of communication are used

3. **Nursing interventions**
    a. Assess comprehension and expression of written and spoken language
    b. Explain to patient and family the extent and pathology of language deficit
    c. Encourage patience when communication difficulties arise
    d. Use strengths when communicating (e.g., gestures, yes/no, pointing, pictures, alphabet board)
    e. Speak slowly; use short phrases
    f. Allow time for patient to respond
    g. Repeat/rephrase questions
    h. Communicate for short periods to avoid tiring and frustrating patient
    i. Collaborate with speech therapist in developing and following through with specific interventions
    j. Involve family in developing and using effective communication techniques

4. **Evaluation of nursing care**
    a. Able to communicate and have needs met
    b. Ability to communicate improves in response to interventions

Impaired Physical Mobility related to weakness or paralysis of one or more body parts

1. **Assessment for defining characteristics**
    a. Limited range of motion
    b. Decreased muscle strength, control, mass, and endurance
    c. Inability to move purposefully in the environment, including bed mobility, transfer, and ambulation

2. **Expected outcomes**
    a. Maintains full joint range of motion and strength
    b. Exhibits no evidence of complications, such as contractures or skin breakdown

3. **Nursing interventions**
   a. Perform range of motion exercises to joints; progress from passive to active as tolerated
   b. Assess motor strength every shift
   c. Encourage independent activity as tolerated
   d. Reposition every 2 hours; maintain functional anatomic alignment; protect bony prominences
   e. Collaborate with physical and occupational therapists in teaching of self range-of-motion, splinting devices, transfer techniques, etc.
   f. Place items within reach of unaffected arm
   g. Involve family in therapy as appropriate
   h. Assess integrity of skin when turning
   i. Up in chair two to four times per day as tolerated per order
4. **Evaluation of nursing care**
   a. Joint mobility is maintained
   b. No evidence of skin breakdown
   c. Absence of contractures

Alteration in Thought Processes related to confusion, short-term memory loss, and short attention span

1. **Assessment for defining characteristics**
   a. Disoriented to time, place, person, and environment
   b. Altered problem-solving abilities
   c. Lack of sequential thought (i.e., unable to remember events as they occurred or in the proper time sequence)
   d. Noncompliance to requests or instructions
   e. Inability to complete simple tasks due to altered attention span
2. **Expected outcomes**
   a. Performs activities of daily living with minimal assistance or guidance
   b. Oriented to environment
3. **Nursing interventions**
   a. Orient to environment frequently
      i. Call patient by name
      ii. Tell patient your name
      iii. Provide tools to help maintain orientation (e.g., calendar, clock, newspapers, radio, TV)
      iv. Keep patient items in same place
   b. Provide simple instructions frequently; assist and encourage as necessary
   c. Protect from injury (e.g., Posey restraint, side rails, call light, bed near nurses' station)
   d. Mobilize as appropriate per orders
   e. Teach and involve family as appropriate

4. **Evaluation of nursing care**
   a. Oriented to environment
   b. Absence of injury
   c. Carries out simple activities of daily living

Ineffective Individual Coping related to situational crisis, loss of control and independence, and change in role

1. **Assessment for defining characteristics**
   a. Verbal manipulation
   b. Inappropriate use of defense mechanisms
   c. Inability to meet basic needs
   d. Inability to meet role expectations
   e. General irritability
   f. Verification of situational crisis
2. **Expected outcomes**
   a. Becomes involved in planning and participating in care
   b. Communicates feelings about present situation
   c. Develops positive ways to deal with illness/deficits
3. **Nursing interventions**
   a. If possible, assign primary nurse to provide continuity and promote development of a relationship
   b. Spend time with patient; allow patient to express fears and concerns. Help develop coping strategies
   c. Explain present and future treatment plan
   d. Encourage participation in care; allow choices
   e. Give feedback about progress
   f. Determine patient's ongoing strengths and values
   g. Include family in planning and implementation
4. **Evaluation of nursing care**
   a. Participates and takes responsibility for aspects of care
   b. Verbalizes feelings about situation
   c. Incorporates effective coping behaviors

Ineffective Family Coping related to disruption of usual family roles, burden of care, and changes in family member's present and future functioning

1. **Assessment for defining characteristics**
   a. Family member(s) expresses concern for future care of patient
   b. Expresses unrealistic expectations of outcome
   c. Expects to see daily improvement
   d. Expresses concern about family's financial, social, and spiritual future
   e. Demanding and manipulative with nursing/medical staff
2. **Expected outcomes**

a. Expresses impact of patient's illness on relationships and family functioning
b. Develops coping strategies to deal with caring for a chronically ill family member

3. **Nursing interventions**
   a. Facilitate family conferences; help family identify key issues and select support services as needed
   b. Encourage use of coping behaviors that have worked previously; help develop new coping strategies
   c. Assist family to develop realistic expectations of current and future functioning of patient, while maintaining an optimistic attitude
   d. Allow family to express feelings of hurt, fear, anger, despair, and guilt
   e. Encourage family members to participate in care when possible
   f. Interpret patient's behavior to family, particularly if bizarre or combative
   g. Refer to professional counseling after consultation with team

4. **Evaluation of nursing care**
   a. Family expresses concerns and describes how they will cope
   b. Demonstrates effective adaptive strategies

PATIENT HEALTH PROBLEMS

Increased Intracranial Pressure

1. **Pathophysiology**
   a. Nondistensible intracranial cavity is filled to capacity with essentially noncompressible contents: CSF, intravascular blood, brain tissue water (interstitial and intracellular fluid)
   b. Monro-Kellie hypothesis states that if volume of one of constituents of intracranial cavity increases, a reciprocal decrease in volume of one or both of the others must occur or an overall increase in ICP will result
   c. Principal spatial buffers that resist increases in ICP are displacement of CSF from cranial vault and compression of low-pressure venous system. Increased CSF absorption may also contribute to spatial compensation
      i. Volume of fluid that can be displaced is finite; an increase in ICP will ultimately occur if volume of intracranial mass exceeds volume of fluid displaced
      ii. Relationship between intracranial volume and pressure has been plotted and an elastance curve (inverse of compliance) constructed (Fig. 3–21). The flat portion of the curve reflects little change in pressure with increases in volume (low elast-

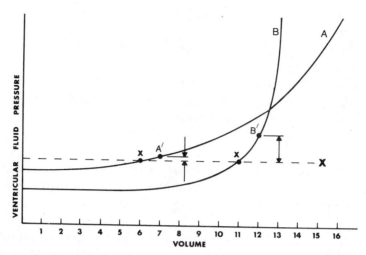

Figure 3–21. Two theoretical volume–pressure curves in different patients. At the same resting pressure (X), addition of 1 unit of volume produces a greater pressure increase on the B curve than the A curve (B′ > A′). (From Mauss, N., and Mitchell, P.: Increased intracranial pressure: An update. Heart Lung 5:920, 1976.)

ance or high compliance), and the steep portion of the curve reflects large pressure changes with small increases in volume (high elastance or decreased compliance). A patient's response to changes in intracranial volume, therefore, depends, in part, on where patient is on volume–pressure curve. Rate of volume change also influences magnitude of ICP change

d. CBF varies with changes in cerebral perfusion pressure (CPP) and diameter of cerebrovascular bed

   i. Increased ICP can increase CBF indirectly by producing cortical vascular dilatation and appears to be principal mechanism responsible for maintenance of CBF in face of rising ICP

   ii. When ICP approaches mean arterial pressure (MAP), CPP decreases to point where autoregulation is impaired and CBF decreases

     (a) When autoregulation is impaired, arterioles passively dilate with increases in arterial blood pressure causing increase in CBF; however, pressure in venous system (capacitance system) also rises, cerebral blood volume increases, and ICP rises further

     (b) Resultant high capillary pressure causes oozing of plasma from vessels and petechial hemorrhages

     (c) Eventually, perfusion pressure can no longer be maintained and CBF gradually falls as ICP increases

   iii. Increases in carbon dioxide tension, and to a lesser extent decreases in oxygen tension, also cause arteriolar dilatation and increases in CBF. Hypoxia and hypercapnia thus lead to intracranial hypertension, especially in patients with unstable intracranial dynamics

e. Herniation syndromes

    i. Tentorial (uncal) herniation: expanding lesions above the tentorium, particularly on one side, force the uncus of the temporal lobe over the medial edge of the tentorium

    ii. Subfalcine herniation: unilateral cerebral lesions can cause a shift of brain tissue from one side to the other, causing the cingulate gyrus to become distorted under the falx cerebri

    iii. Tonsillar (medullary) herniation: displacement of the contents of the posterior fossa, particularly the tonsils of the cerebellum, through the foramen magnum causes brain-stem distortion and potential respiratory and vasomotor collapse

    iv. Central herniation: midline or bilateral lesions of the cerebrum cause it to be displaced downward through the tentorial notch causing pressure on the midbrain. Can progress to tonsillar herniation

f. A supratentorial lesion that causes tentorial herniation compresses the ipsilateral oculomotor nerve and impairs its parasympathetic activity, leading to a larger pupil with a sluggish or absent direct light reflex

g. Increased ICP can also exert pressure on motor and sensory nerve tracts, leading to impairment or loss of function

h. Ischemia of vasomotor center in brain stem may trigger Cushing's reflex, causing rise in systolic pressure, widening pulse pressure, and slowing of pulse. Respiratory rate and pattern may also change

2. Etiology or precipitating factors

a. ICP rises when the volume added to the intracranial cavity exceeds the compensatory capacity. The rate and extent of the increase in ICP depends on

    i. Volume of the mass lesion

    ii. Rate of expansion (i.e., the faster the volume is added, the greater the rise in ICP)

    iii. Total volume within the intracranial cavity

    iv. Intracranial elastance (compliance) (i.e., the capacity for compensation)

b. Increases in brain volume

    i. Mass lesions: subdural, epidural, or intracerebral hematomas, tumors, abscesses, or any other space-occupying lesions

    ii. Cytotoxic cerebral edema: intracellular swelling of neurons and glial cells. Caused by hypoxia or acute hypo-osmolality (water intoxication). Hypoxia causes anaerobic glycolysis and a decreased production of ATP. Because there is insufficient ATP to fuel the sodium–potassium pump, sodium is no longer pumped out of the cell or potassium back into the cell, leading to an accumulation of sodium inside the cell. Water then moves into the cell, causing cellular swelling. Acute hypo-osmolality causes intravascular dilution of osmotically active substances, causing water to move into the cell via osmosis since there is now a greater concentration of solute inside the cell as compared with the extracellular environment. All cells are affected, and swelling of the epithelial cells surrounding the capillaries causes vascular compression and ischemia

   iii. Vasogenic cerebral edema: increase in extracellular fluid space caused by breakdown of the blood–brain barrier, which allows osmotically active molecules, such as proteins, to leak into the interstitium, drawing water from the vascular system and cells into the interstitium. Caused by most types of cerebral injury or insult, including contusion, tumors, or abscesses. Edema is localized around the lesion

  c. Cerebrovascular alterations

    i. Venous outflow obstruction: caused by

     (a) Rotation, hyperextension, or hyperflexion of head; endotracheal or tracheotomy ties too tight. Causes flattening or compression of the jugular veins and inhibits venous return, causing venous engorgement

     (b) Raised intrathoracic and/or intra-abdominal pressures may also lead to impaired venous return. Pressure is transmitted throughout the venous system; therefore, raised intrathoracic or intra-abdominal pressure is transmitted to the jugular veins and impairs venous return. Positive end-expiratory pressure, coughing, vomiting, and Valsalva's maneuver may all cause this phenomenon

    ii. Fluctuations in blood pressure or cerebral perfusion pressure

     (a) Blood pressure that exceeds the limits of autoregulation contributes to increased cerebral blood volume and cerebral edema

     (b) Autoregulation may be impaired, either globally or regionally, by cerebral injury or insult. CBF to affected area of brain is then dependent on blood pressure; that is, CBF increases as the blood pressure rises, contributing to cerebral edema and increased ICP. Conversely, as the blood pressure falls, CBF falls and leads to cerebral ischemia

     (c) Cerebral perfusion pressure less than 40 mm Hg exceeds the cerebrovascular capacity for autoregulation; CBF falls, leading to cerebral ischemia

    iii. Vasodilatation

     (a) Hypoventilation causes hypercapnia and vasodilatation, leading to increased CBF and ICP. Abnormal respiratory patterns, obstructed airway, or excess secretions may all cause carbon dioxide retention

(b) Hypoxia also causes cerebral vasodilatation, although its effects are not significant until the Pa_{O_2} falls below 60 mm Hg. Hypoxia can be caused by the same factors that lead to hypoventilation but may also be produced by pulmonary pathology

(c) Certain anesthetic agents, such as halothane, ketamine, and nitrous oxide, cause cerebral vasodilatation and lead to increased cerebral blood volume and increased ICP and thus should be used with caution in the neurosurgical patient

(d) Other drugs may also cause vasodilatation and must be used with caution in the neurologically compromised patient. These include nitroprusside and curare

d. Increases in CSF volume (hydrocephalus)

   i. Increased production of CSF is a rare cause of increased CSF volume and will not be seen often in clinical practice

   ii. Decreased reabsorption of CSF leading to increased CSF volume is caused in two major ways

     (a) Obstruction of CSF circulation out of the ventricular system—may be caused by mass lesions in or near ventricles or obstruction of basal cisterna at base of brain

     (b) Impaired reabsorption of CSF from subarachnoid space into venous system—may be caused by inflammation of meninges and obstruction of arachnoid villa by debris such as blood cells or bacteria

3. **Nursing assessment data base**

a. Nursing history: consistent with intracranial pathology

b. Nursing examination of patient

   i. Increased ICP may be present with little or no change in clinical presentation, depending on etiology

   ii. Changes in level of consciousness, motor activity, pupillary size or reflexes, cranial nerves, and vital signs from one assessment to another indicate possible increasing ICP

   iii. Papilledema may be present with long-standing intracranial hypertension

   iv. Other signs and symptoms that indicate a change in patient's neurologic status or increased ICP must be evaluated in light of history and clinical presentation

     (a) Increasing headache

     (b) Blurred vision, diplopia, photophobia

     (c) Seizure activity—may be due to head trauma, anoxia, tumors, or electrolyte disorders in acutely ill patient without history of seizure disorders

(d) Vomiting—lesions that produce vomiting are those that involve vestibular nuclei, impinge on floor of fourth ventricle, or (less often) produce brain stem compression secondary to increased ICP

(e) Nuchal rigidity—difficulty or an inability to flex patient's head and complaints of neck pain indicate irritation of meninges, most commonly due to meningitis or subarachnoid hemorrhage

c. Diagnostic study findings

　i. Lumbar puncture: contraindicated by increased ICP. Reliable measure of ICP only if communication between lumbar subarachnoid space and ventricular system is unobstructed

　ii. ICP monitoring

　　(a) ICP—because brain is deformed and displaced easily by mass lesions, it is believed that persistent differences in pressure do not develop within brain substance

　　　(1) CSF pressure—CSF is contained within a closed system, and since pressure is transmitted equally in all directions in fluid, CSF is considered the most accurate indicator of ICP. Choroid plexus pulsations are transmitted to CSF throughout ventricular system and subarachnoid space. The pulsations produce a waveform with the same characteristics as an arterial waveform in the ventricles, although of lower amplitude. The waveform is further dampened in the subarachnoid space and often resembles a venous waveform. Variations coincident with respiratory cycle also occur

　　　(2) Intraparenchymal pressure—recent research has demonstrated a linear relationship between intraventricular and intraparenchymal pressure measured with a fiberoptic transducer-tipped probe

　　　(3) Normally, ICP is less than 20 mm Hg, although pressures between 10 and 20 mm Hg are considered mildly to moderately elevated

　　(b) Indications for ICP monitoring—patients who benefit are those with head trauma, known or suspected hydrocephalus, posterior fossa lesions, or Reye's syndrome. Patients with tumors may benefit from ICP monitoring and control

　　(c) Techniques—the four most common are

　　　(1) Intraventricular. Cannula is inserted into lateral ventricle (usually the anterior horn in nondominant hemisphere) via a twist drill hole through skull. Cannula is connected via a stopcock to fluid-filled pressure tubing to a transducer that is positioned at level of

foramen of Monro (middle of ear may be used as reference)

   a) Advantages—ability to measure CSF pressure directly, drain CSF therapeutically, and withdraw CSF for analysis

   b) Disadvantages—risks of infection, inadvertent loss of CSF, and difficulty in placement of cannula if ventricles are small or displaced

(2) Subarachnoid bolt. Hollow bolt is placed into subarachnoid space through a twist drill hole in skull. Fluid-filled pressure tubing connects the screw to transducer. A fiberoptic transducer-tipped probe may also be placed in the subarachnoid space

   a) Advantage—ability to measure CSF pressure directly increases accuracy of readings

   b) Disadvantages—CSF sampling and drainage from this system are usually not possible. The bolt system needs to be irrigated to keep it patent, and thus the potential for infection is increased. The addition of even a small amount of irrigating solution to the subarachnoid space may increase ICP. Improper placement of either the bolt or the fiberoptic probe results in erroneous measurements. Additionally, fiberoptic probe cannot be re-zeroed once in place

(3) Epidural. Device (e.g., fiberoptic transducer or balloon radio transmitter) is placed between skull and dura, with pressure-sensitive membrane toward dura. Transducer continually balances air pressure in transducer with pressure being applied to dura; it may also be placed subdurally

   a) Advantage—ability to monitor ICP while leaving dura intact. Should protect patient from intracerebral infection although wound, bone, or epidural infections may still occur

   b) Disadvantages—epidural pressure is higher than intraventricular pressure. Accuracy of values is questionable at high ICP levels. Once in place, fiberoptic transducer cannot be zero-balanced or calibrated, further contributing to possibility of inaccurate readings

(4) Intraparenchymal. Fiberoptic transducer-tipped probe is placed into the parenchyma of the brain through a twist drill hole in the skull. This is connected to a monitor that provides an analog readout and can be

interfaced to the standard pressure monitor to visualize a waveform

    a) Advantages—easy to place; not dependent on ventricular size or position

    b) Disadvantage—once in place cannot be re-zeroed. Fiberoptic probe is fragile and may break if bent when transferring patient or in restless patients. Probe may become dislodged if bolt-connection is not tight

4. **Nursing diagnoses**
   a. Alteration in cerebral tissue perfusion related to increased ICP
      i. Assessment for defining characteristics
         (a) Changes in level of consciousness, pupillary size and reaction, motor ability, and vital signs may indicate rising ICP
         (b) Rise in ICP noted on monitor
         (c) See Alteration in Cerebral Tissue Perfusion, p. 366
      ii. Expected outcomes
         (a) Maintains ICP below 20 mm Hg and CPP above 60 mm Hg or as ordered
         (b) Experiences no complications as a result of ICP monitoring
      iii. Nursing interventions
         (a) Interventions necessary to maintain ICP monitoring
            (1) For intraventricular and subarachnoid bolt techniques, ensure a closed system to prevent contamination. Luer-Lok connections should be used. Because system must be opened to obtain CSF specimens and to zero-balance great care must be taken to prevent contamination
            (2) Maintain transducer at level of foramen of Monro
               a) Zero-balance whenever bed or patient's position is changed or if erroneous readings are suspected. Calibrate transducer per ICU protocol
               b) Keep transducer and tubing free of air bubbles to avoid dampening of waveform and inaccurate readings
            (3) Report and record changes in waveform, elevations in pressure, and therapy instituted
               a) Normal ventricular pressure is less than 10 mm Hg with pressures between 10 and 20 mm Hg considered mildly to moderately elevated. Pressures above 20 mm Hg are regarded as severely elevated
               b) Transient increases may occur with suctioning,

coughing, Valsalva's maneuver, inappropriate positioning, or other nursing interventions

   c) Three types of ICP waveforms have been described

      ☐ A waves (also called plateau or Lundberg waves)—elevations of intracranial pressure between 50 and 100 mm Hg, lasting 5 to 20 minutes. They may or may not be associated with clinical manifestations of increased ICP but are associated with advanced stages of intracranial hypertension

      ☐ B and C waves are variations in pressure that correspond to respiratory and arterial pressure changes, respectively, but generally are not considered clinically significant

      ☐ Recent research of ICP waveform analysis demonstrates that there is a relationship between changes in waveform configuration and intracranial compliance and pathologic cause. Research in this area is continuing

(b) Interventions necessary to control ICP

  (1) Facilitate venous return

    a) Elevate head of bed 15° to 30°

    b) Prevent hyperextension, flexion, or rotation of head

    c) If patient has tracheostomy, make sure ties are not too tight

  (2) Limit suctioning to 15 seconds to minimize blood gas alterations. Hyperventilation/hyperoxygenation before and after suctioning may further minimize effects of suctioning

  (3) Assist patient when moving in bed to avoid Valsalva's maneuver

  (4) Therapy is aimed at reducing volume of one or more of the three components of ICP—cerebral blood volume, brain tissue water, or CSF volume

    a) Hyperventilation (usually to Pa_{CO_2} of 25 to 30 mm Hg) causes vasoconstriction and thus reduces cerebral blood volume. Nursing responsibilities include careful respiratory assessment, collaborating with respiratory therapist in maintaining ventilator settings, and monitoring and reporting arterial blood gas values

    b) Diuretics, including mannitol, urea, glycerol (osmotic diuretics), furosemide or ethacrynic acid (loop diuretics), aim at reduction of brain tissue water. Nursing responsibilities include careful monitoring of fluid and electrolyte status

c) In patients with enlarged ventricles, CSF may be drained via intraventricular cannula to reduce CSF volume. Nursing responsibilities include maintaining a closed drainage system, monitoring and recording the amount of CSF drainage, and maintaining the drip chamber at the appropriate level to avoid inadvertent loss of CSF

(5) Glucocorticoids (e.g., dexamethasone or methylprednisolone)—may help control cerebral edema caused by chronic conditions such as tumors, although mechanism is unclear. They are of no proven clinical value in patients with head trauma. Nursing responsibilities include monitoring of glucose levels and protecting the patient from infection

(6) Barbiturate coma (administration of pentobarbital or thiopental in doses and at intervals sufficient to produce complete unresponsiveness and burst-suppression on EEG) has been employed alone and in conjunction with other methods. Barbiturates reduce metabolic activity and may have direct effect on ICP; exact mechanism is not known. Patient must be intubated and on a ventilator; arterial blood pressure must be monitored continuously. Pulmonary artery pressure monitoring is advised. Respiratory, hemodynamic, and metabolic complications may occur. Nursing responsibilities include frequent suctioning and turning (cough reflex is abolished); monitoring hemodynamic parameters; maintaining adequate intravascular volume; monitoring temperature and maintaining core body temperature above 92° F (33° C); monitoring ICP and maintaining below 20 mm Hg; monitoring serum levels of barbiturate being used. (*NOTE:* be careful to identify the specific drug level desired on laboratory slip)

(7) Paralyzing agents (e.g., pancuronium)—also decrease body's metabolic requirements and may be used in conjunction with other therapy. Nursing interventions include monitoring of ICP response, administration of sedatives in awake patients to minimize fear, and maintaining desired level of paralysis

(8) Sedation with small, frequent intravenous doses of morphine sulfate or other sedative drugs may assist in control of ICP in restless or agitated patients.

Because of potential for depressing the level of consciousness, ICP monitoring is advised. Nursing interventions include monitoring of effects of sedatives on level of consciousness and ICP

  iv. Evaluation of nursing care
   (a) ICP monitoring system maintained
   (b) Absence of complications due to ICP monitoring and interventions
   (c) ICP controlled at or below maximal ordered level

Hydrocephalus

1. **Pathophysiology:** in the adult, hydrocephalus occurs as a complication of other pathophysiologic conditions. It is a state in which the production of CSF exceeds the rate of absorption
   a. Communicating (nonobstructive): hydrocephalus occurs when CSF is able to circulate out of the ventricular system but is inadequately absorbed via the arachnoid granulations into the venous sinuses. Inadequate absorption is caused by inflammation of the meninges from blood or bacteria and obstruction of the arachnoid villi by blood cells and the by-products of the breakdown of blood, or by the exudate from a bacterial meningitis
   b. Noncommunicating (obstructive): hydrocephalus is caused by obstruction of the circulation of CSF within the ventricles. Intraventricular masses, such as tumors or cysts, or masses that compress the foramen of Monro, aqueduct of Sylvius, or the foramina of Magendie or Luschka prevent circulation of CSF to the subarachnoid space. The continued production of CSF by the choroid plexus causes accumulation of CSF in the ventricles. The ventricles dilate, causing compression of surrounding brain tissue.
2. **Etiology or precipitating factors**
   a. Tumors or masses in or near ventricles
   b. Subarachnoid hemorrhage
   c. Intraventricular hemorrhage
   d. Meningitis
3. **Nursing assessment data base**
   a. Nursing history of above conditions
   b. Nursing examination of patient
      i. Signs of increased ICP (see p. 379)
      ii. Signs of meningitis (see p. 424)
      iii. Signs of subarachnoid hemorrhage (see p. 413)
   c. Diagnostic study findings
      i. CT scan will reveal enlarged ventricles and may reveal causative factor (e.g., tumor)
      ii. ICP monitoring will reveal elevated ICP

iii. Lumbar puncture is contraindicated in the presence of increased ICP

iv. CSF analysis may reveal erythrocytes and leukocytes and cultures will reveal pathologic organism in patients with meningitis

4. **Nursing diagnoses:** alteration in cerebral tissue perfusion related to increased ICP (see pp. 366, 382)

Scalp Lacerations

1. **Pathophysiology:** because of extensive vascularity of scalp and poor contractility of vessels, lacerations can result in significant blood loss that may cause or contribute to hypovolemia

2. **Etiology or precipitating factors:** associated with trauma to head, with or without skull fractures

3. **Nursing assessment data base**
   a. Nursing history: history of trauma to the head
   b. Nursing examination of patient: bleeding or serous oozing from scalp
   c. Diagnostic study findings: skull x-ray films may reveal presence of fracture and/or fragments of debris imbedded in wound or brain

4. **Nursing diagnoses**
   a. Potential fluid volume deficit related to blood loss from scalp laceration
       i. Assessment for defining characteristics
           (a) Changes in vital signs, e.g., fall in blood pressure, tachycardia, tachypnea
           (b) Fall in hematocrit
           (c) Clinical evidence of blood loss
       ii. Expected outcome: maintains adequate circulating volume
       iii. Nursing interventions
           (a) Estimate amount of blood loss
           (b) Apply direct pressure to control bleeding in less severe lacerations
           (c) Assist physician in suturing extensive lacerations to control bleeding
           (d) Monitor vital signs frequently; record and report results
           (e) Monitor hematocrit
       iv. Evaluation of nursing care
           (a) Vital signs remain stable
           (b) Bleeding from scalp is controlled
   b. Potential for infection related to contaminated scalp laceration
       i. Assessment for defining characteristics
           (a) Purulent drainage from scalp wound
           (b) Accumulation of purulent fluid under wound
           (c) Swelling or redness of and around wound

(d) Fever, tachycardia

(e) Laboratory findings consistent with infection (e.g., elevated leukocyte count)

  ii. Expected outcomes

(a) Maintains wound clean, pink, and free of purulent drainage

(b) Experiences no pathogens in cultures

  iii. Nursing interventions

(a) Shave hair around wound; irrigate with saline or solution of physician's choice

(b) Assist physician with debridement of wound if necessary

(c) Maintain dry, sterile dressings

(d) Inspect wound daily for signs of infection

(e) Monitor vital signs

(f) Monitor cultures as indicated

  iv. Evaluation of nursing care

(a) Absence of wound infection

(b) Cultures sterile

Skull Fractures

1. Pathophysiology

  a. Linear skull fracture

    i. Result of elastic deformation of bone without displacement of bone. Area receiving blow bends inward while area around it bends outward. Fracture begins at area of outbending and extends both toward and away from point of impact

    ii. Of significance if fracture interrupts major vascular channel (e.g., middle meningeal artery or superior sagittal sinus). Fracture could cause vessel injury and lead to intracranial hemorrhage, usually epidural hematoma

  b. Depressed skull fracture

    i. Fracture depresses outer table of bone below inner table of adjacent skull

    ii. If associated with scalp laceration (i.e., open fracture) is considered a surgical emergency

    iii. Bone fragments may lacerate or lodge in brain tissue and may lead to intracranial hematoma or other intracranial pathology

  c. Basal skull fracture

    i. Fracture extends into either anterior, middle, or posterior fossae at the base of the skull

    ii. May cause injury to one or more cranial nerves or could extend into the sinuses and cause tearing of dura with resultant CSF leak that could lead to meningitis

    iii. Posterior fossa fractures frequently result from occipital trauma

2. Etiology or precipitating factors
   a. Caused by trauma to head or penetrating injuries
   b. Motor vehicle accidents, falls, assaults, gunshot or stab wounds, and recreational accidents are leading causes of head trauma
3. Nursing assessment data base
   a. Nursing history
      i. History or evidence of head trauma
      ii. May have had a period of unconsciousness
   b. Nursing examination of patient
      i. Linear skull fracture: may have swollen, ecchymotic, tender area of scalp or scalp laceration
      ii. Depressed skull fracture
         (a) Significant contusion and edema of scalp with laceration (open fracture) or without laceration (closed fracture)
         (b) Neurologic presentation will vary depending on location and extent of cerebral involvement; focal neurologic deficits may be present
         (c) Depressed fractures of frontal bone may injure the olfactory nerve (CN I) causing loss of sense of smell (anosmia)
         (d) Depressed fractures of temporal bone may injure the facial nerve (CN VII), causing ipsilateral facial paralysis, or the acoustic nerve (CN VIII), leading to disturbances in hearing or equilibrium
      iii. Basal skull fractures
         (a) Anterior fossa fractures
            (1) May result in CSF rhinorrhea if dura is torn. Patient may complain of dripping down back of throat
            (2) Pneumocephalus may result from air entering cranium through fractured sinus(es)
            (3) May also result in bilateral ecchymotic eyes owing to bleeding in sinuses—sometimes referred to as "owl's eyes" or "raccoon's eyes"
            (4) Injury to olfactory nerve (CN I) is common
         (b) Middle fossa fractures
            (1) CSF otorrhea occurs if dura is torn and tympanic membrane is ruptured. CSF exits via eustachian tube and CSF rhinorrhea results if tympanic membrane is intact. In this case, tympanic membrane will bulge and patient may complain of difficulty in hearing
            (2) Bleeding with resultant ecchymosis over mastoid bone—commonly referred to as "Battle's sign"
            (3) May also result in cranial nerve injuries
         (c) Posterior fossa fractures that lead to epidural hematomas (the most common traumatic space-occupying lesion of the posterior fossa) may result in signs of increased ICP and/or

cerebellar, brain stem, long tract, or cranial nerve signs. Medullary failure and death may occur
  c. Diagnostic study findings
   i. Laboratory
    (a) Linear or depressed skull fractures—nothing specific to injury
    (b) Basal skull fractures—CSF drainage from nose or ear
   ii. Radiologic
    (a) Skull x-ray series
     (1) Linear or depressed—may be seen on plain films
     (2) Basal—difficult to confirm radiologically, although suggestive radiographic findings include an opaque mastoid or air–fluid level in sinuses
4. **Nursing diagnoses**
  a. Alteration in cerebral tissue perfusion related to increased ICP (see pp. 366 and 382)
   i. Assessment for defining characteristics
    (a) Linear—if fracture crosses a major vascular channel, be alert for signs of increased ICP from intracranial hemorrhage
    (b) Depressed and basal—assess for signs of increased ICP from associated intracranial hemorrhage
   ii. Expected outcome: does not experience increased ICP as a result of undetected intracranial hemorrhage
   iii. Nursing interventions
    (a) Assess neurologic status hourly or more often as patient's condition indicates
    (b) Report and record signs and symptoms of possible increased ICP
    (c) Implement measures to control ICP as ordered
   iv. Evaluation of nursing care
    (a) Signs of increased ICP are recorded and reported promptly
  b. Potential for infection related to CSF leak or abscess formation (see p. 371)
   i. Assessment for defining characteristics
    (a) CSF rhinorrhea or otorrhea
    (b) Presence of open, depressed, skull fracture
    (c) Evidence of penetrating intracranial injury
    (d) Clinical signs of intracranial infection—fever, decreased level of consciousness, nuchal rigidity, increased ICP
    (e) Laboratory signs of infection (e.g., positive CSF cultures, increased leukocyte count)
   ii. Expected outcome: will have no pathogens in cultures
   iii. Nursing interventions
    (a) Monitor for CSF rhinorrhea or otorrhea—clear or slightly

serous drainage from nose or ear in patient with clinical signs of basal skull fracture

 (b) Monitor for signs of intracranial infection

 (c) Assess neurologic status, including nuchal rigidity per unit standards or as patient's condition indicates

 (d) Monitor laboratory data for indications of infections (e.g., CBC, sedimentation rate, cultures)

 (e) Monitor vital signs per unit standards or as patient's condition indicates, particularly temperature

 (f) Basal skull fractures with CSF rhinorrhea or otorrhea

  (1) Do not put anything into nose or ears. This includes tissue, dressings, packing, cotton, suction catheters, nasogastric tubes, oxygen catheters, or cannulas

  (2) Instruct patient not to blow nose and allow fluid to flow freely

  (3) Place only a dry, sterile dressing loosely over ear or as a mustache dressing to absorb drainage

  (4) Prevent Valsalva's maneuver and vigorous coughing to avert further tearing of dura and increased CSF flow

 iv. Evaluation of nursing care: absence of intracranial infection

c. Potential for injury related to cranial defect from depressed skull fracture or cranial nerve damage from basal skull fracture

 i. Assessment for defining characteristics (risk factors)

  (a) Focal neurologic deficits resulting from laceration of brain tissue by bone fragments from depressed skull fracture

  (b) Signs of cranial nerve injury from basal skull fracture

  (c) Signs of cerebellar or medullary dysfunction from posterior fossa fracture and hemorrhage

  (d) Unprotected brain resulting from cranial defects from depressed skull fracture

 ii. Expected outcomes

  (a) Will experience no further brain injury from cranial defect

  (b) Will experience no complications as a result of cranial nerve injury

 iii. Nursing interventions

  (a) Position patient away from cranial defect. Apply protective device as indicated

  (b) Teach patient and family how to protect brain under cranial defect from injury by positioning and protective devices

  (c) Assess cranial nerve function; record and report abnormal findings

  (d) Assess and record signs of cerebellar dysfunction in patients with posterior fossa fractures

      (e) Observe for signs of medullary dysfunction in patients with posterior fossa fractures
   iv. Evaluation of nursing care
      (a) Absence of further injury to brain underlying cranial defect
      (b) Cranial nerve injury is detected

Closed-Head Injuries

1. Pathophysiology

  a. Mild concussion represents temporary neurologic dysfunction but is reversible with no persistent sequelae. May be the result of rotational forces on the brain causing stretching of nerve fibers with subsequent failure of conduction. Repeated mild concussions have cumulative effects. Retrograde amnesia occurs

  b. Classic concussion is also reversible and is associated with loss of consciousness for less than 24 hours, with disorientation and retrograde and post-traumatic amnesia present on return of consciousness
    i. Contusions may occur causing focal deficits
   ii. Although recovery seems complete, subtle psychological, personality, or memory changes may occur
  iii. Pathophysiologic mechanism similar to that of mild concussion, although axonal disruption is more severe and there is global dysfunction of cortical activity

  c. Third level of closed-head injury is diffuse injury with loss of consciousness exceeding 24 hours
    i. Coma may persist for days to weeks with purposeful movements, withdrawal from pain, and restlessness
   ii. Retrograde and post-traumatic amnesia are complicated by disorientation
  iii. Treatment is aimed at preventing complications and controlling ICP and cerebral edema
  iv. Permanent residual neurologic, psychological, or personality changes are common, representing anatomic disruption of neuronal pathways caused by widespread axonal disruption throughout the cerebrum

  d. Fourth level of closed-head injury is diffuse white matter shearing associated with severe mechanical disruption of axons and neuronal pathways in the hemispheres, diencephalon, and brain stem
    i. Coma ensues with signs of brain stem and autonomic dysfunction
   ii. Associated with a 55% or more mortality; survivors have profound residual deficits
  iii. Treatment is supportive and preventive, particularly focusing on ICP and pulmonary complications

2. **Etiology or precipitating factors:** neurologic deficit or loss of consciousness caused by blunt head trauma. Cerebral dysfunction results from bruising, small petechial hemorrhages, or laceration of brain tissue as the brain moves within the cranial vault and across the uneven base of the skull. Neuronal pathways are disrupted
3. **Nursing assessment data base**
   a. Nursing history
      i. Head trauma
      ii. Loss of consciousness or neurologic deficits
   b. Nursing examination of patient
      i. Concussion
         (a) May present with focal neurologic deficit from a concussive blow to a discrete cortical area (e.g., cortical blindness resulting from a blow to the occipital lobe). Alteration in consciousness clears spontaneously within 6 to 12 hours
         (b) Retrograde amnesia for the event and events immediately preceding the trauma usually occurs if there has been loss of consciousness
      ii. Severe injury with contusions
         (a) Signs vary depending on severity of trauma and area of brain involved. Signs can range from minimal weakness, sensory and speech disturbances, to functional loss of areas of brain
         (b) Level of consciousness can range from mild confusion and restlessness, to combativeness and wild thrashing, to coma with little or no response to noxious stimuli. Loss of consciousness usually occurs at the time of injury and lasts for varying periods of time
         (c) Brain stem contusion involves not only coma but also cranial nerve dysfunction and impaired or absent oculocephalic and oculovestibular reflexes. Respiratory and cardiovascular instability are often present
         (d) Flexor and extensor posturing may occur with either massive cerebral injury or brain stem injury
         (e) Cerebral edema may result and is maximal at about 72 hours. May cause increased ICP
   c. Diagnostic study findings
      i. CT scan may reveal cerebral edema or areas of petechial hemorrhages and contusion
      ii. MRI may show disruption of axonal pathways and evidence of diffuse white matter shearing
4. **Nursing diagnoses**
   a. Alteration in cerebral tissue perfusion related to increased ICP (see pp. 366 and 382)

b. Ineffective family coping related to change in patient's present and future functioning and burden of care (see p. 374)
c. Alteration in physical mobility related to spasticity, abnormal flexor, or extensor posturing
    i. Nursing assessment for defining characteristics
        (a) Increased muscle tone
        (b) Flexor or extensor posturing
        (c) Extreme restlessness, agitation
    ii. Expected outcomes
        (a) Exhibits no evidence of complications, such as contractures, skin break down
        (b) Experiences no injury from agitated responses
    iii. Nursing interventions
        (a) Apply restraining devices as necessary to prevent falls or other injury
        (b) Medicate as ordered to control agitation
        (c) Collaborate with physical therapist in maintaining range of motion of joints in patients with spasticity or abnormal posturing
        (d) Assess effects of motor activity on ICP
    iv. Evaluation of nursing care
        (a) Minimal or absent musculoskeletal complications
        (b) Absence of injury from agitated behavior

Intracranial Hematomas

1. **Pathophysiology**
  a. Subdural hematoma (SDH): usually caused by venous bleeding; blood accumulates below dura mater
    i. Acute SDH: signs and symptoms occur within 48 hours after injury
    ii. Subacute SDH: signs and symptoms occur within 2 weeks after injury
    iii. Chronic SDH: clot has organized and a membrane forms around it; may not be readily attributable to trauma, and signs and symptoms may not occur for weeks to months after trauma
  b. Epidural hematoma (EDH): usually caused by arterial bleeding; blood accumulates above the dura mater. Posterior fossa EDHs are usually of venous origin
  c. Intracerebral hematoma (ICH): hemorrhage into brain substance itself
2. **Etiology or precipitating factors**
  a. Any of the three types of hematomas may be caused by trauma to head and are often associated with scalp lacerations, skull fractures,

cerebral contusion, or penetrating head injuries (gunshot wound, stab wound)

b. SDH may occur spontaneously, particularly if patient has a coagulation disorder or is taking anticoagulation medication

c. EDH is often associated with linear skull fractures that cross major vascular channels (e.g., middle meningeal artery, transverse or superior sagittal sinus)

d. ICH may also occur as result of rupture of intracranial aneurysm, arteriovenous malformation, vascular tumor, or vessel due to hypertension

3. **Nursing assessment data base**

a. Nursing history

i. Trauma to head

ii. Loss of consciousness, with or without return to consciousness

iii. SDH or ICH may present varying history

b. Nursing examination of patient

i. SDH

(a) Usually presents with signs of increasing ICP (e.g., decreasing level of consciousness, ipsilateral oculomotor paralysis with contralateral hemiparesis/hemiplegia). May cause ipsilateral hemiparesis

(b) Acute and subacute SDH may present with an alteration in sensorium and progress to unconsciousness shortly after injury

(c) Chronic SDH may present with history of slowly progressing change in behavior that may lead to decrease in consciousness, with or without history of trauma. Often associated with acute or subacute SDH

ii. EDH

(a) Classically presents with short period of unconsciousness followed by lucid interval of varying duration. Rapid deterioration follows and is often initiated by complaints of increasingly severe localized headache, irritability, and restlessness

(b) Signs of increasing ICP usually develop rapidly owing to arterial bleeding (e.g., decreasing level of consciousness, ipsilateral oculomotor paralysis with contralateral hemiparesis/hemiplegia)

(c) Posterial fossa EDH may cause delayed signs and symptoms, including headache, nausea, and vomiting. Cardiovascular or respiratory instability should signal need for CT scanning to rule out EDH

iii. ICH

(a) Signs and symptoms vary with area of brain involved, size of hematoma, rate at which blood accumulates, and amount of associated cerebral edema

    (b) May or may not exhibit signs of increased ICP, in addition to neurologic deficits mentioned earlier

c. Diagnostic study findings

   i. Laboratory findings

     (a) Lumbar puncture (LP) is contraindicated by increased ICP and is rarely indicated in diagnosis of head trauma

     (b) Arterial blood gas analysis may reveal respiratory alkalosis due to spontaneous hyperventilation, or metabolic acidosis if patient is in shock, is hypoxic, or has high level of physical activity (e.g., seizures, combative behavior, or decerebrate posturing—all causing lactic acidosis)

   ii. Radiologic findings

     (a) CT scan will show an area of increased density that indicates presence, location, and extent of intracranial hematomas

     (b) Skull x-ray films

       (1) May reveal associated skull fractures

       (2) In presence of increased ICP, calcified pineal gland or choroid plexus may be shifted from midline

     (c) Cerebral angiogram may reveal avascular mantle with displacement or stretching of vessels (rarely performed)

     (d) Cervical spine x-ray films—may show associated injury

4. **Nursing diagnoses** (see pp. 366–375)

a. Alteration in cerebral tissue perfusion related to increased ICP

b. Impaired gas exchange related to altered oxygen supply or oxygen-carrying capacity

c. Ineffective breathing pattern related to depressed level of consciousness, inadequate airway, and intracranial lesions

d. Ineffective airway clearance related to increased secretions and depressed level of consciousness

e. Potential for infection related to invasive lines

f. Impaired physical mobility related to hemiparesis/hemiplegia

g. Potential fluid volume deficit related to excessive loss (e.g., diuretic therapy, diabetes insipidus)

h. Potential fluid volume excess related to excessive retention of fluid secondary to syndrome of inappropriate ADH secretion

i. Ineffective family coping related to burden of care and change in patient's functioning

Acute Spinal Cord Injury

1. **Pathophysiology**

a. Compression, contusion, or transection of spinal cord can be caused by bony dislocation; fracture fragments; rupture of ligaments, vessels, or intravertebral discs; interruption of blood supply; or overstretching of neural tissue

b. Subsequent histopathologic changes may be result of decreased spinal cord blood flow mediated by loss of autoregulation; progressive edema causing small vessel compression; decreased tissue oxygen levels; or release of vasoactive substances such as dopamine, serotonin, or norepinephrine

2. **Etiology or precipitating factors**

a. Most spinal cord injuries are caused by trauma, including falls, motor vehicle accidents, sports injuries, gunshot wounds, or stab wounds

b. Mechanisms include flexion, hyperextension, and rotational injuries, leading to fracture, dislocation, or vascular injury

c. Disease processes (e.g., tumors, ruptured arteriovenous malformations, infectious processes, or hematomas) may also precipitate acute loss of function

3. **Nursing assessment data base**

a. Nursing history

i. Trauma resulting in acute decrease or loss of function

ii. Acute loss of function without history of trauma (e.g., rupture of arteriovenous malformation, spinal cord tumors)

b. Nursing examination of patient

i. Motor system

(a) Corticospinal tracts—voluntary motor function is controlled by the corticospinal tracts, also called pyramidal tracts

(1) All major muscle groups are tested by first asking the patient to move his extremities. If the patient is able to wiggle his fingers and toes, he is then asked to lift each extremity off the bed

(2) The examiner then applies resistance to each muscle group while the patient attempts to move against this resistance

(3) Each muscle group is evaluated by asking the patient to flex, extend, abduct, and adduct each extremity (Table 3–1)

(b) Grading of motor strength—each muscle group is graded as absent, weak, or strong. More exact grading can be done using the 0 to 5 scale with 0 representing no function whatsoever; 1, trace function (i.e., minimal contraction of the muscle); 2, movement of the extremity in a horizontal plane (i.e., the patient can move but not lift the extremity); 3, the patient is able to overcome gravity with the distal part of the limb; 4, the muscle can work against the

Table 3–1. MUSCLE TESTING FOR MOTOR STRENGTH

Motor Action	Muscle Tested	Spinal Cord Segment
Abduction of arm	Deltoid	C5
Flexion of forearm	Biceps	C6
Extension of forearm	Triceps	C7
Flexion of digits 2, 3, 4, and 5	Flexor digitorum superficialis and profundus	C8
Opposition of metacarpal of the thumb	Opponens policis	T1
Hip flexion	Iliopsoas	L1–2
Knee extension	Quadriceps femoris	L3
Dorsiflexion of foot	Tibialis anterior	L4
Dorsiflexion of big toe	Extensor hallucis longus	L5
Plantar flexion of foot and big toes	Gastrocnemius flexor hallucis longus	S1–2

Reprinted with permission from Nikas, D. L.: Acute spinal cord injuries: Care and complications. In Nikas, D. L. (ed.): The Critically Ill Neurosurgical Patient. Churchill Livingstone, New York, 1982.

resistance provided by the examiner; and 5, normal motor strength (Table 3–2)

(c) Muscle stretch reflexes—evaluation of motor ability includes assessment of both superficial and deep tendon reflexes (Table 3–3). While assessment of reflex functions does not provide specific information regarding motor ability, it does allow for determining the presence of spinal shock and helps to delineate complete from incomplete lesions

ii. Sensory system

(a) Posterior columns (fasciculus gracilis and fasciculus cuneatus)—the posterior columns convey proprioception (position) and vibratory sense as well as some deep-touch sensation. Usually either position or vibratory sense is tested since both functions are carried in the same tracts

(1) Proprioception is tested by asking the patient to close his eyes and to identify whether a finger or toe is moved toward or away from the head

Table 3–2. GRADING OF MOTOR STRENGTH

Grade	Functional Ability
0	No movement
1	Trace muscular contraction
2	Movement in horizontal plane
3	Can overcome gravity
4	Movement against resistance
5	Normal strength

Reprinted from Nikas, D. L.: Pathophysiology and nursing interventions in acute spinal cord injury. Trauma Q. 4[3]:26, 1988, with permission of Aspen Publishers, Inc., © May 1988.

Table 3–3. TENDON AND CUTANEOUS REFLEX TESTING

Deep Tendon Reflexes	Spinal Cord Segment
Biceps	C5–6
Brachioradialis	C5–6
Triceps	C7–8
Finger flexion	C7–T1
Quadriceps (patellar)	L2
Achilles (ankle jerk)	L5–S1–3
Superficial Reflexes	
Upper abdominal*	T7–9
Lower abdominal*	T11–12
Cremasteric*	L1–2
Plantar†	S1–2

*These reflexes are absent in upper motor neuron lesions.

†The Babinski sign is the result of upper motor neuron lesions in response to plantar stimulation.

Reprinted with permission from Nikas, D. L.: Acute spinal cord injuries: Care and complications. In Nikas, D. L. (ed.): The Critically Ill Neurosurgical Patient. Churchill Livingstone, New York, 1982.

    (2) Vibratory sense may be assessed by asking the patient to identify the vibration of a tuning fork placed on bony prominences or soft tissue. Both sides should be assessed

    (3) Deep-touch sensation can be tested by pinching the belly of muscles of each extremity

  (b) Spinothalamic tracts—the anterior and lateral spinothalamic tracts convey pain and temperature sensation as well as light-touch sensation

    (1) Pain perception is tested by asking the patient to close his eyes and gently touching the skin, starting at the toes, with the sharp and dull ends of a safety pin. The patient is asked to distinguish sharp from dull, and the responses are recorded as the sensation is felt in relation to the distance from anatomic landmarks—iliac crest, umbilicus, nipples, or clavicle

    (2) Both sides should be tested, and the appropriate dermatomes determined for both lower and upper extremities with lumbar and cervical lesions, respectively

    (3) A clean safety pin should be used for each patient, and care must be taken not to pierce or scratch the skin

    (4) Temperature perception can be tested with test tubes of hot and cold water. As in posterior column functions, testing of either pain or temperature perception is sufficient because both functions are carried in the same tracts

    (5) Light-touch perception is tested by asking the patient

to identify when he feels a wisp of cotton touch his skin with his eyes closed

iii. Type and extent of lesion

    (a) Complete transection—total loss of sensory and motor function below level of lesion; irreversible

    (b) Incomplete lesion—varying degree of motor and sensory loss below level of lesion; represents sparing of some tracts

        (1) Central cord syndrome—greater motor loss in upper extremities than in lower; varying sensory loss

        (2) Brown-Séquard syndrome (hemisection of cord)—ipsilateral loss of motor, position, and vibratory sense; contralateral loss of pain and temperature sensation

        (3) Anterior cord syndrome—complete motor loss and loss of pain and temperature below level of lesion, with sparing of proprioception, vibratory sense, and touch

        (4) Other incomplete lesions cause partial dysfunction of some or all spinal cord tracts

iv. Level of lesion

    (a) C1–4—quadriplegia with total loss of respiratory function

    (b) C4–5—quadriplegia with possible phrenic nerve involvement owing to edema that results in loss of respiratory function

    (c) C5–6—quadriplegia with gross arm movements; sparing of diaphragm leads to diaphragmatic breathing

    (d) C6–7—quadriplegia with biceps muscles intact; diaphragmatic breathing

    (e) C7–8—quadriplegia with triceps and biceps intact but no function of intrinsic hand muscles; diaphragmatic breathing

    (f) T1–L2—paraplegia with loss of varying amounts of intercostal and abdominal muscle

    (g) Below L2—cauda equina injury; mixed picture of motor-sensory loss, bowel and bladder dysfunction

v. Spinal shock: patients are areflexic with flaccid paralysis immediately after injury—"spinal shock." Spinal shock is a state of transient reflex depression below the level of the lesion. The pathophysiology of spinal shock is incompletely understood, but in part is due to sudden withdrawal of predominantly facilitory influences from higher centers, persistent inhibition from below the lesion acting on extensor reflexes, and axonal degeneration, particularly of axons severed near the cell body. The intensity of spinal shock varies with the level of the lesion, and some distal reflexes may be retained, although diminished, in cervical transection. Spinal shock leads to a flaccid paralysis even though the lesion is of an upper motor neuron type. Once spinal shock has subsided and reflex function returns, the spastic paralysis typical of an upper motor neuron lesion is manifested. Although there is a great deal of variability of reflex return after spinal shock, reflex return is generally in a rostral direction, with anal and bulbocavernous reflexes and response to plantar stimulation occurring earlier. The reflexes innervated by muscles closest to the lesion may never return. The duration of spinal shock varies considerably, lasting from days to weeks or even months; reflex return may be delayed by septic or toxic conditions

   vi. Patient may complain of neck pain or tenderness

  c. Diagnostic study findings

    i. Laboratory findings: CSF analysis if pathology other than trauma

    ii. Radiologic findings

      (a) Spinal series—fractures, dislocation, degeneration will be visualized

      (b) Tomography identifies bony lesion that is difficult to visualize on plain films

      (c) Myelogram may be done if occlusion of spinal subarachnoid space is suspected or pathology is unclear

      (d) CT scan is able to delineate bony lesions or other spinal cord pathology

      (e) MRI is able to delineate both bony deformities and spinal cord pathology

4. Nursing diagnoses

  a. Potential for decreased cardiac output related to sympathetic blockade

    i. Assessment for defining characteristics

      (a) Hypotension—loss of sympathetic outflow caused by spinal cord transection above T5 results in vasodilatation, decreased venous return, and hypotension. It may be further complicated by hemorrhage from associated injuries

      (b) Bradycardia—probably due to sympathetic blockade. It may lead to junctional escape beats or rhythm and rarely to ventricular beats. Is aggravated by hypothermia or hypoxia

      (c) Vasovagal reflex—cardiac arrest induced by suctioning that leads to hypoxia and vagal stimulation

    ii. Expected outcomes

      (a) Maintains systolic blood pressure above 90 mm Hg

      (b) Experiences no bradycardia or arrest during suctioning

    iii. Nursing interventions

      (a) Hypotension—usually self-limiting, but judicious fluid replacement may be necessary (colloid as well as crystalloid may be required). If hypotension is severe, as in multiple trauma, hemodynamic monitoring may be instituted. Vasopressors may be necessary to maintain systolic blood pressure at 90 mm Hg

    (b) Bradycardia—treat with atropine if symptomatic or other dysrhythmias occur. Treat contributing factors (e.g., hypothermia, hypoxemia)

    (c) Vasovagal reflex—oxygenate prior to suctioning; monitor cardiac rate and rhythm

  iv. Evaluation of nursing care

    (a) Cardiac output maintained within normal limits

    (b) Absence of bradycardia and cardiac arrest from vasovagal reflex

b. Alteration in temperature regulation related to poikilothermism

  i. Assessment for defining characteristics: core temperature tends to drift toward ambient temperature and becomes hypothermic or hyperthermic depending on the environmental temperature. This results from interruption of sympathetic pathways to temperature regulating centers in hypothalamus

  ii. Expected outcome: maintains core temperature above 92°F (33°C)

  iii. Nursing interventions

    (a) Ensure cool environment to avoid hyperthermia

    (b) Treat with warming blanket if hypothermic

    (c) Monitor temperature every 2 hours until stable, then per unit protocol

  iv. Evaluation of nursing care: core temperature maintained within normal limits

c. Alteration in tissue perfusion related to venous thrombosis, flaccid paralysis, and decreased venous blood flow

  i. Assessment for defining characteristics

    (a) Venous thrombosis—decreased rate of blood flow and flaccid paralysis contribute to venous stasis in legs and pelvis

    (b) Not possible to detect clinical signs of early venous thrombosis in spinal cord–injured patient since he will not have pain or tenderness in affected extremity

    (c) Observe for late signs of venous thrombosis—redness along course of vein, swelling around inflamed area, warm to touch

    (d) Signs of sudden change in respiratory status may indicate pulmonary embolus

  ii. Expected outcomes

    (a) Does not experience inflammation, redness, or swelling of extremities

    (b) Avoids embolization of thrombi

    iii. Nursing interventions
      (a) Venous thrombosis
        (1) Prophylactic anticoagulation (normal and low dose heparin therapy) has been recommended
        (2) Antiembolic stockings or alternating pressure devices for legs may be ordered
        (3) Recent research has revealed that clinical observation for usual signs of venous thrombosis is often inadequate for lower extremities and of no value in pelvic thrombi. ^{125}I-fibrinogen venogram may aid in diagnosis. A 2-cm or more increase of daily calf and thigh measurements indicates a need for definitive diagnosis
      (b) Pulmonary embolus—prevention and early detection of venous thrombosis is the best means of prevention. It should be suspected in patients who exhibit sudden change in respiratory status
      (c) Range of motion exercises performed three to four times per day
      (d) Mobilization to chair as soon as possible
      (e) Kinetic bed therapy may be employed
    iv. Evaluation of nursing care
      (a) Absence of venous thrombosis
      (b) Absence of pulmonary embolus
  d. Alteration in respiratory function related to paralysis of respiratory muscles, ineffective coughing, and deep breathing
    i. Assessment for defining characteristics
      (a) Hypoventilation—injury below C4 results in diaphragmatic breathing, decreasing tidal volume, and decreased vital capacity. Paralysis of abdominal and intercostal muscles leads to ineffective cough and retention of secretions. Abdominal distention may restrict diaphragmatic excursions
      (b) Pneumonia—collection of secretions in dependent segments of lung caused by immobility, ineffective cough, and decreased vital capacity. Artificial airways offer easy access for infection. Aspiration is a common complication
      (c) Pulmonary edema—usually attributable to overtransfusion of fluids. There have been case reports of apparent neurogenic pulmonary edema with cervical spinal cord injuries, but mechanism is unclear
      (d) Pulmonary embolus—may result from venous thrombosis from pelvis or legs
    ii. Expected outcomes
      (a) Maintains adequate ventilation
      (b) Does not experience pneumonia

(c) Does not experience pulmonary edema

(d) Does not experience pulmonary embolism

iii. Nursing interventions

(a) Hypoventilation—measure vital capacity and tidal volume at regular intervals to detect deterioration. Monitor arterial blood gases. Nasotracheal intubation, using a fiberoptic bronchoscope, and mechanical ventilation may become necessary to facilitate respiratory care

(b) Pneumonia—assist patient with deep breathing and diaphragmatic coughing. Provide adequate humidification to airway to prevent tracheobronchitis. Use sterile suctioning technique. Change respiratory equipment daily or per unit protocol. Monitor sputum with cultures

(c) Pulmonary edema—use hemodynamic monitoring to guide fluid therapy. Chest auscultation will detect presence of rales. Monitor oxygenation status and chest x-ray films

(d) Pulmonary embolus (see p. 98)

iv. Evaluation of nursing care

(a) Adequate ventilation maintained

(b) Pneumonia and pulmonary edema do not occur

(c) Pulmonary embolus does not occur

e. Potential for fluid volume deficit related to gastric dilatation or hemorrhage

i. Assessment for defining characteristics

(a) Abdominal distention

(b) Decreased or absent bowel sounds

(c) Vomiting

(d) Coffee-ground drainage from nasogastric suction

(e) Fall in hemoglobin/hematocrit

(f) Decreased blood pressure

(g) Change in sensorium

ii. Expected outcomes

(a) Does not experience pulmonary complications of gastric dilatation and ileus

(b) Does not experience hemorrhage from Cushing's ulcers or abdominal trauma

iii. Nursing interventions

(a) Gastric dilatation and ileus—inspect abdomen for distention. Insert nasogastric tube and attach to intermittent suction. Monitor amount and quality of output. It is probably caused by loss of central control and can subsequently interfere with diaphragmatic functioning, causing hypoventilation/hypoxia. Vomiting and pulmonary aspiration may occur

(b) Cushing's ulcer—type of stress ulcer seen with CNS injuries. Probably the result of vagal-stimulated gastric acid production and/or ACTH release. Antacids and H_2 receptor antagonists have been recommended in prevention and treatment. Gastric bleeding has been treated with warm and cold saline lavage. Intra-arterial infusion of vasopressin has been used. Gastric surgery may become necessary

    (c) Hemorrhage—secondary to abdominal trauma. Intraperitoneal lavage may be used to detect presence of intra-abdominal hemorrhage. It is difficult to diagnose because of loss of usual clinical indicators (e.g., pain) and may progress rapidly because of loss of sympathetic compensatory mechanisms

    (d) Monitor respiratory status hourly or as patient's condition indicates

    (e) Monitor hematocrit and hemoglobin levels frequently

    (f) Monitor coagulation factors

    (g) Monitor cardiovascular status frequently

    (h) Monitor bowel sounds and abdominal girth frequently

    (i) Monitor gastric output. Check for presence of blood

  iv. Evaluation of nursing care

    (a) Pulmonary complications absent

    (b) Hemorrhage is avoided or detected and treated promptly

f. Urinary retention related to atonic bladder or areflexia

  i. Assessment for defining characteristics

    (a) Bladder distention

    (b) No urine output

    (c) Signs of urinary infection—cloudy urine, foul odor, sediment

    (d) Positive urine cultures

  ii. Expected outcomes

    (a) Maintains adequate urinary elimination

    (b) Maintains sterile urine cultures

  iii. Nursing interventions

    (a) Urinary retention—intermittent or indwelling catheterization is necessary in initial stages due to bladder atony. It may lead to urinary reflux, stone formation, upper urinary tract back pressure, and renal deterioration. Assess for bladder distention

    (b) Urinary tract infections—intermittent catheterization is recommended to decrease incidence. Early detection is essential, since infection can prolong period of spinal shock and may lead to sepsis. Monitor urine cultures. Urinary tract infection may result from urinary retention or catheterization. Assess for signs of infection

  iv. Evaluation of nursing care

      (a) Urinary elimination is adequate

      (b) Absence of urinary tract infection

g. Potential impairment of skin integrity related to immobilization

  i. Assessment for defining characteristics

      (a) Presence of denervated areas. These areas break down faster and heal slower than those with normal nerve supply. Poor circulation may be contributory

      (b) Physical immobility

      (c) Presence of traction

  ii. Expected outcome: experiences no skin breakdown

  iii. Nursing interventions

      (a) Frequent turning (every 1 to 2 hours) and meticulous skin care are essential. Protect bony prominences

      (b) Inspect skin when turning

      (c) Use preventative skin care devices (e.g., padding, pressure mattress, special beds)

      (d) Keep linen dry and free of wrinkles or crumbs

      (e) Involve patient and family in preventative measures

  iv. Evaluation of nursing care: absence of skin breakdown

h. Impaired physical mobility related to paralysis and spasticity

  i. Assessment for defining characteristics

      (a) Muscle atony and wasting—occurs during flaccid paralysis that characterizes spinal shock

      (b) Contractures—may result from spastic paralysis that occurs as spinal shock dissipates

  ii. Expected outcomes (see p. 372)

  iii. Nursing interventions (see p. 373)

      (a) Treat spasticity with proper positioning, range of motion exercises, and drug therapy as ordered (baclofen has been used for spasticity)

      (b) Kinetic beds may be employed

  iv. Evaluation of nursing care (see p. 373)

i. Disturbance in self-concept related to change in body image or role performance

  i. Assessment for defining characteristics

      (a) Verbal responses to change in function

      (b) Nonverbal responses to actual change in function

      (c) Paralysis of body parts

      (d) Inability to perform previous activities

      (e) Loss of independence

      (f) Feelings of powerlessness due to immobility

      (g) Present and future role changes

  ii. Expected outcomes

      (a) Acknowledges change in body image

      (b) Participates in decisions about various aspects of care

        (c) Expresses positive feelings about self

  iii. Nursing interventions

        (a) Accept patient's perceptions of self

        (b) Assess readiness for decision making, then involve in making choices and decisions related to care

        (c) Encourage participation in care

        (d) Allow opportunities for patient to verbalize feelings

        (e) Provide positive reinforcement of efforts to adapt and participate in care

  iv. Evaluation of nursing care

        (a) Acknowledges change in body image

        (b) Participates in decisions about various aspects of care

        (c) Expresses positive feelings about self

j. Powerlessness related to total physical dependency

  i. Assessment for defining characteristics

        (a) Verbal expressions of having no control over situation

        (b) Apathy

        (c) Passivity

        (d) Fear

        (e) Sadness, crying

        (f) Expressions of frustration over inability to perform previous tasks or activities

        (g) Dependency on others may result in irritability, anger, resentment, and guilt

        (h) Depression over physical deterioration

        (i) Reluctance to express true feelings, feeling alienation from caregivers

        (j) Constant requests for routine care beyond requirements

  ii. Expected outcomes

        (a) Able to express feeling of powerlessness

        (b) Participates in planning care

  iii. Nursing interventions

        (a) Encourage patient to express feelings about present situation

        (b) Accept patient's feelings of powerlessness as normal

        (c) Assist in identifying specific areas in which the patient can maintain control

        (d) Begin teaching patient what he must do to maintain health (e.g., drinking adequate fluids to maintain adequate hydration, turning every 2 hours, performing respiratory care activities)

  iv. Evaluation of nursing care

        (a) Expresses feeling of powerlessness

        (b) Participates in planning care

k. Ineffective individual coping related to situational crisis, loss of control and independence, and change in role

l. Ineffective family coping related to burden of care and changes in patient's present and future functioning

Stroke: Patients with stroke are not routinely admitted to critical care units unless they are unstable or have multiple system involvement or definitive therapy is planned

1. Pathophysiology

a. Ischemic-hypoxic brain damage results from decreased cerebral blood flow, either focal or diffuse, which causes hypoxia of cerebral tissues, leading to anaerobic glycolysis

   i. Ischemia induces inhibition of synaptic transmission as a result of neurotransmitter depletion caused by inadequate ATP. It may be reversible

   ii. Subsequently, structural changes of neuronal membranes occur in which high-energy phosphates (e.g., ATP) are depleted and intracellular ionic balances cannot be maintained. Complex biochemical changes occur, further contributing to cellular swelling and neuronal death

b. Occlusive vascular disease

   i. Thrombosis

      (a) Most common cause of stroke

      (b) Lacunar strokes are small irregular areas of infarction and necrosis associated with thrombosis of small arteries of the deep white matter of the brain

      (c) Atherosclerosis of large cerebral vessels causes progressive narrowing leading to progressive levels of deficits. Plaques may embolize to smaller vessels

   ii. Embolus

      (a) May be calcified plaques from extracranial vessels, vegetation from diseased heart valves, fat, air, or tumor fragments. Blood clots from extracranial sources, such as those arising from a diseased heart, are common

      (b) Emboli become lodged at bifurcations of arteries where blood flow is most turbulent. Fragments may become lodged in smaller vessels

c. Hemorrhagic

   i. Accounts for as many as 25% of strokes

   ii. Bleeding into parenchyma of brain, causing irritation of and pressure on cerebral tissues and nerves leading to loss of function and death of neurons

   iii. Hypertensive intracranial hemorrhage usually occurs in the basal ganglia, cerebellum, or brain stem but may affect more superficial areas of the cerebrum

2. Etiology or precipitating factors

a. Thrombosis
  i. Long-standing hypertension
  ii. Diabetes mellitus
  iii. Cardiac disease
  iv. Atherosclerosis
  v. Vascular inflammatory processes
b. Embolus
  i. Cardiac disease
  ii. Extracranial arterial plaques or clots
  iii. Clots produced by other hematologic conditions, such as polycythemia
  iv. Other substances in the vascular system such as air, fat, infectious emboli
c. Hemorrhagic
  i. Usually caused by hypertensive vascular disease
  ii. Ruptured intracranial aneurysms
  iii. Ruptured arteriovenous malformations
  iv. Traumatic intracerebral hemorrhage
  v. Rupture of a vascular tumor
  vi. Systemic hemorrhagic disorders and diathesis

3. Nursing assessment data base

a. Nursing history
  i. Subjective findings
    (a) Patient's chief complaint
      (1) Decreased neurologic function
      (2) Headache
      (3) Seizure (uncommon)
    (b) Other symptoms—reports of prior neurologic symptoms
  ii. Objective findings
    (a) History of etiologic or precipitating factors
    (b) Transient ischemic attacks (TIAs)—an ischemic event that results in reversible short-lived (less than 24 hours but may be only minutes) neurologic deficit such as loss of vision in one eye (amaurosis fugax), numbness or weakness of a hand or leg, dysarthria, or aphasia. Lacunar TIAs generally result in a pure motor or pure sensory deficit lasting more than 1 hour
    (c) Reversible ischemic neurologic deficit (RIND) is a neurologic deficit that lasts more than 24 hours but leaves little or no neurologic deficit
    (d) Family history—vascular or heart disease, diabetes mellitus, hypertension
    (e) Social history
      (1) Cigarette smoking

        (2) Illicit drug use, particularly cocaine

        (3) Heavy alcohol use

        (4) Long-standing stress

    (f) Medication history

        (1) Oral contraceptive use, especially in women at risk (e.g., smokes, has hypertension or migraines)

        (2) All current therapeutic drugs

b. Nursing examination of patient

  i. Inspection

    (a) Main presenting feature in hemorrhagic or embolic stroke is sudden onset of signs and symptoms

    (b) Clinical presentation varies depending on area of brain involved and extent of injury

    (c) Patient with injury to right cerebral hemisphere may exhibit some or all of the following dysfunctions

        (1) Left homonymous hemianopia—blindness in left half of both visual fields

        (2) Left hemiparesis or hemiplegia

        (3) Sensory agnosia

          a) Astereognosis—inability to recognize objects placed in hand without aid of visual clues

          b) Astatoagnosia—inability to determine position of body parts

          c) Tactile inattention—lack of attention to simultaneous stimuli

          d) Anosognosia—unawareness of neurologic deficit (e.g., hemiplegia)

          e) Constructional apraxia—patient does not complete left half of figures he is drawing

          f) Dressing apraxia—inability to dress oneself properly

        (4) Inattention to objects in left visual field and to left auditory stimuli

        (5) Deviation of head and eyes to right

    (d) Patients with injury to left cerebral hemisphere may exhibit some or all of the following dysfunctions

        (1) Right homonymous hemianopia—blindness in right half of both visual fields

        (2) Right hemiparesis or hemiplegia

        (3) Sensory agnosia

          a) Astereognosis

          b) Astatoagnosia

          c) Finger agnosia—inability to identify the finger touched

          d) Right-left disorientation

(4) Aphasia

    a) Expressive—inability to speak or write language or name familiar objects

    b) Receptive—inability to understand spoken (auditory aphasia) or written (visual aphasia-dyslexia) words

    c) Mixed or global—both expressive and receptive language difficulties

(5) Deviation of head and eyes to left

  ii. Palpation: no specific findings

 iii. Percussion: deep tendon reflexes are usually hyperactive indicating upper motor neuron lesion

 iv. Auscultation

    (a) Bruits over carotid arteries may be heard

    (b) Murmurs or irregular rhythm may be heard in cardiac disease

c. Diagnostic study findings

  i. Laboratory

    (a) CSF—may reveal erythrocytes and increased protein after hemorrhage

    (b) Serum glucose—should be checked to rule out hypoglycemic coma and diabetes mellitus

    (c) Clotting profile—check adequacy of clotting

  ii. Radiologic

    (a) CT scan

      (1) Ischemia and infarctions are revealed as areas of decreased absorption or density best seen 24 hours or more after occlusive event

      (2) Hemorrhage appears as an area of increased absorption or density and is seen immediately after the event

    (b) Cerebral angiography—may reveal vessels in spasm, areas of hemorrhage, aneurysms, arteriovenous malformations, or vessels displaced or stretched

 iii. Special

    (a) MRI—will reveal gross changes in cerebral blood flow and areas of edema. It may reveal causative factor depending on etiology

    (b) Many direct and indirect noninvasive tests for detecting carotid artery disease are available. They include spectral phonoangiography, Doppler imaging, and ophthalmodynamometry

    (c) Cerebral blood flow studies

      (1) Positive emission tomography—provides quantitative values for cerebral blood flow, cerebral blood volume,

and brain cell metabolism to define infarction size and location. Test is expensive and not readily available

 (2) Xenon isotope (^{133}Xe) inhalation technique measures flow by regional calculation of the rate of decline in radioactivity by externally placed scintillation detectors

4. Nursing diagnoses

 a. Alteration in cerebral tissue perfusion related to progression of stroke (see p. 366)

  i. Assessment for defining characteristics

   (a) Change in level of consciousness

   (b) Dysrhythmias may be a causative factor

   (c) Hypertension

   (d) Increased motor weakness

   (e) Increased confusion

   (f) Other signs of neurologic dysfunction

  ii. Expected outcome: experiences no worsening of neurologic condition

  iii. Nursing interventions

   (a) Assess neurologic status per unit standards or as condition indicates

   (b) Treat cardiac dysrhythmias per physician's orders

   (c) Record and report neurologic or cardiac changes promptly

   (d) Monitor arterial blood pressure; medicate as ordered

   (e) Administer anticoagulation therapy as ordered—may be employed for stroke of embolic etiology only

  iv. Evaluation of nursing care

   (a) Neurologic changes, even transient, are recorded and reported promptly

   (b) Cardiac dysrhythmias are controlled

 b. Impaired verbal communication related to expressive/receptive dysphasia (see p. 371)

 c. Alteration in thought processes related to confusion, short-term memory loss, and short attention span (see p. 373)

 d. Impaired physical mobility related to hemiparesis/hemiplegia (see p. 372)

 e. Unilateral neglect related to cerebral impairment, usually right hemisphere

  i. Assessment for defining characteristics

   (a) Consistent inattention to stimuli on affected side

   (b) Inadequate self-care

   (c) Positions self inappropriately on affected side

   (d) Attempts to move or get up without assistance for affected side

   (e) Does not look toward affected side

(f) Homonymous hemianopsia

(g) Does not recognize affected body parts as part of body

ii. Expected outcomes

(a) Demonstrates increased awareness of and attention to affected side

(b) Does not experience injury

iii. Nursing interventions

(a) Provide a safe environment by orienting patient, providing good lighting, positioning patient's bed and personal objects in unaffected visual field, keeping side rails up and call light within reach, restraining only if necessary

(b) Protect neglected side during activities

(c) Teach scanning of affected visual field or side

(d) Gradually move objects to affected side; encourage patient to attend to that side

(e) Include family in interventions

iv. Evaluation of nursing care

(a) Attends to and is aware of affected side

(b) Absence of injury

Intracranial Aneurysms

1. **Pathophysiology**
   a. Dilatation of an artery resulting from weakness in media layer and internal elastic laminar layer of arterial wall
   b. Ninety-five per cent of aneurysms occur close to the circle of Willis at bifurcations of the internal carotid, middle cerebral, and basilar arteries and in relation to the anterior and posterior communicating arteries
   c. Most cerebral aneurysms occur in vessels of anterior portion of circle of Willis
   d. High arterial pressures and continuous arterial pulsations lead to ballooning of weakened arterial wall
   e. Rupture of aneurysm can cause intracerebral hematoma and subarachnoid hemorrhage
   f. Clot forms in and around rupture site and inhibits continuing hemorrhage
2. **Etiology or precipitating factors**
   a. May include congenital defects of wall of artery, complicated by degenerative changes
   b. No specific precipitating causes present in all patients
   c. Hypertension is not a major factor in the etiology of aneurysms but is a poor prognostic sign if present after rupture
3. **Nursing assessment data base**
   a. Nursing history

   i. Subjective findings
      (a) Patient's chief complaint—mild to severe headaches
      (b) Other symptoms
         (1) Signs of meningeal irritation—nuchal rigidity, head-ache, photophobia, low back pain
         (2) Altered awareness
         (3) Nausea and vomiting
         (4) Focal neurologic deficit—motor, sensory, speech
  ii. Objective findings
      (a) Presence of etiologic or precipitating factors—hypertension may or may not be present
      (b) Family history—no clear genetic or familial link in all cases, but familial aggregations do occur in a minority of patients
      (c) Social history—no clear correlation with alcohol or illicit drug use, smoking, or other factors known to influence cardiovascular disease, but some studies suggest higher incidence of rupture in these patients
      (d) Medication history—no specific correlations
 b. Nursing examination of patient
   i. Inspection
      (a) Clinical presentation
         (1) Mild to severe headache
         (2) Nausea or vomiting
         (3) Seizures
         (4) Meningismus—nuchal rigidity, headache, photophobia, diplopia; Kernig's or Brudzinski's sign may be present
         (5) Neurologic deficit—motor, sensory, speech
         (6) Altered sensorium
      (b) Physical examination—neurologic examination reveals varying signs and symptoms depending on severity and location of hemorrhage. Aneurysms may be categorized as follows
         (1) Grade I
            a) Alert, no neurologic deficit
            b) Minimal headache
            c) Slight nuchal rigidity
         (2) Grade II
            a) Awake, minimal neurologic deficit (e.g., oculomotor nerve [CN III] palsy)
            b) Mild to severe headache
            c) Nuchal rigidity
            d) No vasospasm
         (3) Grade III

                         a) Drowsiness, confusion, mild focal neurologic deficit
                         b) Nuchal rigidity
                    (4) Grade IV
                         a) Unresponsiveness, hemiplegic
                         b) Nuchal rigidity
                         c) May or may not have vasospasm
                    (5) Grade V
                         a) Comatose—moribund
                         b) Decerebrate posturing
                         c) Vasospasm likely
           ii. Palpation: noncontributory
           iii. Percussion: noncontributory
           iv. Auscultation: noncontributory
     c. Diagnostic study findings
           i. Laboratory: lumbar puncture—not done if signs of increased
              ICP are present. If done, will reveal bloody or xanthochromic
              CSF and elevated CSF protein and cell count. CSF pressure
              may be elevated
           ii. Radiologic findings
                    (a) Cerebral angiogram will usually illustrate size, shape, and
                        location of aneurysm. It may also show spasm of involved
                        vessels and may detect intracerebral hematoma or hydro-
                        cephalus
                    (b) CT scan will reveal intracerebral hematoma and intraven-
                        tricular blood. Hydrocephalus will be evident if present.
                        High-resolution enhanced scan may reveal aneurysm
           iii. MRI will reveal evidence of hemorrhage, hydrocephalus, and
                vasospasm
           iv. Cerebral blood flow studies may reveal decreased flow
  4. **Nursing diagnoses**
     a. Potential for alteration in cerebral tissue perfusion related to re-
        bleeding, vasospasm, hydrocephalus (see p. 366)
           i. Assessment for defining characteristics
                    (a) Sudden change in neurologic status
                    (b) Sudden rise in ICP
                    (c) Drop in cerebral perfusion pressure
           ii. Expected outcomes
                    (a) Maintains stable neurologic status
                    (b) Will not experience rebleeding and vasospasm
                    (c) Will not experience postoperative complications
           iii. Nursing interventions
                    (a) Minimize potential for rebleeding and promote stabiliza-
                        tion of patient
                            (1) Complete bed rest—surgery is usually delayed until

patient's condition has improved to grades I or II. Timing of surgery is controversial

    (2) Elevate head of bed 15° to 30° to promote venous drainage

    (3) Vasospasm may be treated with hypervolemia, hemodilution, hypertension, or calcium channel blockers, individually or in combination

    (4) Ensure quiet, dark environment, especially if patient has photophobia

    (5) Keep patient quiet. Sedatives (e.g., phenobarbital) may be necessary. Avoid restraints

    (6) Take axillary temperatures

    (7) Avoid letting patient strain

    (8) If patient is hypertensive, drugs may be used to control blood pressure, although not necessarily to bring it to normal levels

  (b) Monitor patient's postoperative condition closely

    (1) Frequency of neurologic assessments depends on type of procedure done and status of patient

      a) Carotid clamping—neurologic assessments may be needed as often as every 5 minutes while clamp on artery is being tightened

      b) If a clip is applied to neck of aneurysm, routine postcraniotomy care is required

      c) Wrapping of aneurysm with muslin or other material or embolization of aneurysm may be done if aneurysm cannot be clipped. Routine post-craniotomy care is required

  (c) Prevent seizure activity. Ensure adequate oxygenation and electrolyte balance. Give prophylactic anticonvulsant medications routinely

  (d) Prevent increased ICP

  iv. Evaluation of nursing care

    (a) Accurate recording and reporting of neurologic status and grade

    (b) Absence of rebleeding and/or vasospasm

    (c) Absence of complications of therapy or surgery

b. Fluid volume excess related to hypervolemic, hypertensive, and hemodilution therapy

  i. Assessment for defining characteristics

    (a) Hypertension—systolic blood pressure about 160 mm Hg

    (b) Hematocrit less than 30%

    (c) Adventitious breath sounds (e.g., crackles)

    (d) Increase in central venous or pulmonary capillary wedge pressure readings

(e) ECG changes indicative of cardiac compromise

(f) Peripheral edema

(g) Increased ICP

ii. Expected outcomes

(a) Will not experience cardiac or pulmonary complications

(b) Maintains ICP below 20 mm Hg

iii. Nursing interventions

(a) Monitor ECG continuously

(b) Assess pulmonary status every 1 to 2 hours as patient's condition requires

(c) Monitor hematocrit every 4 to 6 hours or as ordered. Will usually be maintained between 30% and 35%

(d) Monitor blood pressure continuously

(e) Monitor central venous or pulmonary artery pressure continuously. (*NOTE:* Central venous pressure may be adequate in patients with no history of cardiopulmonary disease who are younger than 60 years of age. In those who are at risk or who develop signs of cardiopulmonary compromise, a pulmonary artery catheter is necessary to monitor the effects of hypertensive, hypervolemic therapy.)

(f) Monitor ICP

(g) Monitor electrolytes and osmolality per orders

iv. Evaluation of nursing care

(a) Cardiopulmonary complications are prevented

(b) ICP remains below 20 mm Hg

c. Potential for infection related to invasive lines, monitoring, and therapeutic devices (see p. 371)

d. Other nursing diagnoses may apply if the patient has neurologic deficits (see pp. 371–375)

Arteriovenous Malformation (AVM)

1. **Pathophysiology:** this abnormal vascular network consists of one or more direct connections between the arterial inflow and venous outflow without an intervening capillary network. An AVM is one of five types of CNS vascular abnormalities that can occur. AVMs primarily occur in the supratentorial structures and most frequently involve the vessels of the middle cerebral arterial tree, followed by those of the anterior and then posterior circulation. Grossly, AVMs appear as a tangled mass of dilated vessels. The vessels become passively enlarged over time, secondary to high flow volume and increased venous pressure produced by the AV shunt. The arterial walls become thin over time due to collagenous replacement of the normal smooth muscle component of the media. Saccular aneurysms are found in 10% to 15% of patients with AVMs, most occurring on arteries hemodynamically related to the AVM

2. Etiologic or precipitating factors: congenital lesions developing in the fourth to eighth week of embryonic life

3. Nursing assessment data base
  a. Nursing history
    i. Subjective findings
      (a) Patient's chief complaint
        (1) Intracranial hemorrhage—most common presenting symptom in patients with small AVMs leading to headache and altered consciousness
        (2) Seizures—most common presenting symptom in patients with large AVMs
      (b) Other symptoms
        (1) Headache
        (2) Hydrocephalus is an uncommon presenting symptom but may occur as a result of subarachnoid hemorrhage
        (3) Intellectual deterioration may occur in older patients with large AVMs
    ii. Objective findings
      (a) Presence of etiologic or precipitating factors
      (b) Family history—although there are occasional reports of familial incidence, there is no statistical evidence of a familial or genetic predisposition
      (c) Social history—noncontributory
      (d) Medication history—noncontributory
  b. Nursing examination of client
    i. Inspection
      (a) In absence of hemorrhage, clinical symptoms correlate to the site of the lesions
      (b) Signs of cerebral ischemia
      (c) Signs of increased ICP (see p. 379)
    ii. Palpation: noncontributory
    iii. Percussion: noncontributory
    iv. Auscultation: nonspecific findings but careful monitoring of vital signs is necessary
  c. Diagnostic study findings
    i. Cerebral angiography: most definitive study. Will demonstrate feeding and draining vessels and the size and location of AVM. Will also reveal intracerebral hematoma and cerebral vasospasm
    ii. CT scan—without and with contrast. Will assist in differentiating AVM from tumor or intracerebral hematoma
    iii. MRI—will demonstrate location, size, and effects of AVM, e.g., reduced blood flow to area round AVM; cerebral edema
    iv. Lumbar puncture—contraindicated if increased ICP is known or suspected. If done, pressure may be elevated, especially in

presence of intracerebral hematoma or subarachnoid hemorrhage. CSF will be bloody or xanthochromic

4. **Nursing diagnoses**
   a. Alteration in cerebral tissue perfusion related to increased ICP (see p. 366)
   b. Potential for injury related to seizures (see p. 430)
   c. Potential for infection related to invasive lines (see p. 371)
   d. Other nursing diagnoses may apply if patient has neurologic deficits (see pp. 371–375)

Brain Tumors

1. **Pathophysiology:** brain tumors act as space-occupying lesions and are life threatening because they destroy brain tissue and nerve structures and produce increased ICP. Tumors may be spherical, well delineated, and encapsulated or diffuse, infiltrating masses. The tumor may enlarge owing to cell proliferation, necrosis, edema, or hemorrhage. Tumors cause neurologic symptoms due to compression, invasion, or destruction of brain tissue. The pathophysiologic complications that can occur include cerebral edema, intracranial hypertension, seizures, focal neurologic deficits, hydrocephalus, and hormonal changes. Tumors are classified by histologic features and grade of malignancy (grades I to IV, with IV being the most malignant). Of great clinical and surgical significance is the location and accessibility of the tumor
   a. Glioma: nonencapsulated, infiltrates and displaces brain tissue; arises from neuroglial cells; comprises 40% to 50% of intracranial tumors
      i. Astrocytoma: usually grade I to II but may advance to higher grades (glioblastoma); commonly found in cerebral hemispheres in adults and the brain stem in children. It may also occur in the spinal cord. Survival of patients with grades I to II is more than 7 years with complete removal and less with subtotal removal
      ii. Glioblastoma multiforme: malignant (grade III to IV), occurs throughout cerebral hemispheres, primarily in inferior half. It grows rapidly, invades tissues, and causes edema. Some researchers categorize this tumor as a malignant astrocytoma
      iii. Oligodendroglioma: rare, slow-growing tumor in adults; occurs in cerebral hemispheres, particularly frontal and temporal; grades I to IV. A dense, calcified lesion, it is well circumscribed, subcortical. Seizures are often first symptom
      iv. Ependymoma: arises from cells lining the ventricles and is slow growing. It most commonly occurs in fourth ventricle but can occur throughout ventricular system. It causes obstructive hydrocephalus and increased ICP and may involve cranial nerve

nuclei if tumor invades floor of fourth ventricle. Cerebellar signs such as ataxia and incoordination may occur

    (a) Colloid cyst: arises from ependymal cells, usually between the foramen of Monro and the roof of the third ventricle. It is benign and can be surgically excised

    (b) Choroid plexus papilloma: arises from choroid plexuses, causes increased production of CSF; rare, childhood tumor

  v. Optic nerve glioma: astrocytoma of the optic nerves and optic chiasm. Slow growing tumor may affect hypothalamic function and vision

  vi. Medulloblastoma: highly malignant, grows in vermis of cerebellum; causes obstructive hydrocephalus; most common in young children. Survival is usually less than 5 years but is improved with surgery and chemotherapy

b. Extra-axial tumors: arise from supporting structures of nervous system

  i. Meningioma: arises from meningeal tissues, primarily in area of dura: e.g., along superior sagittal sinus where arachnoid granulations penetrate, sylvian region, sphenoid ridge, and convexity of brain. It is vascular, firm, encapsulated, slow growing, and benign. Prognosis is good unless size or location makes surgery more difficult

  ii. Acoustic neuroma: also called acoustic schwannoma because it arises from Schwann cells of the acoustic nerve (CN VIII). It is sometimes referred to as a cerebellopontine angle tumor because it originates at the junction of the cerebellum and pons. Often affects function of cranial nerves, including acoustic (CN VIII), facial (CN VII), and sometimes trigeminal (CN V), glossopharyngeal (CN IX), and vagus (CN X). Cerebellar signs of incoordination and ataxia may occur. Large tumors may cause hydrocephalus and increased ICP. The tumor is slow growing and benign but may be difficult to remove surgically as it gets larger because of brain stem structures that the tumor may encase

c. Developmental tumors

  i. Hemangioblastoma: slow growing, vascular tumor that develops from embryonic vascular elements and is most frequently found in cerebellum

  ii. Craniopharyngioma: found usually in suprasellar region and believed to arise from pituitary hypophysis. It occurs primarily in children and causes increased ICP, pituitary and hypothalamic dysfunction, and visual disturbance. Although generally benign, it may recur if surgical removal is subtotal

  iii. Chordoma: slow growing, found in both brain and spinal cord, and arises from fetal notochord. It invades bone and is difficult to excise completely

    d. Pituitary tumors

        i. Nonsecreting tumor: chromophobe adenoma—space-occupying lesion that produces endocrine dysfunction by compressing pituitary gland and producing hypopituitarism. It causes compression of optic chiasm and visual changes and represents 90% of all pituitary tumors

       ii. Secreting tumors

          (a) ACTH-secreting tumor—stimulates production of cortisol from adrenal gland and symptoms of Cushing's syndrome

          (b) Growth-hormone secreting tumor—eosinophilic pituitary adenoma. Giantism occurs if tumor develops in childhood; acromegaly occurs if tumor develops in adulthood

    e. Metastatic tumor: metastases most common from breast in women and lungs in men. Primary cancers of gastrointestinal and genitourinary tract may also metastasize. Lesions may be single or multiple or encapsulated or diffuse and affect meninges or brain tissue

2. **Etiology or precipitating factors:** the causes of tumor growth are not fully understood. Theories include an abnormality in the structure or function of one or more genes, the influence of hormones, an angiogenesis factor (a substance in tumor cells that stimulates capillary growth), chemicals, radiation, viruses, trauma, and diet

3. **Nursing assessment data base**

    a. Nursing history

        i. Subjective findings

          (a) Patient's chief complaint

            (1) See nursing examination of patient

            (2) Headache—most common presenting symptom with tumors. It may be generalized or localized, initially worse in morning and eventually more constant, and not as severe as the headaches associated with subarachnoid hemorrhage or migraine

            (3) Seizures—another very common presenting symptom. They may be focal or generalized

            (4) Mental changes and drowsiness

          (b) Other symptoms

            (1) See nursing examination of patient

            (2) Visual changes (caused by chronic intracranial hypertension)

            (3) Vomiting—usually occurs without nausea or abdominal discomfort. It is unrelated to meals, more common in morning, and may be projectile

       ii. Objective findings

          (a) Presence of etiologic or precipitating factors

    (1) Historic symptoms secondary to size and location of tumor (see nursing examination of patient)

   (b) Family history—some tumors may have genetic relationship

   (c) Social history—although diet and exposure to carcinogens is a cause of some types of tumors, there is no conclusive link to most brain tumors (except radiation)

   (d) Medication history—current medications should be identified

 b. Nursing examination of patient: findings are secondary to location of tumor and increased ICP

  i. Frontal lobe tumor

   (a) Inappropriate behavior

   (b) Inattentiveness

   (c) Inability to concentrate

   (d) Loss of self-restraint and social behavior

   (e) Impaired recent memory

   (f) Difficulty with abstraction

   (g) Flat affect

   (h) Expressive aphasia (if lesion in dominant hemisphere)

   (i) Motor weakness

  ii. Parietal lobe tumor

   (a) Hyperesthesia

   (b) Paresthesia—tingling, crawling, burning

   (c) Loss of two-point discrimination

   (d) Astereognosia

   (e) Autotopagnosia

   (f) Anosognosia

   (g) Gerstmann's syndrome—consists of

    (1) Finger agnosia

    (2) Loss of left-right discrimination

    (3) Agraphia

    (4) Acalculia

   (h) Constructional apraxia

   (i) Homonymous hemianopsia

   (j) Unilateral neglect

  iii. Temporal lobe tumor

   (a) Psychomotor seizures

   (b) Homonymous hemianopsia

   (c) Homonymous quadrantopsia

   (d) Receptive aphasia if in dominant hemisphere

  iv. Occipital lobe tumor

   (a) Contralateral homonymous hemianopsia

   (b) Visual hallucinations

   (c) Seizures with a visual aura

      v. Pituitary and hypothalamic region tumor
        (a) Visual defects
        (b) Hypopituitarism
        (c) Headache
        (d) Cushing's syndrome
        (e) Acromegaly
     vi. Ventricular and periventricular tumors
        (a) Hydrocephalus
        (b) Headache
        (c) Change in level of consciousness
    vii. Cerebellar tumor
        (a) Ataxia
        (b) Incoordination
        (c) Dysmetria
        (d) Dizziness
        (e) Nystagmus
   viii. Brain stem tumor
        (a) Cranial nerve deficits
        (b) Cerebellar dysfunction
        (c) Vomiting
  c. Diagnostic study findings
      i. Visual field and fundoscopic examination: reveals papilledema, visual field defects
     ii. Skull x-ray films: may reveal deviation of calcified pineal gland, erosion of bone, calcified areas
    iii. CT scan: without and with contrast enhancement. It reveals size and location of tumor, presence of cerebral edema, hydrocephalus
    iv. Cerebral angiography: reveals vascularity of tumor and vessels that supply it. It may also demonstrate displacement and distortion of uninvolved vessels and formation of new vessels
     v. MRI: will reveal size and location of tumor, vascularity, and cerebral edema
     vi. Other tests may be performed for further differentiation of tumor (e.g., blood flow studies)
    vii. Endocrine studies: abnormally high or low values indicate secreting tumor or destruction of secreting cells

4. Nursing diagnoses (see pp. 366–375)
  a. Alteration in cerebral perfusion related to increased ICP
  b. Impaired gas exchange related to altered oxygen supply or oxygen-carrying capacity
  c. Impaired breathing pattern related to depressed level of consciousness, intracranial pathology, and metabolic imbalance
  d. Ineffective airway clearance related to increased secretions and depressed level of consciousness

e. Potential for fluid volume deficit related to excessive loss and decreased intake
f. Potential for fluid volume excess related to syndrome of inappropriate secretion of ADH
g. Potential for infection related to invasive lines, monitoring, and therapeutic devices
h. Impaired verbal communication related to expressive/receptive dysphasia
i. Impaired physical mobility related to weakness or paralysis of one or more body parts
j. Alteration in thought processes related to confusion, short-term memory loss, and short attention span
k. Potential for injury related to seizures
l. Potential for injury related to infectious process
m. Ineffective individual coping related to situational crisis, loss of control and independence, and change in role
n. Ineffective family coping related to disruption of usual family roles, burden of care, and changes in family member's present and future functioning

Meningitis

1. **Pathophysiology**
   a. Pathologic organisms gain access to subarachnoid space and meninges via bloodstream, sinuses, and middle ear; directly through penetrating injuries, ventriculostomy catheters, and surgical wound contamination; or indirectly as result of cerebral abscess or encephalitis
   b. Exudate forms in subarachnoid space, and inflammation of meninges occurs. There is congestion of tissues and blood vessels
   c. This congestion leads to cortical irritation, and increased ICP may result from hydrocephalus/cerebral edema
   d. Progressive involvement leads to
      i. Vasculitis with necrosis of cortical parenchyma
      ii. Ependymitis or pyocephalus
      iii. Petechial hemorrhage within brain
      iv. Hydrocephalus or subdural hygroma
      v. Cranial nerve neuritis
2. **Etiology or precipitating factors**
   a. Infecting organisms
      i. Virus: enterovirus, mumps virus, herpes virus, arbovirus
      ii. Bacteria
         (a) Most common after neurologic surgery are staphylococci—usually *S. aureus* but also *S. epidermidis*
         (b) Gram-negative enteric bacilli including *Escherichia coli,*

Serratia, Klebsiella, Citrobacter, Proteus, Pseudomonas, and *Acinetobacter*

    (c) *Neissera meningitidis* (meningococcal meningitis)—one of most contagious

    (d) *Haemophilus influenzae*

    (e) *Streptococcus pneumoniae*

    (f) *Mycobacterium tuberculosis*

  b. Sources of infection

    i. Neurologic surgery—contamination during surgery; local wound infection from irrigation systems or drains

    ii. Penetrating head injury—stab wounds, gunshot wounds, depressed skull fractures

    iii. Basal skull fracture resulting in dural tears with CSF leaks

    iv. Otitis media or sinusitis

    v. ICP monitoring devices

    vi. Septicemia, septic emboli

3. Nursing assessment data base

  a. Nursing history

    i. Subjective findings

      (a) Patient's chief complaint

        (1) Headache that has grown progressively worse

        (2) Neck or back pain on flexion

      (b) Other symptoms

        (1) Nausea and vomiting

        (2) Irritability, confusion

        (3) Photophobia

    ii. Objective findings

      (a) Presence of etiologic or precipitating factors—a highly suspect injury, procedure, or pathologic condition

      (b) Family history—noncontributory

      (c) Social history—intravenous drug abuse

      (d) Medications—immunosuppressant drugs such as corticosteroids

  b. Nursing examination of patient

    i. Inspection

      (a) Infectious signs

        (1) Fever

        (2) Tachycardia

        (3) Chills

        (4) Rash—petechiae or purpura most common in meningococcal meningitis

      (b) Meningeal irritation

        (1) Headache

        (2) Nuchal rigidity—resistance to flexion of neck

(3) Brudzinski's sign—adduction and flexion of legs as attempts are made to flex neck

(4) Kernig's sign—after flexing thigh or abdomen, attempts at extending it are met with resistance

(c) Neurologic abnormalities

(1) Decreased level of consciousness

(2) Cranial nerve involvement

a) Optic (CN II)—papilledema may be present; blindness can occur

b) Oculomotor, trochlear, abducens (CN III, IV, VI)—impairment of ocular movement, ptosis and unequal pupils, and diplopia are common findings

c) Trigeminal (CN V)—photophobia

d) Facial (CN VII)—facial paresis

e) Acoustic (CN VIII)—tinnitus, vertigo, deafness

(3) Focal neurologic signs (e.g., hemiparesis/hemiplegia)

(4) Seizures

(d) Complications

(1) Waterhouse-Friderichsen syndrome (adrenal hemorrhage) with resulting hemorrhage and shock—may be seen in fulminating meningococcal meningitis

(2) Disseminated intravascular coagulation

(3) Brain abscess, subdural effusions, encephalitis

(4) Hydrocephalus

(5) Cerebral edema

ii. Palpation: nuchal rigidity

iii. Percussion: deep tendon reflexes will be hyperactive

iv. Auscultation: tachycardia

c. Diagnostic study findings

i. Laboratory findings

(a) CSF—findings depend on type of organism

(1) Elevated protein level seen in most cases; higher in bacterial meningitis than in viral meningitis

(2) Low glucose content seen in most bacterial meningitis—may be normal in viral meningitis

(3) Purulent—turbid but may be clear with some viruses

(4) Cells—predominantly polymorphonuclear leukocytes in bacterial meningitis and lymphocytes in viral meningitis

(b) Cultures—culture CSF, blood, and drainage from sinuses or wounds to identify organism. Ensure that specimens are transported to laboratory immediately since certain organisms require prompt culturing

(c) Nasopharyngeal smear—causative bacteria may be present

       (d) Electrolytes—either hyponatremia or hypernatremia may be seen

    ii. Radiologic findings

       (a) CT scan—usually normal in acute uncomplicated meningitis but may show diffuse enhancement in some types or reveal hydrocephalus

       (b) Skull x-rays films—infected sinuses may be seen; basilar skull fracture may be evident

    iii. Other diagnostic findings—EEG may show generalized slow-wave activity

4. Nursing diagnoses

  a. Alteration in cerebral tissue perfusion related to increased ICP (see p. 366)

  b. Potential for injury related to seizures (see pp. 430–432)

  c. Alteration in comfort, headache, related to meningeal irritation

    i. Assessment for defining characteristics

       (a) Communicates pain perception—headache, pain in neck or back

       (b) Guarding or protective behavior (i.e., unwillingness to move in bed)

       (c) Narrowed focus—altered time perception, withdrawal from social contact

       (d) Facial mask of pain

       (e) Moaning, crying

       (f) Change in vital signs

    ii. Expected outcomes

       (a) Articulates factors that intensify pain, and modifies behavior accordingly

       (b) Expresses a feeling of comfort and relief from pain

    iii. Nursing interventions

       (a) Assess symptoms of pain and administer pain medication as ordered. Monitor and record effectiveness and side effects

       (b) Perform comfort measures to promote relaxation

       (c) Plan activities with patient to provide distraction (e.g., radio, visitors, TV, or reading if able)

       (d) Explain reasons for pain (e.g., nuchal rigidity) to increase pain tolerance

       (e) Manipulate environment to promote periods of uninterrupted rest (e.g., turning down lights)

       (f) Position in comfortable position

    iv. Evaluation of nursing care

       (a) Manipulates factors that intensify pain

       (b) Reports relief of pain from interventions and medication

  d. Hyperthemia related to infectious process

i. Assessment for defining characteristics
   (a) Fever
   (b) Tachycardia
   (c) Tachypnea
   (d) Warm, flushed skin
   (e) Seizures
ii. Expected outcomes
   (a) Maintains temperature below 100.5° F (38.0° C)
   (b) Maintains fluid intake equal to or greater than output
   (c) Does not experience seizures
iii. Nursing interventions
   (a) Monitor temperature every 2 to 4 hours as condition indicates
   (b) Administer antipyretic medications as ordered
   (c) Employ other cooling measures as indicated—remove blankets, tepid water/alcohol sponge, hypothermia blanket
   (d) Monitor systemic responses to fever/infection (e.g., vital signs, respiratory rate, level of responsiveness)
   (e) Prevent skin irritation and breakdown if sponge baths or hypothermia blanket is used
   (f) Administer antibiotic therapy as ordered
iv. Evaluation of nursing care
   (a) Temperature maintained below 100.5° F (38.0° C)
   (b) Adequate fluid intake
   (c) Absence of seizures

Seizures

1. Pathophysiology
   a. Paroxysmal high-frequency or synchronous low-frequency, high-voltage electrical discharge in neurons of cerebral cortex and possibly neurons of the brain stem
   b. Properties of epileptogenic neurons
      i. Generation of autonomous paroxysmal discharges is influenced by synaptic activity
      ii. Increased electrical excitability is present
      iii. Cortical surface is electrically negative to surrounding normal cortex
      iv. Initiation of volleys of high-frequency impulses is caused by depolarization of resting membrane potential
      v. They are able to induce secondary epileptogenic foci in synaptically related areas
   c. Seizure activity may be idiopathic or symptomatic. Idiopathic seizures will usually present in childhood or early adulthood. Recurrent idiopathic seizures are generally referred to as epilepsy. New onset

of seizures indicates a need for diagnostic investigation at any age but is most likely to be a symptom of other neurologic or metabolic pathology when it occurs in the adult

2. **Etiology or precipitating factors**
   a. Idiopathic
   b. Genetic
   c. Perinatal injury
   d. Craniocerebral trauma
   e. Cerebrovascular disease
   f. Infections, particularly of CNS
   g. Cerebral tumors
   h. Metabolic or toxic disorders
   i. Arteriovenous malformations of the brain
   j. Abrupt withdrawal of anticonvulsant medications or chronically used sedatives

3. **Nursing assessment data base**
   a. Nursing history
      i. Subjective findings
         (a) Patient's chief complaint
            (1) Events occurring at onset of seizures
            (2) Frequency and duration of seizures
      ii. Objective findings
         (a) Presence of etiologic or precipitating factors
            (1) Observers' reports of events occurring at onset of attack
            (2) Observers' reports of postictal events
            (3) Duration of disorder and frequency of seizure as reported by family
         (b) Family history—genetic history of seizures
         (c) Social history—use of alcohol or illicit drugs
         (d) Medication—use of prescribed medications; abrupt withdrawal of anticonvulsant medications or chronically used sedatives
   b. Nursing examination of patient
      i. Inspection
         (a) Neurologic examination may reveal possible causative factor (i.e., abnormality that suggests intracranial pathology)
         (b) If seizures are idiopathic, examination will be normal unless patient is in postictal state
         (c) Examination of other body systems may reveal possible causative factors (e.g., signs of electrolyte imbalances, arterial blood gas abnormalities, or other serious illness)
         (d) Clinical presentation
            (1) Generalized

    a) Tonic-clonic (grand mal)
- Tonic-clonic symmetric movements involving whole body
- No focal onset but may have high-pitched epileptic cry at beginning of seizure
- Loss of consciousness; no purposeful actions or responses
- Profuse salivation during seizure
- Apnea and cyanosis may develop, clearing as seizure terminates
- Incontinence is common
- Usually lasts 1 to 5 minutes

    b) Absence (petit mal)
- Brief loss of contact with environment (i.e., absence)
- Patient may exhibit minor motor movements such as drooping or twitching of lips or rolling or turning up of eyes
- Lasts less than 30 seconds; ends abruptly. Patient (usually a child) is generally unaware that anything has happened
- Not usually seen in patients older than 16 years of age; onset occurs before 12 years of age

    c) Myoclonic—sudden, brief, muscular contractions that may occur singly or repetitively; usually involve arms

    d) Akinetic—sudden, brief loss of muscle tone that may be manifest as "drop attacks"

  (2) Partial

    a) Partial seizures with elemental symptomatology
- Motor—focal motor seizures that are confined to specific body parts but may progress and become generalized (commonly termed *jacksonian*); may be associated with *aura*—a sensory phenomenon preceding seizure activity
- Sensory—somatic sensory seizures that patient usually describes as numbness or tingling; may generalize. Special sensory seizures may include visual, auditory, or vertiginous symptoms

    b) Partial seizures with complex symptomatology
- Automatisms or temporal lobe seizures (psychomotor)—may present as simple or elaborate behavioral or sensory alterations. Although behavior appears intentional, patient has amnesia

regarding the seizure, which usually lasts 1 to 5 minutes
□ Visceral or autonomic symptoms
c. Diagnostic study findings
　　i. Laboratory findings: dependent on cause or related pathology
　　ii. Radiologic findings: dependent on intracranial pathology, if any (e.g., tumors, abscesses, hematomas, aneurysms, or arteriovenous malformations)
　　iii. Special: EEG
　　　　(a) May be done under variety of conditions (e.g., sleeping, hyperventilation, photostimulation)
　　　　(b) May be repeated at different times of day or under different conditions
　　　　(c) Abnormal results vary depending on causative pathology but generally reveal localized or diffuse slowing of the pattern when patient is not having a seizure and localized or diffuse increase in EEG activity during seizures. Certain seizures (e.g., petit mal) have characteristic EEG patterns

4. Nursing diagnoses
　a. Potential for injury related to seizure activity
　　i. Assessment for defining characteristics (See Nursing examination of patient for descriptions of types of seizures)
　　ii. Expected outcomes
　　　　(a) Does not experience injuries from seizure activity
　　　　(b) Adheres to medication regimen
　　　　(c) Experiences no toxic effects of anticonvulsant therapy
　　iii. Nursing interventions
　　　　(a) Observe seizure activity; record and report observations
　　　　　　(1) Note time and signs of impending attack
　　　　　　(2) Observe parts of body involved, order of involvement, and character of movements
　　　　　　(3) Check for deviation of eyes and nystagmus; note change in pupillary size
　　　　　　(4) Assess respiratory pattern
　　　　　　(5) Note tonic and clonic stages
　　　　　　(6) During postictal stage
　　　　　　　　a) Ensure adequate airway and check for apparent injury
　　　　　　　　b) Evaluate patient's neurologic status, particularly motor weakness and speech
　　　　(b) Prevent injuries during convulsive seizure activity
　　　　　　(1) Never force anything into mouth
　　　　　　(2) Do not attempt to restrain patient's movements
　　　　　　(3) Remove objects from vicinity that could cause injury

(4) Protect head from injury

(5) Remove restraining or constricting clothing

(c) Improve control of seizure activity

    (1) Monitor and maintain therapeutic plasma levels of anticonvulsant medications; more than one drug may be used at a time. Therapeutic ranges are laboratory specific. General ranges are given

        a) Phenytoin (Dilantin)—generalized or partial seizures. Therapeutic blood level—10 to 20 µg/ml

        b) Phenobarbital—generalized or partial seizures. Therapeutic blood level—20 to 40 µg/ml

        c) Primidone (Mysoline)—generalized and complex partial seizures. Therapeutic blood level—5 to 12 µg/ml

        d) Carbamazepine (Tegretol)—generalized and simple or complex seizures. Therapeutic blood level—8 to 12 µg/ml

        e) Ethosuximide (Zarontin)—petit mal and complex partial seizures. Therapeutic blood level—40 to 90 µg/ml

        f) Clonazepam (Klonopin)—myoclonic and akinetic seizures. Therapeutic blood level—5 to 50 µg/ml

        g) Valproic acid (Depakene)—simple (petit mal) and complex absence seizures. Therapeutic blood level—50 to 100 µg/ml

    (2) Diagnose and treat causative factors (e.g., metabolic disorders, cerebral tumors, or infections)

    (3) Eliminate precipitating factors

        a) Inadequate or inappropriate anticonvulsant medication

        b) Nonadherence to drug regimen

        c) Alcohol abuse

        d) Emotional stress

        e) Lack of proper nutrition or sleep

(d) Combat toxic side effects of drugs

    (1) Obtain serum levels and maintain at therapeutic levels

    (2) CNS dysfunction is most common result of toxicity

    (3) Encourage good oral hygiene to prevent gingival hypertrophy, which commonly occurs with phenytoin therapy

    (4) Many drugs increase or decrease plasma concentration of certain anticonvulsant drugs, particularly phenytoin. Phenytoin may also decrease plasma concentra-

tions of other drugs. Consult a pharmacist for patient on multiple medications
  iv. Evaluation of nursing care
     (a) Accurate recording and reporting of seizure activity
     (b) Absence of injuries due to seizures
     (c) Adequate control of seizure activity
     (d) Absence of toxic effects of anticonvulsant therapy
  b. Knowledge deficit related to anticonvulsant actions and side effects
     i. Assessment for defining characteristics
        (a) Verbalizes lack of information regarding drug regimen
        (b) Unable to relate limitation of activities while taking anticonvulsant
        (c) Unable to list potential side effects
        (d) Requests information about drug therapy
     ii. Expected outcome: verbalizes understanding of drug action, dosage, frequency, limitations of activities, and side effects
    iii. Nursing interventions
        (a) Develop goals for learning with patient
        (b) Include family in teaching
        (c) Select teaching strategies appropriate for patient's individual learning needs and style
        (d) Assist patient in determining how to fit drug therapy into activities of daily living
        (e) Teach effects, side effects, precautions, alterations in activities necessary (e.g., good oral hygiene to prevent gingival hypertrophy when taking phenytoin; avoiding alcohol while on anticonvulsant therapy)
        (f) Teach patient and family what to report to physician regarding seizures or effects and side effects from drug
        (g) Provide name and phone number of resources, agencies, or organizations to contact with questions or problems
     iv. Evaluation of nursing care: verbalizes understanding of drug therapy, side effects, and limitations

Status Epilepticus

1. **Pathophysiology**
   a. Tonic-clonic seizures cause a rapid succession of many action potentials in single cells
   b. Heavy metabolic demand is placed on cells, leading to decline of high-energy phosphates (e.g., ATP) and failure of the sodium–potassium ATPase pump
   c. Cerebral metabolic rate, oxygen and glucose use, and glycolysis increase two to three times normal

    d. Cerebral blood flow increases three to five times normal, owing in part to increased arterial pressure and cerebrovascular dilation

    e. Cellular swelling may occur with prolonged seizures and may be due to the osmotic effects from uptake of increased amounts of metabolic by-products (e.g., lactate, amino acids, ammonia) and failure of the sodium–potassium pump

    f. Systemic metabolic acidosis contributes to cardiovascular collapse

    g. Hyperthermia occurs as a result of increased metabolic activity

2. Etiology or precipitating factors

    a. Withdrawal from anticonvulsant medications

    b. Acute alcohol withdrawal

    c. Electroshock therapy

    d. CNS infections (e.g., meningitis, encephalitis, abscesses)

    e. Brain tumors, particularly in frontal lobe

    f. Acute withdrawal from chronically used drugs that have sedative or depressant effects

    g. Metabolic disorders (e.g., uremia, hypoglycemia, hyponatremia)

    h. Craniocerebral trauma

    i. Cerebral edema

    j. Cerebrovascular disease

3. Nursing assessment data base

    a. Nursing history

        i. Presence of one or more etiologic or precipitating factors

        ii. Seizure activity

    b. Nursing examination of patient

        i. Absence (petit mal): 200 to 300 absences in 24 hours. Rarely occurs; not life threatening

        ii. Epilepsia partialis continua: partial or focal seizures that occur regularly or are continuous. Not usually accompanied by loss of consciousness. May generalize

        iii. Tonic-clonic (grand mal): grand mal seizures that recur, with incomplete recovery between seizures. As seizures repeat, post-ictal interval becomes progressively shorter. Seizures may become continuous. Life-threatening owing to metabolic and physical exhaustion that occurs

        iv. Electrical status: little or no clinical evidence of seizure activity, although EEG shows continuous spike discharges

    c. Diagnostic study findings

        i. Laboratory findings

            (a) Electrolyte abnormalities may be precipitating cause of seizure activity or may result from prolonged seizures. Pay particular attention to sodium and potassium levels

            (b) Blood glucose should be monitored. Hypoglycemia may be precipating cause of seizures or may result from prolonged seizure activity. Glucose consumption is increased during seizures and may lead to hypoglycemia

(c) Arterial blood gases—hypoxia may precipitate or result from seizures. Hypoxia leads to increased lactic acid production and, along with carbon dioxide retention, causes acidosis

(d) Serum levels of enzymes, particularly creatine phosphokinase (CPK), will be elevated after seizure activity

(e) Myoglobinuria is not uncommon after seizures

ii. Radiologic findings: after seizures are controlled, diagnostic studies may be done to find precipitating or complicating cause

iii. Special: EEG will show seizure activity

4. Nursing diagnoses

a. Potential for injury related to metabolic complications of seizure activity

   i. Assessment for defining characteristics

     (a) Respiratory and metabolic acidosis

     (b) Hypoxemia

     (c) Hypoglycemia

     (d) Hyperthermia

     (e) Electrolyte imbalances

     (f) Renal failure

     (g) Death from exhaustion

   ii. Expected outcomes

     (a) Maintains oxygenation and ventilation

     (b) Experiences no complications of drug therapy

     (c) Experiences no complications of status epilepticus

     (d) Maintains seizure-free state

   iii. Nursing interventions

     (a) Establish and maintain patent airway and adequate ventilation

       (1) Endotracheal intubation and controlled ventilation with ventilator may become necessary if seizures cannot be controlled rapidly

       (2) Monitor arterial blood gases frequently, and treat respiratory or metabolic acidosis

       (3) Maintain adequate oxygenation—seizure activity increases oxygen consumption

     (b) Assess causes or contributing factors

       (1) Analyze blood for glucose, sodium, potassium, calcium, phosphorus, magnesium, and blood urea nitrogen since severe imbalance of any of these many precipitate and/or perpetuate seizures

       (2) Obtain toxic screen for drugs (e.g., phencyclidine [PCP], alcohol, lead)

(3) Obtain anticonvulsant drug levels (e.g., barbiturate, phenytoin)

(4) Obtain blood cultures if sepsis is suspected

(5) Complete blood cell count with differential may reveal disorders that are associated with seizures, (e.g., lead poisoning, sickle cell anemia, leukemia)

(c) Stop seizure activity—the following drugs may be used

(1) Lorazepam (Ativan)

a) 4 mg IV. Repeat after 15 minutes if seizures persist. Therapeutic plasma levels are 30 to 60 μg/ml

b) Onset is usually within 15 minutes

c) Respiratory depression may occur but not seen as frequently as with diazepam

(2) Diazepam

a) 10 to 20 mg IV at 5 mg/min. Therapeutic plasma levels are 0.5 μg/ml or greater. Onset of action is almost immediate. Duration of action is 30 to 60 minutes

b) Do not dilute

c) Respiratory and cardiovascular depression may occur

d) Mechanism of action is believed to be enhancement of the neurotransmitter GABA

(3) Phenobarbital

a) 5 to 8 mg/kg IV at 60 mg/min. Therapeutic plasma levels are 20 to 40 μg/ml. Onset of action is 5 to 20 minutes. Duration of action is about 24 hours

b) Depression of blood pressure, respiration, and consciousness may occur

c) Mechanism of action is believed to include increased neuronal threshold to electrical and chemical stimuli, depressed physiologic excitation, enhanced inhibition at the synapse, and reduced calcium uptake by depolarized nerve terminals

(4) Phenytoin

a) 12 to 18 mg/kg IV, no faster than 50 mg/min. Therapeutic plasma levels are 10 to 20 μg/ml. Onset of action is 10 to 20 minutes. Duration of action is 24 hours

b) Administration should be intravenous, as close to infusion site as possible. Line should be flushed with saline or absolute alcohol to preclude precipitation or crystallization with glucose. Because of its basic pH, it should not be given intramuscularly

    c) Monitor ECG continuously for dysrhythmias or conduction changes. Use with caution in patients with heart block or Stokes-Adams syndrome. Hypotension may occur, particularly if drug is given too fast

    d) Major mechanism of action is to decrease intracellular influx of sodium and calcium, blocking neurotransmitter release

   (5) Paraldehyde

    a) 0.1 to 0.15 ml/kg IM every 2 to 4 hours. Give deep IM in 5-ml increments

    b) Particularly effective in alcoholic seizures. May be given if patient is allergic to other drugs

    c) May be given rectally, especially to children

  (d) Monitor and assess condition closely to prevent complications

   (1) Insert nasogastric tube and attach to gastric suction to prevent vomiting and aspiration

   (2) Establish intravenous line for medications

   (3) Monitor cardiac rate and rhythm and arterial blood pressure

   (4) Cardiovascular drugs should be readily available

   (5) Assess neurologic status frequently

   (6) Treat hyperthermia

  (e) Maintain fluid and electrolyte balance

   (1) Maintain accurate intake and output

   (2) Administer glucose solutions intravenously based on blood glucose levels

   (3) Assess electrolytes, calcium, and magnesium levels and renal and liver function

   (4) Myoglobinuria may result from prolonged seizure activity and can lead to renal failure. Treat with fluid and diuretics

  (f) Maintain seizure-free state

   (1) If diazepam is used to stop seizures, anticonvulsant drugs, preferably phenytoin, must be given simultaneously to prevent recurrent seizures

   (2) Phenytoin is often preferred since it does not mask neurologic signs

   (3) Phenobarbital may be used if sedation is not a concern

   (4) General anesthesia may be indicated to control seizures if they cannot be stopped in 2 to 4 hours

  (g) Investigate and treat underlying pathology

   (1) Signs of head trauma

   (2) Signs of drug abuse (e.g., needle tracks)

(3) Diagnostic tests for intracranial pathology (e.g., CT scan, angiography)

(4) Diagnostic tests for conditions that are associated with seizures (e.g., fluid and electrolyte imbalance, leukocyte or erythrocyte abnormalities)

iv. Evaluation of nursing care
   (a) Arterial blood gas values within normal limits
   (b) Seizure activity controlled
   (c) Absence of complications of anticonvulsant therapy
   (d) Absence of complications of status epilepticus
   (e) Maintenance of seizure-free state
   (f) Underlying cause treated, if possible

b. Hyperthermia related to seizure activity
   i. Assessment for defining characteristics
      (a) Fever
      (b) Persistent tonic-clonic seizure activity, focal or generalized
      (c) Tachycardia
   ii. Expected outcome: Maintains temperature below 100° F (38° C)
   iii. Nursing interventions
      (a) Administer antipyretics as ordered
      (b) Tepid sponge bath if hyperthermia persists or temperature greater than 103° F or as ordered
      (c) Stop seizure activity
   iv. Evaluation of nursing care: Temperature maintained below 100° F (38° C)

c. Other nursing diagnoses that may be applicable include (see pp. 367–370)
   i. Impaired gas exchange related to altered oxygen supply
   ii. Ineffective breathing pattern related to depressed level of consciousness and inadequate airway
   iii. Ineffective airway clearance related to increased secretions and depressed level of consciousness
   iv. Potential fluid volume deficit related to excessive loss and decreased intake

Guillain-Barré Syndrome: Also called Landry-Guillain-Barré-Strohl syndrome, polyneuritis, polyradiculoneuritis, infectious polyneuritis

1. Pathophysiology

a. Edema and inflammation of spinal nerve roots, with subsequent demyelination

b. Focal perivascular lymphocytic infiltration occurs within nerve roots, peripheral nerves, and CNS

c. Schwann cells deposit myelin around axon. Myelin insulates axon and is interrupted at 1- to 2-mm intervals by nodes of Ranvier. Impulse of myelinated fibers is conducted from node to node (i.e., saltatory conduction) instead of continuously along axon and thus allows for more rapid impulse conduction. When demyelination occurs, this ability is lost and nerve impulses are conducted more slowly or not at all. In addition, anterior horn cells in spinal cord may undergo chromatolysis (i.e., degeneration). This resolves as edema and inflammation of nerves resolves, and remyelination occurs

d. Demyelination classically begins in distal nerves and ascends symmetrically, resulting in ascending paralysis. This process may halt at any point or may progress to quadriplegia and involvement of motor cranial nerves

e. When demyelination ceases, remyelination occurs slowly, resulting in return of transmission of nerve impulses and restoration of function. Return of function first occurs proximally and proceeds distally, with complete recovery in an overwhelming majority of cases

2. **Etiology or precipitating factors**
   a. Etiology unknown, but an autoimmune disease theory is popular since it explains a mechanism common to a variety of etiologies
   b. A viral infection, such as an upper respiratory tract infection or gastroenteritis, may precede onset of symptoms by 2 to 3 weeks. Vaccination for smallpox, flu, tetanus, or measles has also been associated with the syndrome
   c. Previous surgery and preexisting illnesses (e.g., Hodgkin's disease or systemic lupus erythematosus) have also been associated with syndrome
   d. Many patients have no history of any of these

3. **Nursing assessment data base**
   a. Nursing history
      i. Subjective findings
         (a) Patient's chief complaint—progressive, ascending weakness; mild to moderate sensory changes, primarily tingling and muscle pain
         (b) Other symptoms—mild shortness of breath in early stages
      ii. Objective findings
         (a) Presence of one or more etiologic or contributing factors
         (b) Family history—noncontributory
         (c) Social history—noncontributory
         (d) Medication history—immunosuppressive drugs may complicate course
   b. Nursing examination of patient
      i. Inspection
         (a) Muscle weakness—symmetric involvement (distal muscles most severely affected). Level of paralysis varies greatly; may halt at any level

      (b) Cranial nerve involvement—most commonly dysphagia (glossopharyngeal and vagus nerves [CN IX, X]) and facial weakness (facial nerve [CN VII]); extraocular muscle paralysis (oculomotor, trochlear, abducens nerves [CN III, IV, VI]), masseter muscle paralysis (trigeminal nerve [CN V]), paralysis of the sternocleidomastoid and trapezius muscles (spinal accessory nerve [CN XI]), and paralysis of the tongue (hypoglossal nerve [CN XII]) may occur

      (c) Decreased vital capacity due to weakness of respiratory muscles

      (d) Paresthesias, hyperesthesia, hypalgesia

      (e) Muscle tenderness

   ii. Palpation: noncontributory

  iii. Percussion: depressed or absent deep tendon reflexes

   iv. Auscultation: ANS dysfunction manifested by fluctuation in blood pressure and heart rate

c. Diagnostic study findings

    i. CSF: elevated protein with normal cell count, referred to as "albuminocytologic dissociation" (a classic finding). Protein highest 10 to 20 days after onset

   ii. Radiologic: all normal

  iii. Special: electromyography not generally used during acute stages but may be done during rehabilitation to document nerve regeneration

4. Nursing diagnoses

a. Powerlessness related to total physical dependency (see pp. 406–407)

b. Disturbance in self-concept related to change in body image (see pp. 405–406)

c. Alteration in tissue perfusion related to venous thrombosis (see pp. 401–402)

d. Alteration in respiratory function related to paralysis of respiratory muscles, ineffective coughing and deep breathing (see pp. 402–403)

e. Potential for infection related to invasive lines (see p. 371)

f. Impaired physical mobility related to paralysis (see p. 405)

g. Ineffective individual coping related to situational crisis, loss of control and independence, and change in role (see p. 374)

h. Ineffective family coping related to disruption of usual family roles, burden of care, and changes in family member's present and future functioning (see p. 374)

i. Potential for alteration in cardiac output related to autonomic nervous system dysfunction

    i. Assessment for defining characteristics

      (a) Fluctuations in blood pressure; hypertension more common than hypotension

      (b) Alteration in heart rate—may fluctuate widely

(c) Flushed, warm skin

(d) Vasovagal reflex—suctioning that leads to hypoxia and vagal stimulation may cause severe bradycardia or cardiac arrest

ii. Expected outcomes

(a) Maintains adequate blood pressure and heart rate

(b) Does not experience complications from vasovagal reflex

iii. Nursing interventions

(a) Monitor blood pressure frequently as condition indicates. Use vasoactive drugs to control blood pressure with caution

(b) Bradycardia—treat with atropine if symptomatic

(c) Tachycardia—beta blockers have been used

(d) Vasovagal reflex—oxygenate with 100% oxygen for 3 to 5 minutes prior to suctioning. Limit suctioning time to 15 seconds. Monitor cardiac rate and rhythm during and after suctioning. Atropine may be necessary if oxygenation does not abolish reflex

iv. Evaluation of nursing care

(a) Blood pressure and heart rate within normal limits

(b) Absence of vasovagal reflex

j. Alteration in comfort related to hyperesthesias, paresthesias, deep muscle aches

i. Assessment for defining characteristics

(a) Reports of muscular pain that feels like a "charley horse"

(b) Hypersensitivity of skin that feels like pins and needles, tingling

(c) Reports of sharp, shooting, "electric shock"–like sensations

(d) Facial expression of discomfort (if facial nerve [CN VII] not affected)

(e) Hot flashes caused by ANS dysfunction

ii. Expected outcome—reports discomfort controlled with a combination of analgesics and noninvasive techniques

iii. Nursing interventions

(a) Assess symptoms of pain and administer pain medication as ordered. Monitor and record effectiveness and side effects

(b) Perform comfort measures to promote relaxation (e.g., positioning, rubbing of skin)

(c) Plan activities with patient to provide distraction (e.g., radio, visitors, TV or reading if able)

(d) Explain reason for discomfort (e.g., ANS involvement, peripheral nerve involvement)

(e) Manipulate environment to promote periods of uninterrupted rest (e.g., turning down lights)

(f) Position in comfortable position; reposition often

(g) Involve family in pain control measures

iv. Evaluation of nursing care: reports relief of pain from interventions and medication

k. Potential alteration in nutrition, less than body requirements, related to decreased intake

i. Assessment for defining characteristics

(a) Inability to chew (trigeminal nerve [CN V])

(b) Absent gag reflex, inability to swallow (glossopharyngeal and vagus nerves [CN IX, X])

(c) Facial paralysis (facial nerve [CN VII])

(d) Paralysis of tongue (hypoglossal nerve [CN XII])

(e) Gastric dilatation, ileus

ii. Expected outcomes

(a) Avoids aspiration

(b) Maintains optimal body weight

iii. Nursing interventions

(a) Assess bowel sounds every shift

(b) Weigh patient daily or per unit protocol

(c) Monitor intake and output

(d) Administer prescribed amount of tube feeding when bowel sounds are present

(1) Begin regimen with small, dilute concentrations. Increase volume and concentration as tolerated

(2) Elevate head of bed during infusion

(3) Check feeding tube placement at least once every shift

(4) Give water and juices, as needed, to maintain adequate hydration

(5) Put food coloring in tube feeding to monitor for aspiration

(6) Check for residual every 4 hours

(e) Provide nares care every 4 hours to prevent ulceration and skin breakdown. Tape nasogastric tube to prevent visual obstruction. Use hypoallergenic tape

(f) Change gastrostomy dressing daily or according to institutional protocol

(g) Ensure proper temperature of feeding (room temperature); change tube feeding bags and tubing according to institutional protocols

(h) Auscultate and record breath sounds every 4 hours; report wheezes, rhonchi, crackles, or decreased breath sounds. If aspiration is suspected, stop tube feeding. Keep suction apparatus at bedside, and suction as needed. Turn on side to avoid further aspiration

iv. Evaluation of nursing care

(a) Absence of aspiration
(b) Maintenance of optimal body weight

Myasthenia Gravis: Patients are usually admitted to the critical care unit only if they are in crisis or in the immediate postoperative period. This section will address those situations

1. **Pathophysiology**
   a. Chronic disorder of neuromuscular transmission characterized by abnormal muscular fatigability brought on by activity; improves with rest
   b. Normally, each nerve impulse liberates acetylcholine from nerve terminal causing depolarization (i.e., end-plate potential). Subsequent action potential in turn initiates events that result in muscular contraction
   c. Research implicates a post-synaptic defect as cause. This theory suggests reduction of available acetylcholine receptors at neuromuscular junction brought about by an autoimmune process (i.e., antibodies directed against cholinergic receptors)
   d. Decrease in number of acetylcholine receptor sites leads to reduced amplitude of end-plate potentials and impairment of muscle action potential and impulse transmission, and therefore of muscular contraction

2. **Etiology or precipitating factors**
   a. Etiology unknown: most accepted theory is that it is an autoimmune disorder affecting postsynaptic receptor sites. Significant incidence of thymoma and thymic hyperplasia and association with other autoimmune diseases lends support to this theory
   b. Precipitating factors of crisis
      i. Inadequate anticholinesterase drug levels (myasthenic crisis)
      ii. Overdosage of anticholinesterase drugs (cholinergic crisis)
      iii. Influenza
      iv. Menstrual cycle or pregnancy (especially first trimester)
      v. Certain drugs: quinidine, aminoglycoside antibiotics, procainamide, quinine, phenothiazines, barbiturates, tranquilizers, narcotics
      vi. Emotional stress and anxiety
      vii. Fatigue
      viii. Alcohol
      ix. Surgery

3. **Nursing assessment data base**
   a. Nursing history
      i. Subjective findings
         (a) Patient's chief complaint
            (1) Complaints of feeling tired and weak, especially after sustained activity or late in day

        (2) Improvement in strength and recovery from fatigue after rest

        (3) Complaints of weakness of specific muscle groups with repetitive use

     (b) Other symptoms—increased salivation, abdominal discomfort

   ii. Objective findings

     (a) Presence of etiologic or precipitating factors

     (b) Family history—noncontributory

     (c) Social history—use of alcohol may precipitate crisis

     (d) Medication history

        (1) Certain drugs may precipitate crisis

        (2) Ascertain compliance with medication regimen

b. Nursing examination of patient

   i. Inspection

     (a) Includes asking patient to perform repetitive actions using involved muscle groups, to assess for fatigability

     (b) Other physical signs vary depending on type and number of muscles involved and on severity

        (1) Ptosis

        (2) Diplopia

        (3) Dysphagia

        (4) Jaw weakness, especially with chewing and speaking (dysarthria)

        (5) Hoarseness after talking a few minutes; dysarthria

        (6) Limb weakness—usually symmetric in terms of involvement, although not necessarily in terms of severity

        (7) Respiratory difficulty—decreased vital capacity

   ii. Palpation: noncontributory

   iii. Percussion: noncontributory

   iv. Auscultation: decreased breath sounds

c. Diagnostic study findings

   i. Laboratory: serum antibody tests

     (a) Serum antibody titers are increased

     (b) Normal triiodothyronine (T_3) and thyroxine (T_4) levels rule out thyroid etiology

   ii. Radiologic

     (a) Repetitive nerve stimulation studies—electrical stimulation of nerves at various frequencies leads to progressive decrement of muscle action potentials

     (b) Anticholinesterase tests

        (1) Edrophonium chloride (Tensilon)—injection of 2 mg is given IV, and patient is assessed for improvement in muscle strength. If no reaction within 45 seconds,

repeated doses of 2 to 5 mg may be given at 2-minute intervals until response is obtained, or a total of 10 mg has been given. Duration of drug is about 5 minutes

    (2) Neostigmine—0.5 to 1.0 mg IV may be used if Tensilon test is not conclusive

  (c) Curare test—administration of small doses (nonparalytic doses in normal persons) leads to an abnormally clinically documented increase in weakness. *NOTE:* Not commonly used for diagnosis owing to risk of respiratory collapse. Be prepared to support ventilation

4. Nursing diagnoses

  a. Impaired physical mobility related to muscle weakness

    i. Assessment for defining characteristics

      (a) Muscle weakness that worsens with use

      (b) Diplopia

      (c) Ptosis

      (d) Dysphagia

      (e) Dysarthria

      (f) Difficulty chewing

      (g) Signs of myasthenic or cholinergic crisis

        (1) Changes in vital signs initiated by impending respiratory failure

        (2) Severe generalized weakness

        (3) Urinary incontinence

        (4) Increased secretions

        (5) Increased salivation, sweating, lacrimation (seen in cholinergic crisis)

        (6) Abdominal cramping and diarrhea (seen in cholinergic crisis)

        (7) Blurred vision

        (8) Fasciculations (seen in cholinergic crisis)

    ii. Expected outcomes

      (a) Will not experience complications of decreased neuromuscular function

      (b) Will respond to therapy for myasthenic crisis

      (c) Will respond to therapy for cholinergic crisis

      (d) Will not experience complications from thymectomy

      (e) Will not experience complications from plasmapheresis

    iii. Nursing interventions

      (a) Control symptoms

        (1) Improve neuromuscular transmission

          a) Administer anticholinesterase agents—neostigmine, pyridostigmine, ambenonium chloride (Mytelase)

            ☐ Very important to administer on schedule

        ☐ Carefully note all muscular responses to medications. Atropine may control side effects (e.g., excessive oral secretions or diarrhea) but may mask cholinergic crisis—use with caution

    b) Administer adrenal corticosteroids

        ☐ Corticosteroids are generally indicated in patients not satisfactorily controlled by anticholinesterase medication or thymectomy. Mechanism of action is not precisely known but is believed to be an interruption of autoimmune response

        ☐ Anticholinesterase drugs are regulated as necessary. When patient begins to respond to prednisone, dosage of anticholinesterase drugs can be decreased as tolerated

    c) Although controversial in patients without thymoma, thymectomy has been shown to produce improvement in or remission of symptoms in high percentage of myasthenic patients. Improvement may occur gradually and may not be maximal for as long as 1 to 10 years. Many patients continue to require corticosteroids and/or anticholinesterase medications after thymectomy, although often in smaller amounts

  (2) Anticipate problems of inability to ventilate adequately

  (3) Avoid certain drugs that might precipitate problems (see precipitating factors)

  (4) Prevent aspiration

  (5) Develop method of communication with patient if he is unable to talk. Explain care and procedures to him

(b) Treat myasthenic crisis (inadequate dosage of or tolerance to anticholinesterase drugs)

  (1) Tensilon test may be used to differentiate between myasthenic crisis and cholinergic crisis. If patient's symptoms improve after receiving Tensilon, crisis is myasthenic; if they get worse, it is cholinergic

  (2) Improve neuromuscular transmission by administering anticholinesterase drugs, repeating as necessary. Corticosteroids are usually avoided in crisis

  (3) Monitor and assess muscle strength frequently

  (4) Treat any underlying condition that may have precipitated crisis or may be perpetuating it

(c) Treat cholinergic crisis (overdosage of anticholinesterase drugs)

  (1) Improve neuromuscular transmission by withholding

anticholinesterase drugs, usually for 72 hours while supporting patient
(2) Anticholinesterase drugs are then reinstituted slowly
(3) Cholinergic symptoms may be controlled with medications such as atropine (which carries danger of masking important signs of anticholinesterase overdosage)
(d) Care for patient post thymectomy
(1) Anticholinesterase drugs may be discontinued prior to surgery. Patient will need ventilator support and frequent suctioning to handle secretions
(2) A transcervical or sternal approach may be used. Institute appropriate care after chest surgery (e.g., chest tubes)
(3) Anticholinesterase medications and/or corticosteroids will be reinstituted slowly postoperatively, starting with low doses. Assess response carefully
(4) Monitor respiratory status
(5) Remind patient that full effects of thymectomy may not be apparent for some time
(e) Care for patient undergoing plasma exchange (plasmapheresis)—process of separating blood into component parts for purpose of removing one or more components (in this case, the autoantibodies believed to be the cause of myasthenia gravis)
iv. Evaluation of nursing care
(a) Neuromuscular function maximized; absence of complications
(b) Myasthenic crisis reversed
(c) Cholinergic crisis reversed
(d) Absence of complications post thymectomy
(e) Absence of complications post plasmapheresis
b. Ineffective breathing pattern related to weakness or paralysis of respiratory muscles
i. Assessment for defining characteristics
(a) Bradypnea
(b) Shallow respirations
(c) Decreased tidal volume, vital capacity
(d) Pa_{CO_2} greater than 45 mm Hg
(e) Nasal flaring
(f) Weak cough
(g) Dyspnea
ii. Expected outcome: Maintains Pa_{CO_2} between 35 and 45 mm Hg
iii. Nursing interventions
(a) Monitor pulmonary status as indicated

        (b) Monitor tidal volume (V_T) and vital capacity (V_C)

        (c) Be prepared to assist with intubation and mechanical ventilation

        (d) Maintain Pa_{CO_2} within ordered range

        (e) Chest physical therapy as ordered

     iv. Evaluation of nursing care: Pa_{CO_2} maintained between 35 and 45 mm Hg

  c. Potential alteration in nutrition, less than body requirements related to decreased intake (see p. 441)

  d. Ineffective airway clearance related to increased secretions (see p. 368)

  e. Fluid volume deficit related to plasmapheresis (see p. 403)

  f. Ineffective individual coping related to situational crisis, loss of control and independence, and change in role (see p. 374)

Drug Intoxication

1. **Pathophysiology:** varies with drug(s) ingested, amount of drug(s) ingested, time from ingestion to treatment, and preexisting condition of patient
2. **Etiology or precipitating factors**
     a. Opioids and opiates
       i. Seen most commonly in adolescents and young adults who abuse heroin and methadone
       ii. Children who ingest parents' drugs accidentally
       iii. Health-related personnel and patients who have painful chronic illness and become dependent on narcotics; may be suicide attempt
     b. Barbiturates, sedatives, hypnotics, and tranquilizers
       i. Most commonly taken as a suicide attempt
       ii. Simultaneous ingestion of a number of drugs, often including alcohol
     c. Alcohols
       i. Most commonly seen in alcoholic population
       ii. Frequent concomitant to other drugs in suicide attempt
       iii. Common contributing/coexisting factors in multiple trauma
     d. Disulfiram (Antabuse): alcoholics who drink alcohol while under therapy
     e. Hallucinogens (e.g., LSD, mescaline, psilocybin, hashish, marijuana, cocaine, and PCP) may cause toxicity in inexperienced users or those who may not be aware of purity of drug ingested, inhaled, or injected
     f. Lithium: toxicity may result from overdose or decreased excretion or may be secondary to diuretic-induced hyponatremia
     g. Salicylates
       i. Accidental ingestion, particularly in children with fevers whose

parents either administer increased dosage or decrease the dosage interval

    ii. May also be due to extensive application of products containing methyl salicylate

    iii. Suicide attempt

    iv. Simultaneous ingestion of several drugs containing aspirin

  h. Acetaminophen

    i. Ingestion of greater than recommended dosages, usually over several days

    ii. Ingestion of several drugs containing acetaminophen

  i. Tricyclic antidepressants: accidental ingestion by children, suicide attempts, simultaneous ingestion of these agents with alcohol or other drugs

3. Nursing assessment data base

  a. Nursing history

    i. Subjective findings

      (a) Patient's chief complaint

        (1) See nursing examination of patient

        (2) Psychiatric presentation

      (b) Other symptoms—see nursing examination of patient

        (1) Suspected duration of sleep or coma

    ii. Objective findings

      (a) Presence of etiologic or precipitating factors

        (1) May need to rely on relatives, friends, police, or ambulance personnel for information

        (2) See etiology or precipitating factors

      (b) Family history—may be significant for drug or alcohol abuse, psychiatric history, family discord

      (c) Social history

        (1) Previous suicide attempts

        (2) Reasons for despondency

        (3) Previous illicit drug use

        (4) Time when last seen well

      (d) Medication history

        (1) Usual medications and dosages

        (2) Name of prescribing physician or pharmacy from bottle labels

        (3) Date last prescription filled and amount (number of pills) dispensed

      (e) Other medical problems such as seizures, diabetes, hepatitis, renal disease

  b. Nursing examination of patient

    i. Opioids and opiates

      (a) CNS—analgesia, change in level of consciousness, convulsions

    (b) Respiratory depression, aspiration, or infectious pneumonia

    (c) Hypotension

    (d) Miosis

    (e) Decreased gastric motility

    (f) Infection—local and systemic

    (g) Needle tracks, skin-popping, abscesses

ii. Barbiturates, sedatives, hypnotics, tranquilizers

    (a) CNS impairment, depressed level of consciousness, sometimes excitation

    (b) Hypothermia

    (c) Respiratory depression

    (d) Shock

    (e) Cardiac dysrhythmias

    (f) Gastric irritation may be seen with chloral hydrate overdose

    (g) Pulmonary edema has been reported with meprobamate poisoning

    (h) Methaqualone—hypertonicity, hyperreflexia, myoclonus, and seizures

    (i) Skin vesicles

iii. Alcohols

    (a) Ethanol—depends on serum levels. Varies from slurred speech and muscular incoordination to stupor, hypothermia, hypoglycemia, and seizures to coma, depressed respirations, and hyporeflexia

    (b) Methanol—characterized by CNS depression, metabolic acidosis, visual disturbances ranging from blurring to blindness

    (c) Ethylene glycol—CNS depression; cardiopulmonary complications including pulmonary edema may develop; renal tubular degeneration with renal impairment may occur

    (d) Isopropyl alcohol—CNS depression, areflexia, respiratory depression, hypothermia, hypotension, and gastrointestinal distress

iv. Disulfiram (Antabuse): hypotension, flushing of the face and skin, sensation of heat, diaphoresis, throbbing headache, nausea, vomiting, weakness, and confusion. Severe reactions include cardiovascular collapse

v. Hallucinogens: extreme agitation and anxiety

vi. Cocaine: hyperexcitability, anxiety, headache, hypertension, tachycardia, hyperpnea, tachypnea, fever, nausea, vomiting, abdominal pain, delirium, convulsions, and coma

vii. Phencyclidine (PCP): violent behavior, seizures, rhabdomyolysis, hypertensive crisis, coma, hyperthermia

    viii. Lithium
       (a) Mild—diarrhea, lethargy, weakness, polyuria, polydipsia, nystagmus, and tinnitus
       (b) Severe—hyperreflexia, ataxia, dystonia, confusion, seizures, anxiety, coma, hypotension, renal failure, heart failure
    ix. Salicylates
       (a) Tinnitus, diminished auditory acuity
       (b) CNS involvement—vertigo, vomiting, vasodilatation, hyperthermia, hyperventilation, altered mental status manifested by hallucinations, lethargy, delirium, or stupor
    x. Acetaminophen
       (a) Mild/early stage—may be asymptomatic, gastrointestinal irritation, diaphoresis, pallor
       (b) Hepatotoxicity—manifested 12 hours to 4 days later. Liver function tests increased; right upper quadrant pain may occur. Gradual return to normal may occur
       (c) Hepatic necrosis—gastrointestinal irritation and upset, jaundice, hepatosplenomegaly, hepatic encephalopathy, bleeding diathesis, and hypoglycemia. Acute tubular necrosis may develop. Dysrhythmias and shock have been reported
    xi. Tricyclic antidepressants: characterized by anticholinergic and anti-alpha-adrenergic signs
  c. Diagnostic study findings
    i. Laboratory findings
       (a) Opioids and opiates
          (1) Arterial blood gases—may reveal hypoventilation, hypoxemia
          (2) Electrolytes—may reveal imbalance due to complicating factors (e.g., trauma with blood loss)
          (3) Hematocrit—may be low when hypovolemia is due to trauma
          (4) Leukocyte count with differential—may reveal infection
          (5) Serum glucose—may reveal hypoglycemia
          (6) Serum levels of other drugs and alcohol—high percentage of opiate abusers use more than one drug at a time
          (7) Wound or blood cultures may reveal local or systemic infection
       (b) Barbiturates, sedatives, hypnotics, tranquilizers
          (1) Chromatography of gastric fluid, urine, and/or serum will detect presence of several drugs

(2) Serum levels of phenobarbital of 8 mg/dl and short-acting barbiturates of 3.5 mg/dl are potentially fatal

(3) Fatal doses of other drugs vary

(c) Alcohols

(1) Ethanol—serum levels from 0.05 mg/dl (mild intoxication) to more than 0.5 mg/dl (coma and possible death) may be detected

(2) Methanol—serum levels of 50 to 100 mg/dl indicate severe intoxication, usually with acidosis

(3) Ethylene glycol

a) Serum chemistry reveals metabolic acidosis and renal toxicity

b) Hypocalcemia may occur

c) Urinalysis—may reveal low urine specific gravity, proteinuria, microscopic hematuria, and oxylate crystals

d) Complete blood cell count—polymorphonuclear leukocytes (PMNs) with normal hematocrit

(4) Isopropyl alcohol—acetone present in urine and blood

(d) Phencyclidine (PCP)—may be detected in blood or urine

(e) Lithium

(1) Serum levels about 1.5 mEq/L represent toxicity

(2) Serum chemistries may reveal renal impairment

(f) Salicylates

(1) Arterial blood gas values reveal respiratory alkalosis and metabolic acidosis with serum levels > 40 mg/dl

(2) Electrolytes reveal metabolic acidosis with anion gap

(3) Hypoprothrombinemia and platelet dysfunction

(4) Serum glucose levels may be high or low

(5) Repeated serum levels may be necessary to determine peak level

(6) Urine—excretion of large amounts of bicarbonate, sodium, potassium, and organic acids

(7) CSF glucose levels may be disproportionately low in comparison to serum glucose levels

(8) Coagulation studies (PT, PTT, platelet count) may reveal abnormalities

(9) Liver function tests may reveal coagulation defect or salicylate hepatitis

(g) Acetaminophen

(1) Urine—recovery of metabolic by-products: sulfate conjugate, glucuronide conjugate, mercapturate conjugate, or unchanged

(2) Long plasma half-life indicates liver damage

(3) Serum levels greater than 300 µg/dl at 4 hours and

120 µg/dl at 12 hours are uniformly associated with hepatic damage
    (4) Liver enzymes elevated
    (5) Toxicology screen may reveal multiple drugs ingested
  (h) Tricyclic antidepressants—maximum serum levels occur within 24 hours after ingestion. Level greater than 1 ng/ml is potentially lethal

ii. Radiologic findings
  (a) Opioids and opiates—chest x-ray film may demonstrate pulmonary edema and infectious or aspiration pneumonia
  (b) Tricyclic antidepressants—chest x-ray film may reveal signs of pulmonary edema from congestive heart failure

iii. Special
  (a) Opioids and opiates
    (1) Gastric aspirate may be subjected to toxicologic analysis
    (2) Reversal of depressant effects with 2 mg injection of naloxone
  (b) Methanol—visual testing may reveal impairment or blindness
  (c) Tricyclic antidepressants—ECG changes may be detected, including
    (1) Prolonged QRS complex
    (2) Prolonged PR and QT intervals
    (3) ST segment and T wave abnormalities
    (4) Intraventricular conduction defects
    (5) Bundle branch blocks
    (6) Dysrhythmias

4. Nursing diagnoses

a. Potential for injury related to toxic effects of drugs ingested
  i. Assessment for defining characteristics
    (a) Opioids and opiates
      (1) CNS—respiratory arrest, transverse myelitis, abscesses, postanoxic encephalopathy
      (2) Eyes—metastatic endophthalmitis, toxic amblyopia
      (3) Cardiovascular—bacterial endocarditis, atrial fibrillation, vascular insufficiency, vasculitis, lymphedema, thrombophlebitis
      (4) Pulmonary—aspiration, septic emboli, edema, bronchoconstriction, granulomatous disease, cor pulmonale
      (5) Local and systemic infections, including possible hepatitis
    (b) Barbiturates, sedatives, hypnotics, and tranquilizers
      (1) Hypothermia with resultant dysrhythmias
      (2) Respiratory arrest, pulmonary edema

    (3) Circulatory insufficiency, shock
    (4) Gastric mucosal necrosis
    (5) Cardiac dysrhythmias and conduction changes
    (6) Methaqualone may cause seizures

(c) Alcohols
    (1) Methanol—visual impairment and blindness
    (2) Ethylene glycol—acute renal tubular necrosis, chronic interstitial nephritis
    (3) Isopropyl alcohol—depressed respirations, hypotension, hypothermia, gastric irritation

(d) Hallucinogens—severe agitation and anxiety

(e) Cocaine
    (1) Respiratory arrest
    (2) Seizures
    (3) Coma
    (4) Psychologic dependency

(f) Phencyclidine (PCP)
    (1) Seizures
    (2) Hypertensive crisis
    (3) Rhabdomyolysis
    (4) Cardiac arrest

(g) Lithium
    (1) Renal failure
    (2) Heart failure
    (3) Seizures

(h) Salicylates
    (1) Renal tubular necrosis
    (2) Gastrointestinal hemorrhage, pylorospasm
    (3) Hepatotoxicity

(i) Acetaminophen
    (1) Hepatic failure
    (2) Shock (rare)
    (3) Dysrhythmia (rare)

(j) Tricyclic antidepressants
    (1) Seizures
    (2) Coma
    (3) Dysrhythmias
    (4) ECG changes
    (5) Heart failure
    (6) Shock

ii. Expected outcomes
  (a) Maintains vital organ function
  (b) Does not continue to absorb drug
  (c) Eliminates ingested drug

iii. Nursing interventions

(a) Support vital functions
  (1) Protect patients with CNS depression
     a) Treat hypothermia
     b) Administer naloxone, up to 2 mg IV in patients with respiratory and/or CNS depression
     c) Administer 50 to 100 ml of 50% glucose with thiamine 50 mg IV
     d) Treat seizure activity with appropriate drugs
  (2) Endotracheal intubation if gag and cough reflexes depressed or if gastric lavage is initiated in the lethargic patient. Avoid oropharyngeal airway
     a) Monitor breath sounds and chest x-ray film for aspiration, pulmonary edema
     b) Assess arterial blood gases
  (3) Maintain cardiovascular function
     a) Initiate intravenous line
     b) Treat hypovolemia; initially crystalloids are usually used
     c) Monitor ECG for conduction changes and dysrhythmias, especially in patients with tricyclic antidepressant overdose. Treat those problems that compromise circulation
     d) Assess for and prevent congestive heart failure
  (4) Maintain renal function
     a) Monitor urine for myoglobin; obtain toxicology screen
     b) Maintain urine output
  (5) Monitor hepatic function
     a) Assess liver function tests and enzymes
     b) Measure coagulation times and factors
(b) Identify causative agents
  (1) Urine, gastric contents, and blood for toxicology
  (2) Investigate contributing factors
  (3) Monitor biochemical status
(c) Prevent further absorption of drug
  (1) Gastric lavage—place patient in left lateral decubitus position; insert 30 to 36 F Ewald or Levacuator tube orally
  (2) Obtain abdominal x-ray films to identify coalesced mass of pills in patients whose blood levels continue to rise or who fail to recover. Gastroscopy may be necessary
  (3) Induction of vomiting
     a) Should be done only in alert patients
     b) Syrup of ipecac or apomorphine may be used

        c) Patient should remain sitting; if level of consciousness decreases, remove ipecac by lavage

        d) Do not use ipecac with activated charcoal

        e) Depressant effects of apomorphine may be reversed with naloxone

    (4) Absorption of toxin

        a) Activated charcoal may be given orally or via gastric tube lavage

        b) Small aliquots (e.g., 300 ml) recommended to prevent passage of stomach contents into duodenum

        c) Some clinicians recommend removal of charcoal after a brief time; others maintain that it can absorb drugs from small intestine

(d) Facilitate removal of drug(s)

    (1) Dialysis and hemoperfusion

        a) Useful very early in massive overdose before drug becomes stored in body depots

        b) Not effective with all drugs

        c) Indications include

           ☐ Severe clinical intoxication

           ☐ Ingestion of potentially lethal dose

           ☐ Blood levels in fatal range

           ☐ Impairment of normal route of excretion

           ☐ Presence of toxin that is metabolized to a more noxious substance

           ☐ Progressive clinical deterioration

           ☐ Prolonged coma

           ☐ Underlying pathology that compromises recovery

           ☐ Development of complications

           ☐ Ingestion of agents known to produce delayed toxicity

    (2) Forced osmotic diuresis

        a) May be useful in management of ethanol, methanol, ethylene glycol, and isoniazid overdoses

        b) Water and osmotic agents (mannitol, glucose, and urea) have been used

        c) Monitor patient for fluid overload and electrolyte disturbances

        d) Stabilize cardiopulmonary status prior to initiation

        e) Insert urinary catheter

    (3) Forced alkaline and acid diuresis

        a) Urinary alkalinization with sodium bicarbonate recommended in management of salicylate poison-

ing; monitor acid–base and fluid and electrolyte status carefully
  b) Urinary acidification may be accomplished with ascorbic acid or ammonium chloride. Recommended with amphetamines and PCP; monitor acid–base and fluid and electrolyte status hourly
(4) Other
  a) Acetylcysteine (Mucomyst) orally in treatment of acetaminophen overdose; activated charcoal should not be used simultaneously
  b) Physostigmine may be used to reverse the anticholinergic effects of tricyclic antidepressant overdose; carries risk of cholinergic toxicity
iv. Evaluation of nursing care
  (a) Vital organ functions maintained
  (b) Causative agents identified
  (c) Absorption of drug(s) minimized
  (d) Absorbed drug(s) eliminated
b. Potential for self-directed violence related to drug overdose
  i. Assessment for defining characteristics
    (a) Substance abuse or withdrawal
    (b) Aggressive suicidal behavior
    (c) Real or threatened loss of loved one, memory, prestige, job, health
    (d) Feelings of helplessness, loneliness, hopelessness
    (e) Angry facial expression
    (f) Fear of self
    (g) Vulnerable self-esteem
    (h) Verbalizes dependence on drugs
    (i) Verbalizes suicidal ideation
  ii. Expected outcomes
    (a) Regains psychologic stability
    (b) Verbalizes intention to seek follow-up with mental health professional
  iii. Nursing interventions
    (a) Support the restoration of psychologic well-being
    (b) Approach in a nonjudgmental manner
    (c) Listen carefully to what patient has to say about current situation. Do not challenge
    (d) Demonstrate understanding, but do not reinforce denial
    (e) Supervise administration of prescribed medications
    (f) Make appropriate referrals to mental health professionals
    (g) Provide with information regarding resources (e.g. hot lines, crisis centers, counselors, etc.)
  iv. Evaluation of nursing care

   (a) Psychologic state stabilizes
   (b) Seeks follow-up with mental health professional
c. Impaired gas exchange related to altered oxygen supply or oxygen-carrying capacity (see p. 367)
d. Ineffective breathing pattern related to depressed level of consciousness and metabolic imbalance (see p. 368, omitting references to ICP)
e. Ineffective airway clearance related to increased secretions and depressed level of consciousness (see p. 368, omitting references to ICP)
f. Potential fluid volume deficit related to excessive loss and decreased intake (see p. 369)
g. Ineffective individual coping related to situational crisis, loss of control and independence, and change in role (see p. 374)

Recovery from General Anesthesia

1. **Pathophysiology**
   a. Recovery from inhaled anesthetics is function of alveolar ventilation, solubility coefficient of agent, and duration of anesthesia
   b. Recovery from narcotic-based anesthesia depends on dose given, postoperative renal function, and urine output
   c. Recovery from neuromuscular blocking agents is influenced by nature of agent given, dose, and renal and hepatic function. Also affected by body temperature, acid–base status, electrolyte status, and other drugs (e.g., antibiotics, furosemide)
2. **Etiology or precipitating factors:** depends on preoperative condition, type of surgery, anesthetic agent(s) used, duration of anesthesia, and intraoperative course
3. **Nursing assessment data base**
   a. Nursing history
      i. Subjective findings
         (a) Patient's chief complaint—not applicable
         (b) Other symptoms—previous surgical procedures
      ii. Objective findings
         (a) Presence of etiologic and precipitating factors—dependent on preoperative condition, type of surgery, anesthetic agent(s) used, duration of anesthesia, and intraoperative course
         (b) Family history—malignant hyperthermia
         (c) Social history
            (1) Illicit drug use
            (2) Smoking
         (d) Medication history—current medications, dosage, and frequency

b. Nursing examination of patient
  i. Inspection
    (a) Cough reflexes from the carina, then the larynx, return first
    (b) Swallow and vomiting reflex(es) return next with recovery of pharyngeal muscle tone
    (c) Consciousness returns, along with diminution of respiratory and cardiovascular depression
    (d) Some patients have a period of excitement. Potentiated by preoperative administration of scopolamine, phenothiazines, and barbiturates without narcotics
  ii. Palpation: deep anesthesia results in reduced muscle tone, which increases in postanesthesia phase
  iii. Percussion: deep anesthesia results in absent reflexes that return in the postanesthesia phase
  iv. Auscultation
    (a) Breath sounds diminished
    (b) Blood pressure may be lowered or may fluctuate
c. Diagnostic study findings
  i. Laboratory findings
    (a) Complete blood cell count—may reveal inadequate erythrocyte volume or platelets if blood loss was significant; leukocyte count may indicate infection
    (b) Electrolytes—may reveal imbalances (e.g., sodium, potassium, calcium, magnesium)
    (c) Chemistries—may reveal imbalances, (e.g., blood urea nitrogen, creatinine, glucose)
    (d) Arterial blood gas analysis—may reveal hypoxemia, hypoventilation or hyperventilation, metabolic acidosis or alkalosis
    (e) Clotting studies—may reveal coagulopathy
  ii. Radiologic findings
    (a) Chest x-ray film—may reveal pulmonary edema, pneumothorax, atelectasis, or aspiration pneumonitis
    (b) Other tests may be necessary, depending on type of surgery
4. **Nursing diagnoses**
  a. Potential for injury related to systemic complications secondary to general anesthesia
    i. Assessment for defining characteristics
      (a) Cardiovascular
        (1) Dysrhythmias—hypoxemia, drugs
        (2) Cardiac conduction changes
        (3) Hypotension—may be caused by blood loss, fluid loss, anesthesia, depressant effects of cellular elements, vasodilatation

        (4) Hypertension—caused by pain, hypercapnia, hypoxemia, or fluid overload

    (b) Respiratory

        (1) Hypoxemia—ventilation/perfusion mismatch, shunt, atelectasis

        (2) Hypoventilation or hyperventilation—obtundation, pain

        (3) Pneumothorax

        (4) Pulmonary edema

        (5) Pulmonary embolus

        (6) Aspiration pneumonia

        (7) Atelectasis

    (c) Renal

        (1) Acute tubular necrosis—resulting from sepsis or excessive circulating hemoglobin or myoglobin

        (2) Prerenal oliguria—resulting from hypovolemia, hypoperfusion

    (d) Bleeding

        (1) Loss of vascular integrity

        (2) Disseminated intravascular coagulation

    (e) Nausea and vomiting

    (f) Agitation and pain

    (g) Hypothermia or hyperthermia

    (h) Fluid and electrolyte imbalances

    (i) Persistent neuromuscular blockade

    (j) Anoxic-ischemic brain damage

 ii. Expected outcomes

    (a) Recovers completely from anesthetic agents

    (b) Absence of systemic complications and sequelae

iii. Nursing interventions

    (a) Preoperative assessment of physical and psychologic status of patient will provide baseline data postoperatively

    (b) Anesthesiologist/surgeon should report the following information to the nurse

        (1) Patient's name, age, native language

        (2) Surgical procedure, length of surgery, name of surgeon

        (3) Preoperative medications and anesthestic agent(s) used

        (4) Previous medical history, including medications, allergies, mental status, and communication handicaps

        (5) Intraoperative course, including vital signs, medications, dysrhythmias, and estimated blood loss and replacement

        (6) Monitoring required and problems anticipated from anesthesia and/or surgical procedure

(c) Initial assessment should be carried out by anesthesiologist and nurse on admission to recovery room or ICU

(d) Different anesthetic agents have different durations of action. Effect of each drug given must be assessed (e.g., narcotics given with neuromuscular block agents). Factors that may affect reversal of anesthesia must also be sought (See etiology or precipitating factors)

(1) Assess arousability by calling patient's name

(2) Assess gag and swallow reflexes

(3) Assess for reversal of neuromuscular blockade

  a) Ability to sustain head lifting, eye opening, and hand grasp

  b) Ability to extrude tongue for 5 to 10 seconds

  c) Vital capacity of 10 to 15 ml/kg and inspiratory force of -25 cm H_2O

  d) Neostigmine or pyridostigmine may be given to hasten reversal

(4) Naloxone is given to reverse respiratory depression of opiates, but its duration may be shorter than that of the narcotic. Respiratory depression may recur 30 to 60 minutes after naloxone. Maintain observation

  a) Along with reversal of respiratory depression with naloxone comes pain, coughing, and agitation

  b) Patients who are intubated with respiratory support may be allowed to recover from effects of narcotics without reversal

(e) Continuous monitoring for systemic complications

(1) Respiratory

  a) Measurements of ventilation—V_C, V_T, V_E, V_D/V_T, inspiratory force

  b) Rate, rhythm, use of accessory muscles

  c) Breath sounds, adventitious sounds

  d) Arterial blood gases

(2) Cardiovascular

  a) ECG—rate, rhythm, conduction

  b) Blood pressure via cuff, Doppler, or intra-arterial catheter

  c) Hemodynamic integrity—CVP, PAP, PCWP, CO as necessary

  d) Peripheral circulation and pulses

  e) Heart sounds

(3) Central nervous system

  a) Level of consciousness

  b) Protective reflexes, pupillary reflexes

  c) Motor ability

    d) ICP monitoring as necessary; calculation of cerebral perfusion pressure

    e) Tests for neuromuscular blockade reversal. Note that neuromuscular blockade may be increased by hypothermia, hypermagnesemia, hypercalcemia, inhalation anesthetic agents, almost all antibiotics, furosemide, and renal failure

(4) Temperature

    a) Hypothermia may be caused by cold environments, obtundation of thermoregulatory centers, and vasodilatation

    b) Hyperthermia may be caused by infection or reaction to anesthetic—malignant hyperthermia

(5) Renal

    a) Fluid balance, urine output

    b) Electrolytes

    c) Blood urea nitrogen, creatinine

(6) Gastrointestinal

    a) Nausea and vomiting may be caused by any anesthetic agents

    b) Aspiration most common complication

    c) Opiates stimulate vomiting reflex while obtunding protective reflexes

(7) Pain—should be controlled with opiates if severe

    a) May cause nausea if used alone

    b) Monitor patient for respiratory and cardiovascular depression

    c) Titrate dose to patient response

    d) Barbiturates and phenothiazine drugs should not be used alone (i.e., without an analgesic) in patients who are in pain. Barbiturates and phenothiazines cause increased sensitivity to pain and restlessness

    e) Initially analgesics should be given intramuscularly or intravenously

iv. Evaluation of nursing care

    (a) Returns to preoperative status after anesthesia

    (b) Systemic complications and sequelae prevented and/or treated

b. Potential for hyperthermia related to malignant hyperthermia

  i. Assessment for defining characteristics

    (a) High body temperature (greater than 105.8° F [41° C])

    (b) Marked skeletal rigidity

    (c) Metabolic and respiratory acidosis, frequently with a base deficit of greater than 10 mmol

      (d) Myocardial changes, usually manifested as dysrhythmias

      (e) Marked hyperkalemia

      (f) Muscle breakdown as manifested by gross increases in serum creatine phosphokinase and myoglobinuria

      (g) Family history

  ii. Expected outcomes

      (a) Temperature maintained within normal range

      (b) Experiences no systemic complications

  iii. Nursing interventions

      (a) Monitor temperature frequently in known or suspected susceptible persons

      (b) Administer dantrolene sodium as ordered, usually 2 to 4 mg/kg IV in fast running IV (pH 9–10). May be repeated at 15-minute intervals as necessary, up to 10 mg/kg total

      (c) Monitor electrolytes, particularly calcium and potassium

      (d) Monitor creatine phosphokinase levels

      (e) Monitor urine for signs of myoglobinuria; send specimen for analysis

      (f) Monitor cardiac rate and rhythm

      (g) Monitor arterial blood gases and serum bicarbonate levels

c. Nursing diagnoses that may be applicable should the patient develop complications include

  i. Impaired gas exchange related to altered oxygen supply or oxygen-carrying capacity (see p. 367)

  ii. Ineffective breathing pattern related to depressed level of consciousness, intracranial pathology, and metabolic imbalance (see p. 368)

  iii. Ineffective airway clearance related to increased secretions and depressed level of consciousness (see p. 368)

  iv. Fluid volume deficit related to excessive loss and decreased intake (see p. 369)

  v. Fluid volume excess related to excessive intake (see p. 370)

  vi. Alteration in comfort or pain related to surgical procedure or wound (see p. 426)

References

Adelstein, R., and Watson, P.: Cervical spine injuries. J. Neurosurg. Nurs. 15:65–71, 1983.

Alberico, A. M., Ward, J. D., Choi, S. C., et al.: Outcome after severe head injury: Relationship to mass lesions, diffuse injury, and ICP course in pediatric and adult patients. J. Neurosurg. 67:648–656, 1987.

Batjer, H., Devous, M. D., Seibert, G. B., et al.: Intracranial arteriovenous malformation: Relationship between clinical factors and surgical complications. Neurosurgery 24:75–79, 1989.

Batjer, H., and Samson, D: Surgical approaches to trigonal arteriovenous malformations. J. Neurosurg. 67:511–517, 1987.

Becker, D. M., Gonzalez, M., Gentilli, A., et al.: Prevention of deep venous thrombosis in patients with acute spinal cord injuries: Use of rotating treatment tables. Neurosurgery 20:675–677, 1987.

Black, P. L., Crowell, R. M., and Abbott, W. M.: External pneumatic calf compression reduces deep vein thrombosis in patients with ruptured intracranial aneurysms. Neurosurgery 18:25–28, 1986.

Black, P. M.: Hydrocephalus and vasospasm after subarachnoid hemorrhage from ruptured intracranial aneurysms. Neurosurgery 18:12–16, 1986.

Blount, M., Kinney, A. B., and Luttrell, N.: Myasthenia gravis and Guillain-Barré syndrome. In Nikas, D. L. (ed.): The Critically Ill Neurosurgical Patient. Churchill Livingstone, New York, 1982.

Borovich, B., Braun, J., Guilburd, J. N., et al.: Delayed onset of traumatic extradural hematoma. J. Neurosurg. 63:30–34, 1985.

Bose, B., Northrup, B. E., Osterholm, J. L., et al.: Reanalysis of central cervical cord injury management. Neurosurgery 15:367–372, 1984.

Boss, B. J.: Dysphasia, dyspraxia, and dysarthria: Distinguishing features: I. J. Neurosurg. Nurs. 16:151–159, 1984.

Bracken, M. B., Shepard, M. J., Hillenbrand, K. G., et al.: Methlyprednisolone and neurological function one year after spinal cord injury. J. Neurosurg. 63:704–713, 1985.

Bricolo, A. P., and Pasut, L. M.: Extradural hematoma: Toward zero mortality. Neurosurgery 14:8–12, 1984.

Brown, J. T., ed.: Fluid and Blood Therapy in Anesthesia. Contemporary Anesthesia Practice. F. A. Davis Co., Philadelphia, 1983.

Bucci, M. N., Phillips, T. W., and McGillicuddy, J. E.: Delayed epidural hemorrhage in hypotensive multiple trauma patients. Neurosurgery 19:65–68, 1986.

Camel, M., and Grubb, R. L.: Treatment of chronic subdural hematoma by twist-drill craniostomy with continuous catheter drainage. J. Neurosurg. 65:183–187, 1986.

Carpenter, M. G.: Core Text of Neuroanatomy. Williams & Wilkins, Baltimore, 1983.

Carpenter, R.: Infections and head injury: A potentially lethal combination. Crit. Care Nurs. Q. 10:1–11, 1987.

Chan, R. C., Schweigel, J. F., and Thompson, G. B.: Halo-thoracic brace immobilization in 188 patients with acute cervical spine injuries. J. Neurosurg. 58:508–515, 1983.

Chilton, J., and Dagi, T. F.: Acute cervical spinal cord injury. Am. J. Emerg. Med. 3:340–351, 1985.

Claus-Walker, J., and Halstead, L. S.: Metabolic and endocrine changes in spinal cord injury: II (sections 1 and 2). Partial decentralization of the autonomic nervous system. Arch. Phys. Med. Rehabil. 63:569–580, 1982.

Collins, W. F.: A review of treatment of spinal cord injury. Br. J. Surg. 71:974–975, 1984.

Constantini, S., Cotev, S., Rappaport, Z. H., et al.: Intracranial pressure monitoring after elective intracranial surgery. J. Neurosurg. 69:540–544, 1988.

Cooper, P. R., and Ho, V.: Role of emergency skull x-ray films in the evaluation of head injured patients: A retrospective study. Neurosurgery 13:136–140, 1983.

Cope, D. N., Date, E. S., and Mar, E. Y.: Serial computerized tomographic evaluation in traumatic head injury. Arch. Phys. Med. Rehabil. 69:483–486, 1988.

Cormack, R. S.: Postoperative recovery. In Gray, T. C., Nunn, J. F., and Utting, J. E. (eds.): General Anesthesia. Butterworth & Co., London, 1980.

Corrigan, J. D., and Mysiw, J.: Agitation following traumatic head injury: Equivocal evidence for a discrete stage of cognitive recovery. Arch. Phys. Med. Rehabil. 69:487–492, 1988.

Davne, S. H.: Emergency care of acute spinal cord injury. Am. J. Paraplegia Soc. 6:42–46, 1983.

Dearden, N. M., Gibson, J. S., McDowell, D. G., et al.: Effect of high dose dexamethasone on outcome from severe head injury. J. Neurosurg. 64:81–88, 1986.

Dempsey, R., Rapp, R. P., Young, B., et al.: Prophylactic parenteral antibiotics in clean neurosurgical procedures: A review. J. Neurosurg. 69:52–57, 1988.

Durack, D. T., and Perfect, J. R.: Acute bacterial meningitis. In Wilkins, R. H., and Rengachary, S. S. (eds.): Neurosurgery. McGraw-Hill Book Co., New York, 1985, vol. 2, pp. 1921–1927.

Durward, G. J., et al.: The influence of systemic arterial pressure and intracranial pressure on the development of cerebral vasogenic edema. J. Neurosurg. 59:803–809, 1983.

Eisenberg, H. M., Frankowski, R. F., Contant, C. F., et al.: High-dose barbiturate control of elevated intracranial pressure in patients with severe head injury. J. Neurosurg. 69:15–23, 1988.

Engelke, M. K.: Teaching the patient with a neurologic deficit. J. Neurosurg. Nurs. 15:107–111, 1983.

Faden, A. I.: Pharmacological therapy in acute spinal cord injury: Experimental strategies and future directions. In Becker, V. T., and Povlishock, J. T. (eds.): CNS Trauma Status Report. NINCDS, Bethesda, Md., 1985, pp. 481–485.

Faden, A., Jacobs, T. P., Patrick, D. H., et al.: Megadose corticosteroid therapy following traumatic spinal cord injury. J. Neurosurg. 60:712–717, 1984.

Fegoni, S. F.: Cardiovascular and haemodynamic responses to tilting and to standing in tetraplegic patients: A review. Paraplegia 22:99–109, 1984.

Felley, T. W.: The recovery room. In Miller, R. D. (ed.): Anesthesia. Churchill Livingstone, New York, 1981.

Finn, S. S., et al.: Observations on the perioperative management of aneurysmal subarachnoid hemorrhage. J. Neurosurg. 65:48–62, 1986.

Flamm, E. S., Young, W., Collins, W. F., et al.: A phase I trial of naloxone treatment in acute spinal cord injury. J. Neurosurg. 63:390–397, 1985.

Fleischer, A. S., and Tendall, G. T.: Cerebral vasospasm following aneurysm rupture: A protocol for therapy and prophylaxis. J. Neurosurg. 52:149–152, 1980.

Fowkes, F. R. G., Williams, L. A., Cooke, B. R. B., et al.: Implementation of guidelines for the use of skull radiographs in patients with head injuries. Lancet 2:795, 1985.

Gardner, B. P., Watt, J. W. H., and Krishnan, K. R.: The artificial ventilation of acute spinal cord–damaged patients: A retrospective study of forty-four patients. Paraplegia 24:208–220, 1986.

Garretson, H. D.: Intracranial arteriovenous malformations. In Wilkins, R. H., and Rengachary, S. S. (eds.): Neurosurgery. McGraw-Hill Book Co., New York, 1985, vol. 2, pp. 1448–1458.

Garvey, G.: Current concepts of bacterial infections of the central nervous system: Bacterial meningitis and bacterial brain abscess. J. Neurosurg. 59:735–744, 1983.

Gary, N., and Tresznewsky, O.: Barbiturates and a potpourri of other sedatives, hypnotics, and tranquilizers. Heart Lung 12:122–127, 1983.

Gennarelli, T. A.: Cerebral concussion and diffuse brain injuries. In Cooper, R. R. (ed.): Head Injury. Williams & Wilkins, Baltimore, 1982.

Gennarelli, T. A.: Emergency department management of head injuries. Emerg. Med. Clin. North Am. 4:47–57, 1984.

Gennis, P.: Coma. Top. Emerg. Med. 4:47–57, 1982.

Gentry, L. R., Godersky, J. C., Thompson, B., et al.: Prospective comparative study of intermediate-filed MR and CT in the evaluation of closed head trauma. Am. J. Radiol. 150:673–682, 1988.

Gentry, L. R., Godersky, J. C., and Thompson, B.: MR imaging of head trauma: Review of the distribution and radiopathologic features of traumatic lesions. Am. J. Radiol. 150:663–672, 1988.

Gilbert, V. E., Beals, J. D., Natelson, S. E., et al.: Treatment of cerebrospinal fluid leaks and gram-negative bacillary meningitis with large doses of intrathecal amikacin and systemic antibiotics. Neurosurgery 18:402–406, 1986.

Goldberg, H. I.: Radiology of ischemic cerebrovascular disease. In Wilkins, R. H., and Rengachary, S. S. (eds.): Neurosurgery. McGraw-Hill Book Co., New York, 1985, vol. 2, pp. 1219–1236.

Goldfrank, L., Bresnitz, E., and Weisman, R.: Opioids and opiates. Heart Lung 12:114–122, 1983.

Green, B. A., Marshall, L. F., and Gallagher, T. J.: Intensive Care for Neurological Trauma and Disease. Academic Press, New York, 1982.

Green, D., Rossi, E. C., Yao, J. S. T., et al.: Deep vein thrombosis: Effect of prophylaxis with calf compression, aspirin, and dipyridamole. Paraplegia 20:227–234, 1982.

Grolomund, P., Weber, M., Seiler, R. W., et al.: Time course of cerebral vasospasm after severe head injury. Lancet 1:1173, 1988.

Gronert, G. A., Mott, J., and Lee, J.: Aetiology of malignant hyperthermia. Br. J. Anaesth. 60:253–267, 1988.

Grotenhuis, J. A., Bettag, W., Feibach, B. J., et al.: Intracarotid slow bolus injection of nimodipine during angiography for treatment of cerebral vasospasm after SAH. J. Neurosurg. 61:231–241, 1984.

Gudeman, S. K., et al.: Gastric secretory and mucosal injury response to severe head trauma. Neurosurgery 12:175–179, 1983.

Gwan, K., et al.: Interpretation of nuclear magnetic resonance tomograms of the brain. J. Neurosurg. 59:574–584, 1983.

Haghighi, S. S., Chehrazi, B. B., and Wagner, F. C.: Effect of nimodipine-associated hypotension on recovery from spinal cord injury in cats. Surg. Neurol. 29:293–297, 1988.

Hart, R. G., et al.: Occurrence and implications of seizures in subarachnoid hemorrhage due to ruptured intracranial aneurysms. Neurosurgery 8:417–421, 1981.

Hijdra, A., Vermeulem, M., van Gijn, J., et al.: Rerupture of intracranial aneurysms: A clinicoanatomic study. J. Neurosurg. 67:29–33, 1987.

Hitchon, P. W., McKay, T. C., Wilkinson, T. T., et al.: Methylprednisolone in spinal cord compression. Spine 14:16–22, 1989.

Holliday, P. O., Kelly, D. L., and Ball, M.: Normal computed tomograms in acute head injury: Correlation of intracranial pressure, ventricular size, and outcome. Neurosurgery 10:25–28, 1982.

Hugenholtz, H., and Elgie, R. G.: Considerations in early surgery on good-risk patients with ruptured aneurysms. J. Neurosurg. 58:180–185, 1982.

Husk, G. T.: Seizures. Top. Emerg. Med. 4:59–68, 1982.

Jackson, L. O.: Cerebral vasospasm after an intracranial aneurysmal subarachnoid hemorrhage: A nursing perspective. Heart Lung 15:14–22, 1986.

Jennett, B., and Teasdale, G.: Management of Head Injuries. F. A. Davis Co., Philadelphia, 1981.

Kadowaki, M. H., Watanabe, H., Numoto, M., et al.: Necessity for ICP monitoring to supplement GCS in head trauma cases. Neurochirurgia 31:39–44, 1988.

Kakulas, B. A.: The clinical neuropathology of spinal cord injury: A guide to the future. Paraplegia 25:212–216, 1987.

Kanter, R. K., Weiner, L. B., Patti, A. M., et al.: Infectious complications and duration of intracranial pressure monitoring. Crit. Care Med. 13:837–839, 1985.

Kassell, N. F., et al.: Treatment of ischemic deficits from vasospasm with intravascular expansion and induced hypertension. Neurosurgery 18:101–106, 1982.

Kassell, N. F., and Boarini, D. J.: Patients with ruptured aneurysm: Pre- and postoperative management. In Wilkins, R. H., and Rengachary, S. S. (eds.): Neurosurgery. McGraw-Hill Book Co., New York, 1985, vol. 2, pp. 1367–1371.

Kassell, N. F., and Drake, C. G.: Timing of aneurysm surgery. Neurosurgery 10:514–519, 1982.

Keithley, J. K.: Infection and the malnourished patient. Heart Lung 12:23–27, 1983.

Klauber, M. R., Marshall, L. F., Luerssen, T. G., et al.: Determinants of head injury mortality: Importance of the low risk patient. Neurosurgery 24:31–36, 1989.

Klauber, M. R., Marshall, L. F., Toole, B. M., et al.: Cause of decline in head-injury mortality rate in San Diego County, California. J. Neurosurg. 62:528–531, 1985.

Kusske, J. A.: Cerebral resuscitation in the trauma patient. Prog. Crit. Care Med. 1:147–170, 1984.

Leramo, O. B., Tator, C. H., and Hudson, A. R.: Massive gastroduodenal hemorrhage and perforation in acute spinal cord injury. Surg. Neurol. 17:186–190, 1982.

Lester, M. C., and Nelson, P. G.: Neurological aspects of vasopressin release and the syndrome of inappropriate secretion of antidiuretic hormone. Neurosurgery 8:735–740, 1981.

Lillehei, K. O., and Hoff, J. T.: Advances in the management of closed head injury. Ann. Emerg. Med. 14:789–795, 1985.

Ljunggren, B., Brandt, L., Saveland, H., et al.: Outcome in 60 consecutive patients treated with early aneurysm operation and intravenous nimodipine. J. Neurosurg. 61:864–873, 1984.

Lloyd, L. K., Kuhlemeier, K. V., Fine, P. R., et al.: Initial bladder management in spinal cord injury: Does it make a difference? J. Urol. 135:523–527, 1986.

Lobato, R. D., et al.: Outcome from severe head injury related to the type of intracranial lesion. J. Neurosurg. 59:762–774, 1983.

Lokkeberg, A. R., and Grimes, R. M.: Assessing the influence of nontreatment variables in the study of outcome from severe head injuries. J. Neurosurg. 61:254–262, 1984.

Lougheed, M. G.: Brain resuscitation and protection. Med. J. Aust. 148:458–466, 1988.

Lovely, M. P., and Ozuna, J.: Status epilepticus. In Nikas, D. L. (ed.): The Critically Ill Neurosurgical Patient. Churchill Livingstone, New York, 1982.

Mackenzie, C. F., Shin, B., Krishnaprasad, D., et al.: Assessment of cardiac and respiratory function during surgery on patients with acute quadriplegia. J. Neurosurg. 62:843–849, 1985.

Marshall, L. F., Barba, D., Toole, B. M., et al.: The oval pupil: Clinical significance and relationship to intracranial hypertension. J. Neurosurg. 58:566–568, 1983.

Marshall, L. F., Becker, D. P., Bowers, S. A., et al.: The National Traumatic Coma Data Bank: I. Design, purpose, goals, and results. J. Neurosurg. 59:276–284, 1983.

Marshall, L. F., and Eisenberg, H. M.: ICP monitoring in severe head injury (letter): J. Neurosurg. 67:952–953, 1987.

Marshall, L. F., Knowlton, S., Garfin, S. R., et al.: Deterioration following spinal cord injury. J. Neurosurg. 66:400–404, 1987.

Marshall, L. F., Toole, B. M., and Bowers, S. A.: The national traumatic coma data bank: II. Patients who talk and deteriorate: Implications for treatment. J. Neurosurg. 59:285–288, 1983.

Martuza, R. L.: Neuro-oncology: An overview. In Wilkins, R. H., and Rengachary, S. S. (eds.): Neurosurgery. McGraw-Hill Book Co., New York, 1985, vol. 1, pp. 505–510.

Mass, A. I. R., Braakman, R., Schouten, H. J. A., et al.: Agreement between physicians on assessment of outcome following severe head injury. J. Neurosurg. 58:321–325, 1983.

Mathern, G. W., Martin, N. A., and Becker, D. P.: Cerebral ischemia: Clinical pathophysiology. In Cerra, F. B., and Shoemaker, W. C. (eds.): Critical Care: State of the Art. Society of Critical Care Medicine, Fullerton, Calif., 1987.

McCagg, C.: Postoperative management and acute rehabilitation of patients with spinal cord injuries. Orthop. Clin. North Am. 17:171–182, 1986.

McCarthy, E.: Cardiovascular complications of intracranial disorders. In Nikas, D. L. (ed.): The Critically Ill Neurosurgical Patient. Churchill Livingstone, New York, 1982.

McComb, J. G.: Recent research into the nature of cerebrospinal fluid formation and absorption. J. Neurosurg. 59:369–383, 1983.

McDonald, J. A.: Colloid cyst of the third ventricle and sudden death. Ann. Emerg. Med. 11:365–367, 1982.

McGillicuddy, J. E.: Cerebral protection: Pathophysiology and treatment of increased intracranial pressure. Chest 87:85–93, 1985.

McGraw, C. P., and Howard, G.: Effect of mannitol on increased intracranial pressure. Neurosurgery 13:269–271, 1983.

McKenna, P., Willison, J. R., Phil, B., et al.: Cognitive outcome and quality of life one year after subarachnoid hemorrhage. Neurosurgery 24:361–367, 1989.

McLaurin, R. L., and King, L. R.: Metabolic effects in head injury. In Vinken, P. J., and Bruyn, G. W. (eds.): Handbook of Clinical Neurology: Injuries of the Brain and Skull, Part I. American Elsevier Publishing Co., New York, 1975, pp. 109–131.

McMicken, D. B.: Emergence CT head scans in traumatic and atraumatic conditions. Ann. Emerg. Med. 15:274–279, 1986.

Mendelow, A. D., et al.: A clinical comparison of subdural screw pressure measurements with ventricular pressure. J. Neurosurg. 58:45–50, 1983.

Messeter, K., Nordstrom, C. H., Sundberg, G., et al.: Cerebral hemodynamics in patients with acute severe head trauma. J. Neurosurg. 64:231–237, 1986.

Miller, J. D.: Head injury and brain ischaemia—implications for therapy. Br. J. Anaesth. 57:120–129, 1985.

Mirr, M. P., Jankowski, K., and Taylon, M. A.: Nursing management for barbiturate therapy in acute head injuries. Heart Lung 12:52–59, 1983.

Mitchell, C., and Scott, S.: Total parenteral nutrition: A nursing perspective. Heart Lung 11:426–429, 1982.

Mitchell, P. J.: Intracranial pressure: Dynamics, assessment and control. In Nikas, D. L. (ed.): The Critically Ill Neurosurgical Patient. Churchill Livingstone, New York, 1982.

Mitchell, S. K., and Yates, R. R.: Cerebral vasospasm: Theoretical causes, medical management, and nursing implications. J. Neurosci. Nurs. 18:315–324, 1986.

Mollman, H. D., Rockswold, G. L., and Ford, S. E.: A clinical comparison of subarachnoid catheters to ventriculostomy and subarachnoid bolts: A prospective study. J. Neurosurg. 68:737–741, 1988.

Moossy, J.: Pathology of ischemic vascular disease. In Wilkins, R. H., and Rengachary, S. S. (eds.): Neurosurgery. Mc-Graw Hill Book Co., New York, 1985, vol. 2, pp. 1193–1198.

Moran, J. L.: Latent and manifest hyperosmolal states—two consequences of osmotherapy for head injury. Anaesth. Intensive Care 10:365–369, 1982.

Moser, K. M., and Fedullo, D. F.: Venous thromboembolism, three simple decisions: I. Chest 83:117–121, 1983.

Nagashima, H.: Drug interactions in the recovery room. In Frost, E. A., and Andrews, I. C.: Recovery Room Care. Little, Brown & Co., Boston, 1983.

National Institutes of Health: Diagnostic criterion for Guillain-Barré. JAMA. 240:1709–1711, 1978.

Nelson, P. B., et al.: Hyponatremia in intracranial disease: Perhaps not the syndrome of inappropriate secretion of antidiuretic hormone. J. Neurosurg. 55:938–941, 1981.

Newlon, P. G., and Greenberg, R. P.: Evoked potentials in severe head injury. J. Trauma 24:61–66, 1984.

Nikas, D. L.: Pathophysiology and nursing interventions in acute spinal cord injury. Trauma Q. 4(3):23–44, 1988.

Nikas, D. L.: Critical aspects of head trauma. Crit. Care Nurs. Q. 10:19–44, 1987.

Nikas, D. L.: Prognostic indicators in patients with severe head injury. Crit. Care Nurs. Q. 10:25–34, 1987.

Nikas, D. L.: Resuscitation of patients with central nervous system trauma. Nurs. Clin. North Am. 21:693–704, 1986.

Nikas, D. L.: Neurological assessment of patients with altered states of consciousness. I–III. Focus Crit. Care 10:10–14, 1983; 11:54–58, 1984.

Nikas, D. L.: Acute spinal cord injuries: Care and complications. In Nikas, D. L. (ed.): The Critically Ill Neurosurgical Patient. Churchill Livingstone, New York, 1982.

Nikas, D. L. (ed.): Head trauma. I. The spectrum of critical care. Crit. Care Nurs. Q. 10:1, 1987.

Nikas, D. L. (ed.): Head trauma: II. Nursing issues and controversies. Crit. Care Nurs. Q. 10:3, 1987.

Nikas, D. L. (ed.): The Critically Ill Neurosurgical Patient. Churchill Livingstone, New York, 1982.

Nikas, D. L., and Tolley, M.: Acute head injury. In Nikas, D. L. (ed.): The Critically Ill Neurosurgical Patient. Churchill Livingstone, New York, 1982.

North, J. B., et al.: Phenytoin and postoperative epilepsy: A double-blind study. J. Neurosurg. 58:672–677, 1983.

Ohman, J., and Heiskanen, O.: Effect of nimodipine on the outcome of patients after aneurysmal subarachnoid hemorrhage and surgery. J. Neurosurg. 69:683–686, 1988.

Olson, E., McEnrue, J., and Greenbaum, D. M.: Alcohols and miscellaneous agents. Heart Lung 12:127–130, 1983.

Olson, E., McEnrue, J., and Greenbaum, D. M.: Recognition, general considerations, and techniques in the management of drug intoxication. Heart Lung 12:110–113, 1983.

Orkin, F. K., and Cooperman, L. H.: Complications in Anesthesiology. J. B. Lippincott Co., Philadelphia, 1983.

Orkin, L. R., and Shapiro, G.: Admission assessment and general monitoring. In Frost, E. A., and Andrews, I. C. (eds.): Recovery Room Care. Little, Brown & Co., Boston, 1983.

Ostrup, T. C., Luerssen, T. G., Marshall, L. F., et al.: Continuous monitoring of intracranial pressure with a miniaturized fiberoptic device. J. Neurosurg. 67:206–209, 1987.

Overgaard, J., and Tweed, W. A.: Cerebral circulation after head injury. J. Neurosurg. 59:439–446, 1983.

Overturf, G. D.: Meningitis. Top. Emerg. Med. 4:20–26, 1982.

Owens, W. D., and Spitznagel, E. L.: Anesthetic side effects and complications: An overview. In Owens, W. D. (ed.): Anesthetic Side Effects and Complications: Seeking, Finding, and Treating. Little, Brown & Co., Boston, 1980.

Pacjer, R. J., Sutton, L. N., Rorke, L. B., et al.: Prognostic importance of cellular differentiation in medulloblastoma of childhood. J. Neurosurg. 61:296–301, 1984.

Penny, M. D., Walters, B., and Wilkins, D. G.: Hyponatremia in patients with head injury. Intensive Care Med. 5:23–26, 1979.

Perry, J.: Rehabilitation of the neurologically disabled patient: Principles, practice, and scientific basis. J. Neurosurg. 58:799–816, 1983.

Petrak, R. M., Pottage, J. C., Harris, A. A., et al.: *Haemophilus influenzae* meningitis in the presence of a cerebrospinal fluid shunt. Neurosurgery 18:79–81, 1986.

Plum, F., and Posner, J. B.: Diagnosis of Stupor and Coma. F. A. Davis Co., Philadelphia, 1980.

Powers, S. K., and Edwards, M. S. B.: Prophylaxis of thromboembolism in the neurosurgical patient: A review. Neurosurgery 10:509–513, 1982.

Quandt, C. M., and de los Reyes, R. A.: Pharmacologic management of acute intracranial hypertension. Drug Intell. Clin. Pharm. 18:105–112, 1984.

Rapp, R. P., et al.: The favorable effect of early parenteral feeding on survival in head-injured patients. J. Neurosurg. 58:906–912, 1983.

Raynor, R. B.: Anterior or posterior approach to the cervical spine: An anatomical and radiographic evaluation and comparison. Neurosurgery 12:7–13, 1983.

Reid, A. C., Teasdale, G. M., and McCulloch, J.: The effects of dexamethasone administration and withdrawal on water permeability across the blood–brain barrier. Ann. Neurol. 13:28–31, 1983.

Ricci, M. M.: Intracranial hypertension: Barbiturate therapy and the role of the nurse. J. Neurosurg. Nurs. 11:247–252, 1979.

Ricci, N. M.: Neurological examination and assessment of altered states of consciousness. In Nikas, D. L. (ed.): The Critically Ill Neurosurgical Patient. Churchill Livingstone, New York, 1982.

Ringenberg, B. J., Fisher, A., Urdaneta, L. F., et al.: Rational ordering of cervical spine radiographs following trauma. Ann. Emerg. Med. 17:792–796, 1988.

Robertson, C. S., et al.: Treatment of hypertension associated with head injury. J. Neurosurg. 59:455–460, 1983.

Robinson, R. G.: Chronic subdural hematoma: Surgical management in 133 patients. J. Neurosurg. 61:263–268, 1984.

Ropper, A. H.: In favor of intracranial pressure monitoring and aggressive therapy in neurologic patients. Arch. Neurol. 42:1194–1195, 1985.

Rosenberg, H.: Clinical presentation of malignant hyperthermia. Br. J. Anaesth. 60:268–273, 1988.

Ross, D., Rosegay, H., and Pons, V.: Differentiation of aseptic and bacterial meningitis in postoperative neurosurgical patients. J. Neurosurg. 69:669–674, 1988.

Sack, T.: Prophylactic antibiotics in traumatic wounds. J. Hosp. Infect. 11(suppl.):251–258, 1988.

Sahquillo-Barris, J., Lamarca-Ciuro, J., Vilalta-Castan, J., et al.: Acute subdural hematoma and diffuse axonal injury after severe head trauma. J. Neurosurg. 68:894–900, 1988.

Salminen, C., and Wanski, N.: Central nervous system infections. In Nikas, D. L. (ed.): The Critically Ill Neurosurgical Patient. Churchill Livingstone, New York, 1982.

Sanford, S. J.: Respiratory complications of intracranial disorders. In Nikas, D. L. (ed.): The Critically Ill Neurosurgical Patient. Churchill Livingstone, New York, 1982.

Sang, H.: Microsurgical excision of paraventricular arteriovenous malformations. Neurosurgery 16:293–303, 1985.

Saveland, H., Ljunggren, B., Brandt, L., et al.: Delayed ischemic deterioration in patients with early aneurysm operation and intravenous nimodipine. Neurosurgery 18:146–150, 1986.

Savitz, M. H., and Katz, S. S.: Prevention of primary wound infection in neurosurgical patients: A 10-year study. Neurosurgery 18:685–688, 1986.

Scher, T.: The radiology of pulmonary complications associated with spinal cord injury. S. Afr. Med. J. 62:321–324, 1982.

Schettini, A., Stahurski, B., and Young, H. F.: Osmotic and osmotic-loop diuresis in brain surgery. J. Neurosurg. 56:679–684, 1982.

Seelig, J. M., Becker, D. P., Miller, J. D., et al.: Traumatic acute subdural hematoma. N. Engl. J. Med., 304:1511–1518, 1981.

Selhorst, J. B., Gudeman, S. K., Butterworth, J. F., et al.: Papilledema after acute head injury. Neurosurgery 16:357–363, 1985.

Shui, G. K., Nemoto, E. M., and Nemmer, J.: Dose of thiopental, pentobarbital, and phenytoin for maximal therapeutic effects in cerebral ischemic anoxia. Crit. Care Med. 11:452–459, 1983.

Simard, J. M., and Bellefleur, M.: Systemic hypertension in head trauma. Am. J. Cardiol. 63:32c–35c, 1989.

Sloan, T. B.: Neurological monitoring. Crit. Care Clin. 4:543–557, 1988.

Smith, R. R., and Yoshioka, J.: Intracranial arterial spasm. In Wilkins, R. H., and Rengachary, S. S. (eds.): Neurosurgery. McGraw-Hill Book Co., New York, vol. 2, 1985, pp. 1355–1362.

Snow, R. B., Zimmerman, R. D., Grandy, S. E., et al.: Comparison of magnetic resonance imaging and computed tomography in the evaluation of head injury. J. Neurosurg. 18:45–52, 1986.

Snyder, M. (ed.): A Guide to Neurological and Neurosurgical Nursing. John Wiley & Sons, New York, 1983.

Solomon, R. A., and Stein, B. M.: Surgical management of arteriovenous malformations that follow the tentorial ring. Neurosurgery 18:708–715, 1986.

Soloniuk, D., Pitts, L. H., Lovely, M., et al.: Traumatic intracerebral hematomas: Timing of appearance and indication for operative removal. J. Trauma 26:787–794, 1986.

Spetzler, R. F., Martin, N. A., Carter, L. P., et al.: Surgical management of large AVM's by staged embolization and operative excision. J. Neurosurg. 67:17–28, 1987.

Stanczak, D. E., White, J. G., Gouview, W. D., et al.: Assessment of level of consciousness following neurological insult. J. Neurosurg. 60:955–960, 1984.

Steudel, W. I., Rosenthal, D., Lorenz, R., et al.: Prognosis and treatment of cervical spinal injuries with associated head trauma. Acta Neurochir. Suppl. 43:85–90, 1988.

Stroker, R.: Impact of disability on families of stroke clients. J. Neurosurg. Nurs. 15:360–365, 1983.

Sundberg, G., Nordstrom, C. H., Messeter, K., et al.: A comparison of intraparenchymatous and intraventricular pressure recording in clinical practice. J. Neurosurg. 67:841–845, 1987.

Tanaka, T., Sakai, T., Imura, K., et al.: MR imaging as predictor of delayed post-traumatic cerebral hemorrhage. J. Neurosurg. 69:203–209, 1988

Tans, J., and Poortuliet, D. C. J.: Intracranial volume–pressure relationship in man. J. Neurosurg. 59:810–816, 1983.

Tateishi, A., Sano, T., Takeshita, H., et al.: Effects of nifedipine on intracranial cerebral hemorrhage. J. Neurosurg. 69:82–91, 1988.

Tator, C. H., Duncan, E. G., Edmonds, V. E., et al.: Comparison of surgical and conservative management in 208 patients with acute spinal cord injury. Can. J. Neurol. Sci. 14:60–69, 1987.

Tator, C. H., Rowed, D. W., Schwartz, M. L., et al.: Management of acute spinal cord injuries. Can. J. Surg. 27:289–294, 1984.

Tibbs, P. A., et al.: Diagnosis of acute abdominal injuries in patients with spinal shock: Value of diagnostic peritoneal lavage. J. Trauma 20:55–57, 1980.

Toutant, S. M., Klauber, M. R., Marshall, L. F., et al.: Absent or compressed basal cisterns on first CT scan: Ominous predictors of outcome in severe head injury. J. Neurosurg. 61:691–694, 1984.

Tu, Y. K., Heros, R. C., Candia, G., et al.: Isovolemic hemodilution in experimental focal cerebral ischemia: I. Effects on hemodynamics, hemorheology, and intracranial pressure. J. Neurosurg. 69:72–81, 1988.

Tu, Y. K., Heros, R. C., Karacostas, D., et al.: Isovolemic hemodilution in experimental focal cerebral ischemia: II. Effects on regional cerebral blood flow and size of infarction. J. Neurosurg. 69:82–91, 1988.

Vicaris, S. J.: Ventilatory status early after head injury. Ann. Emerg. Med. 12:145–148, 1983.

Voldby, B., and Enevoldsen, E. M.: Intracranial pressure changes following aneurysm rupture: I. Clinical and angiographic correlations. J. Neurosurg. 58:186–196, 1982.

Voldby, B., and Enevoldsen, E. M.: Intracranial pressure changes following aneurysm rupture: II. Associated cerebrospinal fluid lactic acidosis. J. Neurosurg. 58:197–204, 1982.

Waga, S., Shimosaka, S., and Kojima, T.: Arteriovenous malformations of the lateral ventricle. J. Neurosurg. 63:185–192, 1985.

Wagner, F. C., and Chehragi, B.: Early decompression and neurological outcome in acute cervical spinal cord injuries. J. Neurosurg. 56:699–706, 1982.

Wald, M. A.: Cerebral thrombosis: Assessment and nursing management of the acute phase. J. Neurosci. Nurs. 18:36–38, 1986.

Wallace, M. C., and Tator, C. H.: Failure of blood transfusion or naloxone to improve clinical recovery following experimental spinal cord injury. Neurosurgery 18:428–432, 1986.

Wallace, M. C., and Tator, C. H.: Successful improvement of blood pressure, cardiac output, and spinal cord blood flow after experimental spinal cord injury. Neurosurgery 20:710–715, 1987.

Warren, J. B., Goethe, K. E., and Peck, E. A.: Neuropsychological abnormalities associated with severe head injury. J. Neurosurg. Nurs. 16:30–34, 1984.

Warren, J. B., and Peck, E. A.: Factors which influence neuropsychological recovery from severe head injury. J. Neurosurg. Nurs. 16:248–252, 1984.

Weiner, R. L., and Eisenberg, H. M.: Radiographic evaluation of head injury: Key concepts. Trauma Q. 2:26–39, 1985.

Weir, B.: Intracranial aneurysms and subarachnoid hemorrhage: An overview. In Wilkins, R. H., and Rengachary, S. S. (eds.): Neurosurgery. McGraw-Hill Book Co., New York, 1985, vol. 2, pp. 1308–1329,.

Wermeling, D. P., Blouin, R. A., Poter, W. H., et al.: Pentobarbital pharmacokinetics in patients with severe head injury. Drug Intell. Clin. Pharm. 21:459–463, 1987.

Wilkinson, H. A., Yarzebski, J., Wilkinson, E. C., et al.: Erroneous measurement of intracranial pressure caused by simultaneous ventricular drainage: A hydrodynamic model study. Neurosurgery 24:348–354, 1989.

Wilson, C. B.: A decade of pituitary microsurgery. J. Neurosurg. 61:814–833, 1984.

Yamada, K., Ushio, Y., Hayakawa, T., et al.: Effects of methylprednisolone on peritumoral brain edema. J. Neurosurg. 59:612–619, 1983.

Yano, M., Kobayashi, S., and Otsuka, T.: Useful ICP monitoring with subarachnoid catheter method in severe head injuries. J. Trauma 28:476–484, 1988.

Yonas, H.: Measurement of cerebral blood flow. In Wilkins, R. H., and Rengachary, S. S. (eds.): Neurosurgery. New York, McGraw-Hill Book Co., 1985, vol. 2, pp. 1173–1178.

Yoshino, E., Yamaki, T., Higuchi, T., et al.: Acute brain edema in fatal head injury: Analysis by dynamic CT scanning. J. Neurosurg. 63:830–839, 1985.

Young, H. A., Gleave, J. R. W., Chir, B., et al.: Delayed traumatic intracerebral hematoma: Report of 15 cases operatively treated. Neurosurgery 14:22–25, 1984.

Zuccarello, M., et al.: Epidural hematomas of the posterior cranial fossa. Neurosurgery 8:434–437, 1981.

CHAPTER

The Renal System

June L. Stark, R.N., B.S.N., M.Ed.

PHYSIOLOGIC ANATOMY

Formation of Urine: Involves four processes—filtration, reabsorption, secretion, and excretion

1. **Anatomic structures** (Fig. 4–1)
    a. Cortex
        i. Outermost layer of kidney: the metabolically active portion where aerobic metabolism occurs and where ammonia and glucose are formed
        ii. Site of glomeruli and proximal and distal tubules of nephron
    b. Medulla
        i. Middle layer of kidney: region of glycolytic metabolism that supplies energy for active transport
        ii. Composed of 6 to 10 renal pyramids, formed by collecting tubules and ducts
        iii. Site of deepest part of the long loops of Henle in nephron
    c. Renal sinus and pelvis
        i. Papillae are rounded projections of renal tissues located at the apical ends of renal pyramids positioned with the base facing the cortex and the apices facing the renal pelvis. The apical portion opens into the minor calices.
        ii. Corticomedullary junction: point of division between cortex and medulla formed by the base of the pyramids.
        iii. Renal lobe: composed of a pyramid plus the surrounding cortical tissue
        iv. Calix (calices)

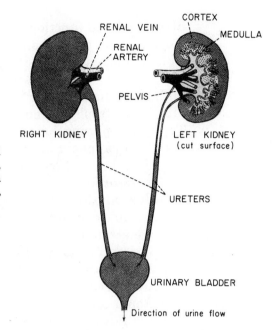

Figure 4–1. The general organizational plan of the urinary system. (From Guyton, A. C.: Textbook of Medical Physiology, 6th ed. W. B. Saunders Co., Philadelphia, 1981.)

    (a) Minor calix wraps around papilla and collects urine flow from collecting duct

    (b) Major calix channels urine from renal sinus to renal pelvis

    (c) Urine flows from renal pelvis to ureter

  d. Nephron: anatomic microscopic structure (Fig. 4–2)

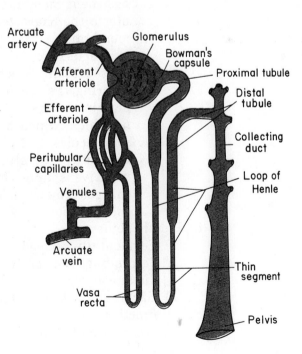

Figure 4–2. The functional nephron. (From Guyton, A. C.: Textbook of Medical Physiology, 6th ed. W. B. Saunders Co., Philadelphia, 1981.)

   i. Structural and functional unit of kidney

  ii. Approximately 1 million in each kidney

 iii. Able to compensate for significant degree of nephron destruction by

    (a) Filtering a greater solute load

    (b) Hypertrophy of remaining functional nephrons

 iv. Types of nephrons, based on location and function in cortex

    (a) Cortical nephrons are located in outer region of cortex and contain short loops of Henle with low capacity for sodium reabsorption

    (b) Juxtamedullary nephrons are located in inner cortex adjacent to medulla. They have long loops of Henle that penetrate deep into medulla and have a greater capacity for concentration of urine because they are sodium-retaining nephrons

  v. Functional segments of nephron

    (a) Renal corpuscle

      (1) Bowman's capsule—a specialized portion of proximal tubule that supports glomerulus

      (2) Glomerulus—a capillary bed

        a) Semipermeable membrane, normally permeable to water, electrolytes, nutrients, and wastes; relatively impermeable to large protein molecules, albumin, and erythrocytes

        b) Composed of three cellular layers—endothelial, basement membrane, and epithelial cells contribute to the characteristic semipermeability of this membrane

        c) Characteristics of cellular layers—endothelial cells contain fenestrations 50 to 100 nm wide, favoring the movement of water and solute. Remaining layers are less porous with openings 1500 nm thick, which may explain impedance of macromolecules

        d) Electrical potential of membrane possesses a negative charge, favoring passage of positively charged molecules and impeding negatively charged molecules such as albumin

    (b) Renal tubules

      (1) Segmentally divided into proximal convoluted tubule, descending loop of Henle, ascending loop of Henle, distal convoluted tubule, and collecting duct

      (2) Each segment has a specific cellular structure and function

        a) Proximal tubule—composed of large epithelial

cells with brush borders surrounded by basement membrane

    b) Descending loop of Henle—thin wall made up of squamous cells

    c) Ascending loop of Henle—lined with cuboidal cells lacking a brush border

    d) Distal tubule—cuboidal and columnar cells lacking a brush border

    e) Collecting ducts—granular appearance with cuboidal cells

2. Physiologic processes

  a. Glomerular ultrafiltration: first step in formation of urine

    i. Characteristics of filtrate

      (a) Normal—protein-free, plasma-like substance with specific gravity of 1.010

      (b) Abnormal—increased permeability of glomerular membrane allows erythrocytes and protein to be filtered into urine. Specific gravity of urine may artificially increase due to the presence of protein or glucose

      (c) Increased amount of serum osmotic substances (glucose, urea) can result in diuresis

    ii. Filtration is determined by pressure and presence of a normal semipermeable glomerular membrane

      (a) Glomerular hydrostatic pressure is 50 mm Hg and favors filtration. This capillary hydrostatic pressure is reflective of cardiac output

      (b) Colloid osmotic pressure of 25 mm Hg and Bowman's capsule pressure of 10 mm Hg oppose hydrostatic pressure and thus oppose filtration

        (1) Colloid osmotic pressure results from oncotic pressure of plasma protein in glomerular blood supply

        (2) Bowman's capsule pressure is reflective of renal interstitial pressure

      (c) Net filtration pressure is derived from the following formula

Glomerular hydrostatic pressure (facilitates)	+50 mm Hg
Colloid osmotic pressure (opposes)	−25 mm Hg
Bowman's capsule pressure (opposes)	−10 mm Hg
Net pressure favoring filtration	+15 mm Hg

    iii. Glomerular filtration rate (GFR)

      (a) Clinical assessment tool to determine renal function

      (b) Definition—volume of plasma cleared of a given substance per minute (may be determined by using endogenous creatinine)

(c) GFR equation

$$\text{GFR} = \frac{(Ux \times V)}{Px}$$

where

x = a substance freely filtered through glomerulus and not secreted or reabsorbed by tubules (e.g., creatinine)
P = plasma concentration of x
V = urine flow rate (ml/min)
U = urine concentration of x

(d) Normal adult GFR is 125 ml/min or 180 L/day
(e) Normal adult urine volume is 1 to 2 L/day; these figures indicate a greater than 99% reabsorption of filtrate
(f) Factors affecting GFR
   (1) Changes in glomerular hydrostatic pressure
      a) Secondary to changes in systemic blood pressure
      b) Variation in afferent or efferent arteriolar tone
   (2) Alterations in oncotic pressure
      a) Dehydration
      b) Hypoproteinemia or hyperproteinemia
   (3) Alterations in Bowman's capsule pressure
      a) Urinary tract obstruction
      b) Nephron destruction due to pathology
      c) Interstitial edema of kidney

b. Tubular functions of reabsorption, secretion, and excretion comprise the following steps in urine formation (Fig. 4–3)
  i. Conversion of 180 L of plasma filtered per day to 1 to 2 L of excreted urine
  ii. Absorption and secretion by two processes
    (a) Passive mechanisms—solute movement without the expenditure of metabolic energy
      (1) Diffusion—solute following either a concentration or an electrical gradient. Influenced by concentration, a solute moves from a solution of higher concentration through a semipermeable membrane to a solution of lower concentration. The electrical gradient causes solute to passively migrate to the opposite charged compartment (e.g., sodium, a positive ion, migrates to a negatively charged compartment, while chloride, a negative ion, moves toward a positively charged compartment)
      (2) Osmosis—water following an osmotic gradient. Influenced by an osmotic agent, water moves from an area of low concentration to an area of higher concentration.

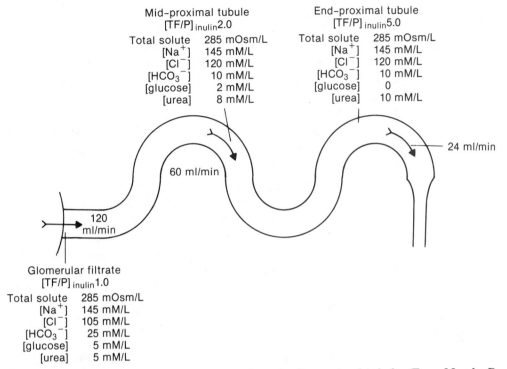

Mid-proximal tubule
$[TF/P]_{inulin}$ 2.0

Total solute	285 mOsm/L
$[Na^+]$	145 mM/L
$[Cl^-]$	120 mM/L
$[HCO_3^-]$	10 mM/L
[glucose]	2 mM/L
[urea]	8 mM/L

End-proximal tubule
$[TF/P]_{inulin}$ 5.0

Total solute	285 mOsm/L
$[Na^+]$	145 mM/L
$[Cl^-]$	120 mM/L
$[HCO_3^-]$	10 mM/L
[glucose]	0
[urea]	10 mM/L

24 ml/min

60 ml/min

120 ml/min

Glomerular filtrate
$[TF/P]_{inulin}$ 1.0

Total solute	285 mOsm/L
$[Na^+]$	145 mM/L
$[Cl^-]$	105 mM/L
$[HCO_3^-]$	25 mM/L
[glucose]	5 mM/L
[urea]	5 mM/L

Figure 4–3. Transport of water and some solutes in the proximal tubule. (From Maude, D. L.: Kidney Physiology and Kidney Disease. J. B. Lippincott Co., Philadelphia, 1977.)

An osmotic agent, such as sodium or mannitol, is a particle that is limited to a compartment

(b) Active mechanisms—ion transport requiring energy (adenosine triphosphate), permits ions to move against a concentration gradient

(c) Maximal tubular transport capacity (Tm)—the active reabsorption mechanisms in the tubule have limited capacity for reabsorption of certain substances. Glucose is a prime example. A plasma glucose level of 375 mg/min, which is the transport maximum (Tm), will reflect no excretion in the urine. However, a plasma glucose level above 375 mg/min will be reflected by glucose excretion or spillage in the urine. A fine point to consider is that the Tm for glucose can vary from one nephron to another. As a result, glucose can sometimes spill into the urine of some individuals at lower serum levels.

iii. Proximal convoluted tubule

(a) Reabsorbs 60% to 80% of filtrate, which remains isotonic to plasma

(b) Major function is active reabsorption of sodium chloride with passive reabsorption of water

(c) Other nutrients reabsorbed are glucose, amino acids, phosphates, uric acid, and potassium
(d) Regulates acid–base balance through reabsorption of bicarbonate (HCO_3^-) and secretion of hydrogen ions (H^+)
(e) Secretes organic acids and foreign substances such as drugs

iv. Loop of Henle
(a) Variations in length depending on type of nephron
(1) Juxtamedullary with long loops
(2) Cortical with short loops
(b) Two distinct segments
(1) Descending segment, the thin limb, permeable to water and impermeable to sodium
(2) Ascending segment, the thick limb, which has active sodium or chloride pump and is impermeable to water
(c) Major function is concentration or dilution of urine, accomplished by countercurrent mechanism that maintains hyperosmolar concentration in the interstitium of the renal medulla

v. Distal convoluted tubule
(a) Receives hyposmotic (or hypotonic) urine from ascending loop of Henle
(b) Major functions are reabsorption of water, sodium chloride, and sodium bicarbonate and secretion of potassium, ammonia, and hydrogen ions
(c) Water permeability at this site is controlled by antidiuretic hormone (ADH), and sodium reabsorption is determined by aldosterone

vi. Collecting duct
(a) Receives urine, which is isotonic to plasma, from distal convoluted tubule
(b) Functions with distal convoluted tubule and is influenced by ADH and aldosterone
(c) Final adjustments of urine are made in this segment before urine enters renal pelvis and progresses to ureter and bladder

Renal Hemodynamics

1. **Renal vasculature**
   a. Specialized arrangement of renal blood vessels reflects interdependence of blood supply with kidney function
   b. Pathway of blood supply
      i. Kidney—aorta → segmented renal arteries → interlobar artery → arcuate artery → interlobular artery → (nephron) → inter-

lobular vein → arcuate vein → interlobar vein → renal vein → inferior vena cava

    ii. Nephron—afferent arteriole → glomerular capillary → efferent arteriole → peritubular capillary → vasa recta adjacent to tubules → interlobular vein → renal vein → inferior vena cava

  c. Juxtaglomerular apparatus: site of renin synthesis

    i. A complex of specialized cells composed of juxtaglomerular cells and macula densa

      (a) Juxtaglomerular cells—enlarged, smooth muscle cells containing granules of inactive renin

      (b) Macula densa—portion of distal tubule making contact with afferent arterioles of its respective glomerulus. These epithelial cells are characteristically "denser" in comparison to other distal tubule cells

    ii. Responds to arterial blood pressure in afferent and efferent arterioles and additionally to the sodium content in the distal tubule

2. **Renal blood flow (RBF) parameters**

  a. Receives 20% to 25% of cardiac output or 1200 ml/min

  b. High flow for low-weight organ (kidneys comprise 0.4% to 0.5% of total body weight)

  c. Translates into a flow rate of 4 ml/g/min to kidney

  d. Oxygen extraction from renal cells is high, but amount is not significant enough to account for flow rate. Rather, the flow is required to support normal renal function

  e. Trends: RBF will be

    i. Higher in males than females

    ii. Increased with age until maturity, then decreased in elderly

    iii. Decreased with exercise

    iv. Increased in supine position

    v. Increased in afternoon and decreased at night

3. **Distribution of RBF**

  a. Renal tissue

    i. Cortex: metabolically active region receiving most of the blood supply (80%)

    ii. Medulla: site of anaerobic metabolism (receives 20%)

  b. Nephrons receive 600 to 650 ml/min of renal plasma flow, which contributes to a GFR of 125 ml/min

4. **Intrarenal autoregulation:** general principles

  a. Mean arterial blood pressure will be maintained in a range of 80 to 180 mm Hg to prevent large changes in GFR

  b. Major site of autoregulation is afferent arteriole

  c. Increase in the renal arterial pressure causes afferent vasoconstriction; decrease in renal arterial pressure causes both afferent and efferent vasoconstriction, producing an increased GFR/RBF ratio

    d. Changes in vascular tone of the efferent arteriole (primarily vaso-constriction) complements efforts to maintain GFR by compensating for reduced blood flow

    e. Autoregulation is essentially absent at a mean arterial pressure of 70 mm Hg or below

5. Neural control

    a. Route of nerve supply: along renal blood vessels

    b. Renal/neurologic intervention is vasoconstrictive

    c. Hypotension results in a decrease in systemic arterial pressure, stimulating the carotid sinus and aortic arch baroreceptors to trigger the sympathetic response and the release of circulating epinephrine

    d. The above sympathetic response decreases both RBF and GFR by vasoconstricting both afferent and efferent arterioles

    e. Other factors that stimulate an increased sympathetic tone are stress, fear, and exercise

    f. Neuronal effect is not the primary factor in autoregulation. This becomes evident when a denervated kidney is successfully trans-planted and still has the ability to compensate for changes in blood pressure

6. Hormonal modulation of RBF (see section on renal regulation of blood pressure, pp. 488–489)

    a. Renin–angiotensin system: a mechanism to sustain systemic blood pressure and plasma volume. It responds to a decreased afferent arteriolar pressure by increasing angiotensin II levels. Angiotensin II vasoconstricts renal blood vessels, particularly the efferent artery, which reduces RBF but increases GFR

    b. Renal prostaglandins: a mechanism to modulate the effects of vaso-active substances on the kidney

7. Pharmacologic effects

    a. Epinephrine and norepinephrine: cause the efferent arteriole to vasoconstrict, leading to a fall in the filtration fraction and a dose-related decrease in RBF

    b. Dopamine: pharmacologic action on RBF is dose related, causing a vasodilatory effect on renal vasculature between a dose of 1 to 3 μg/kg/min IV (optimal dose 3 μg/kg/min). Dosages above 10 μg/kg/min cause renal system vasoconstriction, decreasing RBF and GFR

    c. Furosemide and mannitol: increase GFR initially by increasing blood flow to the kidney and later by decreasing intratubular pressure

Body Water Regulation: Maintenance of volume and concentration of body water content via thirst-neurohypophyseal-renal axis

1. Thirst: regulator of water intake

    a. Thirst center is located in anterior hypothalamus

b. Neuronal cells of this center are stimulated by intracellular dehydration, causing sensation of thirst

c. Role is maintenance of satiety state (i.e., drinking exact amount of fluid to return body to normal hydration state)

2. **Antidiuretic hormone (ADH):** sodium osmoreceptor mechanism for control of extracellular fluid (ECF) osmolality and sodium concentration

a. ADH is synthesized in the paraventricular and supraoptic nuclei of hypothalamus. It then travels along axons of supraopticohypophyseal tract to be stored or released from posterior pituitary. Supraoptic area of hypothalamus may overlap with thirst center, thus leading to an integration of thirst mechanism, osmolality detection, and ADH release

b. Release of ADH occurs during the following circumstances

    i. An increased serum osmolality will stimulate osmoreceptor cells in hypothalamus. (Normal serum osmolality is 285 to 295 mOsm/L.) These cells transmit a message along neurohypophyseal tracts, stimulating ADH release from posterior pituitary

    ii. Volume contraction states, leading to reversal in inhibitory effect on ADH release, are controlled by stretch receptors in left atrium, thus allowing activation of ADH mechanism

c. In presence of ADH, water reabsorption occurs in distal tubule and collecting ducts, resulting in

    i. Production of hypertonic urine

    ii. A hypotonic medullary interstitium

    iii. Eventual correction of contracted ECF

d. Inhibition of ADH secretion occurs when serum osmolality is decreased (as seen during water intoxication)

e. When ADH secretion is inhibited (as above), distal tubule and collecting duct become relatively impermeable to water

    i. Large volumes of hypotonic filtrate will be delivered to collecting duct, resulting in dilute urine

    ii. Final results are excess water loss in comparison to extracellular solute concentration, returning serum osmolality to normal limits

3. **Countercurrent mechanism of kidney:** mechanism for concentration and dilution of urine. It is able to adjust urine osmolality from 50 to 1200 mOsm/L and occurs in juxtamedullary nephron's long loops of Henle and peritubular capillaries of vasa recta. Both anatomic structures are necessary for existence of this mechanism

a. Isotonic glomerular filtrate leaves proximal tubule and enters loop of Henle at 300 mOsm/L

b. Descending limb loop of Henle is permeable to water only. This water is gradually drawn into hypertonic medullary interstitium, resulting in

    i. Gradual increase in osmolality of glomerular filtrate as it becomes dehydrated. At hairpin turn of the loop, osmolality is dramatically increased secondary to removal of water and sodium chloride pumping action. Osmolality can reach 1000 to 1200 mOsm/L

    ii. Medullary interstitium concurrently becomes hypotonic

  c. Thick ascending limb of loop of Henle is permeable to sodium chloride and impermeable to water. Medullary interstitium becomes more hypertonic as its sodium concentration is increased by pumping action at ascending limb

  d. A dilute filtrate reaches distal tubule

    i. In absence of ADH, dilute filtrate is excreted unchanged, resulting in dilute urine with water excretion in excess of solute

    ii. In presence of ADH, water is reabsorbed from dilute filtrate in collecting duct (via mechanism described in section on ADH), resulting in excretion of concentrated urine

Electrolyte Regulation

1. **Sodium regulation:** normal serum concentration is 136 to 145 mEq/L

  a. Sodium is the major extracellular cation and osmotically active solute. Because variation in body sodium can be associated with an exchange of water between intracellular and extracellular compartments, sodium affects ECF volume

  b. Renal reabsorption sites: normal percentages of reabsorbed filtered sodium

    i. Proximal tubule: 65% of filtered sodium

    ii. Loop of Henle: 25% of filtered sodium

    iii. Distal tubule: 6% of filtered sodium

    iv. Collecting duct: 2% to 4% of filtered sodium

  c. Three major factors influence sodium excretion

    i. GFR

    ii. Aldosterone

    iii. "Third factor"

  d. Sodium reabsorption increases at renal tubules during the following conditions

    i. Decreased GFR secondary to renal hypoperfusion (e.g., shock, myocardial infarction): less sodium is delivered to renal tubules and less is excreted

    ii. Aldosterone secretion

      (a) Aldosterone is a mineralocorticoid secreted from zona glomerulosa of adrenal cortex

      (b) Its major effect is to increase renal tubular reabsorption of sodium and to control selective renal excretion of potassium

      (c) Result of aldosterone secretion is an increased quantity of sodium in ECF, which in turn promotes water reabsorption. At same time, potassium ions are secreted into distal tubule and collecting duct to be excreted

(d) Regulating factors for aldosterone secretion are potassium concentration in ECF, renin–angiotensin–aldosterone mechanism, total amount of body sodium, and adrenocorticotropic hormone (ACTH)

iii. Suppression of "third factor": function of "third factor" appears to be promotion of sodium excretion by inhibition of sodium reabsorption along nephron. Therefore, suppression of this factor ensures sodium reabsorption

e. Sodium reabsorption decreases at renal tubules during the following conditions

   i. Increased glomerular filtration rate (e.g., excess ECF volume): effect is increased perfusion to kidneys and therefore increased GFR. More sodium is delivered into renal tubules, and more sodium is excreted through the urine

   ii. Inhibition of aldosterone secretion, resulting in renal sodium excretion

   iii. "Third factor" secretion

   iv. Secretion of ADH: in addition to its role in water balance, ADH may have a secondary effect, enhancing sodium excretion

   v. Action of diuretics, especially loop-affecting diuretics

2. **Potassium regulation:** normal serum concentration is 3.5 to 5.5 mEq/L

   a. Potassium is the major intracellular cation necessary for maintenance of osmolality and electroneutrality of cell

   b. Renal transport sites: potassium is actively reabsorbed in proximal tubule and actively and passively secreted in distal tubule to maintain electroneutrality of urine. This electrical gradient is determined primarily by reabsorption of sodium from urine

   c. Factors enhancing potassium excretion

      i. Increase in cellular potassium

         (a) Elevated cellular levels of available potassium will increase incidence of exchange between sodium and potassium ions. Potassium ions are excreted into urine, and sodium ions are reabsorbed

         (b) Acute metabolic or respiratory alkalosis is a clinical situation that results in movement of potassium ions into cells

      ii. High-volume flow rates in the distal portion of the nephron will increase the number of available potassium ions and thus increase the excretion of potassium. This situation can be created by the effect of osmotic and other diuretics

      iii. Aldosterone, which provides a feedback mechanism for maintenance of ECF potassium ion concentration, functions as follows

(a) Elevation of serum potassium stimulates zona glomerulosa cells of adrenal cortex to secrete aldosterone

(b) Aldosterone acts on distal nephrons and collecting ducts, enhancing retention of sodium and excretion of potassium

(c) Excretion of excess potassium eventually returns patient's potassium concentration to a normal level

3. **Calcium regulation:** normal serum concentration is 8.5 to 10.5 mg/dl

   a. Major functions of calcium ions

      i. Transmission of nerve impulses and muscular contraction

      ii. Role in blood coagulation and activation of clotting mechanism

      iii. Formation of bones and teeth

      iv. Maintenance of cellular permeability

   b. Renal transport sites: 98% of filtered calcium is reabsorbed

      i. Reabsorptive pathways are similar to those used for sodium transport

      ii. Most active reabsorption occurs in proximal tubule

      iii. Other sites include loop (20% to 25%) and distal tubule (10%)

   c. Factors influencing calcium reabsorption

      i. Parathyroid hormone (PTH): decrease in serum calcium stimulates secretion of PTH. PTH stimulates tubular reabsorption of calcium at the distal portion of nephron and stimulates increased phosphate excretion. PTH also mobilizes calcium and phosphate from bone as a further effort to elevate serum calcium levels

      ii. Vitamin D: calcium absorption from the small intestine is dependent on the presence of activated vitamin D (1,25-dihydroxycholecalciferol)

         (a) Activation process—ingestion of ultraviolet light converts 7-dihydrocholesterol in skin to cholecalciferol

            (1) Liver further hydroxylates vitamin D to form 25-hydroxycholecalciferol

            (2) Kidney further hydroxylates to final activated form of vitamin D (1,25-dihydroxycholecalciferol)

         (b) PTH stimulates this activation process

         (c) Reduction in serum calcium level results in decreased urinary calcium excretion. Therefore, activated vitamin D must be available to absorb calcium from small intestine in order to maintain adequate serum calcium levels

      iii. Corticosteroid effect

         (a) Large doses decrease calcium absorption in intestines

         (b) Suspected of interfacing with activation of vitamin D in liver

      iv. Diuretic effect

         (a) These drugs can cause sodium and calcium excretion.

Ultimate effect of reduced serum calcium concentration is decreased excretion

(b) Volume loss—decrease in total body fluid volume, leading to diminished GFR and reduced calcium excretion

4. **Phosphate:** normal serum concentration is 3.0 to 4.5 mg/dl

a. The phosphate ion is located in large quantities in bone, as is calcium. Phosphates play a significant role in intracellular energy-producing reactions. They may also be connected with DNA, RNA, and genetic code information. Phosphates are components of phosphoproteins and phospholipids, which are important constituents of intracellular molecules. Phosphates are used by kidneys to buffer hydrogen ions

b. Renal transport sites: reabsorption of phosphate is an active process that occurs in proximal tubule and is dependent on presence of sodium. Factors influencing phosphate excretion at renal tubule include the following

   i. PTH secretion inhibits proximal tubular reabsorption of phosphates

   ii. Alterations in GFR

      (a) Increased GFR results in decreased reabsorption of plasma phosphates

      (b) Decreased GFR results in increased reabsorption of plasma phosphates

5. **Magnesium:** normal serum concentration is 1.5 to 2.2 mEq/L

a. Magnesium ion is the second major intracellular cation and is a significant factor in cellular enzyme systems and biochemical reactions

b. Renal transport site: reabsorptive process is similar to that for calcium, linked to sodium reabsorption in proximal tubule

c. Factors influencing magnesium reabsorption along renal tubules

   i. Availability of sodium: presence of sodium ion is necessary for this reabsorptive process

   ii. Availability of PTH, although this has a minimal effect on magnesium reabsorption. Mechanisms that stimulate this reabsorptive process are believed to be similar to those used in calcium reabsorption

6. **Chloride:** normal serum concentration is 96 to 106 mEq/L

a. Renal transport sites: reabsorbed with sodium at all sodium absorptive sites in nephron

b. Factors influencing excretion

   i. Acidosis: bicarbonate reabsorbed while chloride is excreted to maintain electrochemical balance

   ii. Alkalosis: bicarbonate excreted while chloride is reabsorbed to maintain electrochemical balance

Excretion of Metabolic Waste Products: A primary role in renal function. It is presently postulated that the kidney excretes over 200 metabolic waste products. The two measured for interpretation of renal function are blood urea nitrogen (BUN) and serum creatinine

1. **Urea:** a nitrogen waste product of protein metabolism that is filtered and reabsorbed along entire nephron
   a. Unreliable measurement of GFR since urea excretion is influenced by
      i. Urine flow (decrease in urine flow rate, such as with volume depletion, may allow for backleak and reabsorption of urea)
      ii. Extrarenal factors such as hypoperfusion states
      iii. Catabolic state as seen with fever, infection, and trauma
      iv. Changes in protein metabolism
      v. Drugs
      vi. Diet
      vii. Gastrointestinal bleeding
   b. Elevation in BUN without an associated rise in creatinine is indicative of
      i. Volume depletion
      ii. Low renal perfusion pressure states
      iii. Increased catabolic process
   c. Elevations of both BUN and creatinine (at a 10:1 ratio) are indicative of renal disease
2. **Creatinine:** a waste product of muscle metabolism
   a. Amount produced each day is proportional to body's muscle mass and occurs at a constant rate
   b. Normal kidney excretes creatinine at a rate equal to the kidney's blood flow or GFR
   c. Creatinine is freely filtered
   d. Combination of equal creatinine production and excretion makes it a reliable assessment for determination of kidney function
   e. Elevation in serum creatinine level can be directly related to a change or deterioration in kidney function

Renal Regulation of Acid–Base Balance: The kidneys regulate acid–base balance by minimizing wide variations in body fluid balance, in conjunction with the appropriate retention or excretion of hydrogen ions. Normal acid–base balance is also regulated by the lungs and the body buffers (serum bicarbonate, blood, and plasma proteins)

1. **Bicarbonate reabsorption**
   a. Most bicarbonate (HCO_3^-) is reabsorbed in proximal tubule, but the process is completed in distal tubule
   b. Bicarbonate is reabsorbed with sodium ions
   c. Bicarbonate reabsorption occurs when filtrate contains more than

28 mEq/L (Tm). This may occur in acidemia and volume contraction (contraction alkalosis)

2. Hydrogen ion secretion

   a. Passive secretion occurs in proximal tubule, and active secretion occurs distally in exchange for sodium ions

   b. Acid is buffered by ammonia (NH_3^+) or phosphate (HPO_4^-) before excretion, providing for hydrogen (H^+) excretion without lowering pH

   c. Hydrogen secretion increases during acidemia and decreases during alkalemia

3. Renal buffers of hydrogen ions

   a. Buffers that are filtered by glomerulus

      i. Bicarbonate is completely reabsorbed (up to 28 mEq/L)

      ii. Phosphate (HPO_4^-) is secreted and then reacts with hydrogen

$$H^+ + HPO_4^{-2} \rightarrow H_2PO_4^{-1}$$

   b. Buffers produced by kidney tubule

      i. Bicarbonate can be synthesized in distal tubule. The process involves excretion of hydrogen into urine at same time that bicarbonate is delivered by ECF with sodium. Hydrogen and bicarbonate both come from distal tubule cell as result of ionization of carbonic acid (H_2CO_3), thus

$$\overset{CA}{H_2CO_3 \rightleftarrows H^+ + HCO_3^-}$$

      ii. Carbonic acid (H_2CO_3) comes from hydration of carbon dioxide (CO_2) via carbonic anhydrase (CA)

$$\overset{CA}{H_2O + CO_2 \rightleftarrows H_2CO_3}$$

      iii. Carbon dioxide (CO_2) is derived from either cellular metabolism or dissolved carbon dioxide in venous blood; thus new bicarbonate can be made in distal tubule from extraurinary sources

      iv. Complete equation

$$\overset{CA}{H_2O + CO_2 \rightleftarrows H_2CO_3 \rightleftarrows H^+ + HCO_3^-}$$

4. Summary of renal response to acidemia

   a. Increased hydrogen ion secretion at distal tubule with an increased excretion of titratable acids (HPO_4^{-2})

   b. All bicarbonate (HCO_3^-) is reabsorbed in proximal nephron

   c. Production of ammonia to accommodate hydrogen ion excretion

$$NH_3 + H^+ \rightleftarrows NH_4^+$$

   d. Urinary pH can be as low as 4.0 owing to excretion of a more acid urine in presence of acidemia

5. **Summary of renal response to alkalemia**
   a. Decreased hydrogen ion secretion in distal tubule
   b. Excess bicarbonate excretion
   c. Decreased production of ammonia
   d. Urine is alkaline with a pH over 7.0

Renal Regulation of Blood Pressure: This regulation involves four mechanisms
1. **Maintenance of volume and composition of ECF**
   a. Normal plasma volume is essential for control of blood pressure
   b. Alterations in plasma volume eventually affect blood pressure
       i. Reduction of plasma volume lowers arterial blood pressure, leading to compensation by vasoconstriction, thus impairing oxygen perfusion
       ii. Expansion of plasma volume results in increased cardiac preload affecting Starling's curve, with ultimate rise in blood pressure
2. **Aldosterone–body sodium balance determines ECF volume:** aldosterone is one of the substances that preserves sodium balance by stimulating renal tubular reabsorption of this ion
3. **Renin–angiotensin–aldosterone system:** a regulatory mechanism to preserve blood pressure and avoid serious volume reduction
   a. Juxtaglomerular apparatus: anatomic unit
       i. Contains inactivated renin granules
       ii. Factors that trigger juxtaglomerular cells to release renin reflect diminished GFR
           (a) Decreased arterial blood pressure in afferent and efferent arteriole
           (b) Reduced sodium content or concentration at distal tubule
           (c) Increased sympathetic stimulation of kidneys
   b. Renin is released from juxtaglomerular cells into afferent arteriole
   c. On entering circulation
       i. Renin acts on angiotensinogen to split away vasoactive peptide, angiotensin I
       ii. Angiotensin I is split to angiotensin II in presence of "converting enzyme" found primarily in lung and liver but also located in kidney and all blood vessels
       iii. Angiotensin II is a potent vasoconstrictor, with potential to cause pronounced vasoconstriction throughout body
   d. Circulatory effect of angiotensin II on arterial blood pressure
       i. Significant constriction of peripheral arterioles
       ii. Venous constriction, a moderate response resulting in reduction of vascular volume
       iii. Renal arteriolar constriction that results in the renal retention

of sodium and water. This expands ECF volume, thus increasing arterial blood pressure

e. Fluid volume response to angiotensin II restores effective circulating volume by

   i. Angiotensin II stimulation of zona glomerulosa cells for release of aldosterone, which enhances renal sodium reabsorption

   ii. Vasoconstriction, to further decrease GFR, leading to sodium reabsorption

   iii. Stimulation of thirst mechanism

4. **Renal prostaglandins:** modulating effect

   a. Unsaturated fatty acids made in presence of oxygen and cyclization of arachidonic acid

   b. Major renal prostaglandins are PGE_2, PGD_2, and PGI_2 types: vasodilators. PGA_2 is vasoconstrictive

   c. Physiologic role: modulation, amplification, and inhibition. The vasoactive substances (angiotensin, norepinephrine, and the bradykinins) stimulate the synthesis and release of prostaglandins. The prostaglandins, in turn, respond by modulating the action of the above vasoactive substances

   d. Prostaglandins cause a diminished or modulated arterial blood pressure and an increase in RBF. This effect is accomplished by arterial vasodilation and inhibition of the distal tubules' response to ADH. The suppressed ADH response leads to sodium and water excretion, which ultimately decreases the effective circulatory volume

   e. Pharmacologic prostaglandin inhibitors are the nonsteroidal anti-inflammatory agents

      i. Salicylic acid

      ii. Ibuprofen (Motrin)

      iii. Indomethacin (Indocin)

      iv. Naproxen (Naprosyn)

Red Blood Cell Synthesis and Maturation

1. **Erythropoietin secretion:** stimulates production of erythrocytes in bone marrow and prolongs life of erythrocyte

2. **Postulated methods for erythropoietin synthesis and stimulus for secretion**

   a. Normal kidneys either produce erythropoietin or synthesize an enzyme that catalyzes its formation

   b. Stimulation for formation is believed to be decreased oxygen delivery to kidney

3. **Erythropoietin deficiency:** primary cause of anemia seen in chronic renal failure, with bleeding as the second most common cause

NURSING ASSESSMENT DATA BASE

Nursing History

1. **Patient Health History**
   a. Previous health problems: indicate presence of or predisposition to renal disease
      i. Kidney disease
      ii. Urinary tract disease
      iii. Cardiovascular disease
         (a) Hypertension—blood pressure control, early diagnosis, and treatment can often prevent or at least halt progress of renal damage. Hypertension also develops in 70% to 80% of patients with advanced renal disease
         (b) Congestive heart failure (CHF)—diuretic-induced hypovolemia and diminished renal perfusion can precipitate renal failure
         (c) Atherosclerosis
      iv. Diabetes mellitus: renal disease due to vascular disease alterations, infection, or neuropathy
      v. Immunologic disorders and allergies
      vi. Pulmonary disease (Goodpasture's syndrome)
      vii. Recent infections (streptococcal infection)
      viii. Recent blood transfusions (history of incompatibility reaction)
      ix. Other: toxemia of pregnancy, renal transplant, anemia, recent surgery, dialysis, drugs and toxins, renal calculi, azotemia, hematuria, and exposure to chemicals or poison (carbon tetrachloride, lead, mercury)
   b. History of specific signs and symptoms
      i. Signs and symptoms of urinary tract disorders
         (a) Dysuria
         (b) Abnormal appearance of urine
            (1) Hematuria (grossly bloody)
            (2) Pyuria (cloudy)
            (3) Biliuria or bilirubinuria (orange)
            (4) Myoglobinuria (usually clear; hematest positive on dipstick)
         (c) Frequency, urgency, hesitancy of urination
         (d) Nocturia (may be due to diabetes insipidus, diabetes mellitus, or congestive heart failure)
         (e) Polydipsia
         (f) Patterns of urine output
            (1) Normal volume (approximately 1500 ml/24 hr)
            (2) Oliguria—less than 400 ml/24 hr
            (3) Anuria—no urine output

        (4) Polyuria—excessive urine output exceeding daily fluid intake

        (5) Nonoliguria—a normal urine volume or excess urine volume in the presence of acute renal failure

    (g) Incontinence

    (h) Fever

    (i) Pain in costovertebral angle; flank or groin pain

  ii. Uremic signs and symptoms

    (a) Nausea and vomiting

    (b) Pruritus and hiccoughing

    (c) Changes in sensorium

    (d) Weakness and fatigue

    (e) Weight loss with muscle wasting

    (f) Edema

    (g) Bleeding

    (h) Asterixis

    (i) Hypertension

    (j) Peripheral neuropathy

    (k) Uremic odor of breath

    (l) Uremic frost of skin (rare)

   (m) Uremic bowel syndrome—observed clinically in patients with end-stage renal disease, associated with intermittent periods of constipation and diarrhea

    (n) Effect of uremia on cognition

        (1) Limited attention span

        (2) Shortened memory

        (3) Diminished response to stimuli

        (4) Altered decision making

        (5) Altered thought processing (i.e., difficulty integrating ideas or concepts)

        (6) Visual disturbances

        (7) Perception—uremia can manifest with unrealistic/inappropriate interpretation of events or environment

    (o) Weight gain/loss

        (1) Patterns of weight gain—reflective of noncompliance with fluid regimen

        (2) Patterns of weight loss—reflective of a deficit in caloric intake and nutritional status

        (3) Dry weight—the ideal weight for patient with renal failure as achieved by a dialysis treatment

    (p) Body image changes associated with uremia/renal disease

        (1) Skin color

        (2) Uremic odor

        (3) Arteriovenous access/Tenckhoff or other catheters

    (4) Edema

    (5) Weight changes

    (6) Donated organ

    (7) Impaired mobility

    (8) Corticosteroid-induced changes—moon face, added fat pads, facial hair

    (9) Self-perception

       a) Focus of control

       b) Feelings of hopelessness, helplessness, and powerlessness

       c) Disorientation to time, place, or person

       d) Change in problem-solving abilities

2. **Family history:** genetic renal disease can account for approximately 30% of all azotemic patients. Thus, determining the risk for genetic transmission of renal disease is valuable for total patient care. The following is a list of genetically transmitted diseases that can cause or precipitate renal disease

  a. Hypertension

  b. Diabetes mellitus

  c. Gout

  d. Malignancy

  e. Polycystic kidney disease/medullary cystic disease

  f. Hereditary nephritis (Alport's syndrome)

  g. Renal calculi

  h. Cardiovascular disease

3. **Social history and habits**

  a. Social history

    i. Psychosocial stressors

      (a) Identify stressors

        (1) Acute/chronic renal disease

        (2) Alterations in life style

        (3) Diminished energy levels

        (4) Altered mobility

        (5) Loss of independence

        (6) Altered role in family and community

        (7) Change in employment

        (8) Altered body image

        (9) Vision of mortality

        (10) Dependence on renal replacement therapy—dialysis, renal transplant

        (11) Organ rejection

        (12) Infection

        (13) Therapeutic restrictions—dietary, fluid

        (14) Activity restrictions

      (b) Recognize expression of stress

            (1) Denial

            (2) Anxiety

            (3) Anger

            (4) Noncompliance/compliance

        (c) Coping

            (1) Describes methods of coping used in the past

            (2) Assess effectiveness of coping strategies

            (3) Assess for adaptation vs. maladaptation

            (4) Signs of maladaptation—chronic depression and expressions of suicide

    ii. Role changes: determine impact of role changes on patient's ability to function

        (a) Role in family—description of family unit structure (hierarchical scheme and roles); determine whether family function is cohesive or dysfunctional

        (b) Identify role changes—often the patient moves from independence reluctantly into an ambivalent role of independence-dependence

        (c) Relation with surrogate dialyzer

        (d) Relation with organ donor

   iii. Sexuality

        (a) Activity prior to renal disease

        (b) Renal dysfunction may contribute to sexual dysfunction

        (c) Hemodialysis has been associated with decreased libido, impotence, and infertility

        (d) Assess return of sexual functioning post transplant

        (e) Aware of sexual dysfunction caused by antihypertensive agents

b. Habits

    i. Dietary habits

        (a) Description of dietary and fluid restrictions

        (b) Pattern of dietary intake—number of meals and nutritional value of intake

        (c) Tolerance of diet—presence/absence of nausea and vomiting; likes/dislikes

        (d) Determine incidence of fluid and electrolyte imbalances

        (e) Complaints of weight loss, increased incidence of infection, diminished energy levels, impaired mobilization, impaired wound healing

    ii. Activity/exercise: relate data to self-care abilities

        (a) Activities of daily living

            (1) Describes normal day

            (2) Describes functional and physical limitations

        (b) Fatigue

            (1) Describes energy level at critical periods during a day

(2) Relates fatigue in terms of activities of daily living, exercise, and leisure times

(c) Mobility

(1) Describes extent of stability on ambulation

(2) Conveys strength/endurance

4. **Medication history**

   a. Nephrotoxic agents

      i. Antibiotic therapy (tetracyclines, aminoglycosides, gentamicin, amphotericin B)

      ii. Analgesic abuse (combination of aspirin and phenacetin)

   b. Diuretics

   c. Cardiac glycosides (digoxin)

   d. Antihypertensives and antiarrhythmic agents

   e. Electrolyte replacement therapy

   f. Immunosuppressives

      i. Corticosteroids

      ii. Azathioprine, cyclophosphamide, antithymocyte globulin (ATG), cyclosporine, OKT_3

Nursing Examination of Patient

1. **Inspection**

   a. Diminished level of consciousness (lethargy, coma)

   b. Skin

      i. Abnormal color: grayish tinge from anemia and yellowish tinge if retained carotenoids are present

      ii. Skin capillary integrity is fragile and, as a result, is easily bruised

      iii. Skin turgor is dependent on age and state of hydration

      iv. Purpura lesions: in some forms of renal failure

   c. Eye: cataracts, periorbital edema

   d. Ear: nerve deafness

   e. Edema

      i. Presence and significance of edema is dependent on amount of water and sodium retained

      ii. Presentation varies from localized edema to anasarca with ascites and pleural effusion

      iii. Edema of renal failure is often related to hypoalbuminemia and can be found in other than dependent areas, such as periorbital tissue

   f. Respiratory rate and pattern: in severe acidosis similar to Kussmaul respiratory pattern seen in diabetic ketoacidosis

   g. Muscle tremors, weakness, and weight loss resulting from generalized debilitation seen with uremic syndrome

   h. Tetany (rare)

      i. Result of severe hypocalcemia or very rapid correction of acidosis (calcium moves into cell in exchange for potassium ions and increased binding of calcium occurs, both contributing to rapid calcium depletion)

      ii. Positive Chvostek's and Trousseau's signs

  i. Asterixis

      i. Indicative of progressive uremic state

      ii. Ask patient to face examiner and raise upper extremities in a fixed hyperextension position. Palms of hands should be visible to examiner, with fingers separated. Positive sign occurs within 30 seconds: irregular movements of wrists and flapping movement of fingers

  j. Fatigue levels

      i. Posture

      ii. Tolerance of examination

      iii. Endurance

  k. Mobility

      i. Movement from lying to sitting

      ii. Movement from sitting to standing

      iii. Extent of ambulation

      iv. Strength

  l. Nutritional status

      i. Measure triceps skinfold thickness

      ii. Normal triceps thickness greater than 25 mm for men and 15 mm for women

      iii. Anemia: pale skin, weakness, signs of shortness of breath

  m. Arteriovenous access

      i. Identify type of access

      ii. Patency

      iii. Observe for redness, tenderness, swelling, and/or drainage

2. **Palpation:** generally performed to determine size and shape of kidney and to check for presence of tenderness, cysts, and masses

  a. Right kidney is easier to palpate than left because its position is lower in the abdomen

  b. Palpate bladder for presence of urine; if bladder is grossly enlarged, suspect bladder neck obstruction

  c. In males, palpate prostate to check size, shape, and potential for infection or cause of obstruction

  d. Palpate flank area to elicit tenderness or pain

  e. Pulse: palpate pulses for a baseline reading and to determine abnormalities

3. **Percussion**

  a. Performed at the costovertebral angles in attempt to elicit various degrees of pain and tenderness: indicative of

      i. Pyelonephritis

      ii. Calculi

     iii. Renal abscess or tumor

     iv. Glomerulonephritis

      v. Intermittent hydronephrosis

  b. If a mass is present, suspect hydronephrosis, polycystic disease, perinephric abscess, or tumor

  c. Percuss abdomen for presence of ascites

4. Auscultation

  a. Listen for aortic and renal artery bruits, heard in flanks or intercostal regions of anterior abdomen

  b. Presence of bruit can be a sign of hypertension, atherosclerosis, or aneurysm

  c. Obtain blood pressure for a baseline reading and to determine abnormalities

Diagnostic Studies

1. Laboratory findings

  a. Blood

      i. Complete blood cell count: hematocrit and hemoglobin levels are reduced reflective of bleeding or a lack of erythropoietin

     ii. Serum creatinine: the most common reference to determine changes in GFR

        (a) A proportional relationship exists between creatinine excretion and creatinine production

        (b) A significant elevation in creatinine is compatible with renal disease and can be correlated with the percentage of nephron damage

     iii. Blood urea nitrogen (BUN)

        (a) Normal BUN to creatinine ratio is 10:1

        (b) Excess in ratio of 20:1, suspect extrarenal problem (dehydration, catabolic state)

        (c) Elevation in both BUN and creatinine results from decrease in GFR

     iv. Serum chemistries (calcium, phosphate, alkaline phosphatase, bilirubin, uric acid, sodium, potassium, chloride, carbon dioxide, magnesium)

      v. Baseline arterial blood gases

     vi. Serum glucose, cholesterol, albumin

    vii. Clotting profile

    viii. Serum osmolality

     ix. Serum protein and albumin: as a reflection of nutritional status or renal disease

  b. Urine

      i. Visual examination for color and clarity

       (a) Clear and colorless with hyposthenuria

       (b) Cloudy when infection is present

       (c) Foamy when albumin is present

  ii. Osmolality (50 to 1200 mOsm/kg)

 iii. Specific gravity (1.003 to 1.030) wide range of normal: this test provides reasonable estimate of urinary osmolality but actually measures density

       (a) Below normal (less than 1.010)—suspect diabetes insipidus, overhydration, or congestive heart failure

       (b) Above normal (greater than 1.030)—suspect proteinuria, glycosuria, presence of x-ray contrast media, or severe dehydration

  iv. Creatinine clearance (CCR)—24-hour urine collection

       (a) Purpose

          (1) To determine presence and progression of renal disease

          (2) Estimation for percentage of functioning nephrons

          (3) For determining specific medication dosages

       (b) Equation

$$\frac{U_{cr} \times V}{P_{cr}} = C_{cr}$$

In 24-hour period

U_{cr} = amount of urinary creatinine excreted

V = urine volume/min

P_{cr} = plasma creatinine level

       (c) In average-sized patients, a satisfactory 24-hour collection always has approximately 1 g of creatinine, regardless of degree of renal function

   v. Culture and sensitivity: check for presence or absence of infection

  vi. pH (normal range 4.0–8.0)

       (a) Average value is 6.0

       (b) Alkaline urine is frequently seen with infection. In the absence of infection, consider renal tubular acidosis if both alkaline urine and systemic acidosis are present

 vii. Glucose: appears in urine when renal threshold for glucose is exceeded

viii. Acetone: seen in urine during starvation and diabetic ketoacidosis. A false-positive result occurs when patient is taking salicylates

  ix. Protein

       (a) Expressed qualitatively as 1+ to 4+

       (b) Diagnostic for presence of glomerular membrane disease such as nephrotic syndrome or for detection of myeloma proteins causing renal failure

    x. Spot urine electrolytes
      (a) Screening test for tubular function
      (b) Measure sodium, potassium, and chloride concentrations
      (c) Assessment of kidney's ability to conserve sodium and concentrate urine
    xi. Urinary sediment
      (a) Casts—precipitation of protein within kidney that takes the shape of tubule in which it originally was formed
        (1) Hyaline casts—entirely protein; small amounts normal in urine. If present in large amounts, suspect significant proteinuria such as albumin or myeloma protein
        (2) Erythrocyte casts—diagnostic for active glomerulonephritis or vasculitis
        (3) Leukocyte casts—indicative of infectious process (e.g., pyelonephritis)
        (4) Granular casts—small number, possibly result of degenerating erythrocyte or leukocyte casts
        (5) Fatty casts containing lipoid material—when seen in abundance, consider lipoid nephrosis or nephrotic syndrome
        (6) Renal tubular casts—seen in acute renal failure
      (b) Bacteria—presence determined by Gram's stain
      (c) Erythrocytes—small numbers normal. In abundance during active glomerulonephritis, interstitial nephritis, malignancies, and infection
      (d) Leukocytes—small numbers normal. Present in infection and interstitial nephritis
      (e) Renal epithelial cells—rarely seen. Present in abundance during acute tubular necrosis, nephrotoxic injury, or kidney allergic reaction
      (f) Crystals—seen in diseases of stone formation or following certain intoxications (e.g., oxalate stones of ethylene glycol)
      (g) Eosinophils—when present in urine, indication of allergic reaction in kidney

2. Radiologic findings

  a. Plain abdominal x-ray film determines position, shape, and size of kidney and identifies calcification in urinary system

  b. Intravenous pyelogram (IVP)
    i. Visualizes urinary tract to diagnose partial obstruction, renovascular hypertension, tumor, cysts, and congenital abnormalities
    ii. Complications: allergic reaction to dye, dehydration
    iii. Contraindicated in presence of

(a) Poor renal function—can further compromise function because of dehydrating effect and nephrotoxicity of IVP dye

(b) Multiple myeloma—IVP dye may potentiate precipitation of myeloma protein in kidney

(c) Pregnancy—abdominal irradiation should be avoided

(d) Congestive heart failure—IVP dye has an acute osmotic effect that can further compromise heart failure by expanding vascular volume and increasing blood return to right side of heart

(e) Diabetes mellitus—rapid deterioration of renal function is commonly seen following IVP in patients with diabetic renal disease

(f) Sickle cell anemia—elevation in renal tissue oncotic pressure from dye can promote sickling and infarction of renal tissue

c. High-excretion tomography: indicated when kidneys cannot be readily visualized on IVP

d. Renal scan: determines renal perfusion and function and can also provide information about obstructions and renal masses

    i. Radioactive dye is taken up by normal kidney tubule cells. Decrease in uptake indicates hypoperfusion due to any cause

    ii. Commonly used to assess status of renal transplants

e. Retrograde pyelography: provides information regarding upper region of urinary collecting system (e.g., obstruction)

f. Retrograde urethrography: provides information about status of urethra

g. Cytoscopy: detects bladder or urethral pathologic processes

h. Renal arteriography (angiography)

    i. Identifies tumors and differentiates type of existing renal or renovascular disease (e.g., renal artery stenosis)

    ii. Complications

        (a) Dye used can be allergenic and cause same complications as IVP dye

        (b) Puncturing of a peripheral artery, with consequent hematoma, embolism, or thrombus formation, is greatest technical risk

i. Voiding cystourethrography: identifies abnormalities of lower urinary tract, urethra, and bladder to determine presence of reflux and residual urine

j. Diagnostic ultrasonography: identifies hydronephrosis, differentiates between solid and cystic tumor, and localizes cysts or fluid collections

k. Computed tomography (CT scan): identifies tumors and other pathologic conditions that create variations in body density (e.g., abscess, lymphocele)

l. Magnetic resonance imaging (MRI)
  i. Improved tissue characterization when compared with CT scan
  ii. Provides direct imaging in several planes, conducive to the detection of renal cystic disease, inflammatory processes, and renal cell carcinoma
  iii. Identifies morphologic changes in renal transplantation
  iv. Detects alterations in blood flow (i.e., slow or absent flow)
m. Chest radiograph
  i. Standard procedure
  ii. Identifies presence of pulmonary disease, pulmonary edema, cardiomegaly, left ventricular hypertrophy, pericardial effusion, uremic lung, Goodpasture's disease, and infections (e.g., tuberculosis or fungal infiltrates)

3. **Kidney biopsy:** most common invasive diagnostic tool
  a. Indicated for renal disease that cannot be definitively diagnosed by other methods
  b. Determines cause and extent of lesions—helpful when planning treatment regimen
  c. Open and closed biopsies
    i. Open: perform if severe anatomic deformities or if "deep specimen" needed for diagnosis of polyarteritis nodosa or dense deposit disease
    ii. Closed: a simple percutaneous procedure
  d. Contraindications to open biopsy: bleeding tendency, hydronephrosis, hypertension, cystic disease, and neoplasms

COMMONLY ENCOUNTERED NURSING DIAGNOSES

Fluid Volume Excess: A state in which an individual experiences increased fluid retention and edema occurring in both acute and chronic renal failure because of the kidney's inability to excrete excess body water. This condition is associated with the presence of oliguria or anuria

1. **Assessment for defining characteristics**
  a. Intake greater than output
  b. Weight gain
  c. Oliguria or anuria
  d. Elevated blood pressure
  e. Edema: peripheral, anasarca, ascites, periorbital, pulmonary
  f. Neck vein distention, elevated central venous pressure
  g. Bounding pulses
  h. Dyspnea, orthopnea
  i. Lung sounds: crackles
  j. Muffled heart sounds

k. Pulmonary congestion on chest x-ray film

l. Decreased hemoglobin and hematocrit

m. Elevated pulmonary artery and wedge pressures

n. Low specific gravity (1.015 or less) dilute urine

o. Dilutional effect on electrolytes

p. Anxiety, restlessness

q. Stupor (seen with water intoxication)

2. **Expected outcomes**

a. Maintains dry weight

b. Normal central venous, pulmonary artery and wedge pressures

c. Free of edema

d. Breath sounds clear bilaterally

e. Maintains normal vital signs

f. Normal mental status

g. Compliant to fluid restriction; intake and output balanced

3. **Nursing interventions**

a. Identify common causes of fluid excess

   i. Expansion of blood volume secondary to renal sodium retention

   ii. Diminished plasma proteins leading to a decrease in plasma oncotic pressure (glomerulonephritis, nephrotic syndrome, malnutrition)

   iii. Increased capillary permeability

b. Document intake and output; compare with daily weights

   i. Consider insensible losses: fluid losses via lungs, skin, and bowel (600 to 800 ml/day)

   ii. Consider oxidative rate: result of fluid liberated from food ingested (carbohydrate metabolism liberates 300 to 350 ml/day)

c. Assess renal function

   i. Urine volume and creatinine clearance

   ii. Urinalysis

   iii. Urine concentration: specific gravity, urine osmolality, spot electrolytes

   iv. 24-hour urine collection for protein evaluation

d. Restrict fluids in overhydration that can be associated with impaired renal function, impaired cardiac function (e.g., congestive heart failure), or syndrome of inappropriate ADH

4. **Evaluation of nursing care**

a. 24-hour intake and output balance is negative or zero

b. Absence of any form of edema: periorbital, peripheral, ascites, or pulmonary edema

c. Absence of adventitious breath sounds

d. Absence of hypertension

e. Compliance with fluid restriction

Fluid Volume Deficit: State in which an individual experiences vascular, cellular, or intracellular dehydration related to actual fluid loss. Volume deficit may occur in the diuretic phase of acute renal failure

1. **Assessment for defining characteristics**
   a. Weight loss
   b. Output greater than intake
   c. Hypotension
   d. Increased pulse
   e. Poor skin turgor
   f. Dry skin and mucous membranes
   g. Thirst
   h. Little or absent neck vein distention
   i. Decreased central venous pressure
   j. Decreased pulmonary artery and wedge pressures
   k. Increased body temperature
   l. Urine output
      i. Polyuric phase: large volume of dilute urine with low specific gravity
      ii. Dehydration with normal renal function: oliguria, a concentrated urine with an elevated specific gravity
   m. Weakness
   n. Stupor (seen with severe hypovolemia)

2. **Expected outcomes**
   a. Normal stable weight
   b. Maintains asymptomatic level of fluid balance
   c. Maintains normal vital signs
   d. Maintains normal central venous, pulmonary artery, and wedge pressures
   e. Urine output restored to within normal limits
   f. Returns to baseline mental status

3. **Nursing interventions**
   a. Identify common causes of fluid deficit
      i. Renal water losses
         (a) Diuretic abuse
         (b) Salt-wasting nephropathies
         (c) Diabetes insipidus (nephrogenic, central)
         (d) Osmotic diuresis (hyperglycemia, urea)
         (e) Postobstruction diuresis
      ii. Gastrointestinal losses
         (a) Diarrhea
         (b) Vomiting
         (c) Nasogastric suctioning
         (d) Fistula/wound drainage
         (e) Blood losses
      iii. Skin
         (a) Skin lesions

          (b) Burns

          (c) Insensible losses

     iv. Third space phenomena

          (a) Intestinal obstruction

          (b) Burns

          (c) Crush injury

          (d) Pancreatitis

  b. Document intake and output; compare with daily weight

  c. Assess renal function

     i. Urine volume and creatinine clearance

     ii. Urinalysis

     iii. Urine concentration: specific gravity, urine osmolality, spot electrolytes

     iv. 24-hour urine collection for protein evaluation

  d. Administer fluid therapy: administer fluids for dehydration that are specific to the type of fluid lost (e.g., gastrointestinal losses, diuretic abuse, fistula drainage)

4. Evaluation of nursing care

  a. 24-hour intake and output balance is positive or zero

  b. Absence of weight loss

  c. Absence of hypotension

  d. Normal urine volume and specific gravity

  e. Maintains or returns to normal mental status

Potential for Electrolyte Imbalance: Hyperkalemia, hyperphosphatemia, hypermagnesemia, hypernatremia, and hypocalcemia—this diagnosis reflects the risk a patient with renal failure has for electrolyte imbalance. A majority of the time the imbalance represents retention of an electrolyte because of the kidneys' inability to excrete solute. In the case of calcium, the imbalance reflects a deficit because of a lack of activated vitamin D and binding with phosphate in the intestines

1. Assessment for defining characteristics

  a. Abnormal neuromuscular function such as irritability, hyporeflexia or hyperreflexia, and seizures

  b. Generalized weakness, malaise, fatigue

  c. Cardiac dysrhythmias

  d. Alteration in mental status

  e. Serum electrolyte abnormalities

2. Expected outcomes

  a. Remains asymptomatic with serum levels of electrolytes within normal limits

  b. Compliant to dietary restrictions

3. Nursing interventions

  a. Identify common causes of electrolyte imbalances

     i. Renal failure

      ii. Nasogastric suctioning

     iii. Vomiting and diarrhea

     iv. Diuretic therapy

      v. Hyperglycemic (osmotic) diuresis

     vi. Massive tissue destruction (in catabolic states with release of hydrogen, potassium, and increase in BUN)

    vii. Acid–base imbalances

   viii. Corticosteroid therapy

     ix. Wound/fistula drainage

      x. Parathyroid disorder

     xi. Adrenal disorder

  b. Recognize presence of electrolyte imbalances

  c. Ensure adequate hydration

  d. Monitor serum and urine electrolyte values

  e. Teach patient dietary prescriptions

  f. Evaluate intake patterns for nutritional value and modification of electrolytes

4. Evaluation of nursing care

  a. Serum electrolyte levels are within normal range or only slightly altered

  b. Absence of symptoms related to electrolyte imbalance

  c. Dietary intake is within prescribed range

Altered Nutrition: Less than body requirements: The state in which an individual experiences an intake of nutrients insufficient to meet metabolic needs. Uremic symptoms and strict dietary restrictions often precede this condition

1. Assessment for defining characteristics

  a. Presence of uremic symptoms

      i. Loss of appetite

     ii. Nausea and vomiting

    iii. General malaise and fatigue

    iv. Foul taste in mouth

  b. Alterations in weight

      i. Loss of weight due to inadequate intake or as a result of dietary restrictions

     ii. Gain in weight due to noncompliance with fluid restriction

  c. Presence of pain or discomfort can diminish appetite

  d. Sore, inflamed buccal cavity secondary to oral candidal infection, common in debilitated person and transplant patient

  e. Anemia

  f. Presence or repeated episodes of infection

  g. Noncompliance with dietary restrictions

  h. Depression

  i. Denial

2. **Expected outcomes**
   a. Intake meets nutritional requirements
   b. Maintains stable, baseline weight
   c. Adequate muscle mass
   d. Normal serum protein and albumin levels
   e. Remains infection free
3. **Nursing interventions**
   a. Identify common causes of inadequate nutritional intake and plan care aimed at etiology
   b. Teach appetite-enhancing measures
      i. Provide oral hygiene prior to meals
      ii. Give small, frequent meals
      iii. Identify food preferences, especially those high in complex carbohydrates and essential amino acids
   c. Teach the essential elements of the renal patient's diet
      i. Essential amino acids and adequate calories
      ii. Adjusted protein and electrolyte intake (sodium and potassium) to avoid uremic symptoms and electrolyte imbalances. Diminished protein intake causes the use of the protein stored in muscles, which leads to body muscle wasting. Providing increased calories can help avoid this situation
      iii. Provide vitamins and iron supplements (folic acid, multivitamins)
   d. Assess for presence of malnutrition
      i. Muscle wasting
      ii. Extreme weight loss
      iii. Frequent infections
      iv. Hypoproteinemia with hypoalbuminemia
      v. Anthropometric measurements: triceps skinfold to assess total body fat and mid-arm circumference to determine lean body mass
   e. Monitor pattern of changes in weight and nutritional intake
   f. Assess for alterations in the coping process expressed as
      i. Anxiety
      ii. Depression
      iii. Dysfunctional denial
   g. Assess for noncompliance with dietary instructions
4. **Evaluation of nursing care**
   a. Weight gain with stabilization pattern
   b. Absence of muscle wasting
   c. Triceps skinfold and mid-arm circumference within normal limits
   d. Serum protein and albumin levels are or approach normal limits
   e. Absence of infection

Potential for Alterations in Blood Pressure: Hypertension: In renal failure the hypertensive state is usually created by the retention of fluid or stimulation of the renin–angiotensin mechanism

1. **Assessment for defining characteristics**
   a. Hypertension defined as a diastolic pressure above 90 mm Hg and a systolic pressure above 140 mm Hg
   b. Headache
   c. Dizziness
   d. Blurred vision
2. **Expected outcomes**
   a. Maintains blood pressure with diastolic pressure below 90 mm Hg and systolic pressure below 140 mm Hg
   b. Absence of symptoms associated with hypertension
   c. Compliant for antihypertensive medications
3. **Nursing interventions**
   a. Identify causes of hypertension
      i. Primary or essential hypertension
      ii. Expansion of plasma volume (e.g., sodium and water retention secondary to renal disease)
      iii. Renin-mediated hypertension
      iv. Pheochromocytoma (rare)
      v. Renal artery stenosis
      vi. Primary hyperaldosteronism
      vii. Coarctation of aorta
      viii. Adrenal cortical hyperfunction
   b. Collaborate with health team to control hypertension
      i. Monitor blood pressure frequently
      ii. Restrict salt and water intake
      iii. Avoid drugs that can elevate blood pressure (such as corticosteroids and sympathomimetic-containing antihistamines)
      iv. Administer diuretics and antihypertensives as appropriate
      v. Diuretic agents
         (a) Indications—treatment of edema and hypertension
            (1) Congestive heart failure
            (2) Renal failure
            (3) Cerebral edema
            (4) Cirrhosis with ascites
            (5) Menstrual edema
            (6) Prior to onset and in the initial stages of oliguric acute renal failure
         (b) Characteristics
            (1) General action—inhibit the active transport of sodium or chloride, resulting in an increase in urine output consisting primarily of sodium and water
            (2) The diuretic effect reduces plasma volume, creating a

continual state of mild hypovolemia. The decrease in effective circulating volume will lower blood pressure

(c) Complications

   (1) Volume depletion

   (2) Hypokalemia (contributing to onset of dysrhythmias)

   (3) Hyperuricemia

   (4) Hyponatremia

   (5) Metabolic alkalosis

   (6) Hypochloremia

   (7) Azotemia

   (8) Hyperkalemia seen with potassium-sparing diuretic

(d) Types of diuretics

   (1) Large volume intake will increase GFR, causing glomerulotubular balance to respond by increasing urine output, resulting in water and electrolyte loss

   (2) Osmotic diuretic—a nonabsorbable solute (mannitol), when present in the tubules, will exert an osmotic effect, causing a water diuresis in excess of sodium chloride. Side effects: blurred vision, rhinitis, rebound plasma volume expansion, thirst, urinary retention, fluid and electrolyte imbalance secondary to diuresis

   (3) Loop diuretics—the most potent diuretics available (furosemide and ethacrynic acid). The primary site of action is the thick segment of the medullary ascending loop of Henle. These diuretics block the reabsorption of sodium chloride, thus contributing to a large diuresis of isotonic urine. Potassium excretion is also enhanced. In addition, they contribute to an increase in RBF by exerting a vasodilatory effect on renal vasculature. Side effects: volume depletion, agranulocytosis, thrombocytopenia, transient deafness, abdominal discomfort, hypokalemia, hypochloremic alkalosis, hyperglycemia. Prolonged use without associated electrolyte replacement results in all other electrolyte imbalances

   (4) Thiazides (hydrochlorothiazide)—sodium reabsorption is inhibited in the ascending loop of Henle and the beginning portion of its distal tubule. Increased potassium excretion is noted, along with a weak carbonic anhydrase inhibitory effect. Side effects: rashes, leukopenia, thrombocytopenia, and acute pancreatitis

   (5) Potassium-sparing diuretics (spironolactone)—these agents are aldosterone inhibitors. The inhibition of aldosterone promotes sodium secretion into the distal tubule and potassium reabsorption, causing a mild

diuresis while protecting the body's potassium level. Potassium-sparing diuretics are usually selected for patients receiving digoxin and diuretic therapy who cannot tolerate low serum potassium levels or when a mild diuretic effect is desirable. Side effects: hyperkalemia, hyponatremia, headache, nausea, diarrhea, urticaria, and gynecomastia or menstrual disturbances

(6) Carbonic anhydrase inhibitors (acetazolamide sodium)—the inhibition of the enzyme, carbonic anhydrase, increases the excretion of sodium by interfering with sodium bicarbonate reabsorption. Therefore, sodium bicarbonate is lost in the urine, creating a hyperchloremic metabolic acidosis. This drug is beneficial when an alkaline urine is desirable. Side effects: hyperchloremic acidosis, renal calculi, rash, nausea, vomiting, and anorexia

(7) Other—any pharmacologic agents that increase both cardiac output and GFR will contribute to the formation of a diuresis. Examples of these agents are the xanthines (theophylline, aminophylline) and digoxin

(e) General nursing considerations in the administration of diuretics

(1) Collaborate with the physician to determine the weight and fluid balance desired at the conclusion of diuretic therapy

(2) Observe for fluid, electrolyte, and acid–base disorders

(3) Maintain intake and output records correlated with daily weights

(4) Monitor serum potassium levels, especially if patient is on digoxin (hypokalemia increases the risk of digitalis toxicity)

(5) Consider administering potent or high doses of diuretics in the early morning or afternoon hours unless a Foley catheter is in place

(6) Monitor blood pressure during aggressive diuresis because hypotension can indicate dehydration and impending circulatory collapse

(7) Advise patient to report the onset of side effects, such as difficulty with hearing

(8) Be aware that a diminished response to diuretics may be related to electrolyte imbalances, particularly hyponatremia, hypochloremia, and hypokalemia

vi. Antihypertensive agents

(a) Indications—to lower and control blood pressure in an

effort to decrease the possibility of hypertensive complications such as cerebrovascular accidents and renal failure

(1) Hypertension—diastolic pressure exceeding 90 mm Hg and/or systolic pressure exceeding 140 mm Hg

(2) Myocardial compromise—indicated in conditions of increased systemic vascular resistance (SVR), since the vasodilator effects of these agents decrease SVR, thus reducing afterload and myocardial work load

(b) Characteristic action

(1) Diminished adrenergic nerve stimulation to vasculature, thus decreasing peripheral resistance

(2) Vasodilatation accomplished by relaxation of the vascular smooth muscle

(3) Reduction of preload secondary to the venous pooling caused by the vasodilatation

(c) Categories of antihypertensives

(1) Sympathetic blockers—inhibition of the sympathetic response can occur at any of three sites: in the central nervous system (clonidine, methyldopa), at the peripheral nerve endings (reserpine, guanethidine), or at the alpha and beta receptor sites (prazosin, propranolol)

  a) The primary effect is achieved through reduction of the SVR as sympathetic vasoconstrictor activity is minimized. However, the beta blockers work by decreasing the cardiac output

  b) RBF may be reduced, causing stimulation of the renin–angiotensin mechanism. This is counterbalanced by the drugs' tendency to cause salt and water retention. This response warrants the use of diuretics in conjunction with sympathetic blockade therapy

(2) Vasodilators—act directly on vessel walls to relax smooth muscle. Therefore, these agents decrease peripheral resistance without interfering with the sympathetic response. The arterioles rather than veins are the site for relaxation. This prevents venous pooling, and cardiac output is maintained

  a) The hypotensive response to these drugs can result in a reflex tachycardia as the sympathetic nervous system response

  b) Renin–angiotensin mechanism is initiated, and salt and water are reabsorbed

  c) The above responses to these agents can be avoided by administering them in conjunction with a diuretic and a beta-blocking drug

    d) Examples of vasodilators are minoxidil, diazoxide, hydralazine, and nitroprusside

    (3) Angiotensin-converting enzyme inhibitor (captopril)—specifically for the patient with renin-mediated hypertension. These agents inhibit angiotensin-converting enzyme, thus preventing the conversion of angiotensin I to angiotensin II

  (d) General nursing considerations in administration of antihypertensive agents

    (1) On admission, obtain baseline blood pressure in three positions (lying, sitting, standing) and in both arms; record if a difference exists

    (2) Maintain a graphic sheet of blood pressure readings. Report any variables that relate to changes in pulse or blood pressure levels (i.e., restlessness, drowsiness, confusion, changes in temperature)

    (3) Schedule antihypertensive doses at regular intervals over a 24-hour period

    (4) Question holding dose prior to hemodialysis

    (5) During initiation or adjustment of antihypertensive, obtain blood pressure immediately prior to administering drug (especially with prazosin hydrochloride [Minipress])

    (6) Routine blood pressure should be obtained within 1 hour of administration

    (7) Establish blood pressure parameters for withholding medications (i.e., if 110/60 mm Hg, then hold dose)

    (8) Observe for symptomatology, relate blood pressure readings, then report

    (9) If postural hypotension occurs, then lying and sitting blood pressure recordings are required, also to be plotted on a graphic sheet

   (10) Be aware if the antihypertensive drugs cause changes in libido. This issue should be addressed, and the patient should be directed to a source for counseling

   (11) Monitor response to antihypertensive therapy. If hypertension is refractory to these medications, further evaluation is necessary—consider the following

    a) Assessment of renin–angiotensin–aldosterone mechanism (i.e., determine plasma renin activity)

    b) Renal artery stenosis

    c) Pheochromocytoma

    d) Surgery—vascular repair of renal artery stenosis or nephrectomy

c. Treat hypotension

      i. Administer fluid challenges with volume expanders (normal saline, albumin, dextran) to increase blood pressure

      ii. If hypotension persists after correcting volume depletion, vasopressors (e.g., dopamine) are indicated

  d. Treat renal hypoperfusion

      i. Restore plasma volume and/or blood pressure in an effort to increase cardiac output. Colloid is the most effective volume expander and consistently increases renal perfusion

      ii. Other agents that may augment RBF are mannitol, dopamine, furosemide, ethacrynic acid, prostaglandin, and bradykinin

4. Evaluation of nursing care

  a. Normal or slightly elevated blood pressure within a range appropriate for the support of renal perfusion

  b. Free of hypertensive symptoms

  c. Demonstrates compliance to antihypertensive medications

Potential for Acid–Base Imbalances: Metabolic Acidosis: A state commonly associated with acute and chronic renal failure caused by the inability of the kidney to excrete hydrogen

1. Assessment for defining characteristics

  a. pH value below 7.35 and bicarbonate level below 22 mEq/L

  b. Kussmaul's respirations

  c. Hypotension

  d. Fatigue

  e. Headache

  f. Cardiac dysrhythmias

  g. Decreased myocardial contractility

  h. Central nervous system depression progressing to coma

  i. Seizures

  j. Chronic acidotic conditions result in skeletal system disorders such as osteitis, fibrosis, and osteomalacia

2. Expected outcomes

  a. Maintains pH within a physiologic range

  b. Maintains normal respiratory and cardiac function

3. Nursing interventions

  a. Identify common causes of metabolic acidosis

      i. Renal failure

      ii. Distal or proximal renal tubular acidosis

      iii. Hyperaldosterone secretion

      iv. Ketoacidosis

      v. Salicylate poisoning

      vi. Diarrhea or fistulas

  b. Assess degree of acidosis

      i. Frequently accompanies renal failure

      ii. Obtain arterial blood gas values

iii. Observe for vague symptomatology: hypoxia secondary to impaired oxygen transport; diminished cardiac output secondary to altered myocardial functioning and impaired effect of catecholamines

iv. Electrolyte imbalances associated with acidosis are hyperkalemia, hyperchloremia, and increased ionized calcium ions

4. **Evaluation of nursing care**
   a. pH level within normal limits
   b. Absence of symptoms associated with metabolic acidosis

Potential for Anemia: Related to a lack of erythropoietin secretion by the kidney

1. **Assessment for defining characteristics**
   a. Shortness of breath on exertion
   b. Pallor
   c. Fatigue and/or muscle weakness, possibly manifested by difficulty completing activities of daily living
   d. Angina
   e. Postural hypotension
   f. Dizziness
2. **Expected outcomes**
   a. Maintains an asymptomatic level of anemia
   b. Able to perform activities of daily living
   c. Compliant with pharmacologic agent and diet
3. **Nursing interventions**
   a. Identify common causes of anemia during renal failure
      i. Suppression of erythropoietin
      ii. Actual blood losses
      iii. Uremic syndrome
   b. Obtain and interpret hematocrit and hemoglobin
   c. Transfuse fresh blood when indicated
      i. Decreases risk of hyperkalemia
      ii. Hypocalcemia can occur from anticoagulants (citrate) present in banked blood
   d. Decrease hepatitis risk
      i. Numerous blood transfusions increase risk of hepatitis B to patient. Non-A, non-B hepatitis, with an incidence of 1.5%, is also related to the frequency of blood transfusions
      ii. Precautions include early recognition of hepatitis antigen–positive persons, followed by isolation measures
      iii. Offer hepatitis B vaccine to staff
   e. Monitor for risk for human immunodeficiency virus (HIV)
      i. Incidence only 0.6% in chronic hemodialysis population
      ii. Use universal precautions as recommended by the Centers for Disease Control (CDC)

f. Treat chronic anemia: therapy includes classic regimen or recently released pharmacologic agent epoietin alfa
   i. Oral iron or Imferon unless patient has excess body iron stores
   ii. Folic acid and pyridoxine (vitamin B_6): important, especially in dialysis patient, since these are dialyzable vitamins. Also indicated in microcytic anemias of folic acid and vitamin B_6 deficiency
   iii. Vitamin B_{12} for vitamin B_{12}–responsive anemia
   iv. Anabolic steroids (e.g., nandrolone decanoate): stimulate erythrocyte formation
   v. Epoietin alfa: recombinant human erythropoietin, which stimulates erythrocyte production and prevents the anemia of chronic renal failure. Drug effect on erythrocytes does not begin until 2 to 6 weeks after administration; as a result, it is not used in acute renal failure

4. **Evaluation of nursing care**
   a. Maintains acceptable hematocrit level (usually 20% to 24% with traditional therapy and 30% to 33% with epoietin alfa therapy)
   b. Completes activities of daily living
   c. Complies with pharmacologic and nutritional supplement therapy

Potential for Uremic Syndrome: The uremic state results from the kidney's inability to excrete toxic waste products. Uremic symptoms occur at BUN levels above 100 mg/dl and/or GFR below 10 to 15 ml/min

1. **Assessment for defining characteristics**
   a. Early uremia
      i. Sensorium change (e.g., loss of attention span, lethargy)
      ii. Nausea, vomiting
      iii. Weight loss and muscle wasting
      iv. Skin changes (pruritus, pale yellow tinge, dryness, ecchymoses)
      v. Uremic fetor
      vi. Edema
      vii. Stomatitis
   b. Progressive uremia
      i. Renal osteodystrophy and soft tissue calcification
      ii. Pericarditis
      iii. Bleeding secondary to platelet dysfunction
      iv. Gastritis
      v. Colitis (rare)
      vi. Constipation
      vii. Skin changes (uremic frost is rare)
      viii. Hyperkalemia and hyponatremia
      ix. Carbohydrate intolerance
      x. Peripheral neuropathy
      xi. Decreased immune response

xii. Pleuritis

xiii. Pulmonary edema

xiv. Hyperparathyroidism (secondary)

xv. Increased rate of atherosclerosis

xvi. Heart murmurs

xvii. Sexual dysfunction and infertility

2. **Expected outcomes**

   a. BUN level maintained below 100 mg/dl or at a level that minimizes uremic symptoms

   b. Stable mental status

   c. Absence of nausea and vomiting

   d. Minimal level of fatigue, as well as other uremic symptoms

3. **Nursing interventions:** based on minimizing azotemia, which will prevent or control uremic symptoms

   a. Prevent dehydration and restrict oral protein intake. Remove blood if present in gastrointestinal tract, since this is another protein source that can be metabolized to ammonia and urea. These two metabolites cannot be handled by diseased kidneys

   b. Consider dialysis to maintain BUN below 100 mg/dl. Each patient develops uremic symptoms at individual levels of BUN. Establish this value for each patient, and strive to maintain the BUN below this level

4. **Evaluation of nursing care**

   a. BUN below 100 mg/dl

   b. Free of or minimized uremic symptoms

   c. Free of lethargy, confusion, or coma

   d. Adequate nutritional and fluid intake, as a result of freedom from nausea and vomiting

Potential for Infection: Infections are the major cause of death in patients with acute renal failure and can seriously compromise the patient with chronic renal failure

1. **Assessment for defining characteristics**

   a. Presence of renal disease

   b. Presence of uremic symptoms

   c. History of repeated infections

   d. Fever and chills

   e. Cough with or without change in sputum

   f. Wound drainage

   g. Cloudy, concentrated urine

   h. Tachycardia and/or hypotension

   i. Alterations in skin integrity, urinary tract, pulmonary, and wound sites

2. **Expected outcomes**

   a. Remains infection free

   b. Infection detected early
3. Nursing interventions
   a. Recognize that patients with renal failure have an impaired immune response
      i. Decreased cellular and hormonal immune responses that may be secondary to uremic toxins
      ii. Reduced phagocytosis by reticuloendothelial system
   b. Implement the following precautions
      i. Obtain urine culture on admission: urinary tract infection (UTI) may be asymptomatic
      ii. Prevent introduction of microorganisms
         (a) Avoid indwelling urinary catheters
         (b) Avoid unnecessary invasive monitoring procedures
      iii. Provide aseptic technique for urinary and intravenous catheter care
      iv. Maintain the BUN at 80 to 100 mg/dl or lower in an effort to minimize susceptibility to infection
      v. Maintain skin integrity: scratching or impaired circulation may precipitate infection, further compromising renal function and increasing severity of uremia by elevating BUN levels. Decrease frequent and unnecessary venipuncture (see also sections on shunt and fistula care, pp. 533 and 534)
      vi. Maintain adequate nutritional intake (protein, calories)
      vii. Institute positive prevention measures (e.g., pulmonary toilet)
      viii. Monitor the environment to decrease cross-contamination between patients
      ix. Use universal precautions
      x. Implement isolation techniques for hepatitis antigen–positive patients receiving hemodialysis: separate machine and consider use of isolation room. These measures are not recommended by the CDC for HIV infection
4. Evaluation of nursing care
   a. Absence of infection
   b. Implementation of preventive measures
   c. Patient achieves optimal level of health

Potential for Bone Disease: Osteomalacia, osteitis fibrosa—chronic hypocalcemia can precipitate hyperparathyroidism, which leads to the mobilization of calcium from the bone. The results are softening of the bone or osteomalacia
1. Assessment for defining characteristics
   a. History of chronic hypocalcemia and/or hyperparathyroidism
   b. Bone pain
   c. Activity intolerance
   d. Fractures

e. Radiologic examination of skull, hands, and feet revealing signs of demineralization

2. **Expected outcomes**
   a. Asymptomatic hypocalcemia
   b. Absence of bone pain and fractures
   c. Maintains ability to ambulate
   d. Compliant with treatment regimen for hypocalcemia

3. **Nursing interventions**
   a. Monitor serum calcium and phosphorus levels and avoid the following
      i. Hypocalcemia: the symptoms of muscle twitching, irritability, and tetany are often masked by the acidemia
      ii. Hyperphosphatemia: stimulates production of parathyroid hormone (PTH) and bone demineralization
   b. Provide pharmacologic therapy to prevent secondary hyperparathyroidism and bone disease
      i. Treatment of hyperphosphatemia can be attempted by dietary restriction, although the more common measure for control is through the administration of antacids that bind dietary phosphates in the intestines. These antacids are composed of an aluminum hydroxide preparation and should be administered to maintain the plasma phosphorus concentration below 5 mg/dl. Side effects of these phosphate binding gels are
         (a) Constipation—sometimes avoided by providing laxatives in conjunction with administration of gels
         (b) Hypophosphatemia
         (c) Aluminum deposits accumulating in fat or brain and other body tissues
      ii. Approaches to vitamin D administration
         (a) Administer large dosages of vitamin D tablets, 50,000 to 125,000 units/day, in an attempt to overcome the vitamin D resistance experienced in renal failure
         (b) Administer dihydrotachysterol, which is a synthetic analogue of vitamin D not requiring 1-hydroxylation in the kidney
         (c) Administer 1,25-vitamin D (the completely activated form) in dosages of 0.25 to 1.0 mg/day
      iii. Calcium supplements can be administered in conjunction with one of the vitamin D preparations
      iv. Explain to the patient the indications for this medication and encourage compliance because avoidance of this medication contributes directly to the development of secondary hyperparathyroidism
      v. Development of secondary hyperparathyroidism presents as hypercalcemia, hyperphosphatemia, and progressive deteriora-

tion of skeletal system. Treatment for uncontrollable hyper-parathyroidism warrants subtotal parathyroidectomy. This treatment will help improve bone disease and may actually curtail some of the uremic symptoms, because PTH has been identified as a significant uremic toxin

4. **Evaluation of nursing care**
    a. Serum calcium level in safe range
    b. Pain free
    c. Compliant with medication therapy

Altered Metabolism of Pharmacologic Agents Related to Renal Failure: A state resulting from the failed kidneys' inability to metabolize and/or excrete medications

1. **Assessment for defining characteristics**
    a. Unusual untoward pharmacologic effects
    b. Enhanced sensitivity to drugs
    c. Retention of the active or toxic metabolites of a medication
    d. Increased azotemia caused by an elevation in metabolic wastes caused by drug usage
2. **Expected outcomes**
    a. Tolerance of pharmacologic therapy
    b. Lack of untoward pharmacologic effects
    c. Minimal to no elevation in BUN
    d. Adequate, prescribed serum drug levels
    e. Stable degree of renal function maintained during pharmacologic therapy
3. **Nursing interventions**
    a. Identify common causes of alterations in the body's use of drugs during renal failure
        i. Distribution of drugs in uremic states
            (a) Decreased stores of body fat affect lipid soluble drugs
            (b) Low cardiac output states—conditions that decrease renal perfusion will limit the amount of drug the kidney is exposed to, thus restricting the degree of renal metabolism and/or excretion of these agents
            (c) Acidemia alters tissue uptake of drugs
            (d) Increased body water has a dilutional effect
            (e) Decreased protein binding occurs during uremia, causing competition by various drugs for tissue binding sites, leading to higher concentration of the unbound drugs
        ii. Specific uremic effects that can alter drug absorption
            (a) Decreased gastrointestinal motility
            (b) Alteration in gastric pH
            (c) Effects on gastrointestinal tract of electrolyte imbalances

(d) Inability of the kidney to excrete or metabolize drugs, or drugs metabolized by liver

(e) Diminished protein binding

   b. General principles for drug administration during renal insufficiency

      i. Reduced drug dosage: essential to be well informed about drugs and dosages administered in relationship to degree of renal failure—mild, moderate, or severe

      ii. Increase intervals between dosages

      iii. Question orders for nephrotoxic agents in order to prevent further renal damage

      iv. Closely observe patient to prevent or assess toxicity due to drug accumulation

      v. Report any untoward signs, especially elevation in serum creatinine, so that drug can be reconsidered, reduced in dosage, or discontinued

      vi. Obtain and monitor serum drug levels, especially in situations requiring a specific drug concentration (e.g., antibiotics, digoxin)

      vii. Administer initial loading doses of drugs that have a long half-life to ensure a more stable serum concentration (e.g., digoxin)

4. Evaluation of nursing care

   a. Patient tolerates pharmacologic therapy

   b. Absence of untoward drug effects

   c. Stable BUN and serum creatinine

   d. Desired serum drug levels

   e. Stable renal function

   f. Compliance with medication

Ineffective Patient and Family Coping: A state created by the stress of renal failure on patient and family

1. Assessment for defining characteristics

   a. Adaptive signs of a patient's ability to cope

      i. Compliance with treatment regimen

      ii. Independence, demonstrates ability to tolerate the restrictions of the dialysis procedure

      iii. Acceptance of role reversal in family and with dialysis staff

      iv. Maintenance or resumption of work

      v. Ability to trust personnel and to relinquish some authority

      vi. Ability to incorporate body image changes into self-concept

   b. Maladaptive signs of a patient's coping

      i. Verbalization of inability to cope or inability to ask for help

      ii. Inability to meet role expectations

      iii. Inability to meet basic needs

      iv. Inability to problem solve

      v. Alteration in societal participation

      vi. Destructive behavior toward self or others

     vii. Unproductive use of defense mechanisms

    viii. Change in usual communication patterns

      ix. Changes in eating patterns: overeating, lack of intake or appetite

       x. Chronic fatigue and/or insomnia

      xi. Alcohol proneness and/or smoking excess

     xii. High rate of illness and/or accidents

    xiii. Muscular tension: frequent neckaches or backaches

    xiv. Chronic anxiety and/or emotional tension

     xv. Poor self-esteem

    xvi. Chronic depression

  c. Maladaptive signs of family coping

       i. Patient expresses or confirms a complaint about family's response to his renal disease

      ii. Family demonstrates a preoccupation with their own personal reaction: fear, anticipatory grief, guilt, anxiety

     iii. Inadequate understanding of patient's condition or therapy that interferes with effective assistance or supportive behaviors

     iv. Withdrawal from communication with patient in time of need

      v. Demonstrates overprotective or underprotective behaviors

2. Expected outcomes

  a. Demonstrates increased independence

  b. Demonstrates increased functional activity

  c. Demonstrates increased social involvement

  d. Appropriately expresses ideas, feelings, and needs

  e. Compliant with treatment regimen

  f. Participates in family activities

  g. Resumes employment

  h. Cooperates with health care personnel

  i. Accepts body image changes as demonstrated through an increased self-esteem

  j. Family provides appropriate support to patient both in stable times and in crisis

  k. Family maintains minimal level of anxiety

  l. Patient and family adjust to role reversal

  m. Seeks support system in times of family crisis

3. Nursing interventions

  a. Identify common causes of stress in the patient and family

       i. Occurrence or exacerbations of acute or chronic illness

      ii. Hospitalization episodes

     iii. Realization of the life-threatening nature of renal disease

     iv. Inability to achieve activities of daily living secondary to fatigue

      v. Restrictions caused by shunt, fistula, or Tenckhoff catheter

      vi. Demands of dialysis schedule

      vii. Reversal in family roles

     viii. Independence vs. dependence conflict

       ix. Effects on sexual behavior and sexuality

        x. Question of maintenance or resumption of work

       xi. Demands of treatment (i.e., dietary restrictions, medication regimen, fluid limitations)

      xii. Onset of complications of renal disease or treatment interventions (e.g., heart disease, neuropathy)

  b. Recognize the psychological consequences of renal disease and its treatment

       i. Denial: the most advantageously used defense mechanism. It is an effective coping mechanism for minimizing the impact of dialysis-related stress

      ii. Depression

     iii. Dependency

     iv. Suicide: believed to be 100 times that of normal population

      v. Sexual dysfunction (loss of libido)

     vi. Other psychosocial problems, family and marital problems, financial problems, significant role reversals

  c. Assess the patient's ability to adapt to the diseased state: a knowledge of the patient's previous responses to stress can provide predictors of how patient will respond to the illness

       i. Gain information about patterns of adaptation and stress by exploring previous responses to failures, illness, and deaths

      ii. Obtain the patient's view of available family support systems

     iii. Describe the patient's present state of satisfaction with medical outcome, spare time activity, self-care abilities, work situation, family life, sexual life, and self

     iv. Determine degree of compliance to treatment regimen (i.e., diet, fluid restriction, dialysis schedule)

  d. Specific nursing interventions directed at supporting adaptation

       i. Orient patient to unit and introduce to personnel and procedures

      ii. Teach the patient about the various treatment alternatives and encourage participation in selection of treatment method

     iii. Provide support systems

        (a) Visits with successfully adjusted patients

        (b) Groups for family members. Patients with supportive families tend to have fewer physical complications, survive longer, and adjust more readily

        (c) Scheduled educational sessions for patients—allows patients to obtain group support

     iv. Functioning within the framework of denial. Educational classes are the most satisfactory means of supplying support to these patients

4. Evaluation of nursing care
   a. Patient demonstrates the following
      i. Willingness to participate in self-care activities
      ii. Participation in social and family activities
      iii. Use of adaptive coping mechanisms such as functional denial
      iv. Increased self-esteem as a measurement of acceptance of body image changes
      v. Cooperation with health care personnel
      vi. Compliance with treatment regimen
   b. Family demonstrates the following
      i. Verbalizes feelings to health care professional and other family members
      ii. Decreased levels of anxiety
      iii. Adaptive change in family roles
      iv. Participates in patient care appropriately
      v. Uses support systems appropriately

PATIENT HEALTH PROBLEMS

Acute Renal Failure: A syndrome of varying etiologies, subclassified into prerenal, renal, and postrenal conditions, resulting in an acute deterioration of renal function. Oliguria or nonoliguria is associated with this disease process; anuria is an uncommon feature. Oliguria is consistent with the presentation of the classic form of acute renal failure (ARF), having a mortality rate of 50% in the critically ill. A slightly higher rate of 50% to 70% is seen in the trauma or postoperative patient. Nonoliguria, a more recently recognized form of presentation, has a better prognosis and a lower mortality rate of 26%

1. Pathophysiology
   a. Prerenal conditions
      i. Physiologic states leading to diminished perfusion to kidney without renal tubular damage
      ii. Effect of diminished pressure to kidney perfusion is
         (a) Decreased pressure to renal artery
         (b) Decreased afferent arterial pressure (below 100 mm Hg), which diminishes forces favoring filtration
   b. Intrarenal conditions
      i. Cortical involvement of vascular, infectious, or immunologic processes
         (a) Causes renal capillary swelling and cellular proliferation, which eventually decreases GFR
         (b) Decreased GFR occurs secondary to obstruction of glomeruli by edema and cellular debris
         (c) Ultimate result is oliguria

ii. Medullary involvement occurs after prolonged ischemia or nephrotoxic injury, specifically to tubular portion of nephron

(a) Tubular necrosis produced is localized into a patchy pattern; extent of damage in nephrotoxic and ischemic injury differs

(1) Nephrotoxic injury affects epithelial cellular layer; this layer can regenerate

(2) Ischemic injury extends sometimes to basement membrane, sometimes involving other parts of nephron and peritubular capillaries. This pattern of damage is crucial, since tubular basement membrane cannot regenerate

(b) Three or four phases of recovery—the classic form of ARF has four phases from onset to oliguria, followed by the diuretic and recovery phases. The nonoliguric form follows only three phases from onset to nonoliguria and then onto the recovery phase. This accounts for the shorter recovery period associated with nonoliguria. Research suggests that the nonoliguric phase is synonymous with the diuretic phase, thus implying that nonoliguric ARF reflects less tubular damage

(1) Onset or initial phase precedes the actual necrotic injury and correlates with a major alteration in renal hemodynamics

a) Associated with a decrease in RBF and GFR

b) Most important factor altering systemic hemodynamics and RBF is a decrease in cardiac output

c) Other mechanisms contributing to the decreased renal perfusion are either an increase in sympathetic activity or an intrarenal angiotensin secretion causing an accentuation of the renal vascular resistance

d) A consistent increase in cardiac output, accomplished during this phase, will produce a consistent increase in RBF. This effect, if sustained, will protect the patient from the impending ARF

(2) Oliguric phase reflects a pathophysiology of four processes

a) Obstruction of tubules by cellular debris, tubular casts, or tissue swelling

b) Total reabsorption or backleak of urine filtration through damaged tubular epithelium and into circulation

c) Tubular cell damage has occurred with the development of necrotic patchy areas. The cell leaks adenosine triphosphate and potassium, and edema is present. There is also an alteration in the mitochondria, and calcium tends to leak into the cell

    d) Renal vasoconstriction continues and may contribute to the decreased GFR

(3) Nonoliguric phase reflects a pathophysiology associated with less tubular damage; symptomatology resembles the diuretic phase

    a) Urine output may exceed 1 L/hr

    b) Solute is present in the urine at approximately 350 mOsm/L

    c) Creatinine clearance as high as 15 ml/min and sodium excretion is low

    d) Hyperkalemia remains a significant problem

    e) Duration of this phase is short, reaching the recovery phase in 5 to 8 days

(4) Diuretic phase signifies that tubular function is returning

    a) Tubular obstruction is relieved, but cellular edema remains as scar tissue forms on necrotic areas

    b) Presents with large daily urine output sometimes exceeding 3 L

    c) This output is due to osmotic-diuretic effect produced by elevated BUN and impaired ability of tubules to conserve sodium and water

(5) Recovery phase

    a) Occurs after gradual improvement of kidney function extending over 3- to 12-month period

    b) Residual impairment in GFR may be the end result

  c. Postrenal conditions: associated with obstruction of urinary collecting system

    i. Partial obstructions: can increase renal interstitial pressure, increasing opposing forces of glomerular filtration. End result is diminished urine output

    ii. Complete obstruction: impediment of urine flow accompanies bilateral kidney involvement. The "back-up" pressure of urine will compress the kidneys

2. Etiology or precipitating factors

  a. Prerenal failure

    i. Hypovolemia secondary to hemorrhage, gastrointestinal losses, and third-spacing phenomena, decreasing ECF volume

    ii. Excessive use of diuretics

    iii. Impaired cardiac function: myocardial infarction, congestive heart failure, acute pulmonary embolism, cardiac tamponade

    iv. Sepsis, progressing to gram-negative shock with vasodilatation

      v. Increased renal vascular resistance resulting from anesthesia or surgery

     vi. Bilateral renal vascular obstruction caused by embolism or thrombosis

  b. Intrarenal failure (cortical involvement)

      i. Acute poststreptococcal glomerulonephritis

     ii. Acute cortical necrosis

    iii. Systemic lupus erythematosus (SLE)

     iv. Goodpasture's syndrome

      v. Bilateral endocarditis

     vi. Pregnancy as seen with abruptio placentae and abortion

    vii. Malignant hypertension

  c. Intrarenal failure (medullary involvement): acute tubular necrosis (ATN) is the most common type of ARF and is the result of nephrotoxic or ischemic injury

      i. Nephrotoxic injury occurs after exposure to nephrotoxic agents, the effects of which are accentuated by dehydration, creating more extensive tubular damage. Examples include

        (a) Antibiotics—aminoglycosides, tetracyclines, penicillins

        (b) Carbon tetrachloride

        (c) Heavy metals—lead, arsenic, mercury, uranium

        (d) Pesticides and fungicides

        (e) X-ray contrast media

     ii. Ischemic injury: during this condition, mean arterial blood flow drops below 60 mm Hg for over 40 minutes. Specific disorders include

        (a) Massive hemorrhage

        (b) Transfusion reaction—tubules are obstructed with hemolyzed erythrocytes

        (c) Septic or cardiogenic shock

        (d) Major trauma or crush injuries

        (e) Postsurgical hypotension

        (f) Postpartum hemorrhage of pregnancy

  d. Postrenal failure: obstructive process can occur anywhere from kidney to urinary meatus

      i. Urethral obstruction

     ii. Prostatic hypertrophy

    iii. Bladder involvement: obstruction, carcinoma, infection, or neurogenic problems

     iv. Ureteral obstruction resulting from renal calculi and edema

      v. Extraureteral problems: abdominal tumor

3. Nursing assessment data base: complete the general assessment for the renal patient described earlier in this chapter, then refer to this section for specific elements concerning ARF

  a. Nursing history: the focus is to collaborate with the physician to establish if a rapidly reversible form of ARF is present. The primary nursing focus is to determine how the patient is coping with the acute failure both physiologically and psychologically

   i. Subjective findings

      (a) Patient's chief complaint—change in the volume or lack of urine output

      (b) Other symptoms—fatigue, lethargy, weakness

  ii. Objective findings

      (a) Etiologic or precipitating factors—collect data necessary to determine etiology of abrupt decrease in renal function, elevated BUN and creatinine levels, and decrease in urine volume

      (1) Prerenal conditions

         a) History of dehydration

         b) History of cardiac failure

         c) History of venacaval obstruction

         d) Profound liver disease (hepatorenal syndrome)

      (2) Intrarenal conditions

         a) Nephrotoxicity—history of exposure to nephrotoxic drugs, either environmental, occupational, or iatrogenic (including aminoglycosides and radiographic contrast media, e.g., IVP dye)

         b) Hypotensive-ischemic catastrophes causing ATN—history of recent surgery, cardiogenic or septic shock, trauma, anesthesia, aortic aneurysm, or severe hemorrhage

         c) Bilateral emboli to both kidneys causing infarction

         d) Glomerular disease—cortical necrosis secondary to pregnancy or anaphylaxis and acute glomerulonephritis occurring after streptococcal infections

         e) Tubular obstruction—occurs with formation of abnormal proteins; seen in multiple myeloma and other obstructive states such as in rhabdomyolysis

      (3) Postrenal conditions (bilateral obstruction)

         a) History of prostatic disease

         b) History of disease of cervix (e.g., malignancy)

         c) History of colonic disease

         d) Bladder malignancy

         e) History of renal calculi with bilateral flank pain and hematuria

         f) History of disease that causes bilateral renal calculi (e.g., leukemia)—results in hyperuricemia and bilateral uric acid stones

         g) Pregnancy

    h) Recent pelvic surgery (hysterectomy or ureteroligation)

    i) Bilateral retroperitoneal disease (e.g., lymphoma, sarcoma, retroperitoneal fibrosis)

   (b) Family history

    (1) Describes the family unit and impact of ARF

    (2) Describes the perception of family member's support of patient

   (c) Social history

    (1) Employment status including type of work and impact of disease on performance or position

    (2) Sexual dysfunction—uremia depresses the libido and sexual function of the patient with ARF. However, since these patients are often hospitalized, this factor may not be an issue unless discharge occurs

   (d) Medication history

    (1) Diuretics—check for excessive use

    (2) Antibiotics—check if taking nephrotoxic antibiotics

    (3) Vasopressors—check if high dosages received; may diminish RBF

   (e) Past hospitalizations

  b. Nursing examination of patient: clinical presentation during first few days of oliguria or nonoliguria is dominated by primary disease process or underlying illness

   i. Inspection

    (a) Neurologic—confusion, lethargy, stupor and neuromuscular involvement including twitching and weakness secondary to metabolic acidosis

    (b) Respiratory—deep, rapid respirations or Kussmaul's respirations secondary to metabolic acidosis

    (c) Cardiovascular—ECG reveals dysrhythmias secondary to electrolyte or cardiac involvement (e.g., congestive heart failure)

    (d) Genitourinary—oliguria defined as less than 400 ml/24 hr or nonoliguria

    (e) Gastrointestinal—weight loss secondary to anorexia, nausea and vomiting, coffee-ground emesis, or melena

    (f) Integument—dry skin, edema, pallor, bruising, uremic frost, and pruritus

    (g) Musculoskeletal—impaired mobility

    (h) Other—examine for signs of local infection such as inflammation, pain, pus, or discolored drainage at a wound site. Systemic infection may present as shaking chills and fatigue

   ii. Palpation

(a) Cardiac—tachycardia, irregular pulse secondary to electrolyte imbalances

(b) Genitourinary—flank pain may be present

iii. Percussion

(a) Bladder—small in oliguria, distended in lower urinary tract obstruction

(b) Abdominal distention—secondary to constipation

iv. Auscultation

(a) Blood pressure may be normal or increased as disease state progresses

(b) Friction rub may indicate uremic pericarditis

(c) Pulmonary rales/crackles associated with pulmonary edema

(d) If on hemodialysis, vascular access—assess for patency by checking bruit or thrill; determine absence of infection

c. Diagnostic study findings

i. Laboratory

(a) Prerenal

(1) Urinary sodium level less than 10 mEq/L

(2) Specific gravity greater than 1.020

(3) Serum BUN elevated in greater proportion than rise in creatinine (greater than the normal 10:1)

(4) Minimal or no proteinuria

(5) Normal urinary sediment

(b) Intrarenal (cortical disease)

(1) Urinary sodium level less than 10 mEq/L

(2) Specific gravity varies

(3) Moderate to heavy proteinuria

(4) Serum BUN and creatinine values elevated

(5) Hematuria

(6) Urinary sediment with erythrocyte casts and leukocytes

(c) Intrarenal (medullary disease)

(1) Urinary sodium level greater than 20 mEq/L

(2) Specific gravity 1.010

(3) Minimal to moderate proteinuria

(4) Serum BUN and creatinine elevated

(5) Urinary sediment with numerous renal tubular epithelial cells, tubular casts, and a rare erythrocyte

(d) Postrenal

(1) Serum BUN and creatinine elevated when complete obstruction present

(2) Bacteriology report significant for a specific organism

(e) Special

(1) Antistreptolysin-O (ASO) titer to diagnose recent

streptococcal infection, which may cause poststrepto-
coccal glomerulonephritis

(2) Antiglomerular basement membrane titers to diagnose
Goodpasture's syndrome, a devastating disease of pulmonary hemorrhage and renal failure

(3) Serum studies for complement components—a fall in
complement levels is seen in active complement-me-
diated glomerulonephritis (e.g., lupus nephritis)

(4) Serum electrophoresis for immunoglobulin levels—
abnormal proteins, as seen in multiple myeloma, can
damage kidneys irreversibly

ii. Radiologic: major reason for urographic studies is to rule out
obstruction as cause of oliguria or anuria. Presence of obstruction must be determined, since its immediate treatment may
reverse symptoms of renal failure

4. **Nursing diagnoses**
   a. Potential for ARF
      i. Assessment for defining characteristics
         (a) Sudden decrease in or cessation of urine output
         (b) Severe dehydration
         (c) Prolonged hypotensive episode
         (d) Presence of septic shock (high incidence of ARF)
         (e) Presence of trauma or burns
      ii. Expected outcomes
         (a) Resolution of ARF
         (b) Resumes renal function (i.e., normal urine output)
         (c) Maintains homeostatic fluid balance
         (d) Maintains blood pressure within normal limits
         (e) Stabilization of septic patient including maintenance of
             adequate renal perfusion
      iii. Nursing interventions
         (a) Monitor for prerenal or onset stage of ATN
            (1) Severe dehydration (hypovolemia) or cardiac failure
               a) Hypotension—renal autoregulation is essentially
                  absent at an arterial pressure of 70 mm Hg or
                  below
               b) Oliguria (occasionally anuria)—the urine is dilute,
                  with a urine osmolality similar to the plasma
                  osmolality and a urinary sodium of 10 mEq/L or
                  less
               c) Renal vasoconstriction—occurs in response to de-
                  creased cardiac output and hypotension as revealed
                  by
                  ☐ A decreased urinary output not responding to
                  intravenous fluid administration

    □ Increased serum renin levels
  (b) Identify patient at high risk for ARF
    (1) Hemodynamically unstable
    (2) Multiple trauma victim
    (3) Burn victim
    (4) Intravenous hemolysis
    (5) Receiving nephrotoxic drugs
    (6) Rhabdomyolysis
    (7) Surgical patients—blood loss, hypotension, and anesthesia can diminish or interrupt RBF
  (c) Monitor arterial and venous blood pressure
  (d) Monitor urine output
  (e) Correct hypotension
  (f) Prevent or minimize causes of prerenal condition (e.g., dehydration, vasodilatation or vasoconstriction, diminished cardiac output)
  (g) Obtain urine and blood specimens for laboratory analysis and interpret results
 iv. Evaluation of nursing care
  (a) Improved renal perfusion and prevention of ATN
  (b) Urine output over 30 ml/hr with normal concentration
  (c) Balanced 24-hour total on intake/output record coincided with daily weight
  (d) Stabilization of primary illness (e.g., sepsis, trauma, or burns)
b. Urinary elimination, altered patterns—oliguria, anuria and nonoliguria, and polyuria are the urinary patterns associated with ARF
 i. Assessment for defining characteristics
  (a) Oliguria—urine output less than 400 ml/24 hr
  (b) Anuria—no urine output
  (c) Nonoliguria—a dilute urine output in a normal volume or a urine volume in excess of the body's need for water
  (d) Polyuria—a large dilute urine output in excess of body water need
 ii. Expected outcomes
  (a) Balanced fluid intake and output
  (b) Physiologic levels of electrolytes
  (c) Return of normal urinary output
 iii. Nursing interventions
  (a) Monitor and record urine output volume
  (b) Assess character of urine—color, clarity, concentration, specific gravity, and odor
  (c) Report changes in the volume or character of the urine output; changes may reflect a recovering kidney. Adjust

therapeutic regimen accordingly, to match the stage of renal recovery

(d) Assess fluid status
(1) Oliguria or anuria—suspect fluid volume excess
(2) Nonoliguria or polyuria—examine for normal hydration or dehydration

(e) Monitor serum electrolytes and assess for the following
(1) Oliguria or anuria—expect retention and accumulation of electrolytes
(2) Nonoliguria or polyuria—expect either accumulation or uncontrolled loss of electrolytes

iv. Evaluation of nursing care
(a) Remains in a zero fluid balance despite the alteration in urine output
(b) Maintains electrolyte balance despite kidney's inability to concentrate the urine
(c) Appearance of normal urine output—volume and concentration

c. Fluid volume excess (see p. 500)
i. Additional assessment for defining characteristics
(a) Compare urinary pattern and fluid balances
(b) Maintain patency of diagnostic arterial or venous lines

ii. Additional expected outcomes
(a) Presence of weight loss or stable weight (as appropriate)
(b) Alert mental status
(c) Dialysis effective in treating fluid imbalances

iii. Additional nursing interventions
(a) Collaborate with physician to establish fluid therapy plan and implement
(b) Implement dialysis for repeated episodes of symptomatic fluid volume overload

d. Fluid volume deficit: a state associated with the diuretic or nonoliguric stage of ARF, which is caused by the excessive loss of urinary volume without adequate volume replacement (see p. 501)
i. Additional assessment for defining characteristics
(a) Presence of diuretic or nonoliguric state

ii. Additional expected outcomes
(a) Stable weight or weight gain
(b) Regains or remains in fluid balance

iii. Additional nursing interventions
(a) Collaborate with physician to establish fluid therapy plan
(b) Implement fluid "push" regimen when appropriate

iv. Additional evaluation of nursing care
(a) Presence of weight gain or stable weight
(b) Alert mental status

e. Potential for uremic syndrome: the uremic syndrome refers to the constellation of symptoms associated with the systemic effects of uremia (see p. 513)

   i. Additional expected outcomes

     (a) Absence of debilitating symptoms (e.g., nausea, vomiting, fatigue)

     (b) Stable on dialysis

  ii. Additional nursing interventions (see p. 514)

     (a) Assess for the presence of uremic symptoms

     (b) Implement conservative measures for controlling BUN

     (c) Initiate dialysis for uncontrollable symptomatic azotemia, acidosis, hypercatabolism, hyperkalemia, and volume overload

     (d) Monitor for indications for hemodialysis

       (1) Acute renal failure

       (2) Chronic renal failure when medications and diet no longer provide effective therapy

       (3) Rapid removal of toxic substances from bloodstream (e.g., alcohol, aspirin, barbiturates, some antibiotics, and other poisons)

       (4) Dialysis to keep BUN under 100 mg/dl to improve survival

       (5) Appearance of uremic pericardial friction rub

     (e) Monitor for contraindications of hemodialysis

       (1) Intolerance to systemic heparinization

       (2) Labile cardiovascular status incompatible with rapid changes in extravascular fluid volume

     (f) Monitor for indications for peritoneal dialysis

       (1) Fluid overload

       (2) Electrolyte or acid–base imbalance

       (3) Acute or chronic renal failure

       (4) Intoxication from dialyzable drugs and poisons

       (5) Peritonitis or pericarditis

       (6) Unavailability of vascular access for hemodialysis (arteriovenous access crisis)

     (g) Contraindications—bleeding disorder, abdominal adhesions, and recent peritoneal surgery

     (h) Monitor for indications/contraindications for continuous arteriovenous hemofiltration (CAVH) and continuous arteriovenous hemodialysis (CAVHD)—a procedure using a hollow-fiber hemofilter capable of rapid fluid removal during hypotensive or low blood flow states

       (1) Conditions of fluid overload or cardiovascular instability requiring a continuous method of fluid removal and/or compensation for azotemia

a) Acute or chronic renal failure

b) Acute pulmonary edema

c) Post cardiac surgery

d) Recent myocardial infarction

e) Ascites

(2) Inability to tolerate the cardiovascular impact of rapid fluid losses that are associated with hemodialysis

(i) Initiate hemodialysis—extracorporeal technique for removing waste products or toxic substances from systemic circulation (Fig. 4–4)

(1) Principles are same as for peritoneal dialysis

(2) Anticoagulation

a) Prior to procedure, heparinization is done to keep blood anticoagulated within hemodialysis machine ("regional heparinization")

b) For patients without complications, 5000 units heparin is administered to start and 2000 units/hr while on machine ("general heparinization"). Dosage may have to be adjusted to meet needs of individual patients

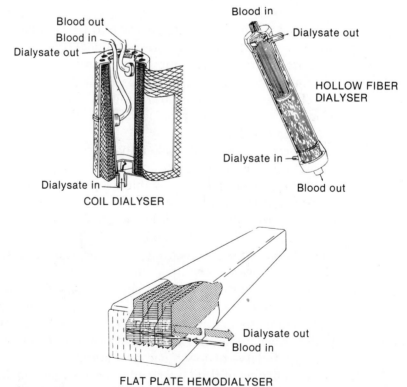

Figure 4–4. Types of hemodialyzers. (From Levine, D. Z.: Care of the Renal Patient. W. B. Saunders Co., Philadelphia, 1983.)

    c) Patients should be monitored closely for signs of bleeding

(3) Shunt care

    a) Auscultate for bruit or palpate for thrill to assess shunt patency

    b) Promptly report any suspicion of clotting, color change of blood, separation of serum from erythrocytes, or absence of pulsations in tubing

    c) Provide adequate hydration to minimize clotting

    d) Change sterile dressing over shunt at least daily. Reinforce dressing as necessary

    e) DO NOT: perform venipuncture, give intravenous therapy, give injections, or take blood pressure with cuff on shunt arm

    f) Instruct patient in self-care of shunt site

(4) Arteriovenous fistula care

    a) DO NOT: perform venipuncture, start intravenous therapy, give injections, or take blood pressure with cuff on arm with fistula

    b) Palpate thrill or auscultate bruit to confirm patency

    c) Avoid circumferential dressings or restrictive clothing

    d) Report bleeding, skin discoloration, drainage, or other signs of infection. Culture drainage

    e) For profuse bleeding, apply a pressure dressing

(5) Femoral vein catheter care

    a) Palpate peripheral pulses in cannulized extremity

    b) Observe for bleeding or hematoma formation. Apply a pressure dressing and notify the physician

    c) Properly position the catheter to avoid dislodgement during the dialysis procedure

    d) If the femoral vein catheter is to be maintained post dialysis, then connect to a pressurized intravenous flow system. Add to the infusion solution a low dose of heparin, usually 500 units/1000 ml. Maintain a secure aseptic dressing to minimize the risk of infection. Discourage ambulation

    e) On removal of the femoral catheter, apply direct pressure to the puncture site for 5 to 10 minutes or the amount of time necessary to cause cessation of bleeding post dialysis (and after its period of heparinization). Complete this procedure with application of a pressure dressing and a period of bed rest

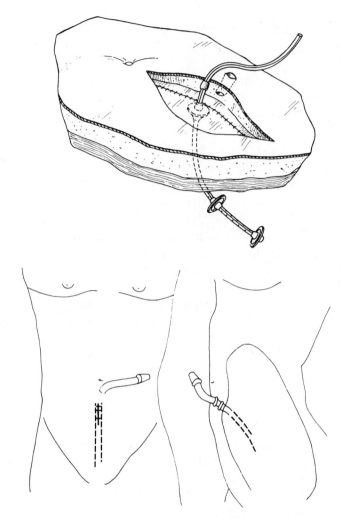

Figure 4–5. Permanent peritoneal catheter in place, showing its position with respect to the different layers of the abdominal wall *(top)*, the anteroposterior position *(lower left)*, and the catheter angle with respect to abdominal wall *(lower right)*. (From Levine, D. Z.: Care of the Renal Patient. W. B. Saunders Co., Philadelphia, 1983.)

    (j) Initiate peritoneal dialysis (Fig. 4–5)
        (1) Principles
            a) Osmosis—movement of water across a semipermeable membrane from area of lesser to one of greater osmolality
            b) Diffusion—movement of molecules from area of higher concentration to one of lower concentration
            c) Filtration—movement of particles through a semipermeable membrane by means of hydrostatic pressure
        (2) Important nursing tasks
            a) Explain procedure to patient—include the duration, limited mobility, and discomfort. Approach varies according to mental status
            b) Weigh patient before and after treatment

c) Prepare equipment using aseptic technique—use automated peritoneal dialysis machine when available since it provides a closed system decreasing the risk of infection

d) Dialysate solution, 1.5%, 2.5%, or 4.25% glucose; select concentration according to desired osmotic gradient necessary for water removal

e) Add medications to dialysate as prescribed
   - ☐ Heparin to prevent clotting in dialysis catheter
   - ☐ Potassium chloride—dosage varies according to serum potassium levels and requirement for digitalization precautions
   - ☐ Antibiotics for treatment of peritonitis
   - ☐ Lidocaine for control of local discomfort (approximately 50 mg/2 L dialysis fluid)

f) Patient must void before procedure is begun to eliminate bladder distention and thus decrease risk of bladder perforation during trocar or Tenckhoff insertion. If unable to void, patient must be catheterized

g) Warm dialysate solution to body temperature

h) Assist physician during trocar insertion

i) First dialysate solution must be drained immediately to determine if catheter is patent—outflow should drain in a steady stream

j) Allow all other infusions to "pool" or "dwell" in abdomen (an average of 20 to 45 minutes) for optimal fluid and electrolyte exchange

k) Drain at end of dwell time and observe characteristics of dialysate outflow
   - ☐ Normal—clear, pale yellow
   - ☐ Cloudy—infection, peritonitis
   - ☐ Brownish—bowel perforation
   - ☐ Amber—bladder perforation
   - ☐ Blood-tinged—common occurrence, first to fourth exchange; if bleeding continues, may indicate abdominal bleeding or uremic coagulopathy

l) Obtain periodic culture and sensitivity of outflow fluid

m) Monitor total body intake and output and maintain records
   - ☐ Follow established therapeutic goal for fluid and electrolyte removal
   - ☐ Measure amount of fluid removed for each ex-

change and record positive and negative balances

n) Monitor vital signs during outflow phase

☐ Anticipate changes in baseline blood pressure and pulse rate and rhythm indicative of impending shock or overhydration

☐ When using hypertonic dialysate (4.25%), expect osmotic effect

☐ Important to monitor glucose levels in all patients, especially in diabetics

(k) Initiate CAVH and CAVHD

(1) Principles of CAVH (Fig. 4–6)

a) Uses the process of hemofiltration, which is the exchange of plasma water and small-sized molecules (such as potassium, BUN, and creatinine) by convection

b) Rate of exchange is dependent on membrane area, fiber diameter, hematocrit, and plasma protein concentration, as well as pressure gradient and blood flow rate

c) CAVHD—incorporates the use of peritoneal dialysis fluid with hemofiltration, thus combining the properties of diffusion with convection. The peritoneal dialysis fluid administration is regulated by

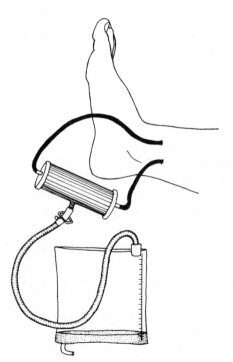

Figure 4–6. Continuous slow ultrafiltration. (From Levine, D. Z.: Care of the Renal Patient. W. B. Saunders Co., Philadelphia, 1983.)

a volumetric pump at 15 ml/min. The dialysis fluid enters the ultrafiltration compartment of the hemofilter and flows in the opposite direction of the blood flow

(2) Overview of method

    a) Prepare patient—explain procedure. Obtain baseline serum studies, clotting time, chemistries, arterial blood gas studies, and complete blood cell count. Administer loading dose of heparin

    b) Prepare hemofilter and connect to arteriovenous access properly

    c) Determine blood flow through hemofilter and resulting ultrafiltration rate and begin fluid replacement therapy

    d) Monitor fluid replacement according to patient's condition and desired rate of filtrate output preventing circulatory collapse

    e) Regulate blood pressure, oncotic pressure, and ultrafiltration compartment to optimize amount of filtrate

f. Potential for electrolyte imbalances (see p. 503): the ARF patient is at risk for a number of electrolyte imbalances, often varying with the phase of ARF

    i. Additional assessment for defining characteristics

      (a) Oliguric phase

        (1) Hyperkalemia

          a) Numbness of extremities to flaccid paralysis

          b) Nausea

          c) Abdominal cramps, diarrhea

          d) Hyperirritable bowel sounds

          e) Oliguria

          f) Tall, peaked T waves and/or widened QRS complex with bradycardia preceding cardiac arrest

          g) Apathy and mental confusion

        (2) Hypocalcemia

          a) Muscle cramps

          b) Abdominal cramps

          c) Tetany to seizures

          d) Laryngeal stridor

          e) Carpopedal spasm

          f) Impaired cardiac contractility with diminished cardiac output

          g) Prolonged ST segment and QT interval

        (3) Hyperphosphatemia—defining characteristics same as for hypocalcemia

(b) Diuretic or nonoliguric phase

    (1) Hypokalemia—results from the loss of potassium in the urine

        a) Malaise to confusion

        b) Muscular weakness progressing to paralysis

        c) Muscle cramps

        d) Nausea and vomiting

        e) Decreased peristalsis to paralytic ileus

        f) Abdominal distention

        g) Polyuria

    (2) Hyperkalemia—seen in early period of nonoliguria

    (3) Hypercalcemia—occurs in patients who have experienced severe rhabdomyolysis

        a) Anorexia

        b) Nausea and vomiting

        c) Lethargy to coma

        d) Headache

        e) Generalized muscle weakness

        f) Deep bone pain

        g) Polyuria and polydipsia

        h) Kidney stones

    (4) Hypophosphatemia—occurs with large amounts of phosphate lost in the urine

ii. Additional expected outcomes

    (a) Asymptomatic or normal levels of electrolytes

    (b) Tolerates therapeutic interventions to correct electrolyte imbalances

    (c) Compliant with preventative measures for control of electrolyte levels

iii. Additional nursing interventions

    (a) Recognize the types of electrolyte imbalances associated with the phases of ARF

    (b) Prevent or practice early detection of electrolyte imbalances

    (c) Collaborate with physician to determine specific therapeutic interventions for each electrolyte imbalance (refer to section on electrolyte imbalances)

    (d) Monitor serum electrolyte levels to assess therapeutic response

    (e) Initiate dialysis for repeated symptomatic electrolyte imbalances

iv. Additional evaluation of nursing care

    (a) Serum electrolyte levels are in a normal or slightly altered range

(b) Absence of symptoms associated with electrolyte imbalance

(c) Compliance with therapeutic regimen

g. Potential for metabolic acidosis: a state created by the acutely failed kidney's inability to excrete hydrogen (see p. 511)

 i. Additional expected outcomes

 (a) Maintains pH within an asymptomatic range

 (b) Tolerates dialysis treatment for correction of metabolic acidosis

 ii. Additional nursing interventions

 (a) Collaborate with physician to establish baseline value for pH

 (b) In emergency situations, administer sodium bicarbonate slowly by intravenous infusion to correct systemic pH

 (c) Be aware that each bolus of sodium bicarbonate contains approximately 54 mEq/50 ml of sodium. Repeated infusions can cause a significant sodium overload that could precipitate pulmonary edema

 (d) Implement dialysis for repeated episodes of symptomatic acidosis

h. Potential for infection: an increased risk of infection is created in ARF by multiple reasons, including primary etiology, uremia, and debilitated, malnourished state. Septic shock is a frequent complication of ARF (see p. 514)

 i. Additional assessment for defining characteristics

 (a) Fever (may be masked) and chills

 (b) Increased leukocyte count

 (c) BUN level over 80 to 100 mg/dl coincides with an increased risk of infection

 ii. Additional expected outcomes

 (a) Remains free of infection

 (b) Infection detected early

 iii. Additional nursing interventions

 (a) Monitor for early signs of septic shock

i. Potential for anemia: the risk for anemia in ARF results from (1) actual bleeding secondary to primary etiology or uremia, (2) lack of erythropoietin, and/or (3) presence of septic shock, which is commonly associated with the onset of disseminated intravascular coagulation (see p. 512)

 i. Additional assessment for defining characteristics

 (a) Actual bleeding

 (1) Positive result of guaiac test of nasogastric drainage, vomitus, stool, or other drainage

 (2) Ecchymotic areas

 (3) Swollen area representative of a collection of blood

(b) Erythropoietin lack—anemia occurring in the absence of any signs of actual bleeding during ARF

(c) Anemia

ii. Additional nursing interventions

(a) Assess for actual bleeding on the onset of anemia

(b) Consider lack of erythropoietin as a cause of anemia

(c) Collaborate with physician to determine the range of hematocrit levels requiring blood transfusions

(d) Assess symptomatology of anemia determining patient's tolerance of this condition

j. Nutrition altered: less than body requirements, a state created by the insufficient intake of nutrients (see p. 504)

i. Additional assessment for defining characteristics

(a) Uncontrollable high BUN levels indicative of hypercatabolic state

ii. Additional nursing interventions

(a) Be aware of factors to consider when determining nutritional needs

(1) Primary disease

(2) Presence of ATN

(3) Presence of catabolism

(4) Predisposition to infection

(5) Presence of fluid and electrolyte imbalances

(6) Presence of acidosis

(b) Assess for presence of hypercatabolism

(1) Repeated elevations of BUN over 100 mg/dl despite the use of routine dialysis

(2) Signs of rapid muscle wasting

(c) Consider usual diet—restricted in protein, sodium, and potassium but including essential amino acids with a high caloric value of 100 g of carbohydrate per day

(d) Be aware that hyperalimentation and daily dialysis have been associated with increased survival rates in ARF, as well as promoting renal tubular cell regeneration. Hyperalimentation requirements include large amounts of amino acids (2 g/day of both essential and nonessential amino acids)

(e) Glucose and lipid solution administered intravenously can also be considered

(f) Monitor serum protein, albumin, hematocrit, and urea levels in conjunction with daily weights to determine effectiveness of nutritional therapy

k. Impaired skin integrity: potential—a state created by uremia effect, malnutrition, and immobility

i. Assessment for defining characteristics

    (a) Dry skin

    (b) Itching

    (c) Bruising

    (d) Uremic frost

    (e) Infection

    (f) Edema

    (g) Presence of wounds and/or skin ulcers

    (h) Changes in skin texture and thickness

  ii. Expected outcomes

    (a) Intact skin

    (b) Presence of wound healing

 iii. Nursing interventions

    (a) Initiate a regimen to keep skin clean, dry, and intact to prevent infection

      (1) Bathe skin daily to remove waste products

      (2) Apply creams or ointments

      (3) Administer medications to relieve itching (e.g., diphenhydramine)

      (4) Use oil in bath to prevent dryness

      (5) Cleanse bruises and open areas to prevent infection

      (6) Monitor for presence of edema

      (7) Avoid tight-fitting shoes or clothing that may create pressure points susceptible to breakdown

    (b) Use aseptic technique during care of wounds

  iv. Evaluation of nursing care

    (a) Dry, clean skin

    (b) Intact skin

    (c) Absence of itching

    (d) Absence of infection

    (e) Healing wounds

l. Sleep pattern disturbance: a state resulting from the critical care environment and the uremic condition

  i. Assessment for defining characteristics

    (a) Frequent interruptions of patient's sleep cycle for monitoring of health status

    (b) Lack of 90-minute periods of sleep

    (c) Patient verbalizes lack of sleep

    (d) Restless during sleep with frequent awakening

    (e) Fatigue, irritability, and lethargy related to sleep deficit

  ii. Expected outcomes

    (a) Three to four 90-minute periods of uninterrupted sleep cycles

    (b) Absence of symptoms of sleep deprivation

 iii. Nursing interventions

    (a) Obtain sleep history (i.e., day or night sleeper)

       (b) Use information acquired in sleep history to develop patient care plan

       (c) Organize care to minimize patient interruptions

       (d) Limit noise in environment

       (e) Allow three to four 90-minute cycles of sleep in a 24-hour period

    iv. Evaluation of nursing care

       (a) Patient receives three to four 90-minute cycles of sleep

       (b) Oriented to time, place, person, and surroundings

       (c) Verbalizes obtaining adequate sleep

m. Knowledge deficit related to ARF: the sudden onset of ARF may be associated with a lack of knowledge

    i. Assessment for defining characteristics: lacks knowledge and/or understanding of the following

       (a) Monitoring equipment in ICU

       (b) Dietary and/or fluid restrictions

       (c) Dialysis machine and process

       (d) Etiology of renal disease

       (e) Prospects for recovery

    ii. Expected outcomes

       (a) Verbalizes basic knowledge of ARF and treatment

       (b) Decreased anxiety as a result of knowledge

    iii. Nursing interventions

       (a) Assess level of readiness to learn

       (b) Assess uremic effects on learning: memory, attention span, thought processing

       (c) Teach patient key points about critical care experience, ARF, and treatment regimen

    iv. Evaluation of nursing care

       (a) Patient conveys basic knowledge of disease process and treatment

       (b) Cooperates with care based on knowledge

       (c) Expresses decreased anxiety

n. Altered metabolism/excretion of pharmacologic agents resulting from the acutely failed kidney's ability to metabolize or excrete medications (see p. 517)

    i. Additional nursing interventions

       (a) Be aware of nephrotoxic agents usually ordered for ARF

          (1) Antibiotics—gentamicin, carbenicillin, and amikacin

          (2) Diuretics—furosemide in large dosages

       (b) Monitor BUN and serum creatinine levels to determine drug effect on renal function

       (c) Monitor serum drug levels

       (d) Observe for and report any untoward drug effects

(e) Collaborate with physician to determine need for modifying pharmacologic administration
    (1) Reduced drug dosage
    (2) Increased intervals between doses

o. Ineffective patient and family coping: the sudden onset of ARF compounds its psychosocial impact (see p. 518)
    i. Assessment for defining characteristics
    ii. Additional expected outcomes
        (a) Maintains minimal level of anxiety
        (b) Cooperates with health care providers
        (c) Exhibits trust of health care providers
        (d) Uses support systems
    iii. Additional nursing interventions
        (a) Identify common causes of stress in the patient
            (1) Sudden, unexpected onset of loss of health
            (2) Uncertainty of future—balance between hope and despair for recovery of renal function
            (3) Body image changes—loss of urine-making ability, arteriovenous or peritoneal access, bruises, changes in skin color and texture
            (4) Long-term hospitalization, including stay in ICU, removes patient from home and work
            (5) Fear for loss of life
    iv. Additional evaluation of nursing care
        (a) Expresses decreased feelings of anxiety
        (b) Participates in care
        (c) Demonstrates trust in caregivers
        (d) Participates during sessions offering psychosocial support

Chronic Renal Failure: A slowly progressive renal disorder culminating in end-stage renal disease. The decline in kidney function correlates with the degree of nephron loss

1. **Pathophysiology:** systemic changes occur when overall renal function is less than 20% to 25% of normal
    a. Bricker's "intact nephron" hypothesis: provides an explanation for the kidney's ability to compensate and preserve homeostasis despite a significant loss (80%) of nephron function. During chronic renal failure (CRF), regardless of etiology, injury occurs to the nephrons in a progressive manner. Significant damage to groups of nephrons will eliminate them from their contributory role in maintaining renal function. The remaining intact nephrons will compensate for the loss of functioning nephrons by cellular hypertrophy. This growth process will enable nephrons to accept larger blood volumes for clearances, resulting in the excretion of greater solute levels; thus compensation results

b. Four stages of CRF: each stage is synonymous with a certain degree of nephron loss
   i. Diminished renal reserve: 50% nephron loss
     (a) Kidney function is mildly reduced, while the excretory and regulatory functions are sufficiently maintained to preserve a normal internal environment. The patient usually is problem free
     (b) The patient's normal serum creatinine value usually will double. A normal value of 0.6 mg/dl will elevate to 1.2 mg/dl, which is still within normal limits
   ii. Renal insufficiency: a 75% nephron loss
     (a) Evidence of impaired renal capacity that appears in the form of mild azotemia, slightly impaired urinary concentrating ability, and anemia
     (b) Factors that can exacerbate the disease at this stage by increasing nephron damage are infection, dehydration, drugs, and cardiac failure
   iii. End-stage renal disease: 90% of the nephrons are damaged
     (a) Renal function has deteriorated so that chronic and persistent abnormalities exist
     (b) Patient requires artificial support to sustain life (dialysis or transplantation)
   iv. Uremic syndrome
     (a) The body's systemic responses to the build-up of uremic waste products and the results of the failed organ system
     (b) Usually described as the constellation of signs and symptoms demonstrated by renal failure
     (c) Symptoms may be avoided or diminished by initiation of early dialysis treatment

2. Etiology or precipitating factors
a. Tubulointerstitial disease or interstitial nephritis
   i. Pyelonephritis, chronic (most common cause)
   ii. Analgesic abuse nephropathy
   iii. Myeloma kidney
   iv. Uric acid renal disease
   v. Hyperkalemic nephropathy
   vi. Cystic disease of kidney
     (a) Congenital multicystic disease
     (b) Polycystic disease
     (c) Medullary cystic disease
     (d) Medullary sponge kidney
   vii. Sarcoidosis
   viii. Immunologic mechanisms (transplant rejection, allergic response, hypersensitivity)
   ix. Radiation nephritis

       x. Idiopathic organ nephritis

      xi. Hypokalemic nephropathy

  b. Glomerulonephropathies

       i. Focal glomerulosclerosis (IgA type antibody: benign and hereditary nephritis)

      ii. Crescentic glomerulonephritis (rapidly progressing)

    iii. Membranoproliferative glomerulonephritis

     iv. Lipoid nephrosis

      v. Membranous glomerulonephritis

     vi. Chronic glomerulonephritis

    vii. Diabetes mellitus—Kimmelstiel-Wilson syndrome

   viii. Systemic lupus erythematosus

     ix. Goodpasture's syndrome

      x. Polyarteritis nodosa

     xi. Wegener's granulomatosis

    xii. Bacterial endocarditis

   xiii. Henoch-Schönlein purpura

  c. Nephrotic syndrome: seen in patients with glomerular or tubular disorders

  d. Renal vascular disorders

       i. Systemic vasculitis (i.e., polyarteritis nodosa, hypersensitivity vasculitis)

      ii. Scleroderma

    iii. Coagulopathies

        (a) Hemolytic-uremic syndrome

        (b) Preeclampsia and pregnancy

        (c) Cortical necrosis

     iv. Thromboembolic disease

        (a) Renal vein thrombosis

        (b) Renal atheroembolus

      v. Sickle cell nephropathy

     vi. Hypertensive nephrosclerosis

        (a) Benign nephrosclerosis

        (b) Malignant nephrosclerosis

        (c) Accelerated nephrosclerosis

  e. Renal cancer

       i. Renal cell carcinoma (most common renal neoplasm)

      ii. Secondary neoplasms such as bronchogenic carcinoma, adenocarcinoma of the stomach and breast, and a variety of other neoplasms. Leukemia and lymphoma may also occur

3. Nursing assessment data base: complete the general assessment for the renal patient described earlier in this chapter; then refer to this section for specific elements concerning CRF

  a. Nursing history: the focus is to determine the stage of CRF and the patient's tolerance of this stage. A history of the patient's experiences with renal replacement therapies is also collected. This information contributes to the formation of a view of how the patient is coping with CRF

   i. Subjective findings
- (a) Patient's chief complaint: fatigue and weakness
- (b) Other symptoms: nausea, vomiting, bone pain, chest pain (pleuritic)

  ii. Objective findings
- (a) Etiologic or precipitating factors: Collect data to determine etiology of the gradual decline in renal function and elevated BUN and creatinine levels. All possibilities must be considered, until the reversible disorders have been considered and eliminated
  - (1) Past examinations reveal pattern of deteriorating renal reserve
  - (2) Unexplained symptoms
    - *a)* General—fever, lassitude, anorexia, edema, nausea, weakness, anemia, headache, tremors, coma
    - *b)* Specific—hematuria, proteinuria, flank pain
  - (3) Pregnancies with recurrent pyelitis, edema, or hypertension
  - (4) Deafness (Alport's syndrome)
  - (5) Chronic urinary tract or renal infections—dysuria, frequency, and polyuria
  - (6) Recent respiratory or skin infection seen in Goodpasture's disease or post-streptococcal infections
  - (7) History of
    - *a)* Diabetes mellitus
    - *b)* Lupus erythematosus
    - *c)* Gout
    - *d)* Arthritis
    - *e)* Hypertension
    - *f)* Amyloidosis
    - *g)* Drug sensitivity
    - *h)* Allergies
    - *i)* Extensive vascular disease
    - *j)* Enuresis past age of 6 years—suggestive of congenital stricture or neurologic anomalies of urinary tract
- (b) Family history
  - (1) Genetic predisposition to actual kidney disorder (polycystic disease, Alport's syndrome, cystinuria, Fanconi's syndrome)
  - (2) Positive for gout, diabetes mellitus, hypertension, vas-

cular disease, lupus erythematosus, arthritis, or heart disease

(3) History of past adjustment to CRF

    a) Family unit and impact of CRF

    b) Perception of family members' support

    c) Role of family in care (e.g., home dialysis)

(c) Social history—employment status: description of present work status and impact of CRF on employment

(d) Medication history—past and current use of

    (1) Diuretics—history of renal response to diuretics

    (2) Antihypertensives—optimal reduction in blood pressure possible; presence of bone marrow suppression or infection; history of past organ rejection

    (3) Immunosuppressives—presence of bone marrow suppression or infection; history of past episodes of rejection

    (4) Use and/or abuse of analgesics, phenacetin-containing compounds, and methysergide

(e) Other

    (1) Uremic symptoms—determine the number and severity of uremic symptoms since this impacts on the course and complications associated with CRF

    (2) Sexual dysfunction—uremia affects the libido and fertility of the CRF patient. The psychological status of the patient (e.g., depression) can compound the sexual dysfunction

    (3) Self-image—alteration may be associated with loss of health and renal function, change in skin texture and color, increased fatigue levels, alteration in ambulation, arteriovenous access, peritoneal dialysis catheter, femoral catheters, edema, bruising, and changes in appearance associated with immunosuppression

    (4) Dietary restrictions—usually 60 g protein, 2 g sodium, and 2 g potassium with fluid restriction. Diet varies per individual case and per source of renal replacement therapy

    (5) Renal replacement therapy

        a) Types—hemodialysis, peritoneal dialysis, continuous ambulatory peritoneal dialysis (CAPD), hemofiltration (CAVH, CAVHD)

b. Nursing examination of patient: clinical presentation—the patient may present at any stage of CRF with symptoms reflecting nephron loss and the compromise of other organ systems

  i. Inspection

    (a) Neurologic—lethargy, confusion, stupor, uremic seizures

(b) Respiratory—deep, rapid respirations or Kussmaul's respirations

(c) Cardiovascular—12-lead ECG changes consistent with uremic pericarditis. Dysrhythmias or cardiac arrest associated with electrolyte imbalances

(d) Genitourinary—normal urine volume to oliguria or anuria

(e) Gastrointestinal—weight loss associated with anorexia and nausea

(f) Integument

    (1) Hypocalcemia with associated signs and symptoms such as tetany, seizures, and numbness and tingling in fingertips, around oral cavity, in nose, and in toes, plus possible ECG changes (prolonged ST segment)

    (2) Alterations in mobility—diminished strength, muscle atrophy, bone pain, change in gait, and edema

    (3) Muscle paralysis secondary to hyperkalemia

    (4) Muscle wasting secondary to malnutrition, particularly protein-deficient diet

ii. Palpation

  (a) Pulse—normal to bradycardia or tachycardia secondary to uremic or electrolyte effects

  (b) Genitourinary

    (1) Palpable masses in both upper quadrants may be indicative of polycystic disease

    (2) Flank pain

    (3) Enlarged prostate

iii. Percussion: bladder size

iv. Auscultation

  (a) Hypertensive blood pressure

  (b) Crackles, rales of pulmonary edema

c. Diagnostic studies

  i. Laboratory findings

    (a) Urinalysis—the following abnormalities may be the first indicators of the presence of renal disease

      (1) Proteinuria—amount exceeding 3 g/24 hr common in glomerulonephropathies and nephrotic syndrome

      (2) Hematuria, gross or microscopic—the presence of this abnormality can also indicate bladder or urinary tract abnormality

      (3) Leukocyte casts and pyuria indicate infection at a site in the urinary tract, particularly when pyuria occurs as a single abnormality. Suspect renal disease when pyuria occurs in conjunction with hematuria, casts, and proteinuria. Eosinophiluria can occur in allergic interstitial nephritis. Lymphocytes are significant in

the renal transplant patient experiencing a rejection episode

(4) Epithelial cells—renal tubular cells with lipid droplets in the cytoplasm are indicative of nephrotic syndrome. Large numbers of these cells are present in glomerulonephritis and pyelonephritis

(5) Casts—provide important diagnostic clues

    a) Erythrocyte casts support hematuria of glomerular origin

    b) Leukocyte casts indicate intrarenal inflammation, often found in pyelonephritis

    c) Mixed leukocyte and erythrocyte casts may be prominent in acute exudative glomerulonephritis

    d) Fatty casts seen in glomerular diseases in conjunction with moderate to heavy proteinuria

    e) Granular casts are common in many diseases

    f) Waxy and broad casts occur in the last stages of renal failure

(6) Urine culture—presence of infection

(7) Urine osmolality—varies with stage of CRF

(8) Creatinine clearance—a decrease in creatinine clearance to 10 to 50 ml/min or a renal reserve of 25% is associated with the onset of renal insufficiency and its symptoms. A creatinine clearance of 10 to 15 ml/min is consistent with end-stage renal disease

(b) Serum results

(1) Creatinine—an inverse relationship exists between serum creatinine, GFR, and the stage of chronic renal failure

    a) Diminished renal reserve—a 50% nephron loss will be reflected by a twice-normal creatinine level of 1.4 to 2.4 mg/dl

    b) Renal insufficiency—a 75% nephron loss causes the serum creatinine level to quadruple, so that an original creatinine value of 1.4 mg/dl will then become 5.6 mg/dl and a creatinine value of 2.4 mg/dl will be 9.6 mg/dl

    c) End-stage renal disease—a 90% nephron loss is synonymous with a serum creatinine value of 10.0 mg/dl or greater

    d) Uremic syndrome—a creatinine value of 10.0 mg/dl or above maintained by some form of dialysis treatment

(2) BUN—the BUN level in CRF correlates well with uremia. Levels over 100 mg/dl are usually associated

with uremic symptoms; therefore it can be used to determine the frequency and duration of dialysis requirements

(3) Increased serum levels of uric acid may suggest gouty nephropathy when there is an elevation out of proportion to the degree of renal failure

(4) Serum triglycerides may be elevated

(5) Glucose tolerance test—to determine presence of carbohydrate intolerance, if patient is symptomatic

ii. Radiologic findings

(a) Intravenous pyelogram

(1) Small kidneys, or one atrophied kidney and one normal size, may indicate bilateral disease. Unilateral disease always causes compensatory hypertrophy of the contralateral kidney

(2) Enlarged kidneys indicate polycystic disease or suggest obstruction

(3) Scarring and altered calices can be suggestive of chronic pyelonephritis or analgesic nephropathy

iii. Renal biopsy: to establish a diagnosis, to determine reversible etiologies, and to establish appropriate therapy

iv. Special: baseline motor nerve conduction velocity studies and long bone x-ray films of skull, hand, and feet determine the development of uremic neuropathy and bone disease

4. **Nursing diagnoses**

a. Fluid volume excess (see p. 500)

i. Additional assessments for defining characteristics

(a) Noncompliance with fluid restriction between dialysis treatments

(b) Ineffective dialysis treatments

ii. Additional expected outcomes

(a) Maintains dry weight

(b) Free of edema

(c) Breath sounds clear bilaterally

(d) Maintains normal blood pressure

(e) Compliant with fluid restriction

iii. Additional nursing interventions

(a) Teach patient the risks of abusing fluid restriction; encourage compliance

(b) Obtain daily weight; determine dry weight

(c) Implement a fluid restriction (amount often equals insensible losses)

(d) Document intake and output validated with daily weights

(e) Assess for the presence of any remaining renal function

(1) Urine volume and creatinine clearance

(2) Urinalysis

(3) Urine concentration—specific gravity, urine osmolality, spot electrolytes

(4) 24-hour urine for protein

(f) Collaborate with the physician to evaluate the effectiveness of dialysis treatments. Consider a more aggressive treatment

(g) Assess for hypertension. Consider severity of hypertension and need for blood pressure control by rapid fluid removal via dialysis

(h) Assess degree of edema and impact on skin integrity

b. Potential for electrolyte imbalance (see p. 503)

i. Additional nursing interventions

(a) Monitor for imbalances affecting cardiac function

(b) Collaborate with physician to determine acute treatment and monitor patient's response

(c) Consider frequent dialysis for repeated imbalances

c. Potential for acid–base imbalances: metabolic acidosis (see pp. 511 and 539)

i. Additional assessment for defining characteristics

(a) Assess degree of acidosis

ii. Additional expected outcomes

(a) Symptom-free pH level

(b) Dialysis implemented for uncontrollable acidosis

iii. Additional nursing interventions

(a) Dialysis and oral sodium bicarbonate provide long-term control

(b) Be aware of method by which dialysis controls acidosis

(1) Acetate or lactate found in hemodialysis and peritoneal dialysis bath is absorbed into the body. These elements enter Krebs' cycle to be converted to bicarbonate

(2) Bicarbonate bath—a specifically adjusted hemodialysis machine that dialyzes with a bath containing bicarbonate. The patient receiving bicarbonate does not have to carry out the metabolic conversion expected with acetate-lactate

d. Potential for anemia: a state caused by the lack or suppression of erythropoietin. Hematocrit maintained at 20% to 33% in general hemodialysis population and above 24% for those with angina (see pp. 512 and 558)

i. Additional assessment for defining characteristics

(a) Hematocrit below 20% for hemodialysis patient, and hematocrit below 24% in hemodialysis patient with history of angina

ii. Additional nursing interventions
   (a) Assess degree of anemia
   (b) Assess degree of uremia since may compound anemia
   (c) Determine baseline hematocrit
   (d) Transfuse fresh packed cells when indicated
      (1) Decrease risk of hyperkalemia
      (2) Hypocalcemia can occur from anticoagulants
   (e) Avoid whole blood (500 ml volume) since it can precipitate pulmonary edema
   (f) Implement precautions for hepatitis and HIV risk
   (g) Epoietin alfa—DNA-recombinant–engineered erythropoietin is an effective replacement agent for erythropoietin. Patients maintain a normal hematocrit with a mild to moderate improvement in exercise tolerance and work capacity, increased aerobic performance, and improved oxygen transport to tissue. Cardiac output and ejection fraction also show improvement. Side effects of epoietin alfa are minimal: higher hematocrits increase blood viscosity, which potentially leads to problems during dialysis treatment, a shortened life of the fistula, hypertension, and limited reuse of dialyzers. These changes are believed to have small consequences in light of the drug's benefits

e. Potential for uremic syndrome (see p. 513)
   i. Additional expected outcomes
      (a) Able to accomplish activities of daily living
      (b) Use of dialysis to modify moderate to severe uremic symptoms
   ii. Additional nursing interventions
      (a) Assess to determine the extent or degree of uremia
         (1) Manifestations of uremic skin changes
            a) Color—pale, abnormal pigmentation resulting from urochrome retention causes yellow to grayish tinge
            b) Bruising and purpura
            c) Change in texture and thickness of skin
            d) Presence of uremic frost (urea crystals)
            e) Pruritus
            f) Infections
            g) Edema
         (2) Manifestations of cardiovascular involvement
            a) Uremic pericarditis—incidence results from the accumulation of uremic toxins
               ☐ Pericardial friction rub
               ☐ Shortness of breath

□ Chest pain—precordial pain, relieved by sitting upright and leaning forward

□ Fever and leukocytosis

□ ECG changes—ST elevations in the leads reflecting the involved epicardial surface may be seen. Some patients with uremic pericarditis present with an atypical ECG pattern for pericarditis

□ BUN—can vary from low to high levels and generally may not reflect the severity of the pericarditis

b) Pericardial effusion—collection of fluid in the pericardial sac

□ Loss of friction rub

□ Increased severity of chest pain

□ Rapid, thready pulse

□ Further increase in venous pressure

□ Hypotension

□ ECG—disappearance of QRS complexes

c) Cardiac tamponade—untreated uremic pericardial effusion and the restriction created by the continual accumulation of fluid in the pericardial sac

□ Hypotension and pulsus paradoxus

□ Increased jugular venous pressure

□ Decreased cardiac output with compression of right atrium and right ventricle

□ Distant heart sounds

d) Pulmonary edema—seen with fluid overload and left ventricular failure

□ Increased left atrial, pulmonary artery, and wedge pressures

□ Shortness of breath with labored respirations

□ Tachycardia

□ Lung sounds—crackles

□ Frothy, pink-tinged sputum

□ Dysrhythmias secondary to hypoxia or heart strain

□ Heart sounds—S_3 diastolic gallop

□ Hypotension and decreased cardiac output

□ Skin cool and clammy

□ Changes in mentation may occur and/or sensation of impending doom

e) Arteriosclerosis—acceleration of vascular changes associated with aging. Major cause of death in hemodialyis population

□ Organ failure commonly associated with the ischemia created by the vascular changes (i.e., angina, myocardial infarction)

□ Hypertension

□ Enhancement and sustained excretion from renin–angiotensin mechanism

f) Symptomatic hyperkalemia (see specific section on this disorder)

g) Hypertension

□ Systolic blood pressure above 140 mm Hg and diastolic reading above 90 mm Hg

□ Prior history of hypertensive disease

□ Fluid overload

□ Elevated peripheral renin levels may be present

□ Hypertensive retinopathy—arteriolar narrowing secondary to vascular changes or spasm

● Grade I—arteriolar narrowing

● Grade II—arteriolar narrowing and arteriovenous nicking

● Grade III—arteriolar narrowing, arteriovenous nicking, plus hemorrhages and/or exudates

● Grade IV—all of the above plus papillary edema

□ Hypertensive encephalopathy—stupor, confusion, restlessness, nausea and vomiting, seizures progressing to coma

(3) Collaborate with health care team in treatment of cardiovascular complications—uremic pericarditis, pericardial effusion, cardiac tamponade, and pulmonary edema

a) Initiate a rigorous schedule for hemodialysis, usually 5 to 7 days during a 2-week period, or until pericarditis or pericardial effusion is alleviated. The goal is to remove uremic toxins and fluid excesses

b) Assist with a pericardiocentesis to relieve restriction of cardiac tamponade. If unsuccessful, consider a pericardial window or pericardiectomy

c) Fluid removal is the main therapeutic goal for pulmonary edema, either by diuretics or usually by dialysis

d) Renal transplantation may be recommended to patients at high risk for accelerated atherosclerotic changes

      ☐ Monitor serum triglyceride levels

      ☐ Provide teaching to reduce other cardiac risk factors

    e) Treat hyperkalemia (as directed in specific section)

    f) Reduce extracellular volume and administer antihypertensives in an effort to normalize blood pressure

(4) Manifestations of pulmonary involvement

    a) Pleural effusion

      ☐ Dyspnea

      ☐ Pleuritic-type chest pain—discomfort on inspiration

      ☐ Fever/malaise

      ☐ Chest x-ray film—fluid collection in dependent regions

      ☐ Lung sounds—decreased or absent breath sounds

    b) Uremic pneumonitis (uremic lung)—associated with fluid overload; in severe cases mimics the picture of adult respiratory distress syndrome

(5) Correct pulmonary involvement by

    a) Initiating frequent dialysis

    b) Providing antibiotics as necessary

    c) Providing pulmonary toilet and preventative pulmonary maintenance therapy

    d) Administering oxygen

    e) Monitoring progress with arterial blood gas analysis and chest x-ray film and correlating results with clinical status

(6) Manifestations of neurologic involvement

    a) Encephalopathy

      ☐ Fatigue

      ☐ Insomnia

      ☐ Shortened attention span and memory

      ☐ More severe symptoms include lethargy to coma and possibly seizures

      ☐ Neuromuscular irritability—tremors, diminished coordination, and asterixis

    b) Peripheral neuropathy

      ☐ "Restless leg syndrome"—usually occurs during bed rest or with limited movement. The patient experiences a vague aching pain that is relieved by movement

      ☐ "Burning" sensation of feet progressing to par-

esthesia and intense pain on dorsal and ventral surfaces of feet
- ☐ Progressing to footdrop and diminished muscle strength
- ☐ Further progression of this disorder leads to a change in gait and possibly paralysis
- ☐ Nerve conduction studies reveal a slowing of nerve conduction velocity and a segmental demyelination of the nerves

(7) Initiate a plan of care to minimize alterations in neurologic status
- *a)* Orient patient as necessary
- *b)* Acquire an awareness of shortened attention span and limited memory
- *c)* Protect from hyperirritability and seizures
- *d)* Correct electrolyte imbalances (hypocalcemia)

(8) Reverse the encephalopathy and minimize the peripheral neuropathy by dialysis
- *a)* Control hypertension and correct hyponatremia because these conditions exacerbate the encephalopathy
- *b)* Monitor parathyroid hormone (PTH) levels because there appears to be a correlation between increases of PTH and exacerbation of neurologic symptoms

(9) Manifestations of endocrine and metabolic involvement
- *a)* Hyperuricemia and gout—accumulation of uric acid
  - ☐ History of uric acid stones may be present
  - ☐ Joint pain and inflammation
  - ☐ Low-grade fever
  - ☐ Hypertension may occur
- *b)* Secondary hyperparathyroidism
  - ☐ Hypercalcemia
  - ☐ Demineralization of bone with associated metastatic calcifications
  - ☐ Bone pain
  - ☐ Pathologic fractures
  - ☐ X-ray films of hands and feet reveal resorption of distal clavicles, areas of demineralization, and subperiosteal bone resorption of the phalanges
- *c)* Hyperlipidemia
  - ☐ Elevations in serum lipid levels—an increase in

type IV lipoprotein is most commonly seen with CRF. Hypercholesterolemia is also seen if the patient is treated with corticosteroids
  □ Onset of complications associated with this disorder (e.g., atherosclerotic heart disease)
  d) Carbohydrate intolerance
  □ Moderate levels of hyperglycemia
  □ Abnormal glucose tolerance test
  □ Elevated insulin levels
  e) Sexual dysfunction
  □ Amenorrhea or abnormal menstruation
  □ Impotence
  □ Infertility
  □ Decreased libido
  □ Diminished testosterone production and reduced ovulation
(10) Collaborate with health care team in treatment of endocrine-metabolic disorders
  a) Administer allopurinol for gout accompanied by hyperuricemia; consider diuretic therapy if kidneys can respond
  b) Monitor serum calcium level and report variations in levels
  c) Recommend hand and feet films at regular intervals to monitor the status of musculoskeletal changes
  d) Consider parathyroidectomy for uncontrollable hypercalcemia or severe bone changes
  e) Adjust dietary intake if possible and administer low-dose corticosteroids in an attempt to decrease serum lipid levels
  f) Dialysis to partially improve a patient's glucose tolerance
  g) Transplantation will normalize most sexual function; dialysis may provide some improvement
  □ Attempt to reduce PTH levels because PTH may contribute to sexual dysfunction
  □ Administer zinc in an attempt to reverse impotence
(11) Manifestations of gastrointestinal involvement
  a) General—anorexia, nausea, vomiting
  b) Uremic bowel—diarrhea or constipation, malabsorption syndrome, weight loss, and fatigue
  c) Peptic ulcer disease—gastric pain and possibly bleeding

(12) Initiate dialysis to begin to alleviate anorexia, nausea, and vomiting, since these are early signs of uremia. In addition
    a) Administer a protein-restricted diet, because a metabolite of protein appears to be responsible for these symptoms
    b) Broad-spectrum antibiotics may be helpful
    c) Administer zinc in an attempt to improve "taste" sensation
    d) Implement antacid therapy for bleeding, gastrointestinal ulceration, or pain; however, use non-magnesium-containing antacids. If this is not possible, then frequent serum magnesium levels must be obtained. An elevation in magnesium would warrant the implementation of dialysis
(13) Manifestations of hematologic involvement
    a) Anemia—a hematocrit of 20% to 25% is associated with the typical pallor of patients with CRF. Observe for dyspnea and chest pain
    b) Platelet function abnormality—decrease in platelet adhesiveness, sometimes accompanied by a mild thrombocytopenia
        ☐ Increased tendency toward bleeding. If bleeding occurs, hematocrit will fall below 20% for reasons beyond renal failure
        ☐ Bruising and purpura
(14) Administer packed cells to maintain an asymptomatic hematocrit, usually in a range of 20% to 24%. Initiate dialysis to minimize uremic effect on platelet function
    a) Iron supplements and folic acid help alleviate anemia
    b) Testosterone and other androgens may reverse the anemia in a select group of patients
(15) Manifestations of musculoskeletal involvement—osteomalacia (renal rickets)
    a) Hypocalcemia with reciprocal hyperphosphatemia
    b) Bone pain
    c) Impaired growth process
    d) Pathologic fractures
    e) Bone changes on x-ray films are rare
(16) Monitor serum calcium levels and administer calcium tablets and 1,25-dihydroxycholecalciferol (or another form of vitamin D) in conjunction with phosphate-binding therapy (Amphogel, Basojel)

(17) Consider conservative management of uremia via diet (protein restriction)

(18) Assess patient for chronic hemodialysis or peritoneal dialysis as a method for uremia control (see p. 514)

(19) Chronic hemodialysis—hemodialysis continues to be the standard to which other treatments for end-stage renal disease are compared. Presently, chronic hemodialysis is available to most patients with end-stage renal disease (see p. 532)

    a) Patient expectations for chronic hemodialysis

        ☐ Maintenance of circulatory access

        ☐ Hemodialysis treatment usually scheduled for three times a week (4 to 5 hours for each treatment). This demanding schedule may interfere with work, family, and personal activities

        ☐ Rigid diet and fluid restrictions

    b) Expectations for home hemodialysis

        ☐ Proper environment—adequate space, plumbing, and hygiene

        ☐ Psychologically prepared—patient demonstrates signs of compliance and adaptation to disease process

        ☐ Physiologically stable—demonstrates ability to physically tolerate dialysis procedure

        ☐ Evidence of established family support system or acceptance of surrogate dialyzer

        ☐ Cognitive ability—demonstrates ability to learn technologic and aseptic skills

(20) Chronic peritoneal dialysis—this procedure follows the same principles and procedures as acute peritoneal dialysis. The differences relate to patient expectations and the regular use of an automated peritoneal dialysis machine, which is frequently called the "cycler"

    a) Patient expectations for peritoneal dialysis

        ☐ Maintenance of Tenckhoff catheter

        ☐ Treatments usually three to four times a week for 10 hours each treatment

        ☐ Dietary and fluid restrictions

    b) Expectations for home peritoneal dialysis (includes continuous ambulatory peritoneal dialysis [CAPD])

        ☐ Proper environment—the treatment requires minimal amounts of space; however, storage area for equipment is necessary. Hygiene is considered

☐ Psychologically prepared—same as for home hemodialysis

☐ Physiologically stable—not as necessary for home peritoneal dialysis since the rapid fluid shifts and dramatic cardiovascular effects are not associated with this treatment

☐ Family support systems are helpful but not essential since most patients dialyze at night, and the family routine may not be disrupted

☐ Cognitive ability—less technologic skill required for peritoneal dialysis; however, proper aseptic technique is essential

(21) Selection criteria for continuous ambulatory peritoneal dialysis (CAPD)

  a) Intact peritoneal cavity without evidence of infection

  b) Presence of adequate visual ability to perform procedures

  c) Presence of manual dexterity to perform procedures

  d) Possession of ability to learn and implement proper hygiene and aseptic technique

  e) Compliance with training sessions and treatment demands

  f) No evidence of

    ☐ Symptomatic lumbar disc disease

    ☐ Familial hypertriglyceridemia

    ☐ Abdominal hernias

    ☐ Psychosocial or environmental limitations

    ☐ Extensive scarring of peritoneal cavity

(22) CAPD—a continuous form of peritoneal dialysis

  a) Knowledge of mechanism of peritoneal dialysis exchange

  b) Patient teaching

    ☐ Treatment effectiveness—replaces 10% of renal function

    ☐ Treatment expectations—exchanges are made 24 hours a day, 7 days a week. Frequency of exchange can vary. Each exchange is for 6 to 8 hours during the day and 8 to 12 hours at night

    ☐ Patient expectations

      ● Permanent Tenckhoff catheter

      ● Completion of rigorous training program

- Self-care
- Strict adherence to treatment schedule resulting in change in life style
- Strict compliance to aseptic technique
- Environmental provisions for storage of dialysis equipment

☐ Complications
- Peritonitis
- Back strain
- Visceral herniation—as a result of increased intra-abdominal pressure
- Obesity—as a result of influx of carbohydrates. Also an improved sense of well-being may increase appetite

☐ Encourage patient to control weight gain
- Increased appetite
- Glucose absorption from dialysate results in additional daily calories

☐ Teach patient to monitor fluid intake
- High serum osmolarity created by glucose absorption may trigger thirst sensation. Direct patient not to respond to this sensation
- Maintenance of intake and output record

☐ Monitor serum electrolytes—values tend to run at low levels (potassium and calcium may both be normal). Possible to decrease dose of phosphate binders, thus preventing constipation

☐ Monitor serum BUN and creatinine to help determine concentration of dialysate (1.5%, 2.5%, 4.25%)
- Removes small, middle, and large molecules, which represent a significant range of possible metabolic toxins responsible for the uremic syndrome
- This form of dialysis is often sufficiently effective to reduce the incidence of uremic complications (neuropathy and skeletal changes)

☐ Record blood pressure response—effectiveness of treatment and volume removal have positive effect on control of hypertension

☐ Recognition of usual elevation in hematocrit during first 3 months. This trend eventually levels off at 10 months. The need for blood transfusions will therefore decrease during this period

(23) Selection criteria for renal transplantation—this treatment has evolved over the past 25 years as an acceptable intervention for CRF. Approximately 4000 patients receive renal transplants each year
    a) Sources of kidney grafts—cadaver donors and living relatives (siblings, parents, or children). The cadaveric donor remains the largest source of donations
    b) Recipient selection criteria
        ☐ Patient has irreversible end-stage renal disease
        ☐ Age 60 and younger
        ☐ Primary etiology of renal disease does not create contraindications
        ☐ No preexisting antibodies
        ☐ No medical or surgical contraindications—vasculature must accommodate transplantation; cardiovascular and pulmonary status can withstand surgery; can tolerate corticosteroid therapy (minimal evidence of gastric ulcers, leukopenia, chronic infection, or psychosis)
        ☐ Functioning bladder and/or urinary tract (no evidence of chronic infection or nephrostomy tube)
        ☐ Psychosocial status—professional evaluation should consider presence of psychosis, severe personality disorder, or history of noncompliance. Any of the above can be contraindications
        ☐ Last-resort alternative—the patient may be accepted based on his inability to participate in other treatment alternatives. This may be due to a lack of vascular access or physical tolerance of the procedure
(24) Renal transplantation (Fig. 4–7)
    a) Possess knowledge of histocompatibility system for self and patient teaching
        ☐ Genetic system that establishes tissue identity and compatibility. This system is responsible for the diversity of each species
        ☐ Major histocompatibility site (locus) on the gene containing the HLA antigens is at chromosome 6
        ☐ HLA antigens (human leukocyte antigens) are found on the surface of all nucleated cells. There are five possible sites for tissue compatibility: HLA-A, HLA-B, HLA-C, HLA-D, and HLA-DR

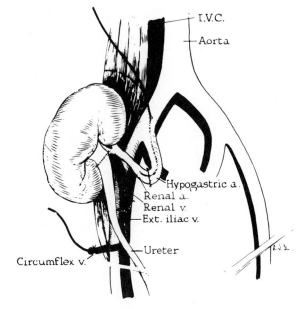

Figure 4–7. Site of renal transplant. (From Friedman, E. A.: Strategy in Renal Failure. Copyright © 1978, John Wiley & Sons, Inc., New York. Reprinted by permission of John Wiley & Sons, Inc.)

□ Individuals possess two antigens (see above listing) from each unit for a total of ten HLA antigens. Five are inherited from each parent

□ D site testing has been correlated with improved graft survival if a D match occurs between donor and recipient in both cadaveric and family-donated transplants

□ A and B site testing is routine, while C has been shown to be antigenically weak

b) Tissue typing

□ ABO blood typing—to determine blood type compatibility between donor and recipient

□ HLA typing—serologic testing for specification of HLA-A, B, and C locus antigen plus lymphocyte-defined typing of the D locus

□ Mixed lymphocyte culture (MLC)—this test reveals the degree of difference between the D loci of donor and recipient

□ Cross match for preformed antibody—the test for the presence of preformed antibody reveals whether the patient has developed cytotoxic antibodies by exposure to blood transfusions, pregnancy, previous transplants, or prior infections. Presence of preformed antibodies significantly decreases the chance of any graft survival. A direct cross-match reaction between donor and recipient leads to a 95% chance of a hyperacute rejection

c) Immunocompetent cells—two kinds of lymphocytes involved in rejection processes

☐ B lymphocytes—for humoral immunity, antibody-producing cells. Responsible for hyperacute rejection and partially involved in acute and chronic rejection

☐ T lymphocytes—cell-mediated immunity involved in acute and chronic rejection. Three types

● T-cell effector—attacks the target organ

● T-cell helper—enhances the function of B cells and results in stimulating a stronger humoral reponse

● T-cell suppressor—suppresses both humoral and cell-mediated immunity. If enhanced, suppressor cells will decrease incidence of rejection

d) Types of rejection

☐ Hyperacute rejection

● Occurs within minutes or hours after surgery

● The renal artery and vein are anastomosed, the clamps are removed, and the kidney first "pinks up," then becomes blue and mottled

● Physiologically, blood flow has been reduced from 300 to 400 ml/min to 30 ml/min owing to the immunologic response of "preexisting antibodies." The occlusion of the renal artery occurs as platelets adhere across the diameter of the vessels, gradually causing ischemia

☐ Accelerated rejection—occurs within the second to fifth day in the immediate postoperative period and physiologically is similar to the hyperacute response

☐ Acute rejection

● Occurs most frequently 2 weeks after transplantation. It can be seen from the first week postoperatively up to 1 year after transplant

● T cells or cellular immunity is the primary mechanism

● Antigen leaves the graft and enters the serum, where it is recognized. On recognition the antigen is incorporated into macrophage RNA. If this type of antigen is ever recognized again, then the macrophage will split open and send the RNA–antigen complex into the serum. Plasma lymphocytes will be able to use the RNA–antigen complex to manufacture specific antibody. The plasma lymphocytes will then travel to the kidney for the immunologic attack

☐ Can usually be reversed by high doses or "pulses" of antirejection medication

   e) Chronic rejection

☐ Occurs at 1 to 5 years post transplant

☐ B-cell or humoral response has a specific antibody production

☐ A slow chronic immunologic response. The gradual deterioration of renal tissue creates a situation similar to CRF

☐ Immunologic response involves primarily the glomerular basement membrane and endothelial layer of the blood vessels

☐ Process cannot be reversed and ultimately will lead to organ failure

  (25) Recognize that alternative renal replacement therapies require essentially complete restructuring of total life style

  iii. Evaluation of nursing care

   (a) Diet or dialysis stabilizes BUN level below 100 mg/dl

   (b) Minimizes alteration in neurologic status

   (c) Maintains adequate cardiac output and improved oxygenation by correcting the uremic effect on the cardiac and pulmonary systems

   (d) Maintains a satisfactory level of ambulation

   (e) Demonstrates ability to achieve self-care activities

   (f) Limits incidence of demineralization of bone, bone pain, and pathologic fractures

   (g) Tolerates hemodialysis or peritoneal dialysis

   (h) Renal transplant replaces renal function

f. Altered nutrition: less than body requirements (see pp. 504 and 540)

  i. Additional nursing interventions

   (a) Assess status of mucous membranes

   (b) Provide mouth care

   (c) Provide small frequent feedings with adequate calories (calorie requirement with normal level of activity is 35 kcal/kg body weight)

   (d) Consider need for restriction of protein, sodium, and potassium

(e) Weigh patient daily and assess degree of muscle wasting; report findings to physician to determine need for changes in diet
g. Alteration in elimination: constipation—a state resulting from the use of phosphate-binding gels and the uremic bowel syndrome
  i. Additional assessment for defining characteristics
    (a) Verbalizes presence of constipation
    (b) Presence of uremic bowel—alternating diarrhea and constipation
    (c) Administration of phosphate-binding gels
  ii. Additional expected outcomes
    (a) Regular bowel evacuation
  iii. Additional nursing interventions
    (a) Administer and/or teach the patient to maintain a diet with increased bulk
    (b) Administer (after assessment of bowel status) stool softeners or consider enemas if patient does not respond to other forms of conservative therapy
    (c) Avoid magnesium-containing laxatives
    (d) Observe consistency, color, frequency, and amount of stool
  iv. Additional evaluation of nursing care
    (a) Verbalizes having regular bowel movements
    (b) Uses routine practices to prevent constipation
h. Potential for infection: a state resulting from the debilitated, uremic condition (see pp. 514 and 539)
  i. Additional nursing interventions
    (a) Evaluation of infection at onset
    (b) Administration of antibiotic therapy
    (c) Assessment of antibiotic dosage (correlation with daily serum creatinine level)
    (d) Encouragement of patient to try to avoid persons with colds, influenza, or other infections
    (e) Use of aseptic techniques during dialysis procedures
    (f) Instruction of patient in how to care for arteriovenous site
  ii. Additional evaluation of nursing care
    (a) Prevention of infection
    (b) Early diagnosis and treatment of infection
i. Lack of knowledge: CRF, dialysis and transplant procedures—a state created from the complexities of CRF, demanding a wide range of patient/family teaching sessions to produce a knowledgeable patient
  i. Assessment for defining characteristics
    (a) Verbalizes lack of knowledge concerning disease process and/or treatment
    (b) Noncompliant with treatments and/or medications
    (c) Lacks participation in self-care activities

  ii. Expected outcomes
   (a) Increased knowledge of CRF, treatment, and medications
   (b) Compliance with treatment expectations
   (c) Participation in care
 iii. Nursing interventions
   (a) Assess knowledge level
   (b) Assess uremic effect on learning
    (1) Decreased attention span
    (2) Diminished memory
    (3) Alteration in thought processes
   (c) Develop teaching plan including reinforcement
   (d) Instruct patient about all aspects of CRF
    (1) Normal renal function and renal disease state
    (2) Fluid management
    (3) Dietary management
    (4) Medications (action, dosage, times)
    (5) Avoidance of infection
    (6) Rest periods to minimize fatigue
    (7) Skin care
    (8) Treatment alternatives; after patient and family acquire knowledge of benefits/disadvantages of each treatment, then support family decision
   (e) Instruct patient/family about dialysis
    (1) Dynamics of hemodialysis or peritoneal dialysis
    (2) Special diet and fluid allowances
    (3) Care of dialysis access
    (4) Need for weight control
    (5) Signs and symptoms of complications such as hypotension, bleeding, infection, and electrolyte imbalance
   (f) Instruct patient/family about transplantation. Initial patient teaching—to assist patient in decision-making process for selection of transplantation as a treatment alternative
    (1) Survival rates
    (2) Patient selection criteria
    (3) Treatment expectations
     a) Antirejection medications
     b) Frequent clinic visits first year
     c) Diet limitations may be necessary
    (4) Benefits—only treatment that provides replacement of renal function
     a) Most pathophysiologic effects of uremia are alleviated (e.g., anemia, sexual dysfunction, osteomalacia)
     b) Allows return to many normal life activities

    (5) Complications
        a) Rejection
        b) Immunosuppressive effects—increased susceptibility to infections, risk of malignancies, esophagitis, peptic ulcer, acute pancreatitis
        c) Surgical complications—are rare because procedure has been perfected. Most common are renal artery stenosis and anastomotic leaks
        d) Ureteral leaks and obstruction; urinary fistulas

(g) Preoperative teaching—general components
    (1) Be ready to report to hospital on request
    (2) Preoperative care to expect
        a) Chest x-ray film
        b) ECG
        c) Blood samples
        d) Bowel prep
        e) Dialysis
        f) Antirejection medications
        g) Anesthesiologist's visit
    (3) Description of surgical procedure (see below)
    (4) Immediate postoperative recovery period—expectations of care
        a) Waken in recovery room
        b) Intravenous therapy.
        c) Foley catheter in place
        d) Pulmonary toilet and oxygen therapy
        e) Wound care
        f) Visitor regulations
        g) Antirejection medications
        h) Renal scan
        i) Cardiac monitor
    (5) Return to transplant unit from recovery room

(h) Surgical procedure—kidney is transplanted into iliac fossa. Revascularization is usually accomplished by anastomosing renal artery to hypogastric artery and renal vein to external iliac vein. The ureter is anastomosed to the recipient's ureter at the pelvis of the kidney (ureteropelvic anastomosis), or donor's ureter can be implanted into the host's bladder (ureteroneocystostomy)

(i) Postoperative teaching—general components
    (1) Ability to maintain own intake and output record
    (2) Ability to obtain and record daily temperature, blood pressure, and weight on wakening
    (3) Knowledge of antirejection medications and side effects

(4) Ability to communicate signs and symptoms of rejection
  a) Fever
  b) Pain, tenderness, redness, and swelling at site of graft
  c) Weight gain
  d) Decrease in urine output
  e) Hypertension
  f) Elevation in serum creatinine level
(5) Activity limitations in first 3 months—avoidance of lifting or strenuous exercise
(6) Avoidance of crowds in first 3 months
(7) Knowledge to report signs and symptoms of infection such as fever or flulike symptoms
(8) Knowledge of diet
(9) Schedule of clinic visits
(j) Antirejection medications
  (1) Corticosteroids—administration begins in preoperative period. Doses are gradually reduced in a manner that varies from unit to unit in an effort to minimize the corticosteroid side effects
    a) Action—anti-inflammatory effect; suppresses production of cytotoxic T cells; affects monocytes, thus preventing stimulation of T cells, and prevents production of a substance (called interleukin-2) that initiates immunologic response
    b) Toxicity
      ☐ High doses create cushingoid effect—roundness of face, increase in fat pads, acne, increased appetite, changes in libido, gastrointestinal bleeding, diabetes mellitus, sodium and water retention, cataract formation, alopecia, and avascular necrosis of bone
      ☐ Predisposition to infection
      ☐ Impaired wound healing
  (2) Azathioprine (Imuran)—begin dosing at 3 mg/kg/day and decrease gradually to 1 mg/kg/day
    a) Action—major effect is to prevent or to deter acute rejection episodes. Prevents the synthesis of DNA/RNA in leukocytes. It may block messenger RNA
    b) Toxicity
      ☐ Bone marrow depression
      ☐ Drug-induced hepatitis/pancreatitis
      ☐ Anemia

☐ Alopecia

☐ Jaundice

☐ Increased incidence of malignancy

(3) Cyclosporine—sometimes administered in conjunction with corticosteroids

   a) Action—results in almost total inhibition of T-cell proliferation, with relatively minor effects on B cells. Shown to be effective in prolonging graft survival, owing to evidence that T-suppressor cells may be spared

   b) Toxicity associated with specific types of lymphomas and nephrotoxicity, also hepatotoxicity

(4) Antilymphocyte globulin (ALG)

   a) Action—depletes circulating T cells, thus suppressing cell-mediated immunity and allograft responses

   b) Toxicity—agranulocytosis/hemolytic response and predisposition to infection

(5) Monoclonal antibodies—experimental (OKT$_3$)

   a) Action—directed at suppressing or inactivating one of two antigen-recognition sites on T cells (T$_2$ or T$_3$)

   b) Toxicity—anaphylaxis, fluid overload

(6) Cyclophosphamide (Cytoxan)—used as a second choice when azathioprine is contraindicated, as in general intolerance of azathioprine or in the presence of liver disease

   a) Action—diminishes the production of antibodies and initiates the destruction of circulating lymphocytes

   b) Toxicity—bone marrow depression, alopecia, cardiotoxicity, anorexia, nausea and vomiting, hemorrhagic cystitis, sterility, nephrotoxicity

  iv. Evaluation of nursing care

    (a) Verbalizes understanding of CRF, treatment, and medication

    (b) Compliance with immunosuppressive agents

    (c) Active participation in care

j. Disturbance in self-concept: body image—a state resulting from the effects of uremia, dependency on treatments, and primary illness other than renal disease

  i. Assessment for defining characteristics

    (a) Verbalizes concern about changes in appearance

    (b) Uremic skin changes/uremic systemic changes

    (c) Protruding abdomen secondary to peritoneal dialysis fluid

   (d) Diminished energy level/decreased exercise tolerance

   (e) Impairment of mobility

   (f) Effect of corticosteroid therapy: moon face, fat padding

   (g) Dependence on renal replacement therapy

   (h) Reduced social involvement

  ii. Expected outcomes

   (a) Adaptation to changes in body image

   (b) Desired amount of social involvement

 iii. Nursing interventions

   (a) Allow patient to express feelings

   (b) Encourage patient to participate in care in order to promote acceptance

   (c) Assess signs of productive versus nonproductive coping

   (d) Encourage maintenance of self-esteem

  iv. Evaluation of nursing care

   (a) Verbalizes acceptance of body image changes

   (b) Participates in self-care

   (c) Demonstrates signs of productive coping

   (d) Participates socially

 k. Sexual dysfunction: state resulting from uremia and its treatments

  i. Assessment for defining characteristics

   (a) Decreased libido

   (b) Impotence

   (c) Amenorrhea

   (d) Infertility

   (e) Verbalization of problem

   (f) Actual or perceived limitation imposed by renal disease

   (g) Altered relationship with significant other

   (h) Change of interest in self and others

  ii. Expected outcomes

   (a) Satisfactory level of sexual functioning

   (b) Resolution of loss of reproductive functioning

 iii. Nursing interventions

   (a) Obtain sexual history

   (b) Plan diagnostic procedures to determine whether a reversible cause of sexual dysfunction is present

   (c) Prepare patient for diagnostic tests

   (d) Advise patient of methods to optimize sexuality (promote personal respect between partners, encourage recognition of individual needs for love and tenderness)

   (e) Consider experimental methods that may improve sexual functioning

   (f) Allow patient to verbalize, providing emotional support for patient and sexual partner

  iv. Evaluation of nursing care

    (a) Verbalizes achievement of a satisfactory level of sexual functioning

    (b) Verbalizes acceptance of loss of reproductive functioning

 l. Ineffective coping patient and family: a state resulting from the multiple stressors of CRF on patient and family (see p. 518)

   i. Additional expected outcomes

    (a) Effective coping of patient and family

    (b) Increased independent participation in social and family activities

   ii. Additional nursing interventions

    (a) Promote adaptation to chronic disease by

     (1) Possessing an awareness of the dialysis patient's most relevant sources of stress

      a) Life threat of renal failure

      b) Demands of dialysis regimen (e.g., dietary and fluid restriction, daily time spent in treatment, medications)

      c) Life-style adjustments—role changes within family unit, loss of employment, marital/sexual problems, financial problems

     (2) Provide support system proven to be effective in counteracting stress of dialysis for patient and family

      a) Patient and/or family social groups

      b) Returning patient to some form of employment to increase level of self-esteem and relieve financial burdens

      c) Use prospective treatment alternatives as source of hope (e.g., transplantation)

Electrolyte Imbalances—Potassium Imbalance: Hyperkalemia: Serum potassium level above 5.5 mEq/L

1. Pathophysiology

 a. Inability of kidney tubules to excrete potassium ions owing to tubular damage, salt depletion, and increased potassium load from injured tissues

 b. Decreased renal perfusion diminishes potassium excretion owing to limited amount of sodium available for exchange with potassium (e.g., in cardiac failure)

2. Etiology or precipitating factors

 a. Acute and chronic renal disease

 b. Increased cellular destruction with potassium release as occurs in burns, trauma, crash injuries, severe catabolism, acute acidosis, intravascular hemolysis, and rhabdomyolysis

 c. Excessive administration/ingestion of potassium chloride

 d. Adrenal cortical insufficiency: hypoaldosteronism

e. Low cardiac output or sodium depletion

f. Acidosis: precipitates the movement of intracellular potassium to the extracellular space

3. **Nursing assessment data base**

a. Nursing history: difficult to obtain specific information leading to the detection of electrolyte imbalances. Suspect imbalances in the presence of renal and endocrine disease, in association with history of excessive loss of body fluid (e.g., vomiting, diarrhea) and in some special situations with drug intoxication (indiscriminate use of electrolyte replacement, hormonal therapy, and vitamins)

   i. Subjective findings

      (a) Patient's chief complaint—lethargy and weakness

      (b) Other symptoms—nausea, abdominal cramps or diarrhea, small urine volumes, or absence of urine output

   ii. Objective findings

      (a) Etiologic or precipitating factors (see above)

      (b) Family history—noncontributory

      (c) Social history—noncontributory

      (d) Medication history

         (1) Potassium chloride supplements to correct potassium losses primarily caused by diuretic therapy

         (2) Kayexalate—a sodium-exchange resin administered as a conservative measure for potassium removal

b. Nursing examination of patient—general: all electrolyte imbalances generally present as evidence of abnormal neuromuscular function such as irritability, hyporeflexia or hyperreflexia, seizures, weakness, and cardiac dysrhythmias

   i. Inspection

      (a) Neurologic—apathy and confusion

      (b) Respiratory—deep rapid respirations when hyperkalemia accompanied by acidosis or shallow respirations as a result of muscle paralysis

      (c) Cardiovascular—dysrhythmias on ECG

      (d) Genitourinary—oliguria

      (e) Gastrointestinal—abdominal cramping

      (f) Musculoskeletal

         (1) Irritability to flaccid paralysis and numbness of extremities

         (2) Fatigue levels

            a) Diminished exercise tolerance

         (3) Mobility

            a) Alterations in mobility caused by muscular weakness

            b) Paralysis

ii. Auscultation: hyperactive bowel sounds, tachycardia, bradycardia

c. Diagnostic study findings

  i. Serum potassium levels exceed 5.5 mEq/L

  ii. ECG: reveals peaked and elevated T waves → widened QRS complex → prolonged PR interval → flattened to absent P wave and ST segment depression → asystole

4. Nursing diagnoses

  a. Electrolyte excess: hyperkalemia

   i. Assessment for defining characteristics

    (a) Dietary or drug noncompliance in renal failure

    (b) Manifestations of hyperkalemia

      (1) Lethargy

      (2) Nausea

      (3) Diarrhea

      (4) Abdominal cramps

      (5) Hyperirritable bowel sounds

      (6) Muscle weakness—beginning in lower extremities and ascending toward trunk and upper extremities. This can lead to paralysis, but respiratory muscles are usually spared

      (7) Numbness and tingling

      (8) Oliguria or anuria

      (9) Tachycardia to bradycardia to cardiac arrest

    (c) Manifestations of myocardial functioning with hyperkalemia

      (1) General—myocardial depressant effect on both conduction and contractility

      (2) Progressive ECG changes and associated symptomatology

        a) Tall peaked T waves

        b) Widening QRS complex with associated bradycardia and hypotension

        c) Disappearance of P wave progressing to idioventricular rhythm to asystole and cardiac arrest

   ii. Expected outcomes

    (a) Maintains asymptomatic level of potassium

    (b) Cardiac function within normal limits

   iii. Nursing interventions

    (a) Initiate cardiac monitoring

    (b) Observe for changes in heart rate and rhythm

    (c) In emergency situations (serum potassium level over 6.5 mEq/L or ECG change indicating severe hyperkalemia) administer

   (1) Glucose, insulin, and sodium bicarbonate intravenously to temporarily drive potassium into cells
      a) Essential to follow up with some other measure (such as Kayexalate and sorbitol administration or dialysis) for permanent removal of potassium
      b) If refractory hyperkalemia occurs, dialysis is indicated
   (2) Calcium chloride or calcium gluconate intravenously to stimulate cardiac contractibility—contraindicated in patients on digoxin
(d) Administer Kayexalate and sorbitol to reverse hyperkalemia
   (1) Action of Kayexalate (a cation-exchange resin)—sodium is "exchanged" 1:1 for a potassium ion in bowel cell wall; therefore, nurse must also assess gain in sodium as well as amount of potassium loss
   (2) Sorbitol, a nonabsorbable sugar, induces an osmotic diarrhea that contributes to potassium loss from the bowel
   (3) Routes of administration—oral or by means of enema. Rectal administration necessitates retention of the Kayexalate solution for at least 30 minutes for maximal effect. In both cases, be certain Kayexalate/sorbitol mixture is expelled, especially postoperatively, since retained Kayexalate can cause bowel obstruction and perforation
(e) Monitor serum potassium levels at frequent intervals
(f) Teach patient of need to remain compliant to potassium restrictions
iv. Evaluation of nursing care
   (a) Serum potassium level below 5.5 mEq/L or in a higher asymptomatic range
   (b) Absence of cardiac complications of hyperkalemia

Electrolyte Imbalances—Potassium Imbalance: Hypokalemia: Serum potassium level below 3.5 mEq/L (frequently associated with other fluid and electrolyte disturbances)
1. **Pathophysiology**
   a. Potassium loss exceeding intake
   b. Alkalosis: stimulates secretion of potassium in distal tubule
   c. Intracellular shifting of potassium
2. **Etiology or precipitating factors**
   a. Alkalosis
   b. Abnormal gastrointestinal losses: nasogastric suction, drainage
   c. Liver disease

    d. Diuretic therapy

    e. Renal tubular acidosis

    f. Increased adrenal corticosteroid secretion or corticosteroid therapy

    g. Laxative abuse or diarrhea

    h. Starvation

    i. Prolonged episode of vomiting

3. Nursing assessment data base

    a. Nursing history: see hyperkalemia for general statement describing the detection of electrolyte imbalance

       i. Subjective findings

         (a) Patient's chief complaint—feeling drowsy, weak with muscle tenderness

         (b) Other symptoms—nausea and constipation

       ii. Objective findings

         (a) Additional etiologic or precipitating factors (see above)

           (1) Dietary indiscretion—episodes either of prolonged dieting without adequate potassium intake or of starvation

           (2) Hyperalimentation without adequate potassium replacement

         (b) Family history: noncontributory

         (c) Social history: noncontributory

         (d) Medication history

           (1) Potassium chloride supplements

           (2) Diuretics—prescribed to treat hypervolemia or to sustain a urine output in the later stages of renal failure may cause potassium loss

    b. Nursing examination of patient

       i. Inspection

         (a) Neurologic

           (1) Drowsiness to coma; malaise, confusion

           (2) Muscle cramping owing to unbalanced electrochemical effect on muscle cell membrane (commonly in the calf muscle)

           (3) Muscular weakness progression to paralysis

         (b) Respiratory—shallow respirations secondary to muscle weakness, possibly progressing to respiratory arrest

         (c) Cardiovascular—dysrhythmia on ECG

         (d) Genitourinary—polyuria

         (e) Gastrointestinal—vomiting

      ii. Palpation: pulses—diminished

     iii. Percussion: noncontributory

     iv. Auscultation

         (a) Heart sounds: irregular rate secondary to dysrhythmias—consider enhanced digitalis effect

   (b) Bowel sounds: diminished secondary to paralytic ileus

   (c) Blood pressure: hypotension

 c. Diagnostic study findings

   i. Serum potassium levels below 3.5 mEq/L

   ii. ECG: reveals depressed ST segments, flat or inverted T wave, presence of U wave, and ventricular dysrhythmias

4. Nursing diagnoses

 a. Electrolyte deficit: hypokalemia

   i. Assessment for defining characteristics (see above)

     (a) Additional manifestations of hypokalemia

       (1) Muscle cramps

       (2) Dizziness

       (3) Nausea and vomiting

       (4) Abdominal distention

       (5) Polyuria (impaired concentrating ability) and polydipsia

     (b) Manifestations of hypokalemic effect on myocardial functioning

       (1) General—increased myocardial excitability or irritability

       (2) Associated dysrhythmias—premature atrial and ventricular contractions, sinus bradycardia, paroxysmal atrial tachycardia, atrioventricular blocks, Wenckebach second-degree atrioventricular block, atrioventricular dissociation, junctional dysrhythmias, and ventricular tachycardia

       (3) Increased incidence of ectopy with digoxin administration

   ii. Expected outcomes

     (a) Maintains serum potassium level above 3.5 mEq/L or within asymptomatic range

     (b) Cardiac function within normal limits

   iii. Nursing interventions

     (a) Provide cardiac monitoring

     (b) Observe for ECG changes and presence of dysrhythmias

     (c) Check serum potassium levels

     (d) Record amount of urine output and estimate degree of potassium lost in drainage (such as from gastric aspirate and diarrhea) to aid in calculating total body potassium balance

     (e) Be aware of signs and symptoms of alkalosis. If present, correction of the alkalosis may correct the hypokalemia

     (f) Administer oral potassium supplements when indicated, diluted to prevent gastrointestinal irritation and to facilitate absorption

(g) Never give potassium chloride rapidly intravenously—large concentrations can precipitate hyperkalemia, producing necrotic effect on vessel wall and possibly inducing ventricular fibrillation

(h) Determine if patient is receiving digitalis or diuretics. Correct potassium losses, since hypokalemia enhances effect of digitalis and can precipitate digitalis toxicity. Hypokalemia can also decrease effectiveness of most diuretics

(i) Emergency treatment
  (1) Slowly administer potassium chloride intravenously while patient is being monitored with ECG in order to observe for dysrhythmias
  (2) Be aware of signs and symptoms of hyperkalemia
  (3) Maintain record of serum potassium levels to assess adequacy of replacement therapy

(j) Follow-up—if patient is on digitalis and diuretics, consider potassium chloride supplement therapy or potassium-sparing diuretics

iv. Evaluation of nursing care
  (a) Asymptomatic serum potassium levels
  (b) Absence of cardiac complications of hypokalemia

Electrolyte Imbalances—Sodium Imbalance: Hypernatremia: Serum sodium level above 145 mEq/L

1. **Pathophysiology**
   a. Increased ECF volume: sodium and water retention
   b. Less total body water in relation to quantity of body sodium, with increased amounts of water loss in comparison to amount of sodium loss

2. **Etiology or precipitating factors**
   a. With normal kidneys: lack of ADH or neurohypophyseal insufficiency (e.g., diabetes insipidus, water loss in excess of salt)
      i. Potassium depletion: causes a concentrating defect in kidney leading to polyuria; thus, water loss can lead to hypernatremic dehydration
      ii. Hypercalcemia: polyuria and dehydration
      iii. Drugs (e.g., osmotic diuretics or increased administration of sodium bicarbonate or sodium chloride solution); also mineralocorticoids, laxatives, and antacids
      iv. Excessive adrenocortical secretion
      v. Loss of thirst mechanism (e.g., in comatose patient)
      vi. Uncontrolled diabetes mellitus with osmotic diuresis secondary to hyperglycemia
   b. Abnormal renal function: inability of renal tubule to respond to

ADH (nephrogenic diabetes insipidus) and decrease in GFR, causing stimulation of aldosterone release

c. Nursing assessment data base: see hyperkalemia for general statement describing the detection of electrolyte imbalance

    i. Subjective findings

        (a) Patient's chief complaint

            (1) Complaints associated with "edematous states" (salt and water retention) and hypoproteinemia, such as in presence of nephrosis or cirrhosis. Patient complains of excessive weight gain and possibly shortness of breath

            (2) Complaints associated with "dehydration states" (sodium retention/water loss) (e.g., extreme thirst, febrile conditions, decreased urine output, dry mucous membranes)

        (b) Other signs and symptoms—muscle weakness and change in volume of urine output

    ii. Objective findings

        (a) Etiologic or precipitating factors

            (1) Presence of hyperadrenocortical secretion

            (2) Absence of thirst mechanism (patients older than age 65 or comatose)

            (3) Diabetes mellitus

            (4) Hypercalcemia

            (5) Episodes of dehydration

            (6) Episodes of overhydration

            (7) Renal tubule disease

            (8) Establish history of dietary abuse, noncompliance to fluid and sodium restriction, or episode of large water volume loss without an equal sodium loss

            (9) Knowledge of hypernatremia; establish presence of past episodes of hypernatremia

        (b) Family history: noncontributory

        (c) Social history: noncontributory

        (d) Medication history

            (1) Laxatives/antacids—containing high sodium content (e.g., sodium bicarbonate)

            (2) Diuretics—promote a greater loss of water than sodium

            (3) Corticosteroids—conserve sodium and waste potassium

        (e) Other

            (1) Dietary restrictions—state diet and fluid restrictions and modification of sodium intake

            (2) Renal replacement therapy—dialysis

        a) Type of dialysis

        b) Tolerance of dialysis

        c) Effectiveness for sodium regulation

  b. Nursing examination of patient

    i. Inspection

      (a) Neurologic—restlessness, irritability, lethargy, confusion to coma, twitching and seizures

      (b) Respiratory—labored breathing associated with pulmonary edema, dyspnea

      (c) Genitourinary

        (1) Oliguria or anuria with dehydration

        (2) Polyuria with osmotic diuresis

      (d) Gastrointestinal—anorexia

      (e) Integument—dry, flushed skin; dry mucous membranes; edematous tongue; pitting edema

      (f) Musculoskeletal—muscle weakness

    ii. Palpation: pulse—thready, weak pulse with increased ECF and tachycardia with decreased ECF

    iii. Percussion: noncontributory

    iv. Auscultation: hypertension with increased ECF and hypotension with decreased ECF

  c. Diagnostic studies: laboratory evaluation

    i. Serum sodium level above 145 mEq/L and elevated hematocrit

    ii. Serum osmolality greater than 295 mOsm/L

    iii. Urine specific gravity greater than 1.030

    iv. Urine osmolality: 800 to 1400 mOsm/L

    v. Urine sodium: greater than 40 mEq/L when hypernatremia due to sodium excess and normal to low sodium value during a water deficit

4. Nursing diagnoses

  a. Electrolyte excess: hypernatremia

    i. Assessment for defining characteristics

      (a) Manifestations of hypernatremia (see above)

        (1) Integument—dry, flushed skin; dry mucous membranes; thirst; edematous tongue

        (2) Neuromuscular—restlessness, irritability, lethargy, confusion to coma, muscle weakness, twitching, seizures, and elevated body temperature

        (3) Cardiovascular—tachycardia, hypertension

        (4) Pulmonary—rales

        (5) Renal—oliguria or anuria, urine osmolality 800 to 1400 mOsm/L, specific gravity greater than 1.030 to 1.035, and urinary sodium value greater than 40 mEq/L

        (6) Other—serum osmolality greater than 295 mOsm/L and serum sodium level greater than 145 mEq/L

    (b) Manifestations of dehydration (water loss only)

        (1) Dry skin and mucous membranes

        (2) Loss of skin turgor

        (3) Warm, flushed, dry skin

        (4) Initial elevated body temperature

        (5) Hypotension with or without postural changes

        (6) Initial response is tachycardia progressing to brady-cardia

        (7) Thirst

  ii. Expected outcomes

    (a) Maintains sodium in normal range or in a high, asymptomatic range

    (b) Maintains normal fluid status

 iii. Nursing interventions

    (a) Monitor for complications of hypernatremia

        (1) If ECF volume (increased sodium and water) is increased, edematous states leading to hypertension, high cardiac output, and pulmonary congestion will occur

        (2) If sodium retention occurs in presence of water loss, severe dehydration leading to hypotension and increased serum osmolality will result in shock and respiratory arrest

        (3) General—neuromuscular involvement can lead to coma, seizures, and death

    (b) For hypernatremia due to excessive water losses

        (1) Goal is to lower plasma sodium level by water replacement

        (2) Administer water in excess of sodium if patient requires volume (D_5W or ½ normal saline or both)

        (3) Monitor serum sodium levels, serum osmolality, and urine osmolality

        (4) Assess hydration status—too rapid correction can lead to acute pulmonary edema

          a) Maintain intake and output record

          b) Maintain weights

        (5) Perform neurologic assessments and correlate with serum sodium levels

    (c) For hypernatremia with sodium retention

        (1) Determine precipitating factors and treat as ordered

        (2) Institute gradual correction by encouraging actual sodium losses by use of diuretics or by administering fluids

   (3) Be aware that too rapid a correction of sodium levels can cause cerebral edema

   (4) Monitor serum sodium level and osmolality plus urine sodium and osmolality levels

   (5) Assess neurologic status

  iv. Evaluation of nursing care

   (a) Asymptomatic sodium level

   (b) Serum osmolality 280 to 295 mOsm/L

   (c) Urine osmolality within normal range

   (d) Normal hydration status

Electrolyte Imbalances—Sodium Imbalance: Hyponatremia: Serum sodium level below 136 mEq/L

1. Pathophysiology

 a. Excess of water relative to amount of sodium in body produces a dilutional effect on sodium concentration

 b. Salt (NaCl) loss in excess of water loss

2. Etiology or precipitating factors

 a. Water excess: excessive water intake without salt and syndrome of inappropriate ADH

 b. Sodium depletion

  i. Diuretics

  ii. Diarrhea

  iii. Nasogastric suction

  iv. Abnormal losses via diaphoresis

  v. Iatrogenic: losses such as in diuretic therapy

  vi. Salt-losing renal diseases: interstitial nephritis

  vii. Hyperglycemia (glucose-induced diuresis)

 c. Congestive heart failure/cirrhosis of liver

  i. Decreased cardiac output increases water retention by kidneys

  ii. Kidneys may retain larger amounts of water in excess of sodium

3. Nursing assessment data base

 a. Nursing history

  i. Subjective findings

   (a) Patient's chief complaint

    (1) Complaints associated with dehydration—thirst and muscle weakness

    (2) Complaints associated with overhydration—edema and muscle weakness

   (b) Other signs and symptoms

    (1) Increased or decreased urine output

    (2) Limitations of accomplishing ADL and other functional and physical limitations (e.g., exercise, ambulation)

  ii. Objective findings

        (a) Etiologic or precipitating factors
           (1) Presence of hypoactive adrenal gland
           (2) Renal tubular disease (sodium-wasting nephritis)
           (3) Aggressive regimen for diuretic therapy
           (4) Prolonged episodes of vomiting or diarrhea
           (5) Establish history of dietary abuse, noncompliance to fluid and sodium intake, or an episode of both water and sodium loss
           (6) Knowledge of hyponatremia; establish presence of past episodes of hyponatremia
        (b) Family history: noncontributory
        (c) Social history: noncontributory
        (d) Medication history
           (1) Diuretics—cause the loss of both sodium and water
           (2) Laxatives—cause a sodium loss via the stool that is greater than the amount of sodium contained in the laxative
        (e) Other
           (1) Renal replacement therapy—dialysis
              a) Type of dialysis
              b) Tolerance of dialysis
              c) Effect on sodium regulation
  b. Nursing examination of patient
    i. Inspection
        (a) Neurologic—malaise, confusion to coma, seizures, headache
        (b) Respiratory—dyspnea with pulmonary edema
        (c) Genitourinary—normal urine output to polyuria
        (d) Gastrointestinal—abdominal cramps
        (e) Integument—poor skin turgor
    ii. Palpation: rapid pulse with water overload
    iii. Percussion: noncontributory
    iv. Auscultation
        (a) Increased or decreased central venous pressure
        (b) Blood pressure may range from hypotension to normal to hypertension
        (c) Rales with fluid overload
  c. Diagnostic study findings: laboratory evaluation
    i. Serum sodium level below 136 mEq/L and decreased hematocrit due to water excess
    ii. Urine volume and urine specific gravity can be normal
    iii. Urine sodium: less than 20 mEq/L if due to a sodium deficit and normal to elevated sodium level if due to water excess

4. Nursing diagnosis
  a. Electrolyte deficit: hyponatremia

    i. Assessment for defining characteristics

      (a) Manifestations of hyponatremia (see above)

        (1) Malaise, confusion to coma

        (2) Headache

        (3) Muscular weakness

        (4) Weight loss

        (5) Poor skin turgor

        (6) Decreased central venous pressure

        (7) Abdominal cramps

        (8) Nausea

        (9) Decreased urinary sodium under 20 mEq/L

       (10) Permanent neurologic changes can occur after experiencing a serum sodium level below 110 mEq/L

      (b) Manifestations of water intoxication

        (1) Headache

        (2) Confusion to delirium

        (3) Seizures

        (4) Weight gain

        (5) Good skin turgor

        (6) Decreased hematocrit

        (7) Decreased BUN

        (8) Increased central venous pressure

        (9) Elevated jugular venous pressure

       (10) Low serum osmolality < 280 mOsm/L

       (11) Normal or increased urinary sodium > 25 mEq/L

       (12) Increased risk of pulmonary edema

   ii. Expected outcomes

      (a) Serum sodium within normal limits or to asymptomatic level

      (b) Maintains normal fluid status

  iii. Nursing interventions

      (a) For sodium and water losses

        (1) Administer diet high in sodium with adequate fluid intake

        (2) Anticipate intravenous replacement with normal saline or hypertonic saline. Watch carefully for pulmonary edema when giving these solutions

        (3) Observe for the reversal of the hyponatremia-caused symptoms

        (4) Obtain serum sodium concentrations to determine effectiveness of therapy, in addition to urine sodium and osmolality

        (5) Monitor neurologic signs and symptoms and report changes in status

        (6) Discontinue diuretics if implicated in etiology

          (7) Maintain intake and output record
     (b) For water intoxication
          (1) Restrict fluid intake (a restriction of 500 ml/day may be appropriate)
          (2) Consider diuretic therapy to aid in the restoration of normal fluid status
          (3) Monitor serum sodium levels to determine if actual sodium replacement is indicated as normal fluid status is restored
          (4) Assess neurologic status, monitoring for signs of improvement
          (5) Do not give hypertonic saline in syndrome of inappropriate ADH secretion. This does not correct basic cause and may precipitate congestive heart failure in susceptible patients
          (6) In syndrome of inappropriate ADH, restrict all water intake because decreased sodium is a result of inability to excrete water normally
   iv. Evaluation of nursing care
     (a) Asymptomatic sodium levels
     (b) Urinary sodium > 30 to 40 mEq/L
     (c) Normal hydration status

Electrolyte Imbalances—Calcium Imbalance: Hypercalcemia: Serum calcium level above 10.5 mg/dl

1. Pathophysiology
   a. Increased mobilization of calcium from bone occurs in primary hyperparathyroidism, immobilization, and thyrotoxicosis
   b. Increased intestinal reabsorption of calcium secondary to large dietary intake and excessive administration of vitamin D
   c. Altered renal tubular reabsorption of calcium

2. Etiology or precipitating factors
   a. Primary hyperparathyroidism seen in adenoma or carcinoma of parathyroids (rare), resulting in increased tubular reabsorption of calcium
   b. Metastatic carcinoma with "osteolytic lesions" and in multiple myeloma; hypercalcemia is result of lesions releasing calcium into plasma
   c. Hypophosphatemia
   d. Immobilization: prolonged bed rest causes calcium to be mobilized from bone, teeth, and intestines
   e. Alkalosis: increases calcium binding to protein; decreases serum calcium levels
   f. Thyrotoxicosis

    g. Excessive doses of vitamin D that increase reabsorption of calcium from intestine

    h. Drugs: chronic thiazide diuretic therapy inhibits calcium excretion

    i. Renal tubular acidosis

3. Nursing assessment data base

    a. Nursing history

       i. Subjective findings

          (a) Patient's chief complaint—lethargy and muscle weakness

          (b) Other signs and symptoms

             (1) Anorexia, nausea, and vomiting

             (2) Increased fatigue

             (3) Increased urine output

             (4) Constipation

      ii. Objective findings

          (a) Etiologic or precipitating factors

             (1) Presence of hyperparathyroidism

             (2) Renal tubular disease

             (3) Presence of hypophosphatemia

             (4) History of prolonged bed rest

             (5) Excessive intake of vitamin D or calcium supplements

             (6) Presence of alkalosis

             (7) Thyrotoxicosis

             (8) Chronic diuretic therapy

             (9) Knowledge of hypercalcemia; establish presence of past episodes

          (b) Family history: noncontributory

          (c) Social history: noncontributory

          (d) Medication history

             (1) Vitamin D—excessive administration will increase calcium absorption from intestines

             (2) Calcium supplements—excessive intake

             (3) Thiazide diuretics—inhibit calcium excretion

    b. Nursing examination of patient

       i. Inspection

          (a) Neurologic—extreme hypercalcemia produces lethargy, confusion to coma, subtle personality changes

          (b) Cardiovascular—if patient is taking digitalis, hypercalcemia may cause an enhanced digitalis effect, which can contribute to dysrhythmias and/or cardiac arrest

          (c) Genitourinary—polyuria, flank/thigh pain associated with renal calculi

          (d) Gastrointestinal—nausea and vomiting may be secondary to hypercalcemia, acting as a stimulus for gastric acid secretion and possible development of peptic ulcer disease.

Inadequate peristalsis is related to hypotonicity of smooth muscle of the bowel, leading to constipation
(e) Musculoskeletal—hypotonicity/weakness of muscles, coma, pathologic fractures, metastatic calcifications affecting extraosseous soft tissue seen in hyperparathyroidism
(f) Other—observe for metastatic calcifications, usually calcium crystals deposited in cornea and visible by slit lamp examination. If extensive, they will be visible to naked eye as band keratopathy (semilunar whitish bands, beginning as "parentheses" at lateral margins of cornea and extending in a band across cornea)
ii. Palpation: noncontributory
iii. Percussion: noncontributory
iv. Auscultation: noncontributory
c. Diagnostic studies
i. Laboratory
(a) Serum calcium level above 10.5 mg/dl
(b) Sulkowitch's urine test for calcium
ii. Radiologic
(a) Renal calculi
(b) Calcium deposits on bone films
(c) Nephrocalcinosis—calcium deposits in renal parenchyma
iii. Special: ECG reveals shortening of ST segment
4. **Nursing diagnoses**
a. Electrolyte excess: hypercalcemia
i. Assessment for defining characteristics (see above)
(a) Additional manifestations of hypercalcemia
(1) Headache
(2) Abdominal pain
(3) Hypertension (occurs in 33% of all cases)
(4) Deep bone pain
(5) Polydipsia secondary to polyuria
(b) Additional manifestations of myocardial functioning with hypercalcemia
(1) ECG changes—shortened ST segment
(2) Increased extracellular levels of calcium create a predisposition to cardiac arrest
(3) Increased incidence of heart block, which may precede cardiac arrest
ii. Expected outcomes
(a) Maintains calcium within normal limits or in asymptomatic range
(b) Cardiac function within normal range
iii. Nursing interventions
(a) Provide cardiac monitoring

   (b) Observe for cardiac involvement
   (c) If administering digitalis, do so cautiously—hypercalcemia enhances action of digitalis and toxicity can result
   (d) Monitor intake and output record and status of renal function
   (e) Anticipate use of therapies to reduce serum calcium level
       (1) Normal saline infusion and diuretics increase GFR and calcium excretion
       (2) Corticosteroids decrease gastrointestinal absorption of calcium
       (3) Mithramycin therapy stimulates bone uptake of calcium
       (4) Oral phosphate binds calcium
   (f) Monitor serum calcium levels to determine effectiveness of therapeutic interventions
   iv. Evaluation of nursing care
       (a) Asymptomatic calcium level
       (b) Absence of neuromuscular or cardiac involvement

Electrolyte Imbalances—Calcium Imbalance: Hypocalcemia: Serum calcium level below 8.5 mg/dl

1. Pathophysiology
   a. Excessive gastrointestinal losses of calcium secondary to diarrhea, effect of diuretics, and increased levels of lipoproteins
   b. Malabsorption syndromes such as vitamin D deficiency and hypoparathyroidism

2. Etiology or precipitating factors
   a. Hypoparathyroidism
       i. Surgical ablation of parathyroids
       ii. Parathyroid adenoma
       iii. Idiopathic
       iv. Depletion of magnesium: needed for effective action of PTH
   b. CRF
       i. Hyperphosphatemia: potentiates peripheral deposition of calcium
       ii. Vitamin D resistance: inability to absorb calcium from intestine, which is vitamin D mediated
   c. Vitamin D deficiency secondary to CRF, hepatic failure, and rickets: "active" vitamin D is necessary for calcium absorption
   d. Chronic malabsorption syndrome resulting from
       i. Magnesium depletion
       ii. Gastrectomy
       iii. Fat diet: fat impairs calcium absorption
       iv. Small bowel disorders: inability to absorb vitamin D

e. Increased thyrocalcitonin: stimulates osteoblasts to prevent calcium entry into serum

f. Malignancy
 i. Osteoblastic metastasis: calcium is consumed for abnormal bone synthesis
 ii. Medullary carcinoma of thyroid: abnormal secretion of thyrocalcitonin

g. Acute pancreatitis: precipitation of calcium in inflamed pancreas and intra-abdominal lipids

h. Hyperphosphatemia: calcium and phosphate bind together and precipitate in tissues
 i. Cytotoxic drugs (cytolysis of bone)
 ii. Increased oral intake of phosphates
 iii. CRF (decreased excretion of phosphate)

3. **Nursing assessment data base**
 a. Nursing history
  i. Subjective findings
   (a) Patient's chief complaint—muscle and abdominal cramps
   (b) Other symptoms
    (1) Bone pain
    (2) Lethargy
    (3) Constipation
    (4) Nausea and vomiting
    (5) Functional and physical limitations (ambulation and exercise)
  ii. Objective findings
   (a) Etiologic or precipitating factors
    (1) Presence of CRF
    (2) Starvation or history of dietary abuse
    (3) Malabsorption syndrome
    (4) Noncompliance to phosphate binders
    (5) Presence of carcinoma with metastasis
    (6) Presence of acute pancreatitis
    (7) Presence of massive infection of subcutaneous tissue
   (b) Family history—noncontributory
   (c) Social history—noncontributory
   (d) Medication history
    (1) Phosphate binders—gels administered in renal failure to bind phosphate in the gut, leaving calcium free to be absorbed
    (2) Vitamin D supplements—promote calcium absorption
    (3) Calcium supplement
    (4) Diuretics—promote renal losses of calcium
   (e) Other—renal replacement therapy
    (1) Type of tolerance

(2) Effectiveness
  b. Nursing examination of patient
    i. Inspection
        (a) Neurologic—lethargy, muscle tremors, and cramps may accompany minor reductions in calcium level
        (b) Respiratory—labored shallow breathing, wheezes, and bronchospasm if respiratory musculature is involved. Neuromuscular irritability can cause airway obstruction and bronchial spasm
        (c) Cardiovascular—dysrhythmias on ECG
        (d) Genitourinary—oliguria or anuria secondary to obstruction caused by renal calculi
        (e) Gastrointestinal—distended abdomen secondary to constipation, diarrhea
        (f) Musculoskeletal—tetany and generalized tonic/clonic seizures develop with severe reductions
        (g) Other—bruising and/or bleeding. Bleeding can occur secondary to changes in clotting mechanism because calcium is necessary for normal clotting
    ii. Palpation
        (a) Chvostek's sign—tap finger on supramandibular portion of parotid gland and observe twitches in upper lip on side of stimulation. This muscle spasm indicates a positive test. False-positive responses can occur
        (b) Pulses—irregular secondary to dysrhythmias
    iii. Percussion—noncontributory
    iv. Auscultation
        (a) Bowel sounds absent secondary to paralytic ileus
        (b) Trousseau's sign—apply blood pressure cuff to upper arm and inflate. If carpopedal spasm results, test is positive; if no spasm appears in 3 minutes, test is negative. Remove cuff and tell patient to hyperventilate (30 times/min). Respiratory alkalosis that develops can also produce carpopedal spasm (positive if occurs)
  c. Diagnostic studies: serum calcium level below 8.5 mg/dl
4. **Nursing diagnoses**
  a. Electrolyte deficit: hypocalcemia
    i. Assessment for defining characteristics (see above)
        (a) Manifestations of hypocalcemia
          (1) Muscle cramps
          (2) Abdominal cramps
          (3) Tetany—early signs include numbness and tingling of extremities and around oral cavity
          (4) Tetany can also progress to seizures
          (5) Laryngeal stridor can predispose to respiratory arrest

(6) Carpopedal spasm

(7) Bleeding abnormality due to decreased prothrombin time (rare)

(8) Increased incidence of fractures

(9) Decreased cardiac output predisposing to cardiac arrest

(10) Positive Chvostek's and Trousseau's signs

(b) Manifestations of myocardial functioning during hypocalcemia

(1) ECG changes—prolonged ST segment and QT interval

(2) Impaired myocardial contractility that can ultimately predispose to cardiac arrest

ii. Expected outcomes

(a) Correct symptomatic hypocalcemia

(b) Prevent cardiac arrest

iii. Nursing interventions

(a) Provide cardiac monitoring

(b) Administer 10% calcium gluconate or calcium chloride slowly intravenously (1 ml/min) for emergency interventions

(1) Monitor for cardiac involvement—decreased cardiac output

(2) Rapid infusion may enhance digitalis or precipitate cardiac arrest

(c) Chronic hypocalcemia necessitates daily oral doses of calcium, usually administered in the range of 1.5 to 3 g/day

(d) If vitamin D deficiency is present, administer vitamin D supplements

(e) If phosphate deficiency is evident, replace phosphates before administering calcium. However, it is usual to see hyperphosphatemia accompanying this imbalance

(f) Monitor serum calcium and phosphate levels

(g) Implement seizure precautions; provide quiet environment

(h) Monitor respiratory status; bronchospasm may precipitate respiratory arrest

(i) Teach patients warning signs of tetany or seizures, and instruct them to inform you at the immediate onset of these symptoms

(j) Monitor therapeutic effectiveness by use of Chvostek's and Trousseau's signs plus ECG

iv. Evaluation of nursing care

(a) Asymptomatic calcium level

(b) Absence of neuromuscular or cardiac involvement

Electrolyte Imbalances—Phosphate Imbalance: Hyperphosphatemia:
Serum phosphate level above 4.5 mg/dl

1. **Pathophysiology**
   a. Inability to excrete phosphate via kidney owing to decrease in GFR to one tenth of normal, or owing to renal failure
   b. Excessive intake due to dietary or cathartic abuse and drugs (cytotoxic agents)
2. **Etiology or precipitating factors**
   a. Acute/chronic renal failure (inability to excrete phosphate)
   b. Hypoparathyroidism: PTH effect on kidney is to cause hypophosphatemia and lower body phosphate
   c. Cathartic abuse or phosphate-containing laxatives and enemas
   d. Cytotoxic agents for neoplasms: serum phosphate increases due to cytolysis (seen in leukemias or lymphomas)
   e. Overadministration of intravenous or oral phosphates
3. **Nursing assessment data base**
   a. Nursing history
      i. Subjective findings
         (a) Patient's chief complaint—muscle cramping
         (b) Other symptoms—seizures, joint pain
      ii. Objective findings
         (a) Etiologic or precipitating factors
            (1) Renal failure
            (2) Presence of vague neurologic complaints
            (3) Seizures of unknown origin
            (4) Metastatic calcifications
            (5) Hypocalcemia
            (6) Noncompliance with use of phosphate-binding gel
         (b) Family history—noncontributory
         (c) Social history—noncontributory
         (d) Medication history—the following are prescribed for hyperphosphatemia and become important when the patient is noncompliant
            (1) Phosphate-binding gels—promote binding of phosphate in intestines, which prevents phosphate absorption
            (2) Calcium supplement—if hypocalcemia accompanies hyperphosphatemia
         (e) Other: renal replacement therapy
            (1) Type and tolerance
            (2) Effectiveness
   b. Nursing examination of patient: presents with vague symptomatology similar to the presentation of hypocalcemia
      i. Inspection
         (a) Neurologic—seizures caused by a chronic phosphate elevation that can depress calcium levels, precipitating the seizure

(b) Musculoskeletal—joint pain secondary to the precipitation of calcium and/or phosphate in soft tissue and joints
   c. Diagnostic study findings
      i. Laboratory: serum phosphate greater than 4.5 mg/dl
      ii. Special: ECG changes comparable with those seen in hypocalcemia (e.g., prolongation of ST segment)
4. **Nursing diagnoses**
   a. Electrolyte excess: hyperphosphatemia
      i. Assessment for defining characteristics: synonymous with assessment parameters provided for hypocalcemia. A natural inverse relationship exists between these two ions, so that hyperphosphatemia leads to a reciprocal hypocalcemia
      ii. Expected outcomes
         (a) Maintains phosphate level within normal limits or within a safe asymptomatic range
         (b) No episodes of tetany or seizures
      iii. Nursing interventions
         (a) Administer aluminum hydroxide gels to bind phosphate in intestines, limiting its absorption and thus reducing serum phosphate levels
         (b) Teach patient purpose of gels (easy to confuse with antacid owing to similarity in drug preparation)
         (c) Monitor serum phosphate and calcium levels to determine effectiveness of therapeutic interventions
         (d) Implement dialysis for rapid correction of hyperphosphatemia if necessary
         (e) Administer acetazolamide to increase urinary phosphate excretion via a normal kidney
      iv. Evaluation of nursing care
         (a) Asymptomatic serum phosphate level
         (b) Absence of neuromuscular symptomatology

Electrolyte Imbalances—Phosphate Imbalance: Hypophosphatemia: Serum phosphate level below 3.0 mg/L
1. **Pathophysiology**
   a. Increased cell uptake to form sugar phosphates occurs during hyperventilation or increased glucose administration (e.g., parenteral hyperalimentation)
   b. Decreased phosphate absorption from bowel
   c. Renal phosphate wasting (loss of proximal tubular function), seen in Fanconi's syndrome and vitamin D–resistant rickets
2. **Etiology or precipitating factors**
   a. Inadequate phosphate intake (seen in chronic alcoholism)
   b. Chronic phosphate depletion: occurs in osteomalacia and rickets
   c. Long-term hyperalimentation lacking in phosphates. Glucose phos-

phorylation uses phosphate and can lead to phosphate depletion if no replacement is available

   d. Hyperparathyroidism: causes renal phosphaturia

   e. Malabsorption syndrome

   f. Abuse or overadministration of phosphate-binding gels

   g. Fanconi's syndrome: loss of phosphates in urine, leading to osteo-malacia (adults)

3. **Nursing assessment data base**

   a. Nursing history

      ii. Subjective findings

         (a) Patient's chief complaint—vague complaints including muscle weakness, muscle wasting, and fatigue

         (b) Other symptoms—confusion, lack of appetite, changes in weight, impaired ambulation

      ii. Objective findings

         (a) Etiologic or precipitating factors

            (1) Presence of metabolic acidosis

            (2) Alcohol abuse without adequate nutritional intake

            (3) Starvation

            (4) Renal failure

            (5) Presence of malabsorption syndrome

         (b) Family history—noncontributory

         (c) Social history—noncontributory

         (d) Medication history

            (1) Phosphate binders—overuse

            (2) Diuretics—prolonged use may (rarely) lead to phosphate depletion

         (e) Other—renal replacement therapy

            (1) Type and tolerance

            (2) Effectiveness

   b. Nursing examination of patient

      i. Inspection

         (a) Neurologic—confusion, malaise

         (b) Respiratory—dyspnea secondary to hypoxia resulting from deficit in erythrocyte phosphate content necessary for 2,3-diphosphoglycerate (2,3-DPG). Shortness of breath can also be the result of cardiac failure

         (c) Genitourinary—decreased urine output secondary to cardiac failure

         (d) Integument—cool skin secondary to decreased cardiac output. Myocardial contractility diminishes owing to the inadequate levels of intracellular phosphates

         (e) Musculoskeletal—muscle weakness and wasting. Symptoms result from acute depletion of intracellular phosphate, which leads to a diffuse muscle-wasting necrosis called rhabdomyolysis. Skeletal changes occur with long-standing hypophosphatemia, which is the result of excessive losses of external phosphate

    ii. Palpation: tachycardia secondary to decrease in cardiac output

    iii. Percussion: noncontributory

    iv. Auscultation

        (a) Hypotension

        (b) Crackles, rales secondary to cardiac failure

  c. Diagnostic study findings

    i. Laboratory: serum phosphate level below 3.0 mg/dl, low serum alkaline pyrophosphate level, high serum pyrophosphate level

    ii. Hypercalcemia and hypercalciuria: indicators of acute phosphate depletion in hyperparathyroidism. PTH increases serum calcium by taking it from bone and decreases serum phosphate by excreting it into urine

    iii. Radiologic: skeletal abnormalities resembling osteomalacia (i.e., pseudofractures characterized by thickened periosteum and new bone formation over what appears to be an incomplete fracture)

4. Nursing diagnoses

  a. Electrolyte deficit: hypophosphatemia

    i. Assessment for defining characteristics (see above)

        (a) Manifestations of hypophosphatemia

            (1) Anorexia

            (2) Malaise

            (3) Muscle wasting and weakness

            (4) Hemolysis and hypoxia—decreased levels of 2,3-DPG

        (b) Manifestations of hypercalcemia (see p. 589). The occurrence of hypophosphatemia creates a reciprocal hypercalcemia

    ii. Expected outcomes

        (a) Asymptomatic serum phosphate level

        (b) No neuromuscular signs of hypophosphatemia

    iii. Nursing interventions

        (a) Treat primary cause of hypophosphatemia

        (b) Replace phosphates intravenously, then orally

        (c) Discontinue phosphate-binding gels

        (d) Monitor phosphate and calcium levels to determine effectiveness of therapy

    iv. Evaluation of nursing care

        (a) Asymptomatic phosphate level

        (b) Absence of neuromuscular involvement

Electrolyte Imbalances—Magnesium Imbalance: Hypermagnesemia:
Serum level above 2.5 mEq/L

1. **Pathophysiology**
   a. Decreased excretion secondary to renal failure
   b. Increased magnesium intake
   c. Acidosis
2. **Etiology or precipitating factors**
   a. Renal failure
   b. Adrenal insufficiency
   c. Excessive intake or administration of magnesium-containing antacid gels or laxatives
   d. Acidotic states (e.g., diabetic ketoacidosis)
3. **Nursing assessment data base**
   a. Nursing history
      i. Subjective findings
         (a) Patient's chief complaint—muscle weakness and fatigue
      ii. Objective findings
         (a) Etiologic or precipitating factors
            (1) Renal failure
            (2) Laxative or antacid abuser
            (3) Presence of adrenal insufficiency
            (4) Presence of diabetes
            (5) Presence of acidosis
         (b) Family history: noncontributory
         (c) Social history: noncontributory
         (d) Medication history
            (1) Laxatives—milk of magnesia or others containing magnesium
            (2) Antacids—containing magnesium hydroxide
   b. Nursing examination of patient
      i. Inspection
         (a) Neurologic—lethargy to coma
         (b) Respiratory—depressed respirations to apnea
         (c) Cardiovascular—bradycardia on ECG
         (d) Musculoskeletal—muscle weakness, loss of deep tendon reflexes, seizures
      ii. Palpation: pulse rate is slow
      iii. Percussion: noncontributory
      iv. Auscultation: hypotension secondary to depressed myocardial contractility can progress to cardiac arrest
   c. Diagnostic study findings
      i. Laboratory serum magnesium level over 2.5 mEq/L
      ii. ECG: peaked T wave similar to that in hyperkalemia
4. **Nursing diagnoses**
   a. Electrolyte excess: hypermagnesemia
      i. Assessment for defining characteristics (see above)

      (a) Sudden onset of vague neuromuscular symptomatology (lethargy, confusion, coma, seizures)

      (b) Depressed respiratory rate

      (c) Cardiac involvement—bradycardia, peaked T wave, or other signs of depressed myocardial contractility

   ii. Expected outcomes

      (a) Serum magnesium level returns to within normal limits

      (b) Absence of neuromuscular and cardiac involvement

  iii. Nursing interventions

      (a) Determine primary cause of hypermagnesemia and intervene

      (b) Consider dialysis and implement if excesses are due to renal failure

      (c) Teach patient to avoid medications containing magnesium

      (d) Observe for respiratory distress and support patient symptomatically while decreasing magnesium level

      (e) If normal renal function, administer diuretics or saline-induced diuresis to encourage magnesium loss. During period of diuresis, maintain intake and output record in an effort to prevent dehydration, which may exacerbate symptoms

      (f) Monitor ECG and neurologic signs

      (g) Monitor serum magnesium levels

      (h) Consider calcium gluconate administration to minimize symptoms of increased magnesium

   iv. Evaluation of nursing care

      (a) Asymptomatic magnesium levels

      (b) Absence of neuromuscular and cardiac complications

Electrolyte Imbalances—Magnesium Imbalance: Hypomagnesemia: Serum level below 1.5 mEq/L

1. Pathophysiology

  a. Decreased intake of magnesium

  b. Diminished intestinal reabsorption

  c. Excess losses in urine or wound or extracellular drainage

  d. Alkalosis (in some instances)

  e. Excessive adrenal corticoid secretions

2. Etiology or precipitating factors

  a. Starvation syndrome

  b. Malabsorption syndrome

  c. Prolonged hyperalimentation without adequate magnesium replacement

  d. Excessive diuretic therapy

  e. Toxemia of pregnancy

  f. Excessive fistula or gastrointestinal losses containing magnesium

(e.g., severe diarrhea, nasogastric suction losses without replacement)

g. Chronic alcoholism

h. Alkalotic states (in some instances)

i. Excessive corticosteroid administration

j. Hypocalcemia

k. Hypoparathyroidism

l. Hyperaldosteronism

m. Ulcerative colitis

n. Hyperthyroidism

o. Acute and chronic pancreatitis

p. Cisplatin treatment for cancer

3. **Nursing assessment data base**

a. Nursing history

i. Subjective findings

(a) Patient's chief complaint—muscle weakness or tremors

(b) Other symptoms—anorexia, nausea, and dizziness

ii. Objective findings

(a) Etiologic or precipitating factors

(1) Starvation

(2) Malabsorption syndrome

(3) History of diuretic usage

(4) Alcohol abuse without adequate nutritional intake

(5) Presence of adrenal disease

(6) Presence of hypocalcemia

(7) History of excessive use of corticosteroids

(8) Recent pregnancy

(b) Family history—noncontributory

(c) Social history—noncontributory

(d) Medication history

(1) Diuretics may cause magnesium wasting

(2) Corticosteroids with an aldosterone component may precipitate hypomagnesemia

(e) Other—renal replacement therapy

(1) Type and tolerance

(2) Effectiveness

b. Nursing examination of patient

i. Inspection

(a) Neurologic—lethargy, confusion, coma

(b) Cardiovascular—dysrhythmias on ECG

(c) Musculoskeletal—hyperirritability, tremors, facial twitching, seizures

ii. Palpation

(a) Pulse—irregular secondary to dysrhythmias or enhanced digitalis effect

(b) Positive Chvostek's sign
  iii. Percussion—noncontributory
  iv. Auscultation
    (a) Blood pressure—normal to decreased if cardiac function altered
    (b) Positive Trousseau's sign
c. Diagnostic study findings
  i. Laboratory: serum magnesium levels below 1.5 mEq/L
  ii. ECG: flat or inverted T waves, possible ST segment depression, prolonged QT interval

4. Nursing diagnoses

a. Electrolyte deficit: hypomagnesemia
  i. Assessment for defining characteristics
    (a) Manifestations of hypomagnesemia
      (1) Vague neurologic symptoms that may have sudden onset without obvious explanations, such as confusion, coma, tremors to tetany, ataxia, psychosis, and seizures
      (2) Anorexia and nausea
      (3) Dizziness
      (4) Muscle weakness
  ii. Expected outcomes
    (a) Serum magnesium level returns to normal
    (b) Free of neuromuscular symptoms (seizures)
  iii. Nursing interventions
    (a) Administer magnesium sulfate 50% solution intramuscularly or intravenously
    (b) Consider administration of calcium gluconate when replacing with large boluses of magnesium. Calcium will retard the effects of sudden reversal to hypermagnesemia
    (c) If hypokalemia occurs simultaneously with hypomagnesemia, then correct magnesium deficit first
    (d) Be aware that hypomagnesemia will enhance digitalis, causing digitalis toxicity
    (e) Correct alkalosis
    (f) Establish seizure precautions
    (g) Monitor serum magnesium levels to determine effects of therapeutic interventions
    (h) Monitor ECG changes
    (i) Consider dietary replacement (seafood, green vegetables, whole grains, and nuts)
  iv. Evaluation of nursing care
    (a) Asymptomatic level of magnesium
    (b) Absence of neuromuscular symptoms

Renal Trauma: Occurs most often in men between the ages of 20 and 40 years

1. **Pathophysiology**: a result of renal tissue trauma
   a. Disruption of the renal system caused by
      i. Nonpenetrating injuries (blunt trauma): accounts for 70% to 80% of all renal injuries
      ii. Penetrating injuries: 20% to 30% of all renal injuries
   b. Classifications of renal injury according to severity
      i. Contusions: comprise approximately 85% of all renal injuries (e.g., subcapsular hematomas, minor cortical lacerations). Hematuria commonly accompanies this injury. Renal collecting system is not involved
      ii. Lacerations: deep renal parenchyma injury (10% of all renal injuries). Damage can involve renal collecting system
      iii. Fractures: extensive lacerations at various sites in the renal parenchyma, with collecting system damage
      iv. Vascular or pedicle injuries: renal arterial intima tears or vessel disruptions. Renal arterial tears cause blood collections between intima and intact media, usually leading to thrombosis, sometimes of the entire vessel's length

2. **Etiology or precipitating factors**
   a. Nonpenetrating renal injuries
      i. Vehicular accident (e.g., impact with dashboard, steering wheel)
      ii. Impact to abdomen or flank after assault or sports injury
      iii. Sudden deceleration or acceleration accidents (e.g., pedestrian-vehicular accident or falls from significant heights). These accidents typically precipitate vascular injuries
   b. Penetrating renal injuries: associated with a high incidence of intraperitoneal visceral injury, hemorrhage, fistulas, and infections
      i. Gunshot wounds
      ii. Stab wounds
      iii. Vehicular accidents
      iv. Industrial accidents
      v. Other sources of trauma

3. **Nursing assessment data base**
   a. Nursing history (acute event)
      i. Subjective findings
         (a) Patient's chief complaint—pain in flank or upper quadrant of the abdomen
      ii. Objective findings
         (a) Etiologic or precipitating factors—history of traumatic incident
         (b) Family history
            (1) Description of family unit
            (2) Adequacy as a support system

  (c) Social history—alcohol or drug abuse

  (d) Medication history—obtain list of medications taken by the patient prior to the trauma

 b. Nursing examination of patient

  i. Inspection

   (a) Abdomen—observe abdomen and flank for symmetry

   (b) Genitourinary

    (1) Observe external genitalia, perineum, and urethral meatus for blood or ecchymosis

    (2) Inspect for type of trauma to provide indicators for the presence of renal injury

     a) High-velocity trauma—contributes to secondary renal necrosis, fistula, hemorrhage, and infection. The presence of significant renal trauma with hemorrhage may require nephrectomy

     b) Low-velocity trauma—associated with low incidence of complications

     c) Nonpenetrating injury should be suspected on description of abdominal, back, or lower chest as the site of trauma

    (3) Signs and symptoms of blunt or penetrating wound in region of kidneys indicating renal injury

     a) Presence of costovertebral angle pain

     b) Renal colic—result of clots obstructing the collecting system

     c) Hematoma over posterior aspect of eleventh or twelfth rib or in flank area (absence of hematoma does not rule out renal injury in 24% of all cases)

     d) Flank mass

     e) Hematuria, gross or microscopic—a common sign suggesting renal injury. However, a correlation does not exist between the degree of hematuria and the extent of the injury

     f) Fractured ribs overlying kidney

     g) Ecchymosis at site of entrance wounds at lateral abdomen and flank

     h) Tenderness in flank or upper quadrant of the abdomen; crepitation or contusion in flank

     i) Retroperitoneal bleeding

  ii. Palpation

   (a) Palpate suprapubic areas and flanks for tenderness, masses, or presence of rib fractures

   (b) Palpate pelvis for fractures

  iii. Percussion: to assist in determining the presence of a collection of fluid or solid material

    iv. Auscultation

        (a) Blood pressure—normal to decreased secondary to blood loss or response to trauma

        (b) Lung sounds—to assess extent of aeration

    v. Other: examine other organ systems for the presence of the following associated injuries concomitant with renal injury (60% to 80% incidence)—liver, colon, lung, spleen, small bowel, stomach, pancreas, duodenum, diaphragm

  c. Diagnostic studies

    i. Laboratory

        (a) Serum

            (1) BUN/creatinine—elevation of BUN indicates the catabolic process in the trauma victim and/or the hypovolemic state. An elevation of both BUN and creatinine levels indicates significant renal involvement

            (2) Hematocrit/hemoglobin—decrease indicates hemorrhage; site must be determined

            (3) Electrolytes—a variety of results may occur. Potassium level usually is elevated secondary to leakage from cells due to trauma, acidosis, or catabolism. The other values will usually reflect a decrease if actual loss has occurred through wound or fistula drainage

        (b) Urine

            (1) Volume—may be diminished if significant renal damage or obstruction and/or hypovolemia are present

            (2) Urinalysis—erythrocytes and protein may be present, but renal trauma can still exist without this response

    ii. Radiologic examination

        (a) Plain film of abdomen—provides an initial radiologic assessment of injury. It can display

            (1) Rib fractures over kidney

            (2) Obliteration of renal or psoas shadow

            (3) Displacement of bowel

        (b) High-dose infusion pyelogram—to establish the status of the uninvolved kidney as well as of the traumatized organ. The direct inspection of the injured kidney will occur at the time of surgery. The results suggestive of renal injury are

            (1) Delayed excretion of dye

            (2) Renal outline enlargement

            (3) Diminished concentration of contrast media level in renal parenchyma—outlines the collecting system and ureters

            (4) If the patient is in shock, radiologic examination should include only the first two studies mentioned

(c) Tomography—particularly helpful when nonpenetrating injury is suspected. Establishes an 80% to 95% accuracy for location and extent of renal parenchymal damage. To perform this examination, the patient must maintain a blood pressure above 90 mm Hg systolic

(d) Ultrasonography—has a minimal value in interpreting nonpenetrating injury. It can determine the renal parenchyma integrity and locate a hematoma's position

(e) Renal scan—determines the status of renal blood flow and the presence of parenchymal injury

(f) Retrograde pyelography—provides minimal information and can contaminate the traumatized victim

(g) Renal angiography—a more precise examination tool when an injury is not clearly defined by other radiologic studies. This procedure would be indicated in cases of continuous bleeding that impairs visualization or causes extravasation of contrast medium

(h) Computed tomography—provides an exact means for the determination of extent of injury

(i) Surgical exploration—a valuable diagnostic tool, usually indicated for all hematomas. If exploration reveals a major laceration, then repair can occur immediately

4. Nursing diagnoses

a. Fluid volume deficit: hemorrhage—stabilize the patient's condition and follow with evaluation of abdomen including urinary tract

  i. Assessment for defining characteristics

    (a) Manifestations of hemorrhage

      (1) Hypotension

      (2) Cool, clammy skin

      (3) Tachycardia

      (4) Dysrhythmias

      (5) Decreased hematocrit and hemoglobin

      (6) Shortness of breath

      (7) Kussmaul breathing

      (8) High incidence of shock

      (9) Evidence of frank bleeding may occur, such as enlarging abdomen

     (10) Restlessness, confusion, lassitude, feelings of impending doom

    (b) Manifestations of hematuria—gross or microscopic

  ii. Expected outcomes

    (a) Remains stable in initial period

    (b) Fluid and blood volume replaced adequately

    (c) Prepared for surgery if indicated

  iii. Nursing interventions

(a) Monitor for complications of renal trauma
  (1) Ileus
  (2) Hemorrhage or rebleeding
  (3) Extravasation of urine (and its associated increased incidence of infection and decreased wound healing ability)
  (4) Sepsis
  (5) Shock
  (6) Impairment or loss of renal function
  (7) Fistula formation
  (8) Perinephric abscess
  (9) Renal abscess
  (10) Late complications—hypertension, hydronephrosis, chronic pyelonephritis, calculus formation, intrarenal calcification
(b) Initial period
  (1) Maintain patent airway
  (2) Provide adequate oxygenation
  (3) Control hemorrhage
  (4) Type and cross-match blood
  (5) Establish multiple intravenous lines in major vessels with at least one line placed centrally
  (6) Correct blood losses
  (7) Reestablish normal fluid balance
  (8) Obtain frequent vital signs
  (9) Maintain blood pressure
  (10) Obtain laboratory data—serum electrolytes, BUN, creatinine, amylase, arterial blood gases, and complete blood cell count
(c) Post minor injury
  (1) Maintain bed rest
  (2) Monitor hematocrit and hemoglobin
  (3) Monitor presence of hematuria
  (4) Obtain vital signs and report any sudden changes
  (5) Provide analgesics
  (6) Administer broad-spectrum antibiotics as prescribed
  (7) Begin ambulation once urine clears of gross hematuria
  (8) Be aware that renal tissue heals from a minor injury within 4 to 6 weeks
(d) Post major injury
  (1) Maintain fluids in immediate postoperative period
  (2) Maintain intake and output record
  (3) Provide analgesics
  (4) Provide preventive pulmonary maintenance therapies
  (5) Administer broad-spectrum antibiotics as prescribed;

renal parenchyma is susceptible to infection secondary to hematuria, ischemia, and urinary extravasation

(6) Obtain urine for culture and analysis

(7) Obtain serum studies for hematocrit, hemoglobin, electrolytes, BUN, and creatinine

(8) Monitor vital signs; hypertension may be a sign of constricting parenchymal fibrosis

(9) Maintain patency of Penrose drain (usually placed in the renal fossa to extrude liquefying hematoma)

(10) Monitor presence of hematuria

(11) Provide adequate nutrition

(12) Ambulate first postoperative day

    iv. Evaluation of nursing care

      (a) Stable vital signs, acceptable arterial blood gas values

      (b) Homeostatic fluid, electrolyte, and protein status

      (c) Injuries managed to prevent complications and promote healing

b. Potential for extravasation of urine

    i. Assessment for defining characteristics

      (a) Midline bulging—result of overdistended bladder

      (b) Lower quadrant distention—indicative of fluid collection

      (c) Lower abdominal pain or mass—resulting from bladder rupture and presence of extravasated urine

      (d) Fluid collection on sides of abdomen or thighs

      (e) Abdominal palpation reveals pain possibly indicative of peritonitis secondary to urine extravasation

      (f) Severe abdominal pain and rebound tenderness may reflect a severe, advancing peritonitis

      (g) Presence of hematuria (not always present)—microscopic or gross

      (h) Anuria (rare)

      (i) Indications for surgery

         (1) Shattered kidney—nephrectomy is indicated

         (2) Vascular injuries

         (3) Deep renal lacerations (controversial)

         (4) Pulsatile hematoma

         (5) Urinary extravasation

         (6) Expanding hematoma

         (7) Necrotic renal parenchyma

         (8) Continually decreasing hematocrit

    ii. Expected outcomes

      (a) Renal and genitourinary integrity restored

      (b) Infection is prevented

      (c) Follow-up care of renal system is obtained

    iii. Nursing interventions

    (a) Assess presence and extent of renal/urinary tract trauma

    (b) Obtain urine sample on admission to emergency department

    (c) Be aware that inability to void warrants catheterization. When catheter cannot be passed due to increased resistance, then radiologic examination of the urinary tract is indicated. Catheters should never be forced, since obstruction is indicative of trauma injury or hematoma

    (d) Blood passage through catheter necessitates removal of catheter. Urology consultation must immediately follow

    (e) Assess urine for presence of hematuria. Hematuria is commonly associated with ruptured bladder

    (f) Observe for signs of extravasated urine (see assessment for defining characteristics above)

    (g) Be aware that extravasated urine contributes to infection (i.e., peritonitis) in the trauma victim. Monitor temperature charts

    (h) Maintain adequate fluid replacement in order to sustain urine output. Hypotension and/or hypovolemia contributes to oliguria or anuria, but these two urinary output patterns may also result from renal trauma. Be aware that massive muscle breakdown secondary to trauma may contribute to rhabdomyolysis, which could cause renal tubular blockage

    (i) Prepare patient for surgery if indicated

    (j) Maintain patency of catheter; constant irrigation may be prescribed

    (k) Offer patient a plan for pain management

    (l) Provide aseptic wound care

    (m) Report any adverse symptoms

iv. Evaluation of nursing care

    (a) Intact renal function

    (b) Patent urinary collecting tract

    (c) Absence of infection

    (d) Healing wound

References

Benson, M., et al.: The role of imaging studies in urinary tract infection. Urol. Clin. North Am. 13:605–626, 1986.

Bowman, M. E., et al.: Effect of tube feeding osmolality on serum sodium levels. Crit. Care Nurse 9(1):9–22, 1989.

Brendan, A. M., et al.: Psychosocial aspects of chronic hemodialysis: The national cooperative dialysis study. Kidney Int. 23:S50, 1983.

Cerilli, G. J.: Organ Transplantation and Replacement. J. B. Lippincott, Philadelphia, 1988.

Chen, H. Y., et al.: A tool for assessing inadequate dialysis. ANNA J. 16:75–79, 1989.

Cogan, M. G., and Garovoy, M. R.: Introduction to Dialysis. Churchill Livingstone, New York, 1988.

Cowan, D. H., et al.: Human Organ Transplantation. Health Administration Press, Ann Arbor, 1987.

Danziger, C. H.: Uremic neuropathy and treatment with renal transplant. ANNA J. 16:67–70, 1989.

DePew, C., et al: Furosemide: Update on a commonly used drug. Crit. Care Nurse 9(2):63–67, 1989.

Erlich, L.: Use of epogen for treatment of anemia associated with chronic renal failure. Crit. Care Nurs. Clin. North Am. 2(1):101–113, 1990.

Foulkes, C. J.: Nutritional evaluation of patients in maintenance dialysis therapy. ANNA J. 15:13–17, 1988.

Frank, D. I.: Psychosocial assessment of renal dialysis patients. ANNA J. 15:207–210, 1988.

Friedman, E. A.: Ethical aspects in renal transplantation. Kidney Int. 23:S90, 1983.

Fuchs, J., and Schreiber, M.: Patient's perceptions of CAPD and hemodialysis stressors. ANNA J. 15:282–285, 1988.

Golper, T. A.: Continuous arteriovenous hemofiltration in acute renal failure. Am. J. Kidney Dis. 6:373–386, 1985.

Green, A., and Claibourne, C.: A nursing challenge: Cytomegalovirus infection in the transplant recipient. Focus Crit. Care 16:349–354, 1989.

Hayward, M. B., et al.: An instrument to identify stressors in renal transplant recipients. ANNA J. 16:80–84, 1989.

Innerarity, S. A., and Stark, J. L.: Fluid and Electrolytes. Springhouse Co., Springhouse, Pa., 1990.

Johnson, D. L.: Nephrotic syndrome: A nursing care plan based on current pathophysiologic concepts. Heart Lung 18:85–93, 1989.

Kee, J. L.: Fluid and Electrolytes with Clinical Application, 3rd ed. John Wiley & Sons, New York, 1982.

Knochel, J. P.: Etiologies and management of potassium deficiency. Hosp. Pract. 22:153–162, 1987.

Kottra, C. J.: Infection in the compromised host: An overview. Heart Lung 12:10–14, 1983.

Kramer, P., et al.: Management of anuric intensive care patients with arteriovenous hemofiltration. Int. J. Artif. Organs 3:225, 1980.

Lancaster, L. E.: Impact of chronic illness over the life span. ANNA J. 15:164–168, 1988.

Lawyer, L. A., et al.: Continuous arteriovenous hemodialysis in the ICU. Crit. Care Nurse 9(1):29–41, 1989.

Leaf, A., and Cotran, R.: Renal Pathophysiology, 3rd ed. Oxford University Press, New York, 1985.

Maher, J. F.: Pathophysiology of renal hemodynamics. Nephron 27:215–221, 1981.

McDougal, W. S.: Renal perfusion—reperfusion studies. J. Urol. 140:1325–1329, 1988.

McDougal, W. S., and Persky, L.: Traumatic Injuries of the Genitourinary System. Williams & Wilkins, Baltimore, 1981.

McFadden, E. A., and Zaloga, G. P.: Calcium regulation. Crit. Care Q. 6:12–21, 1983.

McFarland, H. F.: HIV testing in dialysis units: Preventing the plague. ANNA J. 16:287–289, 1989.

Moore, M. N.: Development of a sleep–awake instrument for use in chronic renal population. ANNA J. 16:15–19, 1989.

Myers, B. D., et al.: Glomerular and tubular function in nonoliguric acute renal failure. Am. J. Med. 72:642–649, 1982.

Myers, B. D., and Moran, S. M.: Hemodynamically mediated acute renal failure. N. Engl. J. Med. 314:97–104, 1986.

Paradiso, C.: Hemofiltration: An alternative to dialysis. Heart Lung 18:282–290, 1989.

Pearlstein, G.: Renal system complications in HIV infection. Crit. Care Nurs. Clin. North Am. 2(1):79–87, 1990.

Penner, B. S., et al.: Renal failure patients: Our perception of their psychological symptoms. Kidney Int. 30:S18, 1988.

Perry, A. G.: Shock complications: Recognition and management. Crit. Care Nurs. Q. 11:1–8, 1988.

Price, C. A.: Continuous arteriovenous ultrafiltration: A monitoring guide for ICU nurses. Crit. Care Nurse 9(1):12, 1989.

Rice, V.: Calcium, the heart and calcium antagonist. Crit. Care Nurse 4(2):30–39, 1982.

Ringoir, S., et al.: Uremic toxins. Kidney Int. 33:S4, 1988.

Rotellar, C.: Acute Renal Insufficiency. Medmaster, Orlando, Fla., 1988.

Sawyer, D. L.: Potential for infection: A nursing diagnosis for the patient with an indwelling catheter. Focus Crit. Care 16:46–52, 1989.

Scheppach, W., et al.: Effects of acetate during regular hemodialysis. Clin. Nephrol. 29:19–22, 1988.

Schneider, N. S., et al.: Continuous arteriovenous hemodialysis. Kidney Int. 33:S159–S162, 1988.

Schrier, R. W.: Manual of Nephrology: Diagnosis and Therapy, 2nd ed. Little, Brown & Co., Boston, 1985.

Schrier, R. W., et al.: Protection of mitochondrial function by mannitol in ischemic ARF. Am. J. Physiol. 247:365–367, 1984.

Sigler, M. H., et al.: Solute transport in continuous hemodialysis: A new treatment for acute renal failure. Kidney Int. 32:562–571, 1987.

Smith, M. F.: Renal trauma: Adult and pediatric considerations. Crit. Care Nurs. Clin. North Am. 2(1):67–77, 1990.

Stark, J. L.: Acute renal failure. In: AACN's Clinical Reference for Critical Care Nursing, 2nd ed. McGraw-Hill Book Co., New York, 1988.

Stark, J. L.: Chronic renal failure. In: AACN's Clinical Reference for Critical Care Nursing, 2nd ed. McGraw-Hill Book Co., New York, 1988.

Stark, J. L.: Renal assessment. In: AACN's Clinical Reference for Critical Care Nursing, 2nd ed. McGraw-Hill Book Co., New York, 1988.

Stark, J. L.: Renal physiology. In: AACN's Clinical Reference for Critical Care Nursing, 2nd ed. McGraw-Hill Book Co., New York, 1988.

Strupp, T. W.: Postshock resuscitation of the trauma victim: Preventing and managing ARF. Crit. Care Q. 11:1–10, 1988.

Thaler, M. K.: Cooperative nursing care for patients using peritoneal dialysis. ANNA J. 15:237–240, 1988.

Vari, R. C.: Induction, prevention, and mechanisms of contrast media–induced acute renal failure. Kidney Int. 33:699, 1988.

Vlchek, D. L.: High efficiency dialysis. Dialysis Transplant 17:128, 1988.

Weiner, M. W., and Adam, W. R.: Magnetic resonance spectroscopy for evaluation of renal function. Semin. Urol. 3:34–42, 1985.

Winkelman, C.: Hemofiltration: A new technique in critical care nursing. Heart Lung 14:265–271, 1985.

Wise, K. L., et al.: Renovascular hypertension. J. Urol. 140:911–924, 1988.

Zaloga, G. P., and Chernow, B.: Magnesium metabolism in critical illness. Crit. Care Q. 6:22–27, 1983.

Zorzanello, M. M.: Preventing acute renal failure in patients with chronic renal insufficiency: Nursing implications. ANNA J. 16:433–436, 1989.

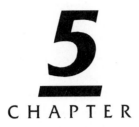

CHAPTER

The Endocrine System

Pamela Miller Gotch, R.N., M.S.N., CDE

PHYSIOLOGIC ANATOMY

Foundational Concepts

1. **Definition of a hormone**
   a. Molecules that are synthesized and secreted by specialized cells. Hormone is released into the blood and exerts biochemical effects on target cells some distance from the site of origin
   b. Hormones control metabolism, transport of substances across cell membranes, fluid and electrolyte balance, growth and development, adaptation, and reproduction
   c. The gastrointestinal tract, heart, liver, lungs, and kidneys produce hormones. These organs are not traditionally considered part of the endocrine system
   d. The brain is an essential part of the endocrine system, regulating the secretions of endocrine glands. Hormones in turn act on the central nervous system to modify its function. Nervous system regulation is achieved through hypothalamic secretion of hormones and through autonomic innervation of endocrine tissues such as the pancreatic islet cells
2. **Chemical structures of hormones**
   a. Peptide or protein hormones: antidiuretic hormone (ADH), thyrotropin-releasing hormone (TRH), insulin, growth hormone (GH), and adrenocorticotropic hormone (ACTH)
   b. Steroids, derived from cholesterol: adrenocortical hormones and gonadal hormones

    c. Amines and amino acid derivatives: norepinephrine, epinephrine, triiodothyronine (T_3), and thyroxine (T_4)

3. **Hormone receptors**
   a. The specificity of hormone action is determined by the presence of a specific hormone receptor on or in the target cell
   b. Receptors are sites on membranes to which hormones can bind
   c. Polypeptide hormones generally bind to receptors on cell surface membranes (membranes that are exposed to the cell's environment)
   d. Steroids and thyroid hormone bind to receptors located chiefly within the cell (nuclear or mitochondrial membranes)
   e. Receptors have two distinct roles: to distinguish a particular hormone from other hormones and to translate the hormonal signal into an appropriate cellular response
   f. Receptors are under regulation. In general, high concentration of a hormone down-regulates (reduces) the number of available receptors
   g. The hormone–receptor complex initiates intracellular events, which ultimately lead to the biologic effects of the hormone acting on that target cell
   h. Receptor abnormalities are known to underlie some pathologic states (e.g., nephrogenic diabetes insipidus, insulin resistance)

4. **Mechanisms of hormone action**
   a. Activation of cyclic adenosine monophosphate (cAMP) (Fig. 5–1)
      i. Hormone binds with a specific receptor on cell membrane of target cell
      ii. After binding, hormone–receptor complex activates adenylate cyclase in cell membrane
      iii. Adenylate cyclase activates conversion of cytoplasmic adenosine triphosphate (ATP) to a cyclic nucleotide, cyclic AMP
      iv. Cyclic nucleotide initiates cellular function
      v. Hormones acting through cyclic AMP are generally protein-type hormones and include thyroid-stimulating hormone (TSH), ACTH, parathyroid hormone (PTH), and ADH
      vi. This process is also known as "second messenger"
   b. Activation of genes (Fig. 5–2)
      i. Lipid-soluble hormone diffuses through cell membrane and enters cytoplasm
      ii. Hormone binds to a specific cytoplasmic receptor
      iii. Hormone–receptor complex diffuses into or is transported into cell nucleus
      iv. Hormone–receptor complex activates specific genes to form messenger RNA (mRNA). mRNA directs new protein synthesis
      v. Hormones acting through gene activation are chiefly steroid hormones and include glucocorticoids, aldosterone, and gonadal hormones
   c. Calcium

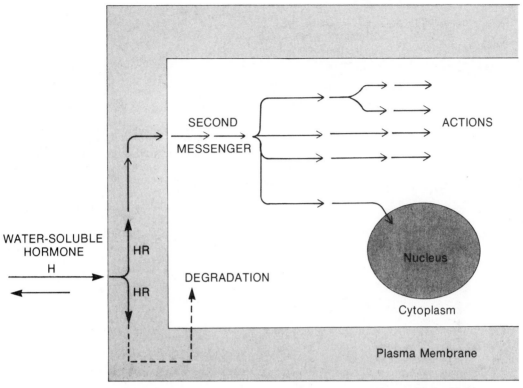

Figure 5–1. Mechanisms of action of water-soluble hormones (peptides and catecholamines; abbreviated *H*), which interact reversibly with receptors on outer surface of target cell. Hormone-receptor complex *(HR)* interacts with one or more membrane components, which, in absence of further participation of hormone, leads to stimulation of a common intracellular pathway (e.g., synthesis of cyclic adenosine monophosphate and activation of protein kinase), which then activates multiple (branched) pathways within the cell. The hormone does not need to enter the cell for expression of hormone action; when it does enter, it is largely for purposes of degradation *(broken line)*. Some effects of these hormones may be modifications of nuclear events, but these are not invariably present and represent only a minority of the events observed. (From Wilson, J., and Foster, D.: Williams Textbook of Endocrinology, 7th ed. W.B. Saunders Co., Philadelphia, 1985.)

      i. Hormones may activate calcium channels in cellular membranes or release calcium from intracellular organelles. Calcium acts as an intracellular messenger

      ii. Calcium exerts its effects by binding to proteins. The calcium–protein complex activates biochemical pathways that lead to cellular responses

5. Feedback control of hormone production

  a. All hormones are under some type of feedback regulation. Feedback control is exerted by cations (calcium on parathyroid hormone), metabolites (glucose on insulin), other hormones (somatostatin on insulin), osmolality (ADH), or extracellular fluid volume (renin-

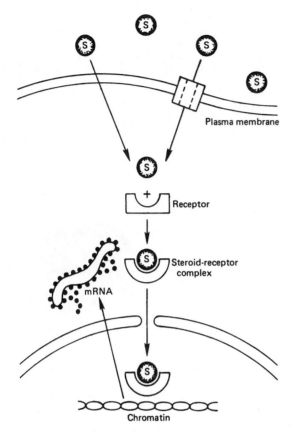

Figure 5–2. Proposed mechanism of steroid hormone action. The steroids enter target cells through diffusion or transport and in the cytoplasm bind to a receptor protein. The steroid–receptor complex is then able to bind to chromatin in the nucleus. New mRNA molecules are transcribed, leading to the synthesis of new protein. (Reproduced, with permission, from Greenspan, F.S., and Forsham, P.H.: Basic and Clinical Endocrinology, 2nd ed. Copyright © 1986, Appleton-Century-Crofts, A Publishing Division of Prentice-Hall.)

angiotensin-aldosterone). Figure 5–3 shows the hypothalamic-pituitary-target organ axis, a classic paradigm for feedback control
 b. Feedback can be positive (low hormone levels stimulating the release of its controlling hormone) or negative (high hormone levels inhibiting the release of its controlling hormone)
 c. Feedback control systems allow self-regulation, preventing the maladaptive consequences of hormonal overproduction

Pituitary Gland

1. **Location:** base of skull in sella turcica of sphenoid bone. It is connected to the hypothalamus by the pituitary stalk, which provides a link between the nervous and endocrine systems (Fig. 5–4)
2. **Composition:** two lobes producing different hormones
 a. Anterior lobe (adenohypophysis)
  i. Comprises 75% of gland
  ii. Secretions controlled by hypothalamic releasing or inhibiting hormones synthesized in hypothalamus
  iii. Hypothalamic hormones are transported to anterior pituitary via hypothalamic-hypophyseal portal vessels in response to stimuli received in the central nervous system

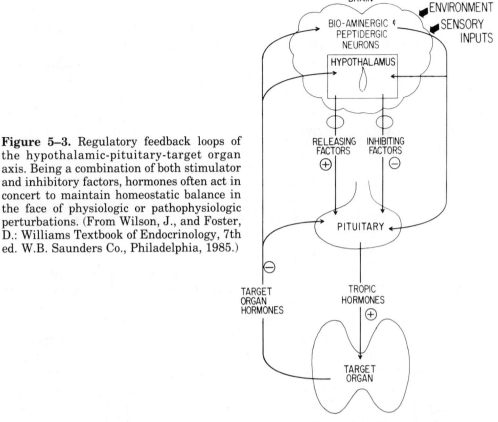

Figure 5–3. Regulatory feedback loops of the hypothalamic-pituitary-target organ axis. Being a combination of both stimulator and inhibitory factors, hormones often act in concert to maintain homeostatic balance in the face of physiologic or pathophysiologic perturbations. (From Wilson, J., and Foster, D.: Williams Textbook of Endocrinology, 7th ed. W.B. Saunders Co., Philadelphia, 1985.)

Figure 5–4. Secretion of hypothalamic hormones. The hormones of the posterior lobe *(PL)* are released into the general circulation from the endings of supraoptic *(SO)* and paraventricular *(PV)* neurons, whereas hypophyseotropic hormones are secreted into the portal hypophyseal circulation from the endings of arcuate *(ARC)* and other hypothalamic neurons. *AL,* anterior lobe; *MB,* maxillary bodies; *OC,* optic chiasm. (Reproduced, with permission, from Greenspan, F.S., and Forsham, P.H.: Basic and Clinical Endocrinology, 2nd ed. Copyright © 1986, Appleton-Century-Crofts, A Publishing Division of Prentice-Hall.)

    b. Posterior lobe (neurohypophysis)
        i. Comprises 25% of gland
       ii. Secretions are controlled by nerve fibers originating in hypothalamus and terminating in posterior pituitary
      iii. Posterior pituitary hormones are synthesized in hypothalamus, travel down nerve tracts in pituitary stalk, and are stored in posterior pituitary. Hormone release occurs following electrical activation of the cell bodies in the nerve tract

3. Anterior pituitary hormones
    a. Growth hormone (GH), also known as somatotropin
        i. Regulation of secretion
          (a) Stimulation—growth hormone–releasing hormone (GRH). GRH is secreted from hypothalamus in response to physical and/or emotional stress, starvation, strenuous exercise, hypoglycemia, anorexia nervosa, and other protein-depleted states
          (b) Inhibition—somatostatin from hypothalamus, postprandial hyperglycemia, and pharmacologic doses of corticosteroids
       ii. Secretion characteristics
          (a) Plasma levels vary throughout day; pulsatile and episodic secretion
          (b) Increased levels occur during early hours of deep sleep. This pattern of GH secretion decreases with age
      iii. Target tissue: cells that are capable of growth
      iv. Physiologic activity
          (a) Increases rate of protein synthesis
          (b) Increases mobilization of fatty acids from adipose tissue (lipolysis)
          (c) Decreases peripheral glucose utilization (insulin-antagonistic effect)
          (d) Stimulates bone and cartilage growth via somatomedins, a family of peptides produced by the liver
          (e) Synergizes with insulin, thyroid hormone, and sex steroids to promote growth
       v. Health disorders resulting from dysfunction
          (a) Excess—gigantism (prepubertal), acromegaly (postpubertal)
          (b) Deficiency—dwarfism (prepubertal)
          (c) Dawn phenomenon—early morning hyperglycemia observed in diabetic patients believed to be due to nocturnal GH surges
    b. Adrenocorticotropic hormone (ACTH), also known as corticotropin
        i. Regulation of secretion
          (a) Stimulation—corticotropin-releasing hormone (CRH) from

hypothalamus. Hypothalamus stimulated by physical and/or emotional stress, hypoglycemia, hypoxia, trauma, surgery, and decreased plasma cortisol levels

   (b) Inhibition—increased plasma cortisol levels will exert a negative feedback on CRH and ACTH. Stress can overcome this negative feedback

  ii. Secretion characteristics

   (a) ACTH has a diurnal pattern

   (b) Highest levels generally occur in early morning (5 to 8 AM), lowest in late evening (10 PM to 2 AM)

   (c) Diurnal pattern is lost during times of intense physical and/or emotional stress

  iii. Target tissue: adrenal cortex

  iv. Physiologic activity: production and release of adrenocortical hormones (glucocorticoids, adrenal androgens, and mineralocorticoids)

  v. Health disorders resulting from dysfunction

   (a) Excess—Cushing's disease

   (b) Deficiency—adrenal insufficiency (chronic), adrenal crisis (acute)

 c. Thyroid-stimulating hormone (TSH), also known as thyrotropin

  i. Regulation of secretion

   (a) Stimulation—thyrotropin-releasing hormone (TRH) from the hypothalamus. Responsiveness to TRH is modulated by the circulating concentration of thyroid hormone

   (b) Inhibition—somatostatin from hypothalamus, increased thyroid hormone levels

  ii. Secretion characteristics

   (a) Episodic or pulsatile secretion

   (b) Hormonal peaks occur during the night

  iii. Target tissue: thyroid gland

  iv. Physiologic activity

   (a) Releases stored thyroid hormone

   (b) Increases iodide trapping in thyroid cells

   (c) Increases synthesis of thyroid hormone

   (d) Increases size, number, and secretory activities of thyroid cells

  v. Health disorders resulting from dysfunction (see Thyroid Gland)

 d. Other anterior pituitary hormones under hypothalamic control

  i. Gonadotropins: luteinizing hormone (LH) and follicle-stimulating hormone (FSH)

  ii. Prolactin (PRL)

4. Posterior pituitary hormones

 a. Antidiuretic hormone (ADH), also known as vasopressin

  i. Regulation of secretion

(a) Stimulation—1% to 2% increase in plasma osmolality stimulates osmoreceptors in hypothalamus. Stimulation causes neurons to transmit impulses to posterior pituitary to release ADH. Other stimulants include hypoxia (via chemoreceptors); reduction in blood volume (10% or greater) via pressure receptors in the atria and pulmonary circulation; reduction in blood pressure via baroreceptors; trauma; pain; and nausea. Pharmacologic agents stimulating release include vincristine, morphine, nicotine, various anesthetics, chlorpropamide, clofibrate, and tranquilizers

(b) Inhibition—from a decrease in plasma osmolality. Pharmacologic agents that inhibit release include ethanol and phenytoin

ii. Target tissue: distal renal tubules and collecting ducts; smooth muscle cells, especially arterioles

iii. Physiologic activity

(a) Increases water permeability in distal renal tubules and collecting ducts, thus controlling extracellular fluid osmolality

(b) In pharmacologic amounts it constricts arterioles

iv. Health disorders resulting from dysfunction

(a) Excess—syndrome of inappropriate ADH secretion (SIADH)

(b) Deficiency—diabetes insipidus

b. Oxytocin

i. Dilatation of lower segment of the uterus, cervix, and vagina causes reflex release of oxytocin. Release is also stimulated by nipple stimulation

ii. Oxytocin stimulates uterine contractions and milk ejection during lactation

Thyroid Gland

1. **Location:** immediately below larynx on either side of and anterior to the trachea
2. **Composition:** two lobes, connected by an isthmus. Distinct cell types produce different hormones
   a. Follicular cells: triiodothyronine (T_3) and thyroxine (T_4)
   b. Parafollicular cells (C cells): located in interstitial tissue between follicles; produce thyrocalcitonin
3. **Regulation of secretion (thyroid hormone)**
   a. Stimulation: TSH stimulates thyroid hormone release. TSH is regulated by TRH from the hypothalamus. Decreased levels of thyroid hormone stimulate TSH and TRH

   b. Inhibition: elevated thyroid hormone levels inhibit TSH and TRH
   c. Thyroid gland stores thyroid hormone in the form of thyroglobulin
      in the follicular lumens
4. **Secretion characteristics**
   a. Ninety percent of thyroid hormone released from the thyroid gland
      is T_4; 10% is T_3. T_3 is more biologically active and has a shorter half-
      life in circulation. Most T_3 is produced extrathyroidally from T_4
   b. Conversion of T_4 to T_3 is blocked by
       i. Severe illness, trauma, malnutrition, anorexia nervosa
      ii. Pharmacologic amounts of glucocorticoids
     iii. Propranolol, propylthiouracil
      iv. Chronic liver disease, chronic renal failure, advanced cancer
   c. Euthyroid sick syndrome (low T_3 and T_4, normal TSH) is believed to
      be an adaptive mechanism designed to protect against excessive
      metabolic activity in the presence of serious illness. The syndrome
      is associated with higher mortality and can be viewed as a poor
      prognostic sign
   d. Most thyroid hormone is bound to plasma protein; free amounts are
      responsible for physiologic activity
5. **Target tissue:** almost all cells
6. **Physiologic activity**
   a. Increases metabolic activity of almost all cells, resulting in increased
      oxygen consumption, increased rate of chemical reactions, and in-
      creased heat production
   b. Stimulates most aspects of carbohydrate, fat, and protein metabolism
   c. Synergizes with insulin, growth hormone, and sex steroids to promote
      growth
   d. Increases metabolism and clearance of various hormones and phar-
      macologic agents
7. **Health disorders resulting from dysfunction**
   a. Excess: hyperthyroidism (chronic), thyroid storm (acute)
   b. Deficiency: hypothyroidism (chronic), myxedema coma (acute)
8. **Thyrocalcitonin** (calcitonin, CT)
   a. Regulation of secretion
       i. Stimulation: from an increase in calcium levels
      ii. Inhibition: from a decrease in calcium levels
   b. Secretion characteristics: 10% increase in calcium concentration
      causes a twofold increase in calcitonin secretion
   c. Target tissue: bone cells
   d. Physiologic activity
       i. Decreases blood calcium by inhibiting calcium mobilization
          from bone and decreasing calcium resorption in kidney
      ii. Decreases phosphate levels by inhibiting bone remodeling;
          increases phosphate loss in urine

e. Health disorders resulting from dysfunction: usually not significant since calcitonin is a relatively weak hypocalcemic agent in humans
f. Is available as a pharmacologic agent and is used to control hypercalcemia of malignancy

Parathyroid Glands

1. **Location:** usually four glands on posterior surface of thyroid gland, located at upper and lower poles of each thyroid lobe. Location can vary depending on embryonic migration
2. **Composition:** chief cells release parathyroid hormone (PTH)
3. **Regulation of secretion**
   a. Stimulation: from a decrease in calcium ion concentration in extracellular fluid
   b. Inhibition: from an increase in calcium ion concentration. Increased level of vitamin D metabolites and hypermagnesemia may also inhibit PTH. Hypomagnesemia can also interfere with PTH secretion
4. **Secretion characteristics**
   a. Hormone levels vary during day; sleep-related surges occur
5. **Target tissue:** renal tubules, gastrointestinal tract, bone
6. **Physiologic activity**
   a. Kidney
      i. Increases renal tubular reabsorption of calcium and magnesium
      ii. Decreases renal tubular reabsorption of phosphate and bicarbonate
      iii. Stimulates formation of 1,25-dihydroxyvitamin D, the active form of vitamin D
   b. Gastrointestinal tract: increases calcium absorption in intestines via 1,25-dihydroxyvitamin D
   c. Bone: larger amounts will increase calcium reabsorption from bone
7. **Health disorders resulting from dysfunction**
   a. Excess: hypercalcemia results from hyperparathyroidism
   b. Deficiency: hypocalcemia results from hypoparathyroidism

Adrenal Glands

1. **Location:** retroperitoneal, at upper poles of each kidney
2. **Composition:** two separate endocrine tissues that produce distinct hormones
   a. Cortex (80% of the gland)
      i. Zona glomerulosa produces aldosterone, the major mineralocorticoid
      ii. Zona fasciculata and zona reticularis produce glucocorticoids (cortisol) and adrenal androgens
   b. Medulla
      i. Secretory cells are in effect postganglionic sympathetic neurons

      ii. Produces catecholamines: epinephrine and norepinephrine
3. Cortical hormones
  a. Glucocorticoids (cortisol, major hormone)
     i. Regulation of secretion
        (a) Stimulation—ACTH. ACTH in turn is secreted in response to CRH from hypothalamus
        (b) Inhibition: cortisol exerts a negative feedback on the anterior pituitary and hypothalamus
     ii. Secretion characteristics
        (a) Episodic secretion, diurnal rhythmicity. Low levels noted in late evening and first several hours of sleep. Rise begins toward awakening. Levels gradually decline throughout the day with fewer secretory episodes
        (b) Diurnal pattern is lost during times of intense physical and/or emotional stress
        (c) Stress responsiveness is abolished by prior high-dose glucocorticoid administration
     iii. Target tissue: almost all cells
     iv. Physiologic activity
        (a) Carbohydrate metabolism
           (1) Increases gluconeogenesis in liver
           (2) Decreases glucose uptake in muscle and adipose tissue (insulin-antagonistic effect)
        (b) Protein metabolism
           (1) Decreases protein stores in all cells except liver
           (2) Decreases protein synthesis and increases protein catabolism, except in liver
           (3) Converts amino acids to glucose in the liver (gluconeogenesis)
        (c) Fat metabolism: promotes lipolysis in adipose tissue
        (d) Synergizes with other hormones, increases tissue responsiveness to other hormones, such as catecholamines and glucagon
        (e) Anti-inflammatory effects include
           (1) Decreased migration of inflammatory cells to sites of injury
           (2) Inhibition of production and/or activity of vasoactive substances
           (3) Prevention of immune response to tissue antigens released by injury
     v. Health disorders resulting from dysfunction
        (a) Excess—Cushing's syndrome
        (b) Deficiency—Addison's disease (chronic), adrenal crisis (acute)
  b. Mineralocorticoids (aldosterone, major hormone)

    i. Regulation of secretion

        (a) Stimulation—renin–angiotensin system acts as a major regulator. Juxtaglomerular cells in kidney produce renin, and renin acts on circulating angiotensinogen to produce angiotensin I. Angiotensin I is converted to angiotensin II. Angiotensin II stimulates aldosterone secretion. Renin is secreted in response to increased activity of the sympathetic nervous system, to a fall in intrarenal arterial pressure, and to a decrease in sodium transport across the renal tubules. Sodium depletion, increases in potassium concentration, and ACTH also stimulate aldosterone release

        (b) Inhibition—decrease in potassium concentration, sodium loading, and increases in plasma volume

    ii. Target tissue: distal renal tubules, sweat glands, salivary glands, and intestines

    iii. Physiologic activity

        (a) Increases sodium reabsorption, indirectly increasing extracellular fluid volume

        (b) Increases potassium excretion

    iv. Health disorders resulting from dysfunction

        (a) Excess—primary aldosteronism, characterized by potassium depletion, extracellular fluid volume expansion, and hypertension

        (b) Deficiency—Addison's disease (chronic), adrenal crisis (acute)

    v. Available as a pharmacologic agent (fludrocortisone)

  c. Adrenal androgens: not of significance in critical care

4. Medullary hormones

  a. Regulation of secretion

    i. Stimulation: fear, anxiety, pain, trauma, hemorrhage, fluid loss, strenuous exercise, extremes in temperature, hypoxia, hypoglycemia, and hypotension. Stimuli are processed in central nervous system, with signals then transmitted to adrenal medulla

    ii. Medullary hormones are first line of defense against stress

  b. Secretion characteristics: 80% of the medullary secretion is epinephrine, 20% is norepinephrine. Norepinephrine is also produced by other sympathetic postganglionic neurons

  c. Target tissue: most cells

  d. Physiologic activity (Table 5–1)

    i. Major insulin antagonists

    ii. Critical in the recovery from insulin-induced hypoglycemia

  e. Health disorders resulting from dysfunction

    i. Excess: pheochromocytoma. Tumor produces epinephrine and/or norepinephrine, causing hypertension

Table 5–1. ADRENERGIC RESPONSES OF SELECTED TISSUES

Organ or Tissue	Receptor	Effect
Heart (myocardium)	β_1	Increased force of contraction
		Increased rate of contraction
Blood vessels	α	Vasoconstriction
	β_2	Vasodilatation
Kidney	β	Increased renin release
Gut	α, β	Decreased motility and increased sphincter tone
Pancreas	α	Decreased insulin release
		Decreased glucagon release
	β	Increased insulin release
		Increased glucagon release
Liver	α, β	Increased glycogenolysis
Adipose tissue	β	Increased lipolysis
Most tissues	β	Increased calorigenesis
Skin (apocrine glands on hands, axillae, etc.)	α	Increased sweating
Bronchioles	β_2	Dilatation
Uterus	α	Contraction
	β_2	Relaxation

Reproduced, with permission, from Greenspan, F. S., and Forsham, P. H.: Basic and Clinical Endocrinology, 2nd ed. Copyright © 1986, Appleton-Century-Crofts, A Publishing Division of Prentice-Hall.

    ii. Deficiency: persons with an intact sympathetic nervous system manifest no clinically significant disability. If autonomic insufficiency includes deficient adrenal medullary epinephrine secretion, the patient will have defects in recovery from insulin-induced hypoglycemia

Pancreas

1. **Location:** lies transversely in left upper quadrant of abdomen, behind the peritoneum and stomach
2. **Composition:** exocrine and endocrine components. Endocrine functions originate from islet cells, which comprise less than 2% of the total pancreatic volume. Sixty-five percent of the islet cells are beta cells, which produce insulin. Glucagon is produced by the alpha cells, and somatostatin and gastrin are produced from the delta cells. Islet cells receive signals from one another and from other hormones and nutrients in the environment surrounding the cells. Islet cell hormones enter portal circulation, producing hormone concentrations higher in portal blood than in peripheral circulation
3. **Insulin**
   a. Regulation of secretion
      i. Stimulation: from increases in blood glucose. Other stimulants include gastrin, secretin, cholecystokinin, (so-called gastrointestinal hormones), and arginine

      ii. Inhibition: alpha-adrenergic effects of catecholamines, somato-statin, and a variety of pharmacologic agents (see diabetic ketoacidosis and hyperglycemic hyperosmolar nonketotic coma)

  b. Secretion characteristics
      i. Hormone levels vary; basal rates exist during times of fasting
      ii. Nutrient-induced surges accompany feeding

  c. Target tissue: many cells including muscle cells, adipose tissue, liver, leukocytes, cartilage, and bone

  d. Physiologic activity
      i. Carbohydrate metabolism
        (a) Increases glucose transport across cell membrane in muscle and fat
        (b) Increases glycogen synthesis in liver and muscle
        (c) Inhibits gluconeogenesis in liver
      ii. Protein metabolism
        (a) Increases amino acid transport across cell membrane
        (b) Increases protein synthesis
        (c) Decreases protein catabolism
      iii. Fat metabolism
        (a) Increases triglyceride synthesis
        (b) Increases fatty acid transport across cell membrane
        (c) Inhibits lipolysis
      iv. Synergizes with thyroid hormone, the sex steroids, and growth hormone to promote growth

  e. Health disorders resulting from dysfunction
      i. Excess: hypoglycemia
      ii. Deficiency: insulin-dependent diabetes mellitus (Type I diabetes)

4. Glucagon
  a. Regulation of secretion
      i. Stimulation: from a decrease in blood glucose. Other stimulants include high protein feeding, pancreozymin, other gastrointestinal hormones, beta-adrenergic effects of catecholamines, and strenuous prolonged exercise
      ii. Inhibition: from an increase in blood glucose and somatostatin

  b. Secretion characteristics: basal level is altered by nutrients, hormones, and neural stimuli. Secretion does not markedly fluctuate in normal persons receiving mixed meals

  c. Target tissue: liver, adipose tissue

  d. Physiologic activity
      i. Increases blood glucose via glycogenolysis and gluconeogenesis
      ii. Increases lipolysis
      iii. Increases amino acid transport to liver and conversion of amino acids to glucose precursors
      iv. Is a major insulin-antagonistic hormone

      v. Critical hormone in the recovery of insulin-induced hypoglycemia

   e. Deficient glucagon production is believed to play a role in defective glucose counterregulation in insulin-induced hypoglycemia in Type I diabetes mellitus

   f. Available as a pharmacologic agent. Used to correct insulin-induced hypoglycemia in the unresponsive person

5. Somatostatin

   a. Present in islet cells, hypothalamus, and gastrointestinal tract

   b. Physiologic activity: inhibits secretion of insulin, glucagon, growth hormone, TSH, and gastrointestinal hormones (gastrin, secretin)

   c. Octreotide acetate: analogue of somatostatin, available for parenteral administration. Decreases the secretion of hormones produced by carcinoid tumors, vipomas, and possibly other endocrine tumors

Gonadal Hormones (Testosterone, Estrogen, Progesterone): Not of significance in critical care

NURSING ASSESSMENT DATA BASE

Nursing History

1. Patient health history

   a. History assists nurse in identifying patient at risk for an endocrine disorder

      i. Presence of pathophysiologic processes that can result in endocrine dysfunction

         (a) Trauma, vascular interruption

         (b) Surgical intervention

         (c) Infection, inflammation

         (d) Autoimmune processes

         (e) Irradiation

         (f) Neoplasms and chemotherapeutic agents and radiation therapy to treat the neoplasm

         (g) Infiltrative disorders

         (h) Acquired immunodeficiency syndrome (AIDS)

      ii. Presence of preexisting chronic endocrine disorder (diagnosed or undiagnosed)

      iii. Evidence of interruption of pharmacologic therapy for a preexisting endocrine disorder

      iv. Presence of an unrelated critical illness in a patient with a preexisting chronic endocrine disorder

   b. Indicators of altered health patterns

      i. Cognitive/perceptual

(a) Personality changes, irritability, emotional lability, lethargy, agitation, attention span deficit, memory impairment
(b) Visual disturbances
(c) Depression, paranoia, delusions, delirium
(d) Changes in level of consciousness
(e) Verbalizations indicate lack of knowledge or misconceptions regarding self-care management

ii. Nutrition/metabolic
(a) Change in weight
(b) Change in appetite
(c) Nausea, anorexia
(d) Polydipsia
(e) Temperature intolerances

iii. Elimination
(a) Diarrhea or constipation
(b) Polyuria or a decrease in urine output
(c) Nocturia
(d) Vomiting

iv. Activity/exercise
(a) Fatigue, weakness
(b) Exercise intolerance
(c) Inability to perform activities of daily living

v. Sleep/rest
(a) Restlessness
(b) Inability to secure adequate sleep

vi. Sexual
(a) Menstrual irregularities
(b) Impotence
(c) Decreased libido
(d) Infertility

vii. Roles/relationships
(a) Discordance in previously stable relationships
(b) Physical and emotional inability to engage in usual role performance

viii. Coping/stress tolerance
(a) Inability to cope
(b) Past/present psychiatric therapy

ix. Health perception/management
(a) Evidence of noncompliance with medical follow-up
(b) Evidence of noncompliance with regimen for managing a preexisting chronic endocrine disorder

2. **Family history**
   a. Presence of endocrine disorders in other family members
3. **Social history**

a. Elderly may be at special risk for developing an endocrine crisis
  i. Gradual decline in physical and mental condition may be wrongly attributed to aging
  ii. Elderly are at risk for dehydration because of diminished thirst mechanism
  iii. Institutionalized elderly may be unable to express their need for water or may be unable physically to obtain water
b. Socially disadvantaged may be at special risk for developing an endocrine crisis since many of the regimens for treating chronic endocrine disorders are costly and require regular medical follow-up

4. **Medication history**
  a. Pharmacologic agents used to treat chronic endocrine disorders
    i. Thyroid hormone
    ii. Antithyroid drug therapy
    iii. Glucocorticoids
    iv. Mineralocorticoids
    v. Insulin
    vi. Oral hypoglycemic agents
    vii. ADH
    viii. Vitamin D, calcium supplements
    ix. Testosterone, estrogen
  b. Pharmacologic agents that may alter endocrine function by either stimulating or inhibiting hormone release or by interfering with hormone action at the target tissue. (See Patient Health Problems for specific discussions)
    i. Tranquilizers, narcotics, anesthetics, sedatives
    ii. Cancer chemotherapeutic agents
    iii. Acetaminophen, phenytoin
    iv. Ethanol, tricyclic antidepressants
    v. Thiazide diuretics, clofibrate, calcium channel blockers
    vi. Lithium, demeclocycline, ketoconazole, rifampin, pentamidine
    vii. Nonsteroidal anti-inflammatory agents
    viii. Glucocorticoids
    ix. Iodine-rich pharmacologic agents (amiodarone, some expectorants, kelp)
  c. Exposure to large iodine loads (contrast materials)

Nursing Examination of Patient

1. **Inspection**
  a. General appearance
    i. Stature
    ii. Fat distribution in relation to sex and maturational level
    iii. Mobility, tremor, hyperkinesis
    iv. Scars, especially neck area

     v. Hair distribution and texture in relation to sex and maturational level

    vi. Change in ring, shoe, or hat size

   vii. Goiter

  viii. Seizure activity

    ix. Presence of medic alert identification

  b. Face

     i. Shape

    ii. Color of skin

   iii. Bone structure

   iv. Hydration status of oral cavity

    v. Periorbital edema

   vi. Eyelid lag, lid retraction, stare

  vii. Conjunctival irritation

 viii. Protruding or sunken eyeballs

  c. Skin

     i. Color, unusual pigmentation

    ii. Texture, temperature

   iii. Tissue turgor, moisture

   iv. Evidence of bruising, striae, thinning, edema

    v. Brittle nails

2. Palpation: neck—enlarged or nodular thyroid gland; palpable thrill over thyroid gland

3. Percussion: abnormal deep tendon reflexes

4. Auscultation

  a. Neck: bruits over thyroid gland

  b. Heart: distant heart sounds, third heart sound

  c. Blood pressure: hypotension, orthostasis

  d. Heart rate and rhythm: tachycardia, bradycardia, dysrhythmias

  e. Respiratory pattern: tachypnea, Kussmaul respirations, acetone odor to breath

  f. Hypoactive bowel sounds

  g. Evidence of pleural/pericardial effusions

5. Additional findings: hypothermia or hyperthermia

Diagnostic Studies in the Critically Ill Patient

1. Laboratory: blood

  a. Electrolytes: sodium, potassium, chloride, calcium, phosphate, magnesium

  b. Glucose, ketoacids, blood urea nitrogen, cholesterol, creatinine, creatine phosphokinase

  c. Plasma osmolality, hematocrit, leukocyte count with differential

  d. pH, P_{O_2}, P_{CO_2}, bicarbonate

  e. Hormone assays

2. **Laboratory:** urine
   a. Electrolytes: sodium, potassium, chloride, calcium
   b. Glucose, ketoacids
   c. Osmolality, specific gravity, pH
   d. Catecholamines, corticosteroids and their metabolites
3. **Radiologic** (assist in identifying precipitating factor)
   a. X-ray films (skull, chest, abdomen)
   b. Scans (thyroid, pancreas)
   c. Computed tomography
   d. Magnetic resonance imaging
   e. Arteriography
   f. Bone mineral densitometry
4. **Electrocardiogram (ECG)**
5. **Visual field testing**
6. **Selective venous sampling**

COMMONLY ENCOUNTERED NURSING DIAGNOSES

Fluid Volume Deficit (Actual or Potential)

1. **Assessment for defining characteristics**
   a. Thirst, dry mucous membranes
   b. Decreased skin turgor
   c. Hypotension, orthostasis, tachycardia
   d. Hemoconcentration
   e. Weight loss
   f. Increased urine output, dilute urine
2. **Expected outcome**
   a. Patient is able to achieve/maintain fluid and electrolyte balance
3. **Nursing interventions**
   a. Monitor hydration status
   b. Monitor electrolyte status
   c. Use flow sheet to document trends in intake, output, vital signs, central venous pressure, urine specific gravity, peripheral perfusion, body weight, laboratory, and other hemodynamic parameters
   d. Administer prescribed fluid and electrolyte therapy
   e. Administer hormone replacement
   f. Provide skin and oral care
   g. See specific discussion presented in sections on diabetes insipidus, diabetic ketoacidosis, and acute adrenal insufficiency
4. **Evaluation of nursing care**
   a. Laboratory parameters are within physiologic range
   b. Vital signs and other hemodynamic parameters are within patient's normal range
   c. Hydration is adequate

Fluid Volume Excess (Actual or Potential)

1. **Assessment for defining characteristics**
   a. Intake greater than output
   b. Weight gain
   c. Third heart sound
   d. Evidence of pulmonary congestion
   e. Deterioration in mental status
   f. Hemodilution
   g. Abnormal electrolyte values
2. **Expected outcome**
   a. Patient is able to achieve/maintain fluid and electrolyte balance
3. **Nursing interventions**
   a. Monitor hydration status
   b. Monitor electrolyte status
   c. Use flow sheet to document trends in intake, output, vital signs, central venous pressure, urine specific gravity, body weight, neurologic status, and laboratory and other hemodynamic parameters
   d. Identify patient at risk for fluid overload. Closely monitor fluid replacement rates in these patients
   e. Assess pulmonary status
   f. Restrict fluids if necessary
   g. Administer pharmacologic agents that assist in fluid excretion
   h. See specific discussion presented in sections on myxedema coma and syndrome of inappropriate ADH secretion
4. **Evaluation of nursing care**
   a. Laboratory parameters are within physiologic range
   b. Hemodynamic parameters are within patient's normal range
   c. Intake approximates output
   d. Patient is alert and oriented

Altered Nutrition, less than body requirements

1. **Assessment for defining characteristics**
   a. Weight loss
   b. Ketosis
   c. Inadequate nutritional intake to meet metabolic demands
   d. Fatigue, weakness
2. **Expected outcomes**
   a. Body weight stabilizes
   b. Patient is able to achieve/maintain normal carbohydrate, fat, and protein metabolism
3. **Nursing interventions**
   a. Provide sufficient calories and vitamins
   b. Administer prescribed pharmacologic therapy aimed at replacing hormone deficiency or preventing hormone excess

c. Obtain daily weight

d. See specific discussion presented in sections on hyperthyroid crisis and diabetic ketoacidosis

4. **Evaluation of nursing care**

As stated above in expected outcomes

Knowledge Deficit

1. **Assessment for defining characteristics**
   a. Verbalizations indicative of lack of knowledge
   b. Inaccurate follow-through of instruction
   c. Statements indicative of misconceptions
   d. Requests for information
2. **Expected outcomes**
   a. Patient/family are able to verbalize self-care knowledge
   b. Patient/family are able to demonstrate self-care skills necessary to implement prescribed regimen
   c. Patient/family are able to verbalize knowledge of self-care practices necessary to prevent recurring endocrine crises
   d. Patient/family are able to explain basic concepts of the health disorder to others
3. **Nursing interventions**
   a. Assess patient/family knowledge of the health disorder and the required self-care
   b. Note precipitating factors
   c. Initiate self-care education for patient and family
   d. Make provisions for continuity in self-care education when patient is transferred to intermediate care unit
   e. Emphasize necessity for long-term medical follow-up
   f. See specific discussions presented in Patient Health Problems
4. **Evaluation of nursing care**

As stated above in expected outcomes

Other Nursing Diagnoses: Discussed under specific Patient Health Problems and include hypothermia, hyperthermia, and ineffective family coping

PATIENT HEALTH PROBLEMS

Diabetes Insipidus

1. **Pathophysiology:** permanent or transient deficiency in synthesis or release of antidiuretic hormone (ADH, vasopressin), osmoreceptor dysfunction, or a decrease in kidney responsiveness to ADH. Deficiency results in an inability to conserve water. In the presence of an adequate

thirst mechanism and a readily available source of fluids, there will be little alteration in fluid balance, although the patient will experience extreme polydipsia and polyuria. If the patient has an impaired thirst mechanism or is unable to secure fluids, dehydration will develop

2. **Etiology or precipitating factors**
   a. Central/neurogenic diabetes insipidus (vasopressin-sensitive)
      i. Familial, idiopathic
      ii. Traumatic: head injury, hypophysectomy, or neurosurgery may lead to disruption of supraoptic axons that travel to pituitary stalk, a loss of osmoreceptor function, and/or damage to the hypothalamic areas that produce ADH
      iii. Neoplasm: craniopharyngioma, leukemia, breast cancer
      iv. Infections: meningitis, encephalitis
      v. Vascular: aneurysm
      vi. Infiltrative disorders (histiocytosis X, sarcoidosis)
   b. Nephrogenic diabetes insipidus (vasopressin-insensitive)
      i. Renal disease: polycystic kidney disease, pyelonephritis
      ii. Multisystem disorders affecting the kidneys: multiple myeloma, sarcoidosis, sickle cell disease
      iii. Familial
   c. Pharmacologic agents
      i. Ethanol and phenytoin: inhibit ADH secretion
      ii. Lithium and demeclocycline: inhibit ADH action in kidney
   d. Insufficient exogenous ADH in the person with diabetes insipidus
3. **Nursing assessment data base**
   a. Nursing history
      i. Subjective findings
         (a) Elimination—polyuria (4 to 16 L/24 hr), nocturia, constipation
         (b) Nutrition—polydipsia, weight loss
         (c) Sleep/rest—lack of adequate sleep since rest is interrupted by need to drink fluids and urinate. Many patients report the need to keep a large container of fluid at their bedside at night
      ii. Objective findings
         (a) Patient health history
            (1) History of head trauma. Recognize that diabetes insipidus may be transient, especially in patients who have experienced head injuries or neurosurgical procedures. Symptomatology may not be evident immediately since some ADH is stored and released from the posterior pituitary or the pituitary stalk
            (2) History of ADH use in past
         (b) Family history—other members have polyuria and polydipsia (familial)

        (c) Social history—recognize that the patient who is unable to maintain fluid balance (impaired thirst mechanism, incapacitated, confused or unable to secure fluids) is at risk for dehydration

        (d) Medication history—use of medications that impair ADH release or action

  b. Nursing examination of patient

    i. Inspection

        (a) Decreased skin turgor, dry skin

        (b) Dry mucous membranes

        (c) Manifestations of dehydration will be evident in those patients who are unable to secure adequate fluids or unable to detect thirst

        (d) Medical identification indicating ADH use

    ii. Auscultation

        (a) Tachycardia; hypotension if the patient has become dehydrated

  c. Diagnostic study findings

    i. Plasma osmolality elevated (greater than 295 mOsm/kg), urine osmolality decreased (less than 500 mOsm/kg). Urine less concentrated than plasma. Urine osmolality can be as low as 30 mOsm/kg

    ii. Hypernatremia

    iii. Urine specific gravity low (1.001 to 1.005)

    iv. Water deprivation test: demonstrates that in the presence of adequate stimulus to ADH release (simple dehydration), kidneys cannot concentrate urine; differentiates psychogenic polydipsia from diabetes insipidus

    v. Vasopressin test: often done with water deprivation test to demonstrate that kidneys can concentrate urine with exogenous ADH; differentiates nephrogenic from central diabetes insipidus

    vi. Low plasma ADH levels in central diabetes insipidus

4. Nursing diagnoses

  a. Actual or potential fluid volume deficit related to inability to conserve water

    i. Assessment for defining characteristics

        (a) Thirst, dry mucous membranes

        (b) Decreased skin turgor

        (c) Hypotension, tachycardia

        (d) Hemoconcentration, plasma hyperosmolality, hypernatremia

        (e) Weight loss

        (f) Increased urine output, dilute urine

    ii. Expected outcome

        (a) Adequate fluid volume is maintained/restored

iii. Nursing interventions
  (a) Administer fluids (oral and/or intravenous)
  (b) Administer replacement therapy (central diabetes insipidus)
    (1) Aqueous Pitressin (intravenous or subcutaneous)—short-acting ADH, useful in transient diabetes insipidus
    (2) Lysine vasopressin (nasal spray)—short-acting ADH. Absorption may be erratic in patients with respiratory infection, rhinitis, or recent transsphenoidal surgery
    (3) Desmopressin acetate (DDAVP)—synthetic ADH (subcutaneous or nasal spray). Longer duration of action, administered once or twice per day
    (4) Vasopressin tannate in oil—duration of 24 to 72 hours; given intramuscularly. Must be warmed and vigorously agitated prior to administration. Not agent of choice, since dose titration is difficult due to prolonged activity
    (5) Observe for water intoxication with all the above agents
    (6) Schedule for replacement therapy is based on observing the duration of the antidiuresis as demonstrated by output
  (c) Administer pharmacologic agents (nephrogenic diabetes insipidus)
    (1) Chlorpropamide—stimulates ADH release and augments renal tubular response to ADH. Observe for hypoglycemia; ensure adequate nutritional intake
    (2) Thiazide diuretics and sodium restriction—mild sodium depletion and reduced solute load will enhance water reabsorption
  (d) Meticulous recording of intake/output, body weight, urine specific gravity, and plasma and urine osmolality. With neurosurgery patients, continue this recording for 7 to 10 days postoperatively since diabetes insipidus can be triphasic (manifestations present, then it appears to resolve only to reappear and be permanent)
  (e) Assist with diagnostic procedures (water deprivation and vasopressin test)
    (1) Secure frequent body weights and vital signs; measure and record urine output
    (2) Secure specimens (urine/blood) at proper times. Inform laboratory personnel of the importance of maintaining the correct sequence of all specimens
    (3) Maintain fluid deprivation for required time interval.

Explain fluid restriction to patient's visitors and all
health care personnel in contact with the patient
- (4) Administer ADH at appropriate time
- (5) Observe for profound dehydration. Water deprivation
test will be terminated if patient experiences 3%
weight loss
- (f) Provide skin and oral care
- (g) Conserve patient's energy by assisting with self-care and
providing frequent rest periods. Nocturia and polydipsia
will interfere with securing adequate rest
- (h) Explain diagnostic procedures to patient/family
- (i) Prevent dehydration by ensuring that patients on long-
term ADH therapy receive adequate fluids and exogenous
hormone replacement when hospitalized
- iv. Evaluation of nursing care
  - (a) Vital signs and other hemodynamic parameters are within
patient's normal range
  - (b) Intake approximates output
  - (c) Laboratory parameters are within normal limits (plasma
and urine osmolality, electrolytes, urine specific gravity)
  - (d) Alert and oriented
  - (e) Patient's normal body weight is restored/maintained
  - (f) Increased moisture observed on oral mucous membranes
  - (g) Skin is warm and dry with good turgor
- b. Potential knowledge deficit regarding self-care management of permanent diabetes insipidus
  - i. Assessment for defining characteristics
    - (a) Patient has newly diagnosed diabetes insipidus
    - (b) Patient did not take medication as prescribed at home
    - (c) Patient unable to state signs and symptoms that require
physician notification
  - ii. Expected outcome
    - (a) Patient/family are able to state regimen for managing
diabetes insipidus post discharge
  - iii. Nursing interventions
    - (a) Initiate medication instruction in those patients with per-
manent diabetes insipidus. Include
      - (1) Purpose, name, dose, schedule of medication
      - (2) Medication administration. Have patient self-admin-
ister nasal spray, if used
      - (3) Importance of adherence
      - (4) Importance of medic alert identification and how to
secure it
    - (b) Instruct patient/family to notify physician of changes in
fluid balance

(1) Evidence of excessive water retention

(2) Evidence of insufficient water conservation (continued or increasing polydipsia or polyuria)

(3) Instruct on proper procedure for obtaining accurate body weight

(c) If patient has preexisting diabetes insipidus and failed to take medication as ordered, explore potential reasons for noncompliance and intervene as necessary

iv. Evaluation of nursing care

(a) Patient/family are able to state purpose, name, dose, and schedule of medication

(b) Patient is able to accurately administer medication

(c) Patient/family are able to state the importance of adhering to the medication regimen

(d) Patient/family are able to identify changes in fluid balance and the need for physician notification

(e) Patient/family are able to state importance of securing medical identification

Syndrome of Inappropriate ADH Secretion (SIADH)

1. **Pathophysiology:** syndrome characterized by plasma hypotonicity and hyponatremia that results from the aberrant or sustained secretion of ADH. There is failure of the negative feedback system, since ADH secretion continues in spite of low plasma osmolality and expanded volume. Dysfunction results in water intoxication

2. **Etiology or precipitating factors**
   a. Central nervous system disorders
      i. Traumatic: skull fracture, subdural hematoma, subarachnoid hemorrhage, cerebral contusion
      ii. Neoplasms
      iii. Infection: meningitis, encephalitis, brain abscess, Guillain-Barré syndrome, AIDS
      iv. Vascular: aneurysm, cerebrovascular accident
   b. Stimulation of ADH release via hypoxia and/or decreased left atrial filling pressure
      i. Pneumonia, tuberculosis, other pulmonary infections, asthma
      ii. Congestive heart failure
      iii. Positive-pressure ventilation
   c. Pharmacologic agents: either increase ADH secretion or potentiate its action
      i. Cancer chemotherapy: cyclophosphamide, vincristine
      ii. Chlorpropamide, acetaminophen, amitriptyline, thiazide diuretics, carbamazepine, pentamidine
   d. Excessive exogenous vasopressin therapy

e. Ectopic ADH production associated with bronchogenic, prostatic, or pancreatic cancer or leukemia

3. **Nursing assessment data base**

   a. Nursing history

      i. Subjective findings

         (a) Cognitive/perceptual—headache, personality change, confusion, irritability, dysarthria, lethargy, impaired memory

         (b) Activity—restlessness, weakness, fatigue, gait disturbances

         (c) Nutrition—nausea, anorexia, vomiting, weight gain

      ii. Objective findings

         (a) Patient health history

            (1) Presence of a precipitating factor

            (2) Recognize that postoperative patients experience situations that stimulate ADH release (pain, stress, nausea, morphine use)

   b. Nursing examination of patient

      i. Inspection

         (a) No evidence of edema

         (b) Muscle twitching

         (c) Seizure activity may be present if severely hyponatremic

      ii. Percussion

         (a) Delayed deep tendon reflexes

   c. Diagnostic study findings

      i. Hyponatremia

      ii. Decreased plasma osmolality

      iii. Urine sodium and urine osmolality elevated (greater than that which is appropriate for the plasma osmolality)

      iv. Inappropriately elevated plasma ADH levels

      v. Normal renal, adrenal, and thyroid function

      vi. Inability to excrete water load

4. **Nursing diagnoses**

   a. Fluid volume excess related to inability to excrete water

      i. Assessment for defining characteristics

         (a) Hyponatremia with plasma hypo-osmolality

         (b) Inappropriately elevated urine osmolality

         (c) Weight gain

         (d) Neurologic changes

      ii. Expected outcome

         (a) Fluid balance is restored to normal

      iii. Nursing interventions

         (a) Recognize subtle, early changes indicative of water intoxication—change in level of consciousness, headache, fatigue, weakness

         (b) Manage fluid therapy

      (1) Fluid restriction (oral and parenteral)—may be based on urine output plus insensible losses. Explain fluid restriction to patient, visitors, and other health care personnel

      (2) Hypertonic sodium chloride infusion may be used in those patients with severe hyponatremia and/or seizure activity. Great caution is advised since fluid overload can worsen and may precipitate heart failure. There is lack of consensus regarding optimal rate of correction of symptomatic hyponatremia. Concern exists as to whether sudden increases in the serum sodium concentration can result in brain damage (osmotic demyelination syndrome) in those patients with chronic hyponatremia who have had time to develop an adaptation to that state

      (3) Diuretics—decrease the effectiveness of ADH. Can cause significant electrolyte losses

      (4) Carefully monitor intravenous infusion rate and urine output in patients at risk

    (c) Administer pharmacologic agents

      (1) Lithium or demeclocycline—interferes with action of ADH at renal tubular level. Demeclocycline is nephrotoxic. Renal function must be monitored.

      (2) Phenytoin—inhibits ADH release

    (d) Administer electrolyte replacement as required

    (e) Meticulous recording of intake/output, body weight, urine specific gravity, hydration, cardiovascular and neurologic status

    (f) Assist with diagnostic studies and explain procedures to patient/family

      (1) Urine and blood specimens for electrolyte studies

      (2) Perform water load test, administer fluids, and collect appropriate specimens

    (g) Administer therapy aimed at precipitating factors

  iv. Evaluation of nursing care

    (a) Intake approximates output

    (b) Laboratory parameters are within normal limits (plasma and urine osmolality, and serum sodium)

    (c) Patient's body weight returns to normal

    (d) Alert and oriented

b. Potential for injury related to impaired cognitive state and physical inactivity

  i. Assessment for defining characteristics

    (a) Cognitive—confusion, impaired memory, irritability, personality change, lethargy

(b) Restlessness, fatigue, weakness

(c) Imposed physical inactivity

(d) Unfamiliar environment and personnel

   ii. Expected outcome

     (a) Remains free from personal injury

  iii. Nursing interventions

     (a) Institute seizure precautions and safety measures such as bed in low position

     (b) Reorient the confused patient. Elicit family's help in doing this

     (c) Prevent complications of immobility (i.e., skin care, repositioning, range of motion exercises)

     (d) Recognize that decreased gastric motility due to hyponatremia, combined with fluid restriction and decreased mobility, may lead to constipation. Tap water enemas are to be avoided since the fluid may be absorbed

   iv. Evaluation of nursing care

     (a) Patient is free from personal injury

Hyperthyroid Crisis (Thyroid Storm, Thyrotoxicosis)

1. **Pathophysiology:** life-threatening emergency characterized by greatly accentuated signs and symptoms of hyperthyroidism. Thyroid hormone levels during a crisis are not significantly more elevated than those found in a hyperthyroid state. Hyperthyroid patients are more sensitive to catecholamines owing to increased number of catecholamine receptors. Hyperthyroid crisis is associated with other acute medical illnesses. The acute medical illness that triggers an outpouring of catecholamines, the preexisting elevated thyroid levels, and increased binding sites available for catecholamines precipitate the crisis. Thyroid hormone–catecholamine interactions result in an increased rate of chemical reactions, increased nutrient and oxygen consumption, increased heat production, alterations in fluid and electrolyte balance, and a catabolic state

2. **Etiology or precipitating factors**
   a. Decompensation of a preexisting hyperthyroid state subsequent to surgery, trauma, infection, diabetic ketoacidosis, toxemia of pregnancy, or other physical stress. Preexisting hyperthyroidism may be caused by Graves' disease (autoimmune thyroid disorder), toxic multinodular goiter, or toxic adenoma
   b. Insufficient provision of antithyroid therapy (hyperthyroid patient who discontinues antithyroid medication and subsequently encounters severe stress)
   c. Post administration of iodine load to a patient who has underlying autoimmune thyroid disease

3. **Nursing assessment data base**

a. Nursing history
   i. Subjective findings
      (a) Cognitive/perceptual—emotional lability, decreased attention span, nervousness, diplopia, blurred vision, complaints of dry scratchy eyes, palpitations. In elderly—apathy or depression. In hyperthyroid crisis—marked changes in mentation including delirium and psychosis
      (b) Activity—weakness, easy fatigability, exercise intolerance, tremor, dyspnea with exertion
      (c) Elimination—diarrhea or frequent bowel movements. Crisis—nausea, abdominal pain, vomiting
      (d) Nutrition/metabolic—in young patients, excessive appetite with weight gain. In elderly, loss of appetite and weight loss. Heat intolerance
      (e) Sleep/rest—inability to secure adequate rest, insomnia, interrupted sleep
      (f) Sexual—decreased libido, menstrual irregularities
      (g) A significant number of patients older than 75 years of age have few if any symptoms
   ii. Objective findings
      (a) Patient health history
         (1) History of treatment with antithyroid medications, radioactive iodine, or thyroid surgery for hyperthyroidism
         (2) Presence of other endocrine disorders
         (3) Exposure to iodine load (dye for cardiac catheterization or lymphangiogram)
         (4) Suspect hyperthyroidism when a febrile patient responds only minimally to conventional cooling measures. Hyperthermia associated with thyroid crisis resembles hypothalamic fever associated with brain injury
      (b) Family history of endocrine disorders, particularly Graves' disease
      (c) Social history
         (1) Family reports discordance in previously stable personal, school, or work relationships
         (2) History of psychiatric treatment for anxiety or depression
      (d) Medication history
         (1) Past or present use of methimazole or propylthiouracil; disruption of an established medication regimen
         (2) Use of antiarrhythmic agents
         (3) Use of iodine-containing medications (amiodarone or expectorants such as Organidin)

b. Nursing examination of the patient
   i. Inspection
      (a) Flushed, diaphoretic skin. Fine, velvety smooth texture to skin; spider telangiectasis
      (b) Moist palms, friable nails, tremor
      (c) Hyperkinesis
      (d) Eyelid lag, retracted lids, staring gaze
      (e) Hair loss
      (f) Exophthalmos may be present. Conjunctiva may be reddened or appear irritated.
      (g) Neck scar may suggest past thyroid surgery
      (h) Dermopathy may be present in Graves' disease (thickening of skin in lower extremities)
   ii. Palpation
      (a) Palpable, enlarged or nodular thyroid
      (b) Impalpable thyroid is common in elderly. Thyroid may be substernal
      (c) The presence of a goiter (enlarged thyroid) does not necessarily indicate thyroid dysfunction
   iii. Percussion
      (a) Hyperreflexia
   iv. Auscultation
      (a) Audible bruits over thyroid gland
      (b) Tachycardia, tachypnea
      (c) Widened pulse pressure
      (d) Increased systolic blood pressure
      (e) Third heart sound
      (f) Evidence of heart failure is common in elderly
   v. Other clinical measurements
      (a) Hyperthermia—100° to 106° F (38° to 41° C)
      (b) Atrial fibrillation common in elderly
      (c) Tachydysrhythmias
c. Diagnostic study findings
   i. Elevated total and free T_3
   ii. Elevated total and free T_4
   iii. Elevated T_3 resin uptake
   iv. Nondetectable TSH
   v. Positive thyroid antibodies in autoimmune thyroid disease (Graves' disease)
   vi. TRH test: performed in equivocal cases. Despite TRH administration, TSH secretion remains suppressed by elevated thyroid hormone levels
   vii. Thyroid-stimulating immunoglobulins present in Graves' disease

     viii. ECG findings: sinus tachycardia, atrial fibrillation, premature ventricular contractions, premature atrial contractions

     ix. Electrolyte levels vary depending on hydration status. May have elevated calcium levels from increased bone resorption

     x. Hyperglycemia may result from insulin resistance, impaired insulin secretion, increased glycogenolysis

4. Nursing diagnoses

  a. Hyperthermia related to accelerated metabolic state secondary to thyroid hormone excess. (Thyroid hormone excess augments sodium–potassium exchange across plasma membranes, increases the turnover of metabolic substrates, and amplifies beta-adrenergic responses.)

    i. Assessment for defining characteristics

      (a) Body temperature 100° to 106° F (38° to 41° C)

      (b) Flushed, warm skin

      (c) Tachypnea

      (d) Tachycardia

      (e) Diaphoresis

      (f) Delirium

    ii. Expected outcome

      (a) Body temperature is restored to normal

    iii. Nursing interventions

      (a) Administer antithyroid medications as ordered

        (1) Propylthiouracil (PTU) or methimazole—inhibits thyroid hormone synthesis. PTU also inhibits conversion of T_4 to T_3 in peripheral tissues. Given orally. Observe for side effects of rash and agranulocytosis

        (2) Iodine-containing medications (sodium iodide, potassium iodide, sodium ipodate)—pharmacologic doses of iodide inhibit release of stored thyroid hormone and retard hormone synthesis

        (3) Glucocorticoids—block conversion of T_4 to T_3

      (b) Administer beta-adrenergic blocking agents, if ordered. These agents block the peripheral effects of excessive thyroid hormone thus alleviating sympathomimetic manifestations. Propranolol and nadolol may block conversion of T_4 to T_3

      (c) Administer antipyretics as ordered. Aspirin is not recommended for fever control since it displaces thyroxine from its carrier protein, increasing the availability of free thyroid hormone. Use acetaminophen

      (d) Use conventional cooling measures (cooling mattress, ice packs). Shivering will increase the metabolic rate and can be controlled with judicious use of chlorpromazine or meperidine

(e) Measure body temperature every hour or use continuous temperature monitoring

(f) Perform frequent neurologic assessments

(g) Supply sufficient fluids and electrolytes to replace losses from diaphoresis

(h) Provide comfort measures appropriate to the febrile patient (frequent change of garments and bed clothing, cool quiet environment)

(i) Because of greatly increased metabolic rate, drug turnover and degradation will be accelerated

(j) If infection is believed to be a precipitator, administer antibiotics

iv. Evaluation of nursing care

(a) Body temperature is restored to normal range

(b) Vital signs and other hemodynamic parameters are within patient's normal range

(c) Awake and oriented

b. Potential for decreased cardiac output related to excessive demands on cardiovascular system due to hyperthermia and increased sensitivity of cardiac catecholamine receptors

i. Assessment for defining characteristics

(a) Dysrhythmias, tachycardia

(b) Hemodynamic parameters indicate impending cardiovascular collapse

(c) Decreasing urine output, hypotension

(d) Deterioration in mental status

ii. Expected outcome

(a) Acceptable cardiac output is restored/maintained

iii. Nursing interventions

(a) Administer beta-adrenergic blocking agents if ordered. Decision to employ these agents is based on the judgment that adrenergic hypersensitivity is playing a key role in the crisis. Monitor respiratory and cardiovascular responses, especially in patients with a history of heart failure or asthma

(b) Perform frequent cardiovascular assessments (heart rate, rhythm, blood pressure, peripheral pulses, and other hemodynamic parameters). Sleeping pulse rate may provide a more accurate assessment of tachycardia

(c) Identify patients at risk for cardiovascular collapse (elderly, those with preexisting coronary heart disease, and those with known cardiac risk factors)

(d) Perform frequent respiratory and neurologic assessments

(e) Record intake and output

(f) Closely regulate fluid replacement

      (g) Provide an environment conducive to rest

      (h) Minimize energy expenditure by assisting patient with activities of daily living

      (i) Interventions for hyperthermia will also diminish the demands on the cardiovascular system

    iv. Evaluation of nursing care

      (a) Hemodynamic parameters are within normal limits

      (b) Vital signs are within patient's normal range

      (c) Free of life-threatening dysrhythmias

      (d) No evidence of heart failure

      (e) Alert and oriented

      (f) Able to tolerate brief periods of physical activity without exhaustion

c. Altered nutrition, less than body requirements, related to hypermetabolic state

    i. Assessment for defining characteristics

      (a) Weight loss

      (b) Inadequate food intake

      (c) Muscle weakness

      (d) Abdominal pain, nausea, vomiting, diarrhea

    ii. Expected outcome

      (a) Stabilization of body weight

    iii. Nursing interventions

      (a) Administer intravenous fluids, electrolytes, B-complex vitamins, and glucose as ordered

      (b) Encourage patient to consume high-calorie diet. Avoid caffeinated beverages and foods that may further stimulate peristalsis

      (c) Provide assistance with eating. Allow sufficient rest periods

      (d) Ascertain patient's food preferences and attempt to incorporate into present meal plan

      (e) Obtain daily weights to monitor progress

      (f) Institute calorie count to quantify nutritional adequacy

      (g) Enlist the assistance of a dietitian to provide meals that are generous in portion and of high biologic quality

      (h) Consider nutritional support if patient is unwilling or unable to eat. Unmet nutritional requirements will result in a protein-depleted state and a patient who is susceptible to infection

      (i) Note glucose levels, since hyperglycemia may result from decreased peripheral and hepatic insulin sensitivity

    iv. Evaluation of nursing care

      (a) Patient's body weight stabilizes (an eventual weight gain may be desirable)

        (b) Calorie count reveals nutritional intake appropriate for current metabolic needs

        (c) Patient is able to consume a well-balanced diet

d. Potential for injury related to impaired cognitive state

  i. Assessment for defining characteristics

        (a) Emotional lability, attention span deficit, delirium, agitation, restlessness, poor judgment

        (b) Unfamiliar environment and personnel

        (c) Weakness

  ii. Expected outcome

        (a) Remains free from personal injury

  iii. Nursing interventions

        (a) Provide interventions to prevent injury (bed in low position, mittens to prevent tube removal)

        (b) Examine environment for possible physical risks and minimize same

        (c) Place patient in as quiet an environment as possible

        (d) Monitor patient's judgment, decision-making abilities, and attention span

        (e) Provide eye protection for the patient with exophthalmos (e.g., eye drops, artificial tears, eye patches)

        (f) Provide emotional support to family

        (g) Supply adequate rest periods

        (h) Assist patient in activities of daily living

        (i) Reorient patient to time, place, person, and circumstance

  iv. Evaluation of nursing care

        (a) Patient is free from personal injury

e. Knowledge deficit regarding hyperthyroidism and its management

  i. Assessment for defining characteristics

        (a) Patient/family request information regarding long-term therapy for hyperthyroidism

        (b) Patient's preadmission behavior suggests inaccurate follow-through with previous instructions regarding hyperthyroidism and its treatment

  ii. Expected outcome

        (a) Patient/family are able to state regimen for managing hyperthyroid state

  iii. Nursing interventions

        (a) Include family or significant others in teaching since patient's attention span deficit may interfere with learning

        (b) Explain symptoms and treatment of hyperthyroidism

        (c) Outline present medication therapy (purpose, name, dose, schedule)

        (d) Encourage continued medical follow-up for definitive treatment (radioiodine therapy or surgery)

(e) Supply written literature if available

(f) Repeat instructions often to compensate for patient's diminished attention span

(g) If patient has known hyperthyroidism in past, assess understanding and past compliance with medications and physician appointments

iv. Evaluation of nursing care

(a) Patient/family are able to state the importance of medical follow-up for hyperthyroidism

(b) Patient/family are able to state purpose, name, dose, and schedule of medication regimen

(c) Patient/family are able to state the importance of adhering to medication regimen post discharge

Myxedema Coma

1. **Pathophysiology:** life-threatening emergency resulting from extreme hypothyroidism. Thyroid hormone insufficiency may result from primary dysfunction of thyroid gland or may be secondary to a dysfunction in hypothalamic-pituitary-thyroid axis. Severe hypothyroidism results in hypometabolism, hypothermia, hypoventilation, and a depressed level of consciousness. The myxedematous state results from the interstitial accumulation of a mucopolysaccharide substance. The substance attracts water, causing a nonpitting type of edema. Myxedema may be evident in skin (puffy face), vocal cords (hoarse voice), middle ear (diminished hearing), or organs such as the heart (pericardial effusion), lungs (pleural effusion), or bowels (paralytic ileus)

2. **Etiology or precipitating factors**

   a. Decompensation of a preexisting hypothyroid state subsequent to infection; loss of blood volume; exposure to cold; administration of sedatives, anesthetics, narcotics, or psychotropic drugs; or other physical stress. Preexisting hypothyroidism may result from thyroidectomy, destruction of thyroid gland post radioactive iodine therapy for hyperthyroidism or Hashimoto's thyroiditis (autoimmune thyroiditis), or from dysfunction within the hypothalamic-pituitary axis (hypophysectomy, pituitary irradiation, pituitary infarction)

   b. Insufficient provision of exogenous thyroid hormone (hypothyroid patient who discontinues replacement therapy, critically ill patient who has preexisting hypothyroidism but does not receive continued replacement therapy while hospitalized)

3. **Nursing assessment data base**

   a. Nursing history

   i. Subjective findings

   (a) Cognitive/perceptual—sluggishness, impaired memory, lethargy, depression, paranoia, delusions. Crisis—coma

        (b) Activity—fatigue, exercise intolerance, inability to perform repetitive or prolonged muscular activity

        (c) Elimination—constipation, abdominal distention

        (d) Nutrition/metabolic—cold intolerance, weight gain despite decreased appetite

        (e) Sexual—decreased libido, menstrual irregularities

  ii. Objective findings

      (a) Patient health history

        (1) History of treatment with thyroid hormone or prior treatment of hyperthyroidism with radioactive iodine

        (2) History of other endocrine disorders

        (3) Past exposure to head/neck irradiation

        (4) Consider the diagnosis of hypothyroidism if cardiovascular collapse occurs when a hypothermic patient is placed on a warming blanket

      (b) Family history of endocrine disorders such as Graves' disease, Hashimoto's thyroiditis, or Type I diabetes mellitus

      (c) Social history

        (1) Family reports gradual change in patient's behavior. Hypothyroidism is common and is very insidious in older adults and may be manifested by memory impairment or confusion

        (2) Family reports snoring with daytime somnolence. Obstructive sleep apnea can be caused by upper airway obstruction due to myxedematous swelling

      (d) Medication history

        (1) Past or present use of levothyroxine or desiccated thyroid; disruption of an established medication regimen

        (2) Lithium carbonate—blocks thyroid hormone synthesis and release. In a susceptible patient (goiter or positive thyroid antibodies) it can cause hypothyroidism

        (3) Ingestion of iodide (kelp, iodine-containing cough preparations, amiodarone) in susceptible patients can cause hypothyroidism by blocking hormone synthesis

b. Nursing examination of patient

  i. Inspection

      (a) Puffy appearance, periorbital edema, faint yellow tinge to skin. Cool, pale dry skin

      (b) Thick tongue, deep husky voice

      (c) Dry, coarse hair

      (d) Thick, brittle nails

      (e) Neck scar may indicate prior thyroid surgery

      (f) Seizure activity

ii. Palpation
(a) Goiter may be present
iii. Percussion
(a) Delay in deep tendon reflexes
iv. Auscultation
(a) Distant heart sounds
(b) Bradycardia
(c) Diastolic hypertension
(d) Hypoactive bowel sounds
v. Other clinical measurements
(a) Hypothermia (94° F [34.4° C] or less). Nurse may suspect thermometer malfunction.
c. Diagnostic study findings
i. Decreased T_3 and T_4 levels
ii. Decreased T_3 resin uptake
iii. Hyponatremia
iv. Decreased plasma osmolality
v. Increased P_{CO_2}, decreased P_{O_2}, decreased pH
vi. Hypoglycemia, anemia, elevated creatine phosphokinase, and carotene levels
vii. Increased cholesterol, hyperlipoproteinemia
viii. Increased TSH levels (primary hypothyroidism)
ix. Thyroid antibodies may be present in autoimmune thyroid disease
x. ACTH stimulation test: before treating hypothyroidism adrenal gland competency must be assured. Thyroid hormone therapy in the presence of adrenal insufficiency might precipitate adrenal crisis
xi. X-ray films: cardiomegaly
xii. ECG: bradycardia, low voltage, prolongation of QT interval

4. Nursing diagnoses
a. Hypothermia related to deficient thermogenesis secondary to decreased metabolic rate associated with profound hypothyroidism
i. Assessment for defining characteristics
(a) Body temperature below 94° F (34.4° C)
(b) Decreased level of consciousness
(c) Bradycardia
(d) Marked peripheral vasoconstriction as evidenced by cool, dry, pale skin
ii. Expected outcome
(a) Body temperature is restored to normal
iii. Nursing interventions
(a) Administer intravenous thyroxine (T_4) or T_3 as ordered
(b) Implement measures to gradually rewarm the patient

(warm room, extra blankets). Aggressive rewarming by external methods may precipitate vascular collapse

(c) Monitor temperature every hour or use continual temperature monitoring

(d) Assess vital signs, other hemodynamic parameters, neurologic status, and peripheral perfusion

(e) Because of greatly decreased metabolic rate, drug turnover and degradation will be delayed

(f) Administer glucocorticoids as ordered. Thyroid replacement may aggravate preexisting adrenal insufficiency. If adrenal status is unknown, support patient with intravenous glucocorticoids

(g) Provide skin care, oral care, and passive range of motion exercises

(h) Take measures to prevent infection. Patient's response to infection will not include fever

iv. Evaluation of nursing care

(a) Body temperature is restored to normal range

(b) Vital signs and other hemodynamic parameters are within patient's normal range

(c) Awake and oriented

b. Ineffective breathing pattern related to reduced central ventilatory drive and respiratory muscle weakness

i. Assessment for defining characteristics

(a) Hypercapnia

(b) Hypoxia

(c) Depressed level of consciousness (somnolence, confusion, coma)

ii. Expected outcome

(a) Hypoxemia is resolved or is improved with oxygen supplementation or mechanical ventilatory support

iii. Nursing interventions

(a) Administer thyroxine (T_4) or T_3 as ordered. Decreased ventilatory response may be secondary to hypothermia. Thyroxine assists with thermogenesis and thus can help improve ventilatory responsiveness

(b) Assess respiratory rate, pattern, chest movements, and neurologic status

(c) Auscultate lungs and heart

(d) Monitor vital signs and other hemodynamic parameters

(e) Note peripheral perfusion

(f) Institute respiratory assistance as soon as it becomes evident that such is required. Interventions to reverse hypoxia and hypercapnia will enhance myocardial contractility, preventing cardiovascular collapse

    (g) Avoid pharmacologic agents that depress the ventilatory drive

    (h) Closely monitor blood gas values

    (i) Administer oxygen, encourage deep breathing, assist with repositioning, remove secretions as necessary

    (j) Ensure adequate nutritional intake (oral, enteral, or parenteral) to prevent further respiratory muscle weakness

    (k) Implement measures to prevent infection. Hypothyroid patients are susceptible to bacterial infections. Patient will not demonstrate usual response to infection such as fever or tachycardia

    (l) As condition improves, monitor patient's response to performing self-care. If activity intolerance is noted, assist with activities of daily living

  iv. Evaluation of nursing care

    (a) Blood gas values within acceptable limits

    (b) Vital signs are within patient's normal range

    (c) Hemodynamic parameters are within normal limits

    (d) Awake and alert

c. Potential for fluid volume excess related to inability to excrete water load

  i. Assessment for defining characteristics

    (a) Intake greater than output

    (b) Hyponatremia with hypo-osmolality

    (c) Weight gain

    (d) Evidence of heart failure

  ii. Expected outcome

    (a) Fluid overload is prevented/corrected

  iii. Nursing interventions

    (a) Closely monitor patient's fluid status. Hypothyroid patients have difficulty handling a water load

    (b) Fluid restriction may be necessary to reverse hyponatremia

    (c) If severe hyponatremia and/or seizure activity is present, small infusions of hypertonic sodium chloride may be necessary. Great caution is advised since fluid overload can worsen and may precipitate heart failure

    (d) Institute seizure precautions

    (e) Meticulous recording of intake/output, body weight, hydration, and cardiovascular and neurologic condition

    (f) Auscultate lungs and heart

    (g) If patient requires digitalization, maintenance dose will be lower than usual owing to prolonged drug degradation rate

  iv. Evaluation of nursing care

  (a) Intake approximates output
  (b) Vital signs and other hemodynamic parameters are within patient's normal range
  (c) Laboratory parameters are within normal limits (osmolality, sodium)
  (d) No evidence of heart failure
d. Knowledge deficit regarding hypothyroidism and its management
  i. Assessment for defining characteristics
    (a) Patient/family requests information regarding long-term therapy for hypothyroidism
    (b) Patient's preadmission behavior suggests inaccurate follow-through with previous instruction regarding hypothyroidism and its treatment
  ii. Expected outcome
    (a) Patient/family are able to state regimen for managing hypothyroidism
  iii. Nursing interventions
    (a) Include family or significant other in teaching since patient's memory deficit and decreased energy may interfere with learning
    (b) Explain symptoms and treatment of hypothyroidism
    (c) Outline present medication schedule (purpose, name, dose, schedule)
    (d) Encourage continued medical follow-up since dosage may need adjustment
    (e) Supply written literature if available
    (f) If patient had preexisting hypothyroidism, assess understanding and past compliance with medication and follow-up appointments
  iv. Evaluation of nursing care
    (a) Patient/family are able to state purpose, name, dose, and schedule of thyroid medication
    (b) Patient/family are able to state the importance of adhering to the medication post discharge

Hypoparathyroidism and Hyperparathyroidism

1. **Pathophysiology:** parathyroid gland dysfunction or production of a tumor-derived PTH-related peptide is associated with disturbances in calcium and phosphorus balance. See Chapter 4 for further discussion of pathophysiology of calcium–phosphorus imbalances
2. **Etiology or precipitating factors**
  a. Hyperparathyroidism
    i. Primary hyperparathyroidism is due to an adenoma of a parathyroid gland (80% of cases) or hyperplasia of the glands

     ii. Secondary hyperparathyroidism is an adaptive increase in PTH secretion associated with health disorders in which there is chronic hypocalcemia. Such disorders include chronic renal failure, osteomalacia, and intestinal malabsorption syndromes. See Chapter 4

  b. Humoral hypercalcemia of malignancy

     i. Tumor is secreting PTH-related peptide, a specific hormone with homology (structural similarity) to PTH

     ii. Associated with squamous cell carcinomas of lung, head, and neck; hypernephroma; ovarian cancer

  c. Hypoparathyroidism

     i. Congenital absence of parathyroid glands

     ii. Surgical removal (or surgical damage) of the parathyroid glands (thyroidectomy, radical neck surgery)

     iii. Autoimmune

     iv. Hypomagnesemia: interferes with PTH secretion. Hypomagnesemia is associated with gastrointestinal malabsorption or alcoholism

3. Nursing assessment data base: Chapter 4. Diagnostic study findings include laboratory measurements of intact PTH, vitamin D levels (25-hydroxyvitamin D and 1,25-dihydroxyvitamin D), total and ionic calcium, phosphorus, magnesium, and urinary cyclic AMP

4. Nursing diagnoses

  a. Hypercalcemia: see Chapter 4. Interventions include hydration and possible administration of loop diuretics. Treatment for humoral hypercalcemia of malignancy may include calcitonin, glucocorticoids, diphosphonates, or plicamycin (mithramycin)

  b. Hypocalcemia: see Chapter 4. Interventions include administration of calcium, vitamin D (ergocalciferol, dihydrotachysterol, or calcitriol), and magnesium

Acute Adrenal Insufficiency (Adrenal Crisis)

1. Pathophysiology: a life-threatening emergency in which there is a deficiency of mineralocorticoids and/or glucocorticoids. Insufficiency may result from primary dysfunction of adrenal glands or may be secondary to a dysfunction in the hypothalamic-pituitary-adrenal axis. Deficiency results in fluid and electrolyte imbalances

2. Etiology or precipitating factors

  a. Primary adrenal insufficiency (usually glucocorticoid and mineralocorticoid deficiency). Adrenal gland dysfunction results from

     i. Adrenal tissue destruction caused by hemorrhage, fungal infections, metastatic tumor invasion, infarction

     ii. Adrenalectomy

      iii. Autoimmune destruction of adrenal cortex (Addison's disease). Occurs in 80% of cases

      iv. Various deficiencies in enzymes necessary for adrenocortical hormone synthesis

      v. Pharmacologic agents that impair corticosteroid production or increase its metabolic clearance

      vi. AIDS

  b. Secondary adrenal insufficiency (glucocorticoid deficiency; mineralocorticoid usually not significantly affected since the major regulator is the renin–angiotensin system). Dysfunction within hypothalamic-pituitary axis results from

      i. Tissue destruction caused by large pituitary tumors, central nervous system tumors, infarction (postpartum necrosis, pituitary apoplexy), head trauma, infiltrative disorders, infection (tuberculosis), and radiation therapy

      ii. Surgical removal (hypophysectomy)

  c. Abrupt withdrawal of corticosteroid therapy in the steroid-dependent patient

  d. Inadequate provision of exogenous corticosteroids in the highly stressed patient who either has suppression of the hypothalamic-pituitary-adrenal axis (pharmacologic use of corticosteroids) or has been receiving physiologic (replacement) doses of corticosteroids. A twofold to threefold increase in dosage should be undertaken during stressful situations followed by a gradual tapering as the stress resolves

3. Nursing assessment data base

  a. Nursing history

      i. Subjective findings

        (a) Cognitive/perceptual—confusion, disorientation, abdominal pain, arthralgias, myalgias

        (b) Activity—weakness, easy fatigability, malaise

        (c) Elimination—vomiting, diarrhea

        (d) Nutrition—anorexia, nausea, weight loss

        (e) Sexual—decreased libido

      ii. Objective findings

        (a) Patient health history

          (1) History of precipitating factor

          (2) Presence of other endocrine disorders (hypothyroidism, Type I diabetes)

          (3) Symptoms of chronic adrenal insufficiency—undue fatigue, general malaise, anorexia, weakness, intermittent nausea and vomiting, diarrhea

          (4) Presence of medical identification indicating corticosteroid use

          (5) AIDS

(b) Family history of endocrine disorders

(c) Medication history

(1) Current or past corticosteroid use. More than 20 mg of hydrocortisone or its equivalent, given for longer than 7 to 10 days, has the potential for suppressing the hypothalamic-pituitary-adrenal axis. Recovery may take 2 to 12 months or longer

(2) Silent adrenal hemorrhage has been documented with anticoagulant therapy

(3) Ketoconazole and the anesthetic etomidate can interfere with steroid biosynthesis. Can precipitate a crisis in patients with marginal adrenal reserve

(4) Rifampin—increases metabolic clearance rate of corticosteroids

b. Nursing examination of patient

i. Inspection

(a) Dry skin, dry mucous membranes

(b) Hyperpigmentation especially noticeable on elbows and knees but also on creases of hand and buccal mucosa; seen in primary adrenal insufficiency where ACTH levels are high

(c) Vitiligo often associated with autoimmune endocrine disorders such as Addison's disease

(d) Decreased body hair

ii. Auscultation

(a) Tachycardia

(b) Hypotension, orthostasis

iii. Other clinical measurements

(a) Fever

c. Diagnostic study findings

i. Hyponatremia, hyperkalemia, fasting hypoglycemia, azotemia, eosinophilia

ii. Low plasma cortisol levels. Normal cortisol levels may be abnormal in the highly stressed patient

iii. ACTH stimulation test: confirms the presence of adrenal insufficiency

iv. Plasma ACTH levels elevated in primary adrenal insufficiency and low or normal in secondary adrenal insufficiency

v. Plasma aldosterone levels decreased in primary adrenal insufficiency

vi. ECG may reflect hyperkalemia

vii. Thyroid hormone levels should be measured since other pituitary hormones (TSH) may also be deficient

4. **Nursing diagnoses**

a. Fluid volume deficit related to adrenocortical hormone deficiency

    i. Assessment for defining characteristics
      (a) Thirst, dry mucous membranes
      (b) Decreased skin turgor
      (c) Hypotension, orthostasis, tachycardia
      (d) Azotemia
      (e) Nausea, vomiting, diarrhea
      (f) Electrolyte abnormalities
   ii. Expected outcome
      (a) Fluid volume and electrolyte balances are restored
  iii. Nursing interventions
      (a) Administer intravenous fluids and electrolytes (usually glucose in normal saline). Initial fluids will be administered rapidly
      (b) Administer scheduled doses of intravenous cortisol. Hydrocortisone supplies glucocorticoid activity and also has some sodium-retaining properties
      (c) Monitor central and peripheral perfusion
      (d) Monitor fluid balance, body weight
      (e) Monitor heart rate and rhythm
      (f) Provide skin and oral care
      (g) Share information regarding possible precipitating factors with the physician
      (h) Explain diagnostic procedures to patient/family
      (i) Prevent crisis by ensuring that patients at risk receive adequate exogenous corticosteroids when confronted with a severe stress state (e.g., patient on long-term corticosteroid therapy who is scheduled for surgery)
   iv. Evaluation of nursing care
      (a) Vital signs and other hemodynamic parameters are within patient's normal range
      (b) Hydration is restored to oral mucous membranes
      (c) Absence of orthostasis
      (d) Normal skin turgor
      (e) Electrolytes are within normal limits
b. Potential knowledge deficit regarding long-term corticosteroid management
    i. Assessment for defining characteristics
      (a) Patient/family request information regarding long-term corticosteroid use
      (b) Patient's preadmission behavior suggests inaccurate follow-through with previous instructions regarding corticosteroid management
      (c) Patient/family are unable to verbalize appropriate stress state management
   ii. Expected outcome

(a) Patient/family are able to state self-care actions necessary to prevent recurrence of crisis

iii. Nursing interventions

(a) Initiate medication instruction

(1) Purpose, name, dose, schedule

(2) Importance of adherence

(3) Importance of medical identification and how to secure same

(b) Instruct patient/family in stress state management

(1) Define stress (tooth extraction, surgery, cold, flu, fever)

(2) Instruct patient to temporarily increase the glucocorticoid dose (collaborate with physician regarding specific amounts)

(3) Instruct patient to inform all health care providers of corticosteroid use

(4) If vomiting occurs and patient is unable to retain oral dose, instruct patient/family to immediately notify physician or go to an emergency department so that parenteral hydrocortisone may be administered. Many families are instructed to use parenteral hydrocortisone at home

(c) Instruct patient/family in importance of gradual corticosteroid tapering (if appropriate). If corticosteroids are discontinued, patient should be advised to continue to carry medical identification for up to 1 year after discontinuation of the corticosteroid.

(d) Instruct previous corticosteroid users to seek medical attention in event of a severe stress state. Patients who have been on long-term corticosteroids should receive glucocorticoids during periods of stress for at least 1 year after the drugs have been discontinued, unless the hypothalamic-pituitary-adrenal axis has been shown to be stress responsive

iv. Evaluation of nursing care

(a) Patient/family are able to state purpose, name, dose, and schedule of corticosteroid regimen

(b) Patient/family are able to state importance of adhering to medication schedule

(c) Patient/family are able to verbalize stress state management

(d) Patient/family are able to state importance of securing medical identification

(e) Patient/family are able to identify situations that warrant physician notification

Diabetic Ketoacidosis (DKA)

1. **Pathophysiology:** life-threatening emergency resulting from relative or absolute insulin deficiency. Usually associated with increased levels of insulin-antagonistic hormones (glucagon, cortisol, catecholamines, and growth hormone). Insulin deficiency and insulin-antagonistic hormone excess result in the following metabolic alterations (Fig. 5–5)
    a. Carbohydrate
        i. Decreased peripheral glucose use in cells that require insulin for glucose entry (fat and muscle)
        ii. Overproduction of glucose by liver (gluconeogenesis)
    b. Fat
        i. Increased lipolysis due to lack of inhibition of lipases
        ii. Fatty acids are released in amounts that exceed liver's ability to metabolize. Fatty acids are partially oxidized to ketoacids
        iii. Ketoacid excess is accentuated by decreased peripheral use
    c. Protein: increased catabolism
    d. Other pathophysiologic processes include
        i. Osmotic diuresis due to hyperglycemia results in intracellular and extracellular fluid volume deficits and electrolyte losses (sodium, chloride, potassium, magnesium, phosphate)
        ii. Metabolic acidosis due to accumulation of ketoacids and possible accumulation of lactic acid secondary to diminished perfusion
        iii. Hyperkalemia as potassium is displaced from intracellular to extracellular space in acidosis. A total body deficit results, since potassium is lost during osmotic diuresis
        iv. Depressed level of consciousness results from hyperosmolality, cellular dehydration, ketoacid accumulation, acidosis, and possible impaired oxygen dissociation since glycosylated hemoglobin binds oxygen more tightly

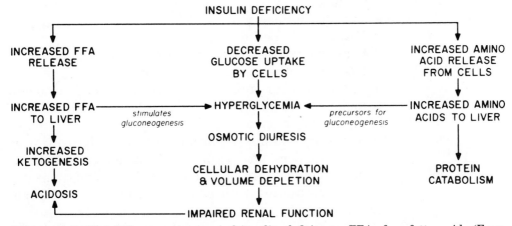

Figure 5–5. Metabolic consequences of insulin deficiency. *FFA,* free fatty acid. (From Skillman, T.: Diabetic ketoacidosis. Heart Lung 7:596, 1978.)

2. **Etiology or precipitating factors**
   a. Inadequate secretion of endogenous insulin (newly diagnosed Type I insulin-dependent diabetes)
   b. Insufficient exogenous insulin (established diabetic who reduces or misses insulin doses)
   c. Unmet increased requirements for insulin due to physical and/or emotional stress (infections, trauma, growth spurts, surgery, other acute illnesses, psychosocial difficulties). Stress is associated with increased secretion of insulin-antagonistic hormones: epinephrine, cortisol, glucagon, growth hormone, and, in pregnancy, placental hormones. Fever and the self-imposed fasting and dehydration that often accompany minor sick day episodes will raise insulin-antagonistic hormone levels.
   d. Medications that interfere with insulin secretion and/or action
      i. Thiazide diuretics: possibly decrease insulin release from pancreas secondary to hypokalemia
      ii. Glucocorticoids: increase gluconeogenesis
      iii. Phenytoin: decreases insulin release from pancreas
      iv. Sympathomimetics: stimulate glycogenolysis; inhibit insulin release
      v. Diazoxide: inhibits insulin release

3. **Nursing assessment data base**
   a. Nursing history
      i. Subjective findings
         (a) Cognitive/perceptual—blurred vision, abdominal pain, depressed level of consciouness (lethargy → coma)
         (b) Activity—fatigue, weakness
         (c) Elimination—polyuria, nocturia, nausea, vomiting, abdominal bloating and cramping
         (d) Nutrition—polydipsia, polyphagia, abrupt weight loss
      ii. Objective findings
         (a) Patient health history
            (1) History of Type I diabetes mellitus
            (2) Symptoms of hyperglycemia prior to admission
            (3) History of other endocrine disorders
            (4) Can also occur in Type II diabetic patients who are under severe stress
         (b) Family history of endocrine disorders
         (c) Social history—family reports psychosocial difficulties or that patient does not comply with established diabetes self-care regimen. At least one third of admissions for DKA are associated with educational deficits or psychosocial distress
         (d) Medication history—use of insulin in the past. Use of a

continuous insulin infusion device in which flow rate has been disrupted

b. Nursing examination of patient
  i. Inspection
    (a) Flushed, dry skin
    (b) Dry mucous membranes
    (c) Decreased skin turgor, sunken eyeballs
    (d) Medical identification indicating presence of diabetes
  ii. Auscultation
    (a) Tachycardia
    (b) Hypotension
    (c) Tachypnea, Kussmaul respirations, acetone odor to breath
    (d) Rales/rhonchi may not be evident in a dehydrated patient with a pulmonary infection
  iii. Other clinical measurements
    (a) Afebrile even when infection is present
c. Diagnostic study findings
  i. Elevated plasma and urine glucose levels (plasma glucose >300 mg/dl)
  ii. Arterial pH below 7.3; decreased bicarbonate levels (<15 mEq/L)
  iii. Positive serum and urine ketoacids
  iv. Azotemia
  v. Electrolyte levels vary, often initially hyperkalemic despite marked total body deficit
  vi. ECG may reflect hyperkalemia

4. **Nursing diagnoses**
a. Fluid volume deficit related to osmotic diuresis induced by hyperglycemia. Deficit worsened by vomiting and/or inadequate oral intake
  i. Assessment for defining characteristics
    (a) Thirst, dry mucous membranes
    (b) Decreased skin turgor
    (c) Hypotension, orthostasis, tachycardia, weak thready pulse
    (d) Hemoconcentration
    (e) Output greater than intake
    (f) Weight loss
  ii. Expected outcome
    (a) Fluid volume and electrolyte balance are restored
  iii. Nursing interventions
    (a) Administer intravenous fluids and electrolytes as ordered via an infusion pump. Fluids will initially be administered rapidly. Solutions will include sodium chloride and potassium replacement. Hypophosphatemia also occurs in DKA. Replacing phosphate may help restore plasma buffering

capacity. Overaggressive phosphate replacement can result in hypocalcemia

    (b) Intake and output

    (c) Assess vital signs, other hemodynamic parameters, and neurologic status

    (d) Obtain body weight

    (e) Facilitate the maintenance of skin integrity

    (f) Facilitate adequate oral hygiene

    (g) Encourage oral fluids as tolerated

    (h) Inform physician of evidence of inadequate perfusion

    (i) If deterioration is noted in neurologic status, promptly inform physician. This may signal the development of cerebral edema

    (j) Assess for evidence of fluid overload. Slow infusion rate and consult with physician

    (k) Maintain flow sheet of laboratory and hemodynamic parameters

  iv. Evaluation of nursing care

    (a) Vital signs and other hemodynamic parameters are within patient's normal range

    (b) Laboratory parameters are within normal limits (plasma osmolality, blood urea nitrogen, electrolytes)

    (c) Hydration is restored to oral mucous membranes

    (d) Normal skin turgor

b. Altered nutrition, less than body requirements, related to catabolic effects of insulin deficiency and stress hormone excess

  i. Assessment for defining characteristics

    (a) Loss of weight despite polyphagia

    (b) Ketosis

    (c) Fatigue, weakness

    (d) Hyperglycemia, glucosuria

  ii. Expected outcome

    (a) Normal carbohydrate, fat, and protein metabolism is restored

  iii. Nursing interventions

    (a) Administer rapid-acting human insulin (regular insulin)

      (1) Continuous intravenous insulin infusion, often preceded by a small intravenous bolus. Use an infusion pump. Flush at least 50 ml of solution through tubing before connecting to patient to saturate binding sites on plastic tubing

      (2) Intramuscular insulin injections every 1 to 2 hours, often preceded by a small intravenous bolus

      (3) Intravenous insulin per closed-loop insulin infusion device (Biostator)

(4) Subcutaneous insulin injections if peripheral perfusion is adequate. Response will not be as prompt as with intravenous insulin

(b) Perform blood glucose testing. Use bedside blood glucose monitoring if patient's blood glucose level is within the meter's established ranges. If above the meter's range, send blood to laboratory for glucose value determinations

(c) Measure urine ketones

(d) Maintain flow sheet documenting laboratory parameters

(e) Offer foods and fluids as tolerated

(f) Secure daily weight

(g) Switch to subcutaneous insulin 1 to 2 hours before stopping the continuous insulin infusion to prevent the recurrence of ketosis and accelerated hyperglycemia

(h) Assess and document the presence of nausea, vomiting, and/or abdominal pain. DKA may mimic an acute surgical abdomen

(i) Assess and document any abdominal distention. Note the presence of bowel sounds

(j) Advance foods and fluids gradually as patient can tolerate

(k) Administer antibiotics if precipitator is an infectious process

iv. Evaluation of nursing care

(a) Blood glucose decrement of 75 to 100 mg/dl/hr

(b) Blood glucose stabilized at 150 to 200 mg/dl

(c) Absence of persistent ketosis

(d) Patient is able to tolerate oral feedings

(e) Body weight stabilized (eventual weight gain may be desirable)

c. Acid–base imbalances related to accumulation of ketoacids secondary to insulin deficiency and stress hormone excess

i. Assessment for defining characteristics

(a) Acetone odor to breath

(b) Tachypnea, Kussmaul respirations

(c) Positive serum/urine ketones

(d) Decreased pH and bicarbonate levels

(e) Initial hyperkalemia

(f) Depressed level of consciousness

ii. Expected outcome

(a) Acid–base balance is restored

iii. Nursing interventions

(a) Assess respiratory pattern noting rate, acetone odor, Kussmaul respirations, or tachypnea

(b) Assess neurologic status

(c) Intravenous fluids and insulin are the primary therapies for correction of acidosis

(d) Administer sodium bicarbonate if ordered. Bicarbonate currently recommended in severe acidosis only (pH 7.1 or below). Excessive use of bicarbonate can precipitate hypokalemia and may prolong the comatose state by abruptly altering the oxygen dissociation curve

(e) Measure urine ketones

(f) As acidosis and volume deficits are being corrected, be alert for hypokalemia

(g) Note and promptly report laboratory and/or clinical evidence of increasing acidosis

iv. Evaluation of nursing care

(a) pH, bicarbonate, and potassium levels are within normal limits

(b) Serum/urine is negative for ketones

(c) Respiratory rate and pattern are within normal limits

(d) No acetone odor is detected on breath

d. Potential hypoglycemia related to insulin therapy and a decrease in circulating insulin-antagonistic hormones

i. Assessment for defining characteristics

(a) Blood glucose level less than 50 mg/dl

(b) Signs and symptoms indicative of hypoglycemia (see section on hypoglycemic episode pp. 669–670)

ii. Expected outcome

(a) Blood glucose is maintained at or above 80 mg/dl

iii. Nursing interventions

(a) Assess for the signs and symptoms of hypoglycemia

(b) If patient is an established diabetic, secure information regarding past experiences with hypoglycemia (causes, symptoms, most effective treatment).

(c) Instruct patient and family in the signs and symptoms of hypoglycemia. Instruct them to report any evidence of hypoglycemia promptly to the nurse.

(d) Plan interventions for prevention of hypoglycemia since hypoglycemia can precipitate dysrhythmias and extend infarcts

(1) Monitor the trend of laboratory data, especially blood glucose levels

(2) Keep physician informed of the trend evidenced in laboratory and clinical data

(3) Expect to switch intravenous fluids to one containing glucose when the blood glucose level is 250 mg/dl. The infusion rate for insulin will also be decreased at this point

    (e) If hypoglycemia occurs, provide the patient with at least 15 g of a quick-acting carbohydrate (60 calories) such as apple juice or sweetened carbonated beverage

    (f) If level of consciousness is depressed and patient cannot tolerate oral feedings, notify the physician for an order to administer glucagon or intravenous glucose (10% or 50%)

    (g) Perform a bedside blood glucose measurement any time the nurse, patient, or family suspects hypoglycemia

    (h) Document and inform the physician of any episode of hypoglycemia

    (i) After treatment of a suspected hypoglycemic episode, monitor patient's response to the carbohydrate source provided

    (j) Provide milk and crackers to afford the patient protection from a recurrence of hypoglycemia

  iv. Evaluation of nursing care

    (a) Blood glucose level is above 100 mg/dl

    (b) Absence of signs and symptoms of hypoglycemia

    (c) Patient/family are able to state at least three symptoms of hypoglycemia

    (d) Patient/family are able to state the need to immediately notify the nurse if hypoglycemia is suspected

e. Potential knowledge deficit regarding home management of hyperglycemia

  i. Assessment for defining characteristics

    (a) Patient is unable to state appropriate sick day management

    (b) Patient discontinued insulin and/or home monitoring before admission

    (c) Patient delayed notifying health care team about deteriorating condition

    (d) Patient has newly diagnosed Type I diabetes mellitus

    (e) Patient unable to state troubleshooting guidelines in the event of sustained unexplainable hyperglycemia while using continuous subcutaneous insulin infusion device

  ii. Expected outcome

    (a) Patient/family are able to state self-management knowledge and skills necessary to prevent recurrence of DKA

  iii. Nursing interventions

    (a) If an established diabetic, identify precipitating factors by securing data regarding

      (1) Home medication regimen. Inquire about the date, time, type, and dose of last diabetic medication. Inquire about appearance of insulin bottle

      (2) Presence of any possible infection (especially genitourinary, pulmonary, or skin)

       (3) Presence of other stressors such as a recent severe emotional upset

       (4) Food and fluid intake 24 hours prior to admission

       (5) Past history of a hyperglycemic crisis and the circumstances surrounding the crisis

       (6) Duration of present illness

       (7) Results of recent home urine or blood glucose testing prior to admission

       (8) Results of ketone testing prior to admission

       (9) Attempts to contact health care team

      (10) Evidence of insulin infusion device malfunction (if used)

  (b) Document findings regarding possible precipitating events and share with physician

  (c) If precipitating factors point to a self-care knowledge or skill deficit, or to noncompliance with the self-care regimen, refer to diabetes educator on transfer from ICU. Share precipitators with the education team

  (d) Instruct patient/family in causes, symptoms, and treatment of hyperglycemia

  (e) Instruct patient/family on sick day management. Include the importance of insulin administration, frequent glucose monitoring, and the importance of ketone testing and fluid replacement

  (f) Reinforce importance of physician notification

iv. Evaluation of nursing care

  (a) Patient/family are able to identify two causes of hyperglycemia

  (b) Patient/family are able to state the impact of infection on blood glucose levels

  (c) Patient/family are able to state three symptoms of hyperglycemia

  (d) Patient/family are able to describe sick day management

  (e) Patient/family are able to state the importance of continuing the prescribed insulin regimen

  (f) Patient/family are able to identify situations that require prompt notification of health care provider

Hyperglycemic, Hyperosmolar Nonketotic Coma (Hyperglycemic, Nonacidotic Diabetic Coma)

1. **Pathophysiology:** life-threatening emergency characterized by extreme hyperglycemia, hyperosmolality, severe dehydration, minimal ketosis, and alterations in neurologic status. Pathophysiologic processes include (Fig. 5–6)

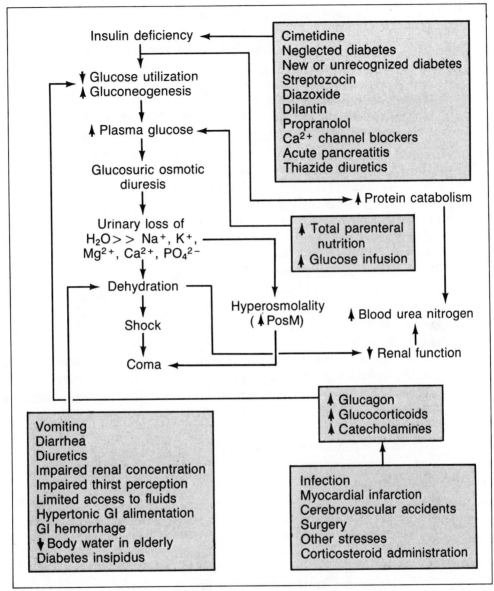

Figure 5–6. Pathogenesis of hyperosmolar nonacidotic uncontrolled diabetes. (From Matz, R.: Hyperglycemic hyperosmolar nonacidotic coma: Not a rare event. Clin Diabetes 6:31, 1988. Reproduced with permission of the American Diabetes Association, Inc.)

  a. Relative insulin deficiency that impairs glucose transport across the cell membrane. Sufficient insulin may be present to inhibit lipolysis or ketogenesis in the liver, but not enough to control hyperglycemia
  b. Hyperosmolality results from the hyperglycemia and the hypernatremia that frequently accompany this state. Hyperosmolality may impair insulin secretion, promote insulin resistance, and inhibit free fatty acid release from adipose tissue

    c. Fluid shifts occur from intracellular to extracellular space to offset increasing plasma osmolality

    d. Osmotic diuresis due to hyperglycemia results in extracellular fluid volume deficits

    e. Electrolyte losses (sodium, chloride, phosphate, magnesium, potassium) occur with osmotic diuresis

    f. Severe intracellular and extracellular fluid volume deficits decrease glomerular filtration, which reduces the kidneys' ability to excrete the glucose load. This adds to the hyperglycemia and hyperosmolality

    g. Neurologic abnormalities result from cellular dehydration due to hyperosmolality

2. **Etiology or precipitating factors**

    a. Inadequate insulin secretion and/or action (newly diagnosed Type II, non-insulin-dependent diabetes). Some patients have no history of diabetes mellitus

    b. Majority of patients are elderly and suffer from dehydration. Elderly have a lower total body water content, which compromises their ability to buffer changes in osmolality. Elderly also have a decreased sense of thirst and therefore do not readily seek fluids to replenish body water stores

    c. Other major illnesses either precipitate or hasten the development of this crisis via increased glucose production secondary to stress hormone excess and inadvertent dehydration. Illnesses include sepsis, pancreatitis, stroke, uremia, burns, acute myocardial infarction, and gastrointestinal hemorrhage

    d. Nonketotic coma has been associated with the following medications

        i. Thiazide diuretics: possibly decrease insulin release from pancreas secondary to hypokalemia

        ii. Glucocorticoids: increase gluconeogenesis and cause peripheral insulin resistance

        iii. Phenytoin: decreases insulin release from pancreas

        iv. Sympathomimetics: stimulate glycogenolysis, inhibit insulin release

        v. Diazoxide: inhibits insulin release

        vi. Chlorpromazine, sedatives, cimetidine, calcium channel blockers, propranolol, immunosuppressive agents: may inhibit insulin release or interfere with insulin action

    e. High caloric parenteral and enteral feedings could present a glucose load that exceeds patient's ability to metabolize

3. **Nursing assessment data base**

    a. Nursing history

        i. Subjective findings

            (a) Cognitive/perceptual—blurred vision, depressed level of consciousness (lethargy → coma), confusion, restlessness, aphasia

   (b) Activity—weakness, fatigue
   (c) Elimination—polyuria, nocturia
   (d) Nutrition—polydipsia, polyphagia. Polydipsia may not be
       prominent in elderly
 ii. Objective findings
   (a) Patient health history
       (1) History of Type II diabetes or impaired glucose toler-
           ance in the past
       (2) Symptoms of hyperglycemia prior to admission
   (b) Family history of Type II diabetes
   (c) Social history
       (1) Condition often presents in the elderly patient whose
           family gives a history of a protracted, gradual deteri-
           oration in the person's physical and mental condition
       (2) Patient at risk includes persons who cannot gain ready
           access to fluids or who cannot recognize or express
           their need for water
   (d) Medication history
       (1) Use of insulin or oral hypoglycemic agent in past;
           disruption of established medication regimen
       (2) Recent introduction of a medication known to elevate
           glucose levels and/or resist insulin action
       (3) Preadmission medications include pharmacologic
           agents that suggest cardiovascular or renal disease.
           Crisis is more common in late middle-aged and elderly
           persons with preexisting renal or cardiovascular dis-
           ease
 b. Nursing examination of patient
   i. Inspection
     (a) Dry, flushed skin, tenting skin
     (b) Decreased skin turgor (will not be evident in elderly)
     (c) Dry mucous membranes, parched lips and tongue
     (d) Seizure activity, hemiparesis, nystagmus
  ii. Auscultation
     (a) Tachycardia
     (b) Hypotension
     (c) Shallow, rapid respirations
     (d) Rales/rhonchi may not be evident in severely dehydrated
         patient with a pulmonary infection
 c. Diagnostic study findings
   i. Elevated plasma glucose levels (plasma levels often over 1000
      mg/dl)
  ii. Azotemia, hemoconcentration, elevated serum creatinine
 iii. Electrolyte levels vary with state of hydration. Hypernatremia
      is usually present and contributes to the hyperosmolality

iv. Plasma hyperosmolality (>330 mOsm/kg). Plasma osmolality can be calculated by using the following equation

$$1.8 \, (Na + K) + \frac{Glucose}{18} + \frac{BUN}{2.8}$$

v. Absence of significant ketosis
vi. pH ≥ 7.30; bicarbonate ≥ 15 mEq/L. Acidosis, if present, is usually due to lactic acid or renal dysfunction

4. **Nursing diagnoses**
   a. Fluid volume deficit: refer to discussion in section on diabetic ketoacidosis. Fluid deficits are usually greater than with ketoacidosis. Hypotonic, balanced crystalloid solutions are usually employed. Because these patients tend to be older and many have underlying heart disease, monitor for evidence of heart failure with rapid fluid replacement
   b. Altered nutrition, less than body requirements: refer to discussion in section on diabetic ketoacidosis. Intravenous route for insulin administration is preferred because of poor peripheral perfusion in these severely dehydrated patients
   c. Potential hypoglycemia: refer to discussion in diabetic ketoacidosis
   d. Potential for impaired peripheral tissue perfusion related to dehydration, hyperviscosity, and increased platelet adhesiveness and/or aggregation
      i. Assessment for defining characteristics
         (a) Cool extremities
         (b) Unequal extremity temperature
         (c) Diminished peripheral pulses
         (d) Extremity pallor
      ii. Expected outcomes
         (a) Color, temperature, and pulse quality in lower extremities are equal bilaterally
         (b) Negative Homans' sign
      iii. Nursing interventions
         (a) Assess and document the status of the circulation in the lower extremities, including color, temperature, and quality of bilateral peripheral pulses
         (b) Assess for signs and symptoms indicative of thrombus formation, such as positive Homans' sign, localized redness, swelling, tenderness, or increased warmth
         (c) If elastic stockings are used, remove stockings for 30 minutes every shift and assess extremities
         (d) Perform active or passive range of motion exercises
         (e) Avoid constricting garments or positions that may impede circulation

(f) Report evidence of thrombus formation promptly to physician. Place patient on bed rest pending physician's orders

(g) Provide adequate foot care, including foot inspection, lotion, and prevention of foot injury

iv. Evaluation of nursing care: as stated in expected outcomes

e. Potential ineffective family coping related to gravity of illness, and/or inadequate knowledge regarding illness and treatment

i. Assessment for defining characteristics

(a) Family describes preoccupation with personal reaction to situation (fear, anticipatory grief, guilt, anxiety)

(b) Family describes inadequate understanding of illness and its treatment

ii. Expected outcomes

(a) Family is able to verbalize feelings and concerns

(b) Family is able to use health care providers for information and support

(c) Family is able to state basic rationale associated with treatment

iii. Nursing interventions

(a) Elicit concerns of family

(b) Explain basic rationale of treatment plan to family

(c) Explain the precipitating factors and the circumstances surrounding admission to the hospital

(d) Keep family informed of patient progress and plan of care

(e) Provide basic information in response to questions regarding long-term management of diabetes

(f) Provide family with the opportunity to participate in patient's care

(g) Discuss usual reactions to acute illness such as guilt, anxiety, and grief

(h) Use communication techniques that confirm the legitimacy of feelings, both positive and negative

(i) Encourage family to draw on other support systems such as clergy and friends

iv. Evaluation of nursing care: as stated in expected outcomes

Hypoglycemic Episode

1. **Pathophysiology:** decrease in plasma glucose level to 50 mg/dl or below. Glucose production (feeding and/or liver gluconeogenesis) lags behind glucose utilization. Results in changes in level of consciousness (glucose is the preferred fuel of the central nervous system) and a rise in counterregulatory (insulin-antagonistic) hormones—glucagon, epinephrine, cortisol, and growth hormone

2. **Etiology or precipitating factors**

   a. Insulin therapy
      i. Insulin dose greater than body's current requirements
      ii. Sudden rotation of sites from hypertrophied area to one with unimpaired absorption
      iii. Change in species of insulin from animal source to human insulin
   b. Sulfonylurea therapy
      i. Oral hypoglycemic agents, especially those that have prolonged activity (chlorpropamide)
      ii. Additional factors (nutritional, activity) usually also present
   c. Insufficient caloric consumption
      i. Missed meal or snack
      ii. Delayed meal or snack
      iii. Insufficient nutritional prescription
      iv. Decreased intake due to nausea, vomiting, anorexia
      v. Interrupted enteral tube feedings
      vi. Delayed gastric emptying in patients with autonomic neuropathy (gastroparesis)
   d. Strenuous physical exercise that is uncompensated by an increase in food intake or a decrease in insulin dose
   e. Potentiation of hypoglycemic medications
      i. Renal insufficiency delays drug degradation, thus potentiating and prolonging the effect
      ii. Liver dysfunction delays drug degradation and excretion. Impaired hepatic gluconeogenesis and glycogenolysis will increase the risk of hypoglycemia
      iii. Medications that potentiate the action of sulfonylureas (phenylbutazone, large doses of salicylates, sulfonamides)
   f. Excessive alcohol intake, ingested in the unfed state, inhibits liver gluconeogenesis
   g. Decreased requirements for exogenous insulin resulting from
      i. Recovery from stress (e.g., infections, trauma). Relief from stressors decreases the levels of insulin-antagonistic hormones, thus decreasing the need for insulin
      ii. Weight loss decreases insulin resistance
      iii. Immediate postpartum period: sudden reduction in anti-insulin effects of placental hormones
      iv. Glucocorticoid dose decrease
   h. Pentamidine: hypoglycemia secondary to pancreatic islet cell necrosis, which results in inappropriately high plasma insulin concentrations
   i. Other health problems
      i. Adrenal insufficiency and hypopituitarism: insufficient glucocorticoids to stimulate gluconeogenesis

ii. Severe liver disease: inadequate glycogen stores and impaired liver gluconeogenesis

iii. Pancreatic islet cell tumor: inappropriate insulin secretion

3. Nursing assessment data base

a. Nursing history

i. Subjective findings

(a) Cognitive/perceptual—headache, impaired mentation, inability to concentrate, inappropriate behavior, irritability, nervousness, visual disturbances, paresthesias, palpitations, dizziness. Prolonged hypoglycemia can lead to irreparable brain damage

(b) Activity—fatigue, lethargy

(c) Nutrition—hunger, nausea

(d) Sleep/rest—nocturnal hypoglycemia is manifested by poor sleep quality, nightmares, restless sleep, headache on arising, nocturnal diaphoresis

ii. Objective findings

(a) Patient health history

(1) History of diabetes mellitus

(2) Recent change in medication regimen, meal patterns, and/or activity level

(3) Some patients with insulin-dependent diabetes mellitus have defective glucose counterregulation (impaired glucagon and epinephrine responsiveness to hypoglycemia). These patients have few if any symptoms of hypoglycemia and have impaired recovery

(b) Medication history

(1) Regular insulin can be associated with a rapid fall in glucose levels and may prompt more adrenomedullary symptoms. Intermediate-acting insulins or continuous insulin infusion devices may prompt a more gradual drop in plasma glucose, thus producing central nervous system symptoms (neuroglycopenia)

(2) Patients on beta-adrenergic blocking agents (propranolol) may not exhibit adrenomedullary symptoms. Beta-adrenergic blocking agents can also impair recovery from hypoglycemia by inhibiting glycogenolysis

b. Nursing examination of patient

i. Inspection

(a) Cool, clammy skin

(b) Pallor

(c) Tremors

(d) Medical alert jewelry or wallet card indicating current insulin or oral hypoglycemic agent use

ii. Palpation

 (a) Tachycardia
 iii. Other clinical measurements
 (a) Tachydysrhythmias
 c. Diagnostic study findings
 i. Plasma or capillary blood glucose level less than 50 mg/dl
4. **Nursing diagnoses**
 a. Actual or potential hypoglycemia related to disparity between available fuel (glucose) and circulating insulin levels
 i. Assessment for defining characteristics
 (a) Subjective and objective indicators as previously stated
 (b) Physical and diagnostic findings as previously stated
 ii. Expected outcome
 (a) Plasma/capillary glucose is restored to or remains within normal range
 iii. Nursing interventions
 (a) Identify patient at risk for hypoglycemia
 (b) If patient is an established diabetic, secure information regarding past experience with hypoglycemia (causes, symptoms, most effective treatment). Record on care plan
 (c) Determine plasma or capillary glucose level in any patient exhibiting symptomatology
 (d) Provide 10 to 20 g of carbohydrate if hypoglycemia occurs. The following contain 15 g
 (1) 4 oz sweetened carbonated beverage
 (2) 4 oz unsweetened fruit juice
 (3) 1 tablespoon honey
 (4) 1 cup skim milk
 (5) Glucose gels or tablets (see package directions for amount)
 (e) Provide parenteral source of glucose if patient is unable to swallow
 (1) Intravenous glucose (50%)
 (2) Glucagon (intramuscularly or subcutaneously); will not be effective in patients with depleted liver glycogen stores
 (f) Inform physician of episode
 (g) Observe patient closely until completely recovered
 (h) Remeasure glucose level 20 to 30 minutes after treatment. Treat again if necessary
 (i) Assess cardiovascular and neurologic systems during and after the episode. Hypoglycemia has the potential for causing dysrhythmias and extending infarcts
 (j) After acute episode is corrected, supply additional nutrients to avoid recurrence (milk or cheese and crackers, or intravenous glucose if necessary)

    (k) Institute measures to correct the cause of the episode

    (l) Instruct patient who is receiving insulin or oral hypoglycemic agents on the signs and symptoms of hypoglycemia and the need to report such promptly to the nurse

    (m) Plan interventions to prevent hypoglycemia

        (1) Monitor trends in glucose values and confer with physician regarding dose adjustments

        (2) Schedule diagnostic studies and procedures to avoid meal or snack interruptions

        (3) Inform physician of a decrease in patient's appetite

        (4) Note worsening of renal insufficiency. Confer with physician regarding dose adjustment

    (n) Prolonged interventions will be necessary for patient on chlorpropamide who is recovering from hypoglycemia

    (o) Maintain flow sheet. Document food intake, plasma or capillary glucose levels, and diabetes-related medications

  iv. Evaluation of nursing care

    (a) Plasma/capillary glucose is within normal range

    (b) Absence of signs and symptoms of hypoglycemia

    (c) Patient is able to state three symptoms of hypoglycemia

    (d) Patient is able to state need to immediately notify the nurse if hypoglycemia is suspected

b. Potential knowledge deficit regarding hypoglycemia management and prevention

  i. Assessment for defining characteristics

    (a) Patient/family request information regarding causes, symptoms, treatment, and prevention of hypoglycemia

    (b) Patient is unable to state causes, symptoms, treatment, and prevention of hypoglycemia

    (c) Precipitating event for hypoglycemic episode suggests patient/family have inadequate knowledge of hypoglycemia and its management

  ii. Expected outcome

    (a) Patient/family are able to state causes, symptoms, treatment, and prevention of hypoglycemia

  iii. Nursing interventions

    (a) Instruct patient and family in causes, symptoms, treatment, and prevention of hypoglycemia

    (b) If patient was admitted because of a severe hypoglycemic episode, secure data regarding possible precipitating factors

        (1) Home medication dosage

        (2) Food, fluid, and alcohol intake prior to admission

        (3) Past experience with hypoglycemia—causes, symptoms, and most effective treatment

(4) Results of recent home blood glucose testing

(5) Activity level before admission

(6) Any recent decline in renal function

(7) Other medications taken at home

(8) Appearance of insulin injection sites (hypertrophy)

(9) Insulin administration technique

(10) Recent change in species of insulin preparation

(c) Document findings regarding possible precipitating factors and share with physician

(d) If precipitating factors point to self-care knowledge or skill deficit, or to noncompliance, refer to agency's diabetes educator

(e) If patient exhibits impaired counterregulation or hypoglycemia unawareness, consider instructing family on use of glucagon

(f) Urge patient to wear medical identification

(g) Urge patient to carry simple carbohydrate at all times

(h) Reinforce the importance of performing home blood glucose monitoring

iv. Evaluation of nursing care

(a) Patient/family are able to identify two causes of hypoglycemia

(b) Patient/family are able to state four symptoms of hypoglycemia

(c) Patient/family are able to state type and amount of three different foods that may be used to treat hypoglycemia

(d) Patient/family are able to state the importance of carrying simple carbohydrate at all times

(e) Family is able to describe when and how to use glucagon

(f) Patient/family are able to state three measures to prevent hypoglycemia

(g) Patient/family are able to perform home blood glucose monitoring

References

Alberti, K., Gill, G., and Elliott, M.: Insulin delivery during surgery in the diabetic patient. Diabetes Care 5 (suppl 1):65–77, 1982.

Aron, D.: Endocrine complications of the acquired immunodeficiency syndrome. Arch. Intern. Med. 149:330–333, 1989.

Boehm, T.: Hyperglycemia in critical care medicine. Crit. Care Q. 6:43–60, 1983.

Bornemann, M., and Holfedt, F.: Insulin-induced hypoglycemia in type I diabetics. Diabetes Educ. 10:13–16, 1984.

Buckalew, V.: Hyponatremia: Pathogenesis and management. Hosp. Pract. 21:49–58, 1986.

Burtis, W., Wu, T., Insogna, K., and Stewart, A.: Humoral hypercalcemia of malignancy. Ann. Intern. Med. 108:454–457, 1988.

Butts, D.: Fluid and electrolyte disorders associated with diabetic ketoacidosis and hyperglycemic hyperosmolar nonketotic coma. Nurs. Clin. North Am. 22:827–836, 1987.

Byyny, R.: Preventing adrenal insufficiency during surgery. Postgrad. Med. 67:219–225, 1980.

Clements, R., and Vourganti, B.: Fatal diabetic ketoacidosis: Major causes and approaches to their prevention. Diabetes Care 1:314–325, 1978.

Cooper, D., and Ridgway, E.: Clinical management of patients with hyperthyroidism. Med. Clin. North Am. 69:953–971, 1985.

Evangelisti, J., and Thorpe, C.: Thyroid storm: A nursing crisis. Heart Lung 12:184–193, 1983.

Felig, P., Baxter, J., Broadus, A., and Frohman, L.: Endocrinology and Metabolism. McGraw-Hill Book Co., New York, 1987.

Fisher, K., Lees, J., and Newman, J.: Hypoglycemia in hospitalized patients. N. Engl. J. Med. 315:1245–1250, 1986.

Germon, K.: Fluid and electrolyte problems associated with diabetes insipidus and syndrome of inappropriate antidiuretic hormone. Nurs. Clin. North Am. 22:785–796, 1987.

Gilliland, P.: Endocrine emergencies. Postgrad. Med. 74:215–226, 1983.

Gotch, P.: Hyperglycemic crisis: A standard care plan. Dimens. Crit. Care Nurs. 2:262–270, 1983.

Gotch, P.: Teaching patients about adrenal corticosteroids. Am. J. Nurs. 81:78–81, 1981.

Greenspan, F., and Forsham, P.: Basic and Clinical Endocrinology. Lange Medical Publications, Los Altos, Calif., 1986.

Hamburger, S.: Diagnosis and management of diabetic ketoacidosis: Selected aspects. Crit. Care Q. 2:53–60, 1979.

Hamburger, S., and Rush, D.: Syndrome of inappropriate secretion of antidiuretic hormone. Crit. Care Q. 3:119–129, 1980.

Havlin, C., and Cryer, P.: Hypoglycemia: The limiting factor in the management of insulin-dependent diabetes mellitus. Diabetes Educ. 14:407–411, 1988.

Hellman, R.: The evaluation and management of hyperthyroid crises. Crit. Care Q. 3:77–92, 1980.

Husband, D., Alberti, K., and Julian, D.: Methods for the control of diabetes after acute myocardial infarction. Diabetes Care 8:261–267, 1985.

Johndrow, P., and Thornton, S.: Syndrome of inappropriate antidiuretic hormone. Focus Crit. Care 12:29–34, 1985.

Johnson, D.: Metabolic and endocrine alterations in the multiply injured patient. Crit. Care Nurse Q. 11:35–41, 1988.

Johnson, D.: Pathophysiology of thyroid storm: Nursing implications. Crit. Care Nurse 3:80–86, 1983.

Johnston, J.: Management of diabetic ketoacidosis. Clin. Diabetes 3:121–123, 1985.

Jordan, R.: Endocrine emergencies. Med. Clin. North Am. 57:1193–1213, 1983.

Kenner, C., Guzzetta, C., and Dossey, B.: Critical Care Nursing: Body–Mind–Spirit. Little, Brown & Co., Boston, 1985.

Kitabchi, A., Matteri, R., and Murphy, M.B.: Optimal insulin delivery systems in diabetic ketoacidosis and hyperglycemic hyperosmolar nonketotic coma. Diabetes Care 5 (suppl. 1):78–87, 1982.

Kitabchi, A., and Murphy, M.B.: Diabetic ketoacidosis and hyperosmolar hyperglycemic nonketotic coma. Med. Clin. North Am. 72:1545–1563, 1988.

Klein, I., Trzepacz, P., Roberts, M., and Levey, G.: Symptom rating scale for assessing hyperthyroidism. Arch. Intern. Med. 148:387–390, 1988.

Kyner, J.: Diabetic ketoacidosis. Crit. Care Q. 3:65–75, 1980.

Ladenson, P., Levin, A., Ridgway, E., and Daniels, G.: Complications of surgery in hypothyroid patients. Am. J. Med. 77:261–266, 1984.

Lancaster, L.: Renal and endocrine regulation of water and electrolyte balance. Nurs. Clin. North Am. 22:761–772, 1987.

Matz, R.: Hyperosmolar nonacidotic uncontrolled diabetes: Not a rare event. Clin. Diabetes 6:25–30, 1988.

McMillan, J.: Preventing myxedema coma in the hypothyroid patient. Dimens. Crit. Care Nurs. 7:136–144, 1988.

Meek, J.: Myxedema coma. Crit. Care Q. 3:131–137, 1980.

Moses, A., and Notman, D.: Diabetes insipidus and syndrome of inappropriate antidiuretic hormone secretion. Adv. Intern. Med. 27:73–100, 1982.

Moss, J., and DeLawter, D.W.: Diabetic ketoacidosis: Effective low-cost treatment in a community hospital. Pract. Diabetol. 7:3–9, 1988.

Nicoloff, J.: Thyroid storm and myxedema coma. Med. Clin. North Am. 69:1005–1017, 1985.

Niedringhaus, L.: A nursing emergency . . . Acute adrenal crisis. Focus Crit. Care 10:31–36, 1983.

Oliver, R., and Jamison, R.: Diabetes insipidus: A physiologic approach to diagnosis. Postgrad. Med. 68:120–131, 1980.

Peden, N., Braaten, J., and McKendry, R.: Diabetic ketoacidosis during long-term treatment with continuous subcutaneous insulin infusion. Diabetes Care 7:1–5, 1984.

Poyss, A.: Assessment and nursing diagnosis in fluid and electrolyte disorders. Nurs. Clin. North Am. 22:773–783, 1987.

Rosenstock, J., and Raskin, P.: Surgery: Practical guidelines for diabetes management. Clin. Diabetes Rev. 1:181–188, 1987.

Sanford, S.: Dysfunction of the adrenal gland: Physiologic considerations and nursing problems. Nurs. Clin. North Am. 15:481–498, 1980.

Schade, D., and Eaton, R.P.: Pathogenesis of diabetic ketoacidosis: A reappraisal. Diabetes Care 2:296–306, 1979.

Schade, D., and Eaton, R.P.: Prevention of diabetic ketoacidosis. JAMA 242:2455–2458, 1979.

Schimke, R.: Adrenal insufficiency. Crit. Care Q. 3:19–27, 1980.

Schira, M.: Steroid-dependent states and adrenal insufficiency: Fluid and electrolyte disturbances. Nurs. Clin. North Am. 22:837–841, 1987.

Skillman, T.: Diabetic ketoacidosis. Heart Lung 7:594–602, 1978.

Slag, M., Morley, J., Elson, M., Crowson, L., Nuttall, F., and Shafer, R.: Hypothyroxinemia in critically ill patients as a predictor of high mortality. JAMA 245:43–45, 1981.

Sneid, D.: Hyperosmolar hyperglycemic non-ketotic coma. Crit. Care Q. 3:29–43, 1980.

Spaulding, S., and Lippes, H.: Hyperthyroidism: Causes, clinical features and diagnosis. Med. Clin. North Am. 69:937–951, 1985.

Sterns, R.: Severe symptomatic hyponatremia: Treatment and outcome. Ann. Intern. Med. 107:656–664, 1987.

Tibaldi, J., Barzel, U., Albin, J., and Surks, M.: Thyrotoxicosis in the very old. Am. J. Med. 81:619–622, 1986.

Tzagournis, M.: Acute adrenal insufficiency. Heart Lung 7:603–609, 1978.

Urbanic, R., and Mazzaferri, E.: Thyrotoxic crisis and myxedema coma. Heart Lung 7:435–447, 1978.

Wake, M., and Bresinger, J.: The nurse's role in hypothyroidism. Nurs. Clin. North Am. 15:453–467, 1980.

Watts, N., Gebhart, S., Clark, R., and Phillips, L.: Postoperative management of diabetes mellitus: Steady-state glucose control with bedside algorithm for insulin adjustment. Diabetes Care 10:722–728, 1987.

Wilson, J., and Foster, D.: Williams Textbook of Endocrinology, 7th ed. W.B. Saunders Co., Philadelphia, 1985.

Winters, B.: Nursing implications of hyperosmolar coma. Heart Lung 12:439–446, 1983.

Zucher, A., and Chernow, B.: Diabetes insipidus and the syndrome of inappropriate antidiuretic hormone release. Crit. Care Q. 6:63–74, 1983.

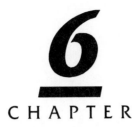

CHAPTER

The Hematologic System

Bonnie Mowinski Jennings, R.N., D.N.Sc. LTC, AN

PHYSIOLOGIC ANATOMY

Bone Marrow

1. **Bone marrow is the production site** of erythroid, myeloid, thrombocytic, and some lymphoid components of the blood as well as platelets
   a. Several different morphologically distinct cells evolve during the maturation process (Fig. 6–1)
   b. Only certain differentiated cells will be discussed here. The reader should consult a hematology text for more complete details
2. **Average adult has 3 kg of bone marrow,** or 30 to 50 ml of bone marrow per kilogram of body weight; about half is active in hematopoiesis while the other half is adipose and vascular tissue
3. **Location of bone marrow**
   a. Most is in the shafts of long bones because of their size, but it is not usually functional. During periods of increased demand (i.e., hemorrhage, hemolysis), active hematopoietic production may recur in long bones
   b. In adults, the functioning marrow is in vertebrae, skull, ilium, clavicle, ribs, sternum, pelvic and shoulder girdles, and proximal epiphyses of long bones
4. **Blood cell development**
   a. All blood cells originate from pluripotential stem cells (also known as colony-forming units)

The opinions or assertions in this chapter represent the views of the author and are not to be construed as official or as reflecting the views of the Department of the Army or the Department of Defense.

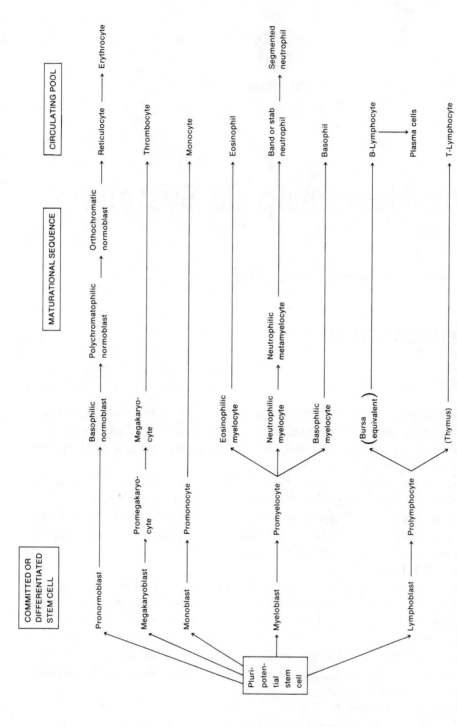

Figure 6–1. Theory of formation and maturation of blood cells (hematopoiesis). (Reproduced with permission from Price, S., and Wilson, L.: Pathophysiology, 2nd ed. New York, McGraw-Hill Book Co., 1986; copyrighted by The C. V. Mosby Co., St. Louis.)

b. Pluripotential stem cells become unipotential stem cells, which are committed to differentiating into the various cell lines; each cell line appears to have its own specific unipotential stem cell

Lymphatic Tissue

1. **Lymph:** pale, yellow interstitial fluid that diffuses through lymphatic capillary walls; increases when interstitial pressure rises, thus forcing more fluid into the lymph system
    a. Returns proteins and fat from the gastrointestinal tract and certain hormones to the blood
    b. Reduces edema by returning excess interstitial fluid to the blood
    c. Compared with blood, lymph
        i. Also contains lymphocytes, granulocytes, enzymes, and antibodies
        ii. Is deficient in erythrocytes, platelets, and fibrinogen
        iii. Coagulates very slowly
2. **Lymphatic capillaries** are thin-walled, endothelially lined vessels that are somewhat larger than blood capillaries; they are irregular in diameter
3. **Lymphatic vessels** (formed by lymphatic capillaries)
    a. Ultimately carry all lymph either to right lymphatic duct or to thoracic duct
    b. Do not supply nonvascular structures (e.g., cartilage)
4. **Lymph ducts**
    a. Right lymphatic duct: short duct formed by several tributaries that carry lymph from right side of head, neck, and thorax; right upper extremity; right lung; right side of heart; and right, upper surface of diaphragm
    b. Thoracic duct: largest of all lymphatic ducts; carries lymph from all other parts of the body
    c. Large ducts drain into subclavian veins and return lymph to blood circulation
5. **Lymph nodes:** small, flat, round-to-bean-shaped organs of varying sizes located along lymph vessels. Internally, they have a spongelike structure through which granulocytes, macrophages, and lymphocytes pass and return to the blood
    a. Sites of some B- and T-lymphocyte distribution and production
    b. Filter bacteria and foreign particles carried by lymph
    c. Distribution: found throughout body, both superficial and deep. Superficial nodes can be palpated; deep nodes must be visualized on radiographic examination
        i. Head and neck
            (a) Superficial—preauricular, posterior auricular, occipital,

tonsillar, submental, superior cervical, posterior cervical, supraclavicular
    (b) Deep—submaxillary, deep cervical, infraclavicular
    ii. Upper extremities: all superficial
        (a) Axillary—lateral, central, subscapular (posterior), pectoral (anterior)
        (b) Epitrochlear
    iii. Mediastinal: all deep
    iv. Abdominal: both superficial and deep
    v. Lower extremities: all superficial—inguinal, femoral, popliteal
6. **Thymus**
    a. Pink-gray, flat, bilobed gland located in the anterosuperior mediastinum below the thyroid
    b. Size changes with age: grows rapidly during fetal development until 2 years of age, then grows slowly until puberty, after which it slowly involutes
    c. Each lobe is packed with lymphocytes that are most dense in the cortex
    d. Very vascular with a unique three-layered structure. For lymphocytes to leave the thymus, they must pass through a barrier composed of an epithelial sheath, connective tissue space, and endothelium. Material entering the thymus must cross through the same layered barrier in reverse order
    e. Controls cellular immunity and most T-lymphocyte function and production
7. **Bone marrow:** produces lymphocytes
8. **Spleen**
    a. White pulp (lymphoid) compartment contains immunoglobulin-synthesizing cells that produce antibodies
    b. Primarily concerned with humoral immunity and B-lymphocyte function

Erythrocyte Production and Destruction

1. **Erythrocyte series:** developmental line of red blood cells (RBCs) leading to mature RBCs (see Fig. 6–1)
    a. Reticulocytes: erythrocyte precursors useful in assessing erythrocyte production (normally 1% to 2% in peripheral blood)
        i. Capable of maturing into erythrocytes within 24 to 48 hours of release into circulation
        ii. Increased numbers of reticulocytes (reticulocytosis) indicates increased bone marrow activity, usually indicating increased blood loss (gastrointestinal hemorrhage) or hemolysis
    b. Erythrocytes: mature cells, released to circulation because storage capacity of bone marrow is limited. Normal life span is 120 days

    c. Primary task of RBCs is to transport oxygen from the lungs to the tissues; RBCs also help maintain acid–base balance through a series of intracellular buffers

    d. RBC membrane: composed of two structures

        i. Innermost structure: a thick and spongelike substance to which hemoglobin attaches

        ii. Outer membrane: a thin, pliable substance on which antigens for major blood groups A, B, and Rh are located (absence of antigenic material results in blood group O)

2. **Erythropoiesis:** production of RBCs; requires energy

    a. Regulation

        i. Largely determined by relationship of cellular oxygen requirements and general metabolic activity

        ii. Stimulated by hypoxemia

        iii. Production controlled by erythropoietin, a hormone synthesized in the kidney

    b. Nutritional requirements

        i. Nutrients (iron, vitamin B_{12}, folic acid) are necessary for erythrocyte and hemoglobin synthesis

        ii. Deficiencies in nutrients result in decreased erythropoiesis and lack of maturation of erythrocytes

    c. Hemoglobin synthesis (hemoglobin is the major component of RBCs): takes place in bone marrow

        i. Iron and a specific porphyrin molecule combine to form the heme molecule; heme then combines with globin, another protein

        ii. Many different types of globin are responsible for producing the different varieties of hemoglobin: some common types are normal adult hemoglobin (HbA); fetal hemoglobin (HbF), which can be fully saturated with oxygen at a lower partial pressure; and the hemoglobin unique to sickle cell disease (HbS)

3. **Hemolysis:** destruction of RBCs; can occur extravascularly or intravascularly

    a. Destruction of immature RBCs occurs in either bone marrow itself or other hematopoietic organs, primarily the liver and spleen (i.e., culling and pitting effect of spleen removes misshapen erythrocytes from circulation; it also removes unwanted parts of RBCs, returning altered and undamaged cells to circulation)

    b. Destruction of senescent RBCs occurs in the liver and spleen

    c. Extravascular hemolysis: removal of normal and abnormal RBCs; occurs in organs with large numbers of reticuloendothelial cells (e.g., spleen, liver) and, to some extent, bone marrow

    d. Intrinsic mechanisms resulting in premature destruction of erythrocytes

      i. RBC membrane abnormalities such as paroxysmal nocturnal hemoglobinuria

      ii. Hemoglobin abnormalities such as HbS in sickle cell disease

      iii. Abnormal metabolic factors intrinsic to the erythrocyte: most commonly glycolytic enzymatic defects such as glucose-6-phosphate dehydrogenase (G6PD)

  e. Extrinsic factors contributing to premature destruction of erythrocytes

      i. Physical trauma (e.g., heart valves)

      ii. Antibodies

      iii. Infectious agents and toxins

  f. Hematopoietic cells catabolize hemoglobin released from erythrocytes that have been destroyed in the spleen. The iron is then returned to the bone marrow for reuse

  g. Erythrocyte destruction increases bilirubin production

Leukocytes: The Phagocytic and Immunologic Systems

1. **Granulocytes (myeloid series):** also known as polymorphonuclear leukocytes (PMNs or polys); have large, easily stained, visible granules in their cytoplasm; active phagocytes (see Fig. 6–1)

  a. Neutrophils

      i. Largest component of circulating white blood cell (WBC) mass (39% to 79%)

      ii. Most actively phagocytic of the granulocytes

      iii. Production

        (a) Originate from precursor cells in the bone marrow. Bone marrow reserve is about ten times the quantity of neutrophils in tissues and body cavities

        (b) Immature form—known as "bands"

          (1) Lack complete phagocytic ability

          (2) Increase in bands in the circulation is a characteristic response to an acute infection

          (3) Shift to the left—the standard laboratory procedure for reporting WBCs is in order of maturity, with less mature forms of WBCs usually printed on the left side of the written report. Hence, the presence of immature cells, either bands or even earlier WBC precursors commonly seen in severe infections, is referred to as a shift to the left

        (c) Mature form—known as segmented neutrophils or "segs"

          (1) Phagocytic; active in inflammation and tissue damage

          (2) Once mature, neutrophils are released into the blood for distribution to the tissues; they are either in the circulating granulocyte pool (CGP) or marginal gran-

ulocyte pool (MGP), where they adhere to walls of capillaries

(d) Neutropenia—condition in which circulating neutrophil values are reduced below normal

(e) Neutrophilia—condition in which circulating neutrophils are present in larger than normal amounts

iv. Destruction

(a) Lost from the blood via the gastrointestinal tract, pulmonary secretions, urine, mouth, and into the tissues

(b) Movement into the tissues is stimulated by pathogens or antigen–antibody reactions or inflammation of any kind

b. Eosinophils

i. Comprise 0% to 5% of the WBC mass

ii. Weak phagocytic activity; strong chemotactic response in detoxifying allergens

iii. Production

(a) Increased in allergic conditions, parasitic infections, drug reactions, and infections

(b) Eosinophilia—when eosinophils are present in larger than normal numbers

(c) Use of corticosteroids can greatly reduce the number of eosinophils

c. Basophils

i. Comprise 0% to 2% of granulocytes

ii. The granules in these cells contain heparin and histamine, which are important in that they both prevent clot formation and play a vital role in systemic allergic reactions

iii. Production: increased in allergic responses, hypersensitivity reactions, chronic inflammation, and some myeloproliferative disorders

2. **Mononuclear phagocytes (monocytes and macrophages):** like granulocytes, these WBCs are also phagocytic (see Fig. 6–1)

a. Monocytes

i. Comprise 3% to 8% of circulating leukocytes

ii. Most monocytes leave the circulation and become tissue macrophages

iii. Have phagocytic activity (ability to capture foreign material or antigens) in response to inflammation and chemotactic stimuli

iv. Corticosteroids diminish the function of monocytes

b. Macrophages

i. Long life span: possibly months or years

ii. Have greater phagocytic ability than PMNs or monocytes

iii. Fixed macrophages (histiocytes)

(a) Located within body structures: bone marrow, Kupffer cells of liver, lung, lymph nodes, and the spleen (the spleen contains more macrophages per gram of tissue than any other organ)

 (b) Phagocytize microorganisms as well as cellular and non-cellular debris

 iv. Free or mobile macrophages

  (a) Found at sites of inflammation and in peritoneal, pleural, and synovial fluids

  (b) Migrate as monocytes from blood through endothelial membrane of vascular system to trap and localize material for phagocytosis

  (c) Work with lymphocytes during immune responses

3. **Lymphocytes (lymphoid series):** the immune component of WBCs; responsible for cellular and humoral immunity (the latter is involved with antibody production) (see Fig. 6–1)

 a. Comprise 10% to 40% of the WBC mass

 b. Development of the immune system

  i. Multipotential, undifferentiated stem cells exist in the fetus; they develop in several distinct ways depending on the kind of specialized epithelia they contact

  ii. The epithelia of the thymus and bursa equivalents in humans (now believed to be in the bone marrow) provide the environment for differentiation (Fig. 6–2)

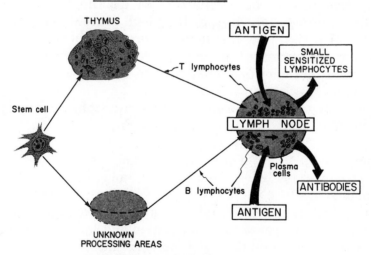

Figure 6–2. Formation of antibodies and sensitized lymphocytes by a lymph node in response to antigens. This figure also shows the origin of *thymic* (T) and *bursal* (B) lymphocytes that are responsible for the cell-mediated and humoral immune processes of the lymph nodes. (From Guyton, A. C.: Textbook of Medical Physiology, 6th ed. W. B. Saunders Co., Philadelphia, 1981, p. 75.)

    iii. Lymphoid stem cells that migrate through the thymus differentiate into specialized thymus-dependent lymphocytes, known as T lymphocytes, or T cells. These cells mediate cellular immune responses

    iv. Lymphoid stem cells that mature via the bursa differentiate into thymus-independent, bursa-equivalent lymphocytes known as B lymphocytes or B cells that further differentiate into plasma cells. Plasma cells produce antibodies, known as immunoglobulins, that mediate humoral immunity

c. Types of lymphocytes

    i. T lymphocytes: mediate cellular immunity

      (a) Comprise 65% to 85% of all lymphocytes

      (b) Sensitized on recognizing foreign tissue by antigen receptors on the T-lymphocyte surface, therefore must be developed by each person

      (c) More resistant to radiation, corticosteroids, and certain chemical immunosuppressants than B lymphocytes

      (d) Functional subtypes have been identified

        (1) Cytoxic or killer T lymphocytes kill target cells directly or indirectly by producing lymphokines

        (2) Helper T lymphocytes produce lymphokines and assist B lymphocytes with antibody production

        (3) Suppressor T lymphocytes modulate the overall immune system by diminishing B-lymphocyte and possibly T-lymphocyte activity

        (4) Memory T lymphocytes—respond to challenges by previously enountered (familiar) antigens

    ii. B lymphocytes: mediate humoral immunity

      (a) Comprise up to 35% of circulating lymphocytes; B-lymphocyte concentrations are higher in tissues

      (b) Immunity can be transferred by serum; surface receptors are present on B lymphocytes that regulate immune response to certain antigens; they also affect histocompatibility genes that regulate synthesis of antigens important to successful tissue transplantation

    iii. Plasma cells: activated or sensitized B lymphocytes

      (a) Fully differentiated B lymphocytes that produce antibodies (immunoglobulins) in the presence of antigen

      (b) Synthesize and release all classes of immunoglobulins (antibodies)

    iv. Null cells

      (a) The remainder of the lymphocytes. These cells lack distinctive markers for classification

      (b) Usually 10% or less of lymphocytes

      (c) Natural killer cells are an example of null cells and are important in the body's immune response to cancer. These cells do not need prior exposure to antigens for activation

4. **Cellular immunity** (T-lymphocyte mediated, delayed hypersensitivity reactions)
   a. Develops more slowly than reactions mediated by antibodies
   b. T lymphocytes are programmed to recognize a person's own tissue (basis of rejection phenomenon); immunity resides in the cell itself
   c. T lymphocytes, once exposed to a foreign substance, are sensitized to recognize those foreign antigens ("memory")
   d. When a foreign antigen enters the body, it attracts circulating T lymphocytes; the T lymphocytes surround the antigen and interact with it, thus becoming sensitized
   e. T lymphocytes release soluble proteins called lymphokines, substances that act as mediators of the cellular immune response. Examples of lymphokines are
      i. Mediators that affect macrophages
         (a) Chemotactic factors—attract macrophages and granulocytes to area of antigen
         (b) Migration inhibition factor (MIF)—prevents migration of macrophages from the area of the antigen
         (c) Macrophage activation factor (MAF)—enhances functioning of macrophages
      ii. Mediators that affect lymphocytes
         (a) Transfer factor (TF)—changes nonsensitized T lymphocytes to sensitized T lymphocytes
         (b) Interleukin-2 (IL-2)—promotes antibody production by B lymphocytes and acts on other lymphocytes
      iii. Mediators that affect tissue cells
         (a) Lymphotoxin (LT)—assists in antigen destruction
         (b) Interferon—interferes with viral growth
   f. Clinical manifestations of cellular immunity
      i. Cutaneous delayed hypersensitivity
      ii. Contact allergy
      iii. Immunity to intracellular parasites: viruses, protozoa, fungi
      iv. Allograft rejection
      v. Graft-versus-host disease
      vi. Tumor immunity and immune surveillance
      vii. Autoimmune diseases (related to decreased levels of T-suppressor lymphocytes)
5. **Humoral immunity:** involves B-lymphocyte recognition of specific antigens
   a. Antibody (immunoglobulin) response
      i. Complex process in which macrophages and helper T lymphocytes are also involved
      ii. When antigen is recognized, B lymphocytes are activated, thus

becoming plasma cells; plasma cells make antigen-specific antibodies (immunoglobulins)

    iii. Antibody levels are not as high after the first encounter with an antigen as they are after the second exposure (anamnestic response)

b. Immunoglobulins (antibodies)

    i. IgG: the major immunoglobulin in humans (75% of total); circulates in fluid and tissues

        (a) Major influence is against bacterial disease; some effect on viruses and fungi

        (b) Functions in anamnestic responses (i.e., those that have immunologic memory from prior encounters with antigens)

        (c) Is major immunoglobulin in commercial gamma globulin

        (d) Is able to cross placenta, providing early form of natural immunity for newborns (until 6 months)

    ii. IgA: 15% of total; found on mucosal surfaces of the respiratory, genitourinary, and gastrointestinal tracts

        (a) Present in most body secretions

        (b) Prevents adherence of antigens to the mucosal surface

    iii. IgM: 10% of total; located intravascularly

        (a) Like IgG, IgM is most influential against bacterial disease with some effect on viral disease

        (b) First antibody formed following exposure to an antigen, but its concentration diminishes rapidly as that of IgG increases

        (c) Does not cross placenta; an elevation of IgM in newborns indicates a viral or bacterial intrauterine infection or mother/child (ABO) incompatibility

    iv. IgD: 1% of total

        (a) Activates B lymphocytes to plasma cells, the key immunoglobulin-producing cell

        (b) Major surface immunoglobulin of peripheral blood lymphocytes

    v. IgE: 0.002% of total; attaches to most cells that are responsible for symptoms of allergic reactions such as the so-called wheal-flare reaction

c. Blood groups: systems to describe type of antigens on surface of RBCs

    i. ABO system

        (a) Basis of four blood groups (phenotypes), depending on presence or absence of A and B antigens

        (b) Antibodies that react with A or B antigens are found when the corresponding antigen is absent from RBC surface

(B antibodies are found in group A blood because B antigens are absent)
- (c) The four ABO blood groups are
  - (1) O—known as universal donor; genotype OO; has no A or B antigens on RBCs; serum contains both anti-A and anti-B antibodies; common in 47% of population
  - (2) A—genotypes AA and AO; has A antigens on RBCs; serum contains anti-B antibodies; common in 41% of population
  - (3) B—genotypes BB and BO; has B antigens on RBCs; serum contains anti-A antibodies; common in 9% of population
  - (4) AB—known as universal recipient; genotype AB; has both A and B antigens on RBCs; serum contains neither anti-A nor anti-B antibodies; common in 3% of population
- (d) Agglutination—basis for cross-matching blood; depends on presence of a serum antibody that reacts with antigens on RBCs
  - (1) Occurs in group A blood when B antigens are introduced, because anti-B antibodies react with B antigen
  - (2) Indicates incompatibility when RBCs of donor and recipient are exposed to one another
- ii. Rh-Hr system: includes several Rh antigens; most potent is RhD
  - (a) Historically, persons were considered Rh positive if their RBCs agglutinated when mixed with rabbit serum that had been immunized by RBCs of the rhesus monkey. Those whose blood did not agglutinate were considered to be Rh negative. Terms *Rh positive* and *Rh negative* imply presence or absence of D, respectively, because this is the most immunogenic of the Rh antigens
  - (b) Antibody acting against Rh-Hr antigen is not generally in serum. Antibody associated with A and B antigens is in serum
  - (c) Antibody against Rh-Hr antigen is formed when an Rh-negative person is sensitized to Rh-positive blood, usually as a result of transfusion therapy or maternal-fetal sensitization
- d. Cold agglutinins: antibodies that cause erythrocytes to coagulate when blood plasma temperature is below normal body temperature
  - i. Relatively rare disease found in patients with chronic autoimmune hemolytic anemia; usually associated with lymphoproliferative diseases and, occasionally, *Mycoplasma* infections, cirrhosis, severe anemia, hemolytic anemia, or chronic disease

ii. When receiving cold blood, patients with chronic illnesses should be observed carefully for symptoms of cell hemolysis resulting from incompatibility of recipient and donor cold agglutinins

iii. Bank blood must be warmed before administering to patients who have cold agglutinins. Do not overheat blood, as proteins may be denatured; therefore, temperature to which blood should be heated must be specifically ordered

e. Coombs' test

   i. Used to determine presence of hemolyzing antibodies (e.g., Rh factor antibodies in Rh-negative person)

  ii. Coombs' serum is prepared from rabbit serum sensitized against human globulins

 iii. Types of Coombs' tests

    (a) Direct—detects antibodies (IgG) attached to RBCs

    (b) Indirect—detects antibodies (IgG) in serum

6. Complement system: enzymatic reactions leading to antigen destruction by lysis

a. Consists of 20+ serum proteins (not antibodies); there are 11 principal proteins labeled C1 to C9 (C1 has three subunits)

b. The proteins can be activated or fixed in two ways

   i. Classic pathway: stimulated by antigen–antibody interaction resulting in multiple effects that help the body limit damage by the invading organism

    (a) Opsonization and phagocytosis—neutrophils and macrophages engulf the bacteria to which antigen–antibody complexes are attached

    (b) Lysis—rupture cell membrane of invading organism

    (c) Agglutination—changes in cell surface of invading organisms so they adhere to one another

    (d) Neutralization of viruses—reduce virulence of viruses

    (e) Chemotaxis—increased migration of neutrophils and macrophages to region of antigen

    (f) Activation of basophils—release of histamine to induce local tissue reactions that inactivate or immobilize the antigen

    (g) Inflammation—hyperemia, leakage of proteins and coagulation of proteins to prevent invading organism from moving through tissues

  ii. Alternate pathway

    (a) Activation of complement without antigen–antibody reaction

    (b) Slower process than classic pathway but is a first-line defense because it does not depend on an antigen–antibody reaction

      (c) The same final products are formed as in the classic pathway

7. **Consequences of immune responses**
   a. Immediate hypersensitivity reaction
      i. Cytotoxic: results in damage to a target cell because a complement-fixing antibody is directed against a surface antigen of that cell (e.g., acute hemolytic transfusion reaction)
      ii. Anaphylactic: antigen–antibody interaction results in chemical mediators acting at secondary sites (particularly smooth muscle and vascular tissue) producing hypotension and shock
   b. Subacute hypersensitivity reaction
      i. Depends on immune complex deposits, activation of complement, and infiltration of PMNs
      ii. Arthus lesions: a local skin reaction. Serum sickness results when reaction is systemic
   c. Delayed hypersensitivity reaction: mediates reactions such as those seen with tuberculin skin testing and allograft rejection

8. **Inflammation:** sequential tissue reaction to injury involving leukocytes; beneficial and desirable because it neutralizes the inflammatory agent, removes necrotic debris, and establishes a suitable environment for repair and healing. Events of inflammation occur chronologically as follows
   a. Vascular response
      i. Transient vasodilation of venules and immediate increase in vascular permeability. Helps leukocytes get to site of inflammation. Involves chemical mediators such as histamine, serotonin, and bradykinin
      ii. Increased capillary permeability, local increases in hydrostatic pressure, and increased oncotic pressure of proteins in interstitium lead to edema
   b. Cellular response
      i. Changes in blood flow and margination
         (a) As blood flow into inflamed area increases and fluid leaks into interstitium, blood becomes more viscous and flow slows within the affected area
         (b) Leukocytes leave the main circulation to marginate and stick along the blood vessel lining
      ii. Chemotaxis: an attractive force that is exerted on circulating WBCs to enhance leukocyte movement to the site of injury
      iii. Emigration: leukocytes (first neutrophils followed by monocytes and, much later, lymphocytes) emigrate through vessel walls in ameboid fashion passing through the junctions between endothelial cells
      iv. Phagocytosis: capturing antigens for presentation to lymphocytes; major function of neutrophils and macrophages; triggers

an immune response, helping to prevent or retard infectious agents from entering the host

    (a) Recognition—phagocytes distinguish foreign cells from normal autologous elements and attach to the foreign particles. Attachment is facilitated by various interactions at the cell membrane (i.e., electrical charge, serum proteins, receptor sites)

    (b) Engulfment—once foreign particles are recognized, phagocytes flow their pseudopods around the particle to be engulfed (i.e., bacteria). Eventually, the particle is taken into the phagocytes' cytoplasm where it is enveloped in a vesicle that pinches off from the cell membrane

    (c) Killing and degradation—killing is an energy-dependent event

        (1) Bacterial killing is accelerated in aerobic conditions, whereas phagocytosis does just as well in either an aerobic or anaerobic environment

        (2) Intracellular chemical events augment bacterial killing. Lactic acid accumulation can reduce pH to 4.0 or less. Bactericidal products from oxygen consumption (H_2O_2, superoxide hydroxyl radical) are generated

  v. Isolation of inflammatory process: may lead to abscess formation, thus limiting spread of microorganisms

    (a) Abscess is filled with pus that contains living bacteria and proteolytic enzymes that can digest dead and living tissue

    (b) Abscess may open by spontaneous rupture or by planned surgical incision and drainage

  c. Bone marrow response: release of more cells into circulation to keep up with the increased demand for neutrophils and macrophages

  d. Wound healing

    i. Regeneration: replacing lost cells and tissue with cells of the same type

    ii. Repair: replacing lost cells by connective tissue; usually results in scar formation; involves macrophages that clean up the debris and fibroblasts that patch the damage

Hemostatic Mechanisms

1. Vascular

  a. Reflex vasoconstriction: arteries constrict when cut, thus reducing blood flow to injury both by restricting vessel size and by pressing the endothelial surfaces together

  b. Larger vessels require collagen support for proper hemostasis. Defective collagen production results in increased capillary fragility

2. Platelets (also called *thrombocytes*; major function is hemostasis)

a. Production
   i. Site: bone marrow
   ii. Precursor cell: megakaryocyte
   iii. Circulating platelets comprise about two thirds of the total platelet mass; the other third is in extravascular sites such as the spleen
   iv. Life span is 9 to 12 days
   v. Regulation
      (a) Because of constancy in platelet count, a regulatory substance called thrombopoietin (like erythropoietin) is postulated
      (b) Also believed that platelet mass, rather than number, regulates production
      (c) Spleen is involved, but exact mechanism is not yet known
      (d) Iron is needed for normal thrombopoiesis
b. Destruction
   i. Spleen sequesters one third of all platelets
   ii. Survival is not predictable; therefore, both random destruction and senescence dictate fate
   iii. Platelet counts are expected to rise after splenectomy and with acute blood loss
c. Properties of platelets
   i. Adhesiveness: stickiness; ability to attach to blood vessel walls or other surfaces
   ii. Aggregation: adhering to one another, which leads to the ability to form clumps
d. Hemostatic response
   i. Drastic changes in platelet characteristics are activated by exposure to collagen in an injured vessel, which initiates a repetitious cycle that leads to platelet plug formation
   ii. Adherent platelets release adenosine diphosphate (ADP), which enhances aggregation
   iii. As platelets degranulate, they release substances (platelet factor 3, serotonin, epinephrine) that facilitate coagulation
   iv. Degranulation also stimulates release of adenosine diphosphate (ADP) that enhances adhesiveness and aggregation, thus augmenting platelet plug formation
e. Platelet performance: depends on
   i. Qualitative features—platelets need the proper characteristics to function (i.e., adhesiveness and aggregation). Drugs such as alcohol (ETOH), aspirin, and quinidine interfere with qualitative features
   ii. Quantitative features: sufficient numbers to do the job
      (a) Surgery can be tolerated with counts as low as $50,000/\mu l$

(b) Spontaneous hemorrhage may occur with values of 20,000 to 30,000/μl

(c) Intracerebral hemorrhages occur when count diminishes to 10,000/μl

f. Platelet disorders can be either acquired or congenital and either quantitative (increased or decreased in number) or qualitative (abnormal function)

g. Thrombocytopenia: decreased numbers of platelets. Major causes are

i. Diminished production of platelets from bone marrow lesions secondary to drugs, disease, or aplastic anemia

ii. Increased destruction of platelets from drug-induced (e.g., quinidine) antibodies, autoimmunity (e.g., idiopathic thrombocytopenic purpura [ITP]), viral disease, or disseminated intravascular coagulation (DIC)

iii. Hypersplenism: often secondary to portal hypertension; results in increased sequestration of platelets in spleen

h. Thrombocytosis: increased numbers of platelets (usually defined as more than 450,000/μl; may lead to excessive thrombosis or excessive bleeding due to abnormal functioning of an excessive number of platelets

3. **Plasma clotting factors:** lead to formation of a fibrin clot

a. Labeled with both Roman numerals and names (i.e., prothrombin and factor II are the same)

b. Consist of proteins, lipoproteins, and calcium

c. Produced in the liver (except factor VIII, the synthesis of which is poorly understood)

d. Factors II, VII, IX, and X are vitamin K dependent

e. Circulate in inactive form until stimulated to initiate clotting through one of two pathways. Once either pathway is stimulated, it progresses in a cascade sequence until activating the common pathway (Fig. 6–3)

f. Pathways that initiate clotting

i. Intrinsic system: initiated by contact activation following endothelial injury (i.e., "intrinsic" to the circulation itself)

(a) Factor XII initiates processes of intrinsic system when it contacts collagen in a damaged vessel wall

(b) Other components of the intrinsic system, in order, include several kinins, factors XI and IX, platelet factor 3, calcium, and factor VIII

ii. Extrinsic system: initiated by lipoproteins, known as tissue thromboplastin, which are released from injured tissue (i.e., "extrinsic" to the circulation)

(a) Factor VII is the plasma protein in the extrinsic system that converges with the common pathway

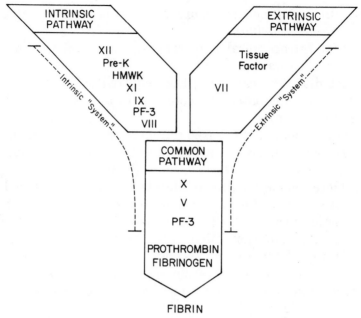

Figure 6–3. Pathways of coagulation. The terms *intrinsic system* and *extrinsic system* are widely used with reference to the reactions indicated by dashed lines. The following abbreviations are used: PF-3, platelet factor 3; Pre-K, prekallikrein; HMWK, high molecular weight kininogen. (From Wintrobe, M. M., et al.: Clinical Hematology, 8th ed. Lea & Febiger, Philadelphia, 1981, p. 418.)

      (b) Calcium ions must be present for the reaction to occur between tissue factor and factor VII

  g. Common pathway: that part of coagulation cascade that is activated by either the intrinsic or extrinsic pathway

     i. Platelet factor 3 (PF3) and calcium react with factors X and V to accelerate clotting and activate prothrombin

    ii. Prothrombin is converted to thrombin (most powerful enzyme in coagulation process) by prothrombin activator complex

    iii. Thrombin acts on fibrinogen to form soluble fibrin or fibrin monomer

    iv. Fibrin is essential portion of a clot; soluble until polymerized by factor XIII, which converts it to a stable (insoluble) fibrin clot

4. Anticoagulant mechanisms in normal system: to maintain blood in fluid state

  a. Fibrinolytic system: clot-lysing activities maintain blood in fluid state

     i. Plasminogen is inert precursor of plasmin

    ii. Plasmin works to lyse fibrin clots

      (a) Attacks either fibrin or fibrinogen

(b) Splits clots into smaller elements called fibrin split products (FSPs) or fibrin degradation products (FDPs)

   iii. FSPs: when increased, predispose patient to bleed

    (a) Destructive effect of FSPs on fibrin in platelet plug

    (b) Impair platelet aggregation, reduce prothrombin, and interfere with polymerization of fibrin

  b. Antithrombin system: defends against excessive clotting. For example, antithrombin III inactivates thrombin; it is synthesized by the liver

NURSING ASSESSMENT DATA BASE

Nursing History: Hematologic evaluation is very dependent on obtaining a thorough history

1. **Family history:** there is a known genetic influence in certain hematologic conditions, thus establishing familial patterns. May be positive for
   a. Jaundice
   b. Anemia
   c. Bleeding disorders: predisposition to bleed (as in hemophilia) and to clot (as in polycythemia)
   d. Malignancies
   e. Hereditary RBC dyscrasias such as sickle cell disease
2. **Patient health history**
   a. Surgery
      i. Splenectomy
      ii. Tumor removal
      iii. Prosthetic heart valves
      iv. Small bowel resection (duodenum is site of iron absorption) or partial or total gastrectomy (removes parietal cells, thus reducing intrinsic factor)
      v. Response to dental extractions
   b. Allergies
      i. Multiple transfusions with blood or blood products
      ii. Known allergies and allergic reactions (including anaphylaxis)
   c. Medical problems
      i. Anemia
      ii. Malabsorption syndrome
      iii. Mononucleosis
      iv. Liver or spleen disorders
      v. Recurrent infections
      vi. Problems with wound healing
      vii. Prolonged or excessive bleeding
      viii. Vitamin K deficiency

  d. Symptoms
    i. General: fatigue, weakness, headache, chills, fever, weight loss, heat intolerance, night sweats, poor wound healing, apathy, lethargy, malaise, pain
    ii. Specific
      (a) Skin—prolonged bleeding, bruising easily, petechiae, pruritus, jaundice, pallor, erythroderma, cyanosis, lesions
      (b) Eyes—visual disturbances, blindness
      (c) Ears—vertigo, tinnitus
      (d) Nasopharynx and mouth—epistaxis, dysphagia, gingival bleeding, sore tongue, persistent hoarseness
      (e) Neck—nuchal rigidity
      (f) Lymph nodes—swelling, tenderness
      (g) Chest—pulmonary emboli, exertional dyspnea, palpitations, angina pectoris, orthopnea, presence of prosthetic heart valves, respiratory tract infections, cough, hemoptysis, sternal tenderness, chest pain
      (h) Gastrointestinal—anorexia, abdominal fullness/belching, melena or hematochezia, hematemesis, liver disease, ulcers, abdominal pain, diarrhea, constipation, masses, alcohol abuse
      (i) Genitourinary—hematuria, menorrhagia, amenorrhea, bladder dysfunction, urinary tract infections
      (j) Nervous system—confusion, headache, ataxia, paresthesias, syncope, irritability, sensory loss, impaired consciousness
      (k) Back and extremities—pain in joints, back, shoulders, or bone

3. Social history and habits
  a. Exposure to radiation: occupational or multiple radiotherapy treatments
  b. Occupational exposure to chemicals (e.g., benzene, lead)
  c. Dietary
    i. May give insight to causes of erythrocyte deficiencies: iron, vitamin B_{12}, folic acid are provided by food and are needed for erythrocyte development
    ii. Alcohol consumption: calories are derived from ETOH, which may diminish desire for food, thus reducing intake of essential nutrients and vitamins. Liver damage from ETOH may affect clotting. ETOH may impair platelet function and RBC production
  d. Sexuality
    i. Sexual preference (i.e., same sex, bisexual)
    ii. Multiple partners
    iii. Safe sex practices
  e. Intravenous drug use

4. **Medication history**
    a. Agents used to treat existing hematologic conditions
        i. Erythrocyte problems: iron (oral and parenteral), vitamin B_{12}, pyridoxine, folic acid
        ii. Bleeding disorders: cryoprecipitate, anticoagulants
        iii. Antineoplastic agents
        iv. Antiviral agents
        v. Immune system reconstitution (i.e., interferon, interleukin-2)
    b. Agents used to treat nonhematologic problems that may exert a negative effect on bone marrow
        i. "Allergy" medication
        ii. Analgesics
            (a) Aspirin
            (b) Analgesics that contain aspirin (i.e., Ascodeen, Empirin, Empirin with Codeine, Percodan)
            (c) Anti-inflammatory agents—glucocorticoids (i.e., ACTH, prednisone), phenylbutazone (Butazolidin)
        iii. Antibiotics
            (a) Trimethoprim-sulfamethoxazole (Bactrim, Septra)
            (b) Chloramphenicol (Chloromycetin)
        iv. Anticonvulsant: carbamazepine (Tegretol)
        v. Antidysrhythmics: quindine sulfate, procainamide, phenytoin (Dilantin, also an anticonvulsant)
        vi. Antifungals: amphotericin B
        vii. Antihypertensives: methyldopa (Aldomet)
        viii. Antituberculins: p-aminosalicylic acid (PAS), isoniazid (INH)
        ix. Diuretics: chlorothiazide (Diuril)
        x. Immunosuppressives: azathioprine (Imuran)
        xi. Oral contraceptives and diethylstilbestrol
        xii. Sympathomimetics: epinephrine (Adrenalin)

Nursing Examination of Patient

1. **Inspection**
    a. Pallor or flushing of mucous membranes and palmar creases
    b. Pallor of nail beds and conjunctivae
    c. Cyanosis
    d. Jaundice of skin, sclera, mucous membranes (best evaluated in daylight)
    e. Bleeding
        i. Purpura, petechiae, ecchymoses
        ii. Mucosal bleeding
        iii. Gingival bleeding
        iv. Retinal hemorrhages and exudates
        v. Hemorrhage from any orifice

    f. Excoriated skin

    g. Leg ulcers

    h. Brownish skin discoloration

    i. Gingival and mucosal ulceration

    j. Tongue texture smooth: color may be beefy red

    k. Neuromuscular alterations

        i. Pain and touch sensation

        ii. Position and vibratory sensation

        iii. Tendon reflexes

2. Palpation

    a. Superficial lymph nodes: evaluate for

        i. Location

        ii. Size in centimeters

        iii. Tenderness

        iv. Fixation: movable or fixed

        v. Texture: hard, soft, or firm

    b. Sternal tenderness

    c. Rib tenderness

    d. Joint mobility and tenderness

    e. Bone tenderness

    f. Liver

    g. Spleen

3. Percussion

    a. Diaphragmatic excursion

    b. Hepatomegaly

    c. Splenomegaly

4. Auscultation

    a. Murmurs

    b. Bruits: carotid, cardiac, hepatic

    c. Rubs: pericardial, pleural, hepatic

    d. Tachycardia

    e. Widened pulse pressure

    f. Bowel sounds

Diagnostic Studies

1. Laboratory

    a. Blood

        i. Complete blood count (CBC) with differential and peripheral smear

            (a) RBC count

                (1) Count of the total number of circulating RBCs, the oxygen transporting component of the blood

                (2) Normal—females, 3.8 to 5.2 $\times$ $10^6/\mu l$; males, 4.4 to 5.9 $\times$ $10^6/\mu l$

     (3) Reduced in anemia and hemorrhage

     (4) Increased in chronic hypoxemia or at high altitudes

(b) Hemoglobin (Hb)

     (1) Measures the oxygen-carrying capacity of the erythrocyte and gives them their color

     (2) Normal—females, 11.7 to 15.7 g/dl; males, 13.3 to 17.7 g/dl

(c) Hematocrit (Hct)

     (1) Compares volume of RBCs with volume of plasma; measured as percent of total RBC volume

     (2) Normal—females, 34.9% to 46.9%; males, 39.8% to 52.2%

(d) Red cell indices

     (1) Mean corpuscular volume (MCV)—measures average size (volume) of RBCs. Normal—80 to 100 fl

     (2) Mean corpuscular hemoglobin (MCH)—measures the average weight of Hb in an RBC. Normal—26.6 to 34 pg

     (3) Mean corpuscular hemoglobin concentration (MCHC)—measures average percent (concentration) of Hb in a single RBC. Normal—31.4 to 36.3 g/dl

(e) Peripheral smear—enables more exact evaluation of blood cell size, shape, and composition. Especially useful in evaluating anemias

(f) WBC count

     (1) Measures total number of leukocytes

     (2) Normal—3,500 to 11,000/μl

        a) Elevated—leukocytosis

        b) Reduced—leukopenia

(g) Differential

     (1) Measures the percentage that each type WBC contributes to the total. Normal values are presented followed by the term for elevation of the WBC type

     (2) Neutrophils—39% to 79% (1500 to 7500/μl); neutrophilia; (The term *neutropenia* refers to a reduced number of cells; reduced values are primarily a concern with neutrophils because of their function and the amount they contribute to the total WBC count.)

     (3) Eosinophils—0% to 5% (0 to 500/μl); eosinophilia

     (4) Basophils—0% to 2% (0 to 200/μl); basophilia

     (5) Monocytes—3% to 8% (0 to 1000/μl); monocytosis

     (6) Lymphocytes—10% to 40% (1000 to 4500/μl); lymphocytosis

(h) Absolute counts of each type of leukocyte are more important than total and differential counts because each leukocyte type is a separate cell system with unique functions, controls, and responses to disease. Derive absolute counts by multiplying the percentage of the cell type by the total WBC count and dividing by 100

  (i) Platelet count—measures quantitative features (number of circulating platelets). Normal—150,000 to 400,000/μl

  ii. Reticulocyte count: reticulocytes are young RBCs; their count assesses the responsiveness and potential of the bone marrow to respond to bleeding or hemolysis. Normal—0.5% to 1.5% of RBC count

 iii. Erythrocyte sedimentation rate (ESR or sed rate)

   (a) Nonspecific, general screening test that measures amount of RBCs that settle in 1 hour. Normal—females, 1 to 20 mm/hr; males, 1 to 13 mm/hr

   (b) Elevated in many conditions, including acute and chronic inflammation, malignancy, myocardial infarction, end-stage renal disease

 iv. Bleeding time: time needed for a standard skin wound to stop bleeding; assesses platelet function. Normal—1 to 9.5 minutes

  v. Prothrombin time (PT): assesses the extrinsic coagulation system by measuring factor VII and the common pathway (X, V, II or prothrombin, and I or fibrinogen). (Prothrombin, VII, and X are vitamin K dependent and are depressed by oral anticoagulants.) Normal—12 to 15 seconds

 vi. Partial thromboplastin time (PTT): tests the intrinsic coagulation system by measuring the kinins, factors XII, XI, IX, and VIII, as well as the common pathway (prolonged by heparin). Normal—25 to 38 seconds

 vii. Thrombin time (TT): reflects time for thrombin to convert fibrinogen to a stable fibrin clot. When prolonged, coagulation is inadequate owing to decreased thrombin activity. Normal—10 to 15 seconds

viii. Fibrinogen: increased values may reflect a hypercoagulable state; elevation also occurs in inflammatory conditions. Decreased values reflect a predisposition to bleed. Normal—200 to 400 mg/dl

 ix. Fibrin split products (FSPs): a measure of the fibrinolytic system. When FSPs are elevated, fibrinolysis is excessive, which may lead to excessive bleeding. Normal—none, but 1 to 10 FSPs may be present without impairing coagulation

  x. Specific factor assays: measure amounts of each of the various plasma proteins (e.g., II, V, VII)

 xi. Serum protein electrophoresis: to assess immunoglobulins

 xii. Serum bilirubin: measures extent of RBC destruction or ability

of the liver to excrete. Indirect values rise with hemolytic disorders
- (a) Total—0.3 to 1.3 mg/dl
- (b) Direct—0.1 to 0.3 mg/dl
- (c) Indirect—0.1 to 1.0 mg/dl

xiii. Serum iron: reflects amount of iron (Fe) in serum. Normal—50 to 150 µg/dl

xiv. Total iron-binding capacity (TIBC): measures the level of transferrin, the serum protein that transports Fe. Normal—250 to 410 µ/dl

xv. Coombs' test: differentiates types of hemolytic anemias and detects immune antibodies
- (a) Direct—measures antibodies (IgG) attached to RBCs. Normal—negative
- (b) Indirect—measures antibodies (IgG) in the serum. Normal—negative

xvi. Blood typing

xvii. Rh factor determination

xviii. Human leukocyte antigens (HLA): genetically transmitted determinants of tissue histocompatibility; basically found on all cells in the body. Used clinically in tissue-typing for transplants, paternity testing, and diagnosing various diseases (e.g., ankylosing spondylitis, multiple sclerosis, myasthenia gravis, subacute thyroiditis, Hodgkin's disease, acute lymphocytic leukemia)

xix. T_4 cell count (helper cells): primary cell in immune system that is infected and killed by human immunodeficiency virus (HIV); important variable in staging HIV infections. Normal—800 cells/mm^3

xx. T_4/T_8 ratio (helper/suppressor T cell): intact immune system has more helper cells than suppressor cells; this ratio is reversed in persons with many conditions, including HIV infection. Normal—ratio of 1.8

xxi. HIV antibody screening (retrovirus test): to detect antibodies specific to HIV; only present if previously infected but absence does not rule out the viral infection because sufficient time must elapse following infection for antibodies to develop; does not indicate immunity as does antibody screening for polio; the antibody screen is *not* diagnostic for HIV
- (a) Enzyme-linked immunosorbent assay (ELISA)—subject to error; up to 10% false-positive results
- (b) Western blot—much more specific with lower incidence of error; part of Walter Reed classification system

b. Urine

i. Routine urinalysis

      ii. Bence Jones protein assay: electrophoretic detection of a small protein, Bence Jones, common in multiple myeloma. Normal—negative

      iii. Hematest

  c. Stool specimen for guaiac test

2. Radiologic

  a. Routine chest radiograph

  b. Radiographs of other areas as indicated by history and physical examination (e.g., spine, flat abdomen)

  c. Lymphangiography to visualize the lymph system radiographically after dye injection: useful in assessing retroperitoneal nodes

  d. Scans: liver/spleen or bone evaluation done radiographically after the injection of radioisotope; may also use computed tomography (CT) scans

3. Biopsies

  a. Bone marrow: aspiration and needle core biopsy of the fluid bone marrow for pathologic examination

  b. Lymph node: removal of lymph tissue for histologic study

4. Skin tests: serve as a barometer of immune functioning because they can manifest evidence of delayed hypersensitivity; defects in skin test response may be seen in later stages of HIV infection; complete absence of delayed hypersensitivity reactions is known as anergy

COMMONLY ENCOUNTERED NURSING DIAGNOSES

Activity Intolerance related to disease or treatment

1. Assessment for defining characteristics

  a. Reports of fatigue or weakness

  b. Abnormal vital signs; tachycardia or hypotension

  c. Exertional discomfort or dyspnea

  d. Inability to perform activities of daily living

  e. ECG changes (i.e., dysrhythmias or ischemia)

  f. Exertional discomfort or dyspnea

2. Expected outcomes

  a. Activity/rest pattern supports feelings of restedness

  b. Patient participates in activities of daily living (bathing, hygiene, dressing, grooming, feeding, toileting) to the greatest extent possible

  c. Vital signs are within an acceptable range of patient's baseline values

3. Nursing interventions

  a. Plan care to alternate periods of rest and activity; strive for a 1:3 rest/activity ratio

b. Assist patient with activities of daily living as needed
c. Place objects within patient's reach to reduce physiologic demands brought on by exertion
d. Reduce demands placed on patient (i.e., limit number of visitors, phone calls, surrounding noise, and repeated interruptions by hospital personnel)
e. Monitor vital signs as indicants of activity tolerance (e.g., pulse < 100; respirations $\leq$ 20)

4. **Evaluation of nursing care**
a. Patient expresses a sense of feeling rested
b. Vital signs remain within patient's normal limits
c. Patient's self-care needs are met
d. Activities involving grooming, toileting, feeding and bathing are completed without fatigue, tachycardia, or hypotension

Potential for Impaired Gas Exchange (i.e., hypoxemia) related to anemia, hemoglobin abnormalities, or blood loss

1. **Assessment for defining characteristics**
a. Tachycardia
b. Tachypnea
c. Hemoglobin less than 10 g/dl
d. Hemoglobin saturation less than 75%
e. Pa_{O_2} less than 50 mm Hg
f. Diminished mental status (i.e., confusion, restlessness, irritability, somnolence)

2. **Expected outcomes**
a. Hemoglobin values return to normal
b. Hypoxemia resolves
c. Heart and respiratory rates are within preestablished normal limits

3. **Nursing interventions**
a. See interventions under activity intolerance
b. Reduce fear and anxiety to minimize oxygen demand
c. Administer supplemental oxygen as ordered
d. Transfuse with blood products as ordered
e. Change position slowly; evaluate dizziness resulting from cerebral hypoxia
f. Position patient to optimize ventilation–perfusion match

4. **Evaluation of nursing care**
a. Heart rate does not exceed patient's baseline by more than 20 beats/min
b. Respiratory rate remains within normal limits ($\leq$ 20 breaths/min)
c. Hemoglobin returns to normal ($\geq$12 g/dl)
d. Pa_{O_2} returns to normal range

Potential Fluid Volume Deficit related to nausea and vomiting or fever

1. **Assessment for defining characteristics**
   a. Decreased urine output
   b. Concentrated urine
   c. Decreased venous filling
   d. Hemoconcentration
   e. Hypotension
   f. Tachycardia
   g. Loss of skin turgor
   h. Altered mental status
2. **Expected outcomes**
   a. Maintains heart and respiratory rates within baseline normal limits
   b. Maintains blood pressure within an acceptable range of normal
   c. Maintains adequate urine output (>30 ml/hr)
   d. Demonstrates normal skin turgor and venous filling
3. **Nursing interventions**
   a. Administer blood products, fluids, and vasopressors as ordered
   b. Monitor oral intake
   c. Monitor urine output and other volume losses (e.g., vomiting, diarrhea)
   d. Assess excretions for gross or occult blood
   e. See interventions under activity intolerance and impaired gas exchange
4. **Evaluation of nursing care**
   a. Vital signs are within normal limits for patient
   b. Blood products administered without incidents
   c. Urine output is maintained at 30 to 50 ml/hr
   d. Excretions are hematest negative

Potential for Impaired Skin Integrity related to activity intolerance, disease, or treatment

1. **Assessment for defining characteristics**
   a. Mechanical irritation (i.e., restraints)
   b. Radiation therapy
   c. Physical immobility
   d. Excretions and secretions (especially incontinence)
   e. Deficient nutritional state
   f. Skeletal prominence
   g. Poor skin turgor
   h. Immunologic deficiencies
2. **Expected outcomes**
   a. Maintains skin integrity
   b. Experiences no tissue trauma

    c. Reduced pressure to integument

    d. Maintains adequate circulation to integument

3. Nursing interventions

    a. Turn patient at least every 2 hours during the day and every 4 hours at night according to a specific schedule

    b. Use protective devices (e.g., eggcrate mattress, alternating air pressure mattress) on the bed

    c. Assess skin for redness, especially over bony prominences and pressure points at least each shift, preferably each time patient is turned

    d. Keep skin clean and dry

    e. Massage skeletal prominences with nondrying lotion after turning patient

    f. Progressively mobilize and ambulate patient as soon as possible

4. Evaluation of nursing care: skin remains intact

Potential for Impaired Tissue Integrity related to interventions

1. Assessment for defining characteristics: damaged or destroyed tissue resulting from excessive invasive procedures

2. Expected outcomes

    a. Maintain tissue integrity

    b. No evidence of petechiae, ecchymoses, purpura, or hematoma

3. Nursing interventions

    a. Reduce the number of venipunctures and initiate intravenous therapy judiciously; consider use of alternate venous access devices; avoid intramuscular and subcutaneous injections

    b. Reduce friction when doing mouth care (i.e., soft-bristle toothbrush, cotton swabs, mild mouthwash)

    c. Evaluate integrity of orifices through which supportive devices/tubes pass: nares, mouth, urethra, anus

    d. Use an electric rather than straight-edged razor for shaving to reduce accidental cuts

    e. If trauma-related bleeding occurs, apply local pressure with dry, sterile dressing for 5 to 10 minutes, or until bleeding is controlled

    f. Reduce frequency of blood pressure readings using a cuff sphygmomanometer and alternate extremities used for readings

    g. Despite danger of bleeding, recognize value of arterial line for pressure monitoring and, when appropriate, blood specimen acquisition

    h. Pad side rails and other firm surfaces, especially if patient is combative or at risk for seizure activity

    i. Be extremely gentle in patient contact (i.e., moving)

4. Evaluation of nursing care: no evidence of tissue trauma or bleeding to include petechiae, ecchymoses, purpura, or hematoma

Potential for Impaired Oral Mucous Membrane Integrity related to treatment, disease, nausea, vomiting, or anorexia

1. **Assessment for defining characteristics**
   a. Coated tongue
   b. Dry mouth
   c. Stomatitis
   d. Oral lesions or ulcers
   e. Reduced or absent salivation
   f. Leukoplakia
   g. Hyperemia
   h. Vesicles
   i. Hemorrhagic gingivitis
2. **Expected outcomes**
   a. Pink, moist, lesion-free oral mucosa, tongue, and lips
   b. No inflammation, lesions, crusts, or hardened debris
   c. No evidence of infection
   d. Patient can swallow and talk without discomfort
   e. Nutritional intake is not compromised by oral discomfort on ingestion
3. **Nursing interventions**
   a. Remove dentures daily; determine if they fit properly
   b. Assess oral mucosa daily for defining characteristics
   c. Distinguish stomatitis (inflammation of the oral mucosa) from candidiasis, which is also known as monoliasis or thrush (subacute—soft white patches on mucosa; chronic—dry, red buccal mucosa); administer nystatin (Mycostatin), an antifungal agent, as ordered
   d. Use mouthwash every 2 hours (baking soda, H_2O_2, normal saline, diphenhydramine hydrochloride [Benadryl] elixir) for comfort
   e. Use soft-bristle toothbrushes, toothettes, or an irrigating syringe to cleanse mouth; avoid lemon and glycerin swabs
   f. For discomfort, apply topical anesthetics: viscous lidocaine (Xylocaine), oral antiseptic anesthetic (Chloraseptic), oxethazaine
   g. Apply petroleum jelly to lips to moisten
4. **Evaluation of nursing care**
   a. Mucosa, tongue, and lips are pink, moist, and intact
   b. No evidence of inflammation, lesions, crusts, hard debris, or infection
   c. Patient can swallow and talk without discomfort
   d. Food intake is not impaired by oral discomfort on ingestion

Anxiety related to disease, hospitalization, or treatment

1. **Assessment for defining characteristics**
   a. Patient expresses feelings of increased tension, apprehension, helplessness, fear, distress, jitteriness

b. Sympathetic nervous system stimulation (i.e., tachycardia, hypotension, superficial vasoconstriction, pupil dilation)

c. Restlessness

d. Insomnia

e. Poor eye contact

f. Hand tremors

g. Voice quivering

2. **Expected outcomes**

a. Verbalizes and demonstrates a reduced anxiety level

b. Demonstrates effective coping behaviors

3. **Nursing interventions**

a. Monitor anxiety

b. Maintain calm, safe environment

c. Encourage involvement in activities, including self-care, when possible

d. Assist patient to identify sources of concern

e. Assist patient to identify feelings engendered by anxiety

f. Help patient to identify and mobilize adaptive coping behaviors

g. Teach relaxation techniques

4. **Evaluation of nursing care**

a. Absence of characteristics and behaviors commonly seen in anxiety

b. Demonstrates effective coping ability

Potential for Infection related to disease or treatment

1. **Assessment for defining characteristics**

a. Loss of skin/mucous membrane integrity

b. Lowered WBC count, especially neutropenia ($<1500/\mu$l)

c. Exposure to pathogens and endogenous microorganisms

d. Fever (temperature $> 100.4°$ F [$38°C$])

e. Potential infectious processes (e.g., cough, reddened areas)

2. **Expected outcomes**

a. Free from signs and symptoms of infection

b. Receives minimal exposure to both potential pathogens and endogenous microorganisms

3. **Nursing interventions**

a. Recognize signs of infection

   i. Assess oral temperature every 4 hours; report elevations greater than $100.4°$ F ($38°C$) to physician. (Fever is a very significant finding in leukopenic patients—when white cells are decreased, classic signs of inflammation may not be manifested; therefore, only fever may occur.)

   ii. Administer acetaminophen as an antipyretic *after* the fever is evaluated; avoid using aspirin if patient is thrombocytopenic

iii. Assess etiology of local and systemic manifestations of infection (i.e., chills, complaints of being cold in warm environment, sore throat, persistent cough, chest pain, burning on urination, rectal pain)

iv. Use proper skin preparation technique for initiating and maintaining intravenous lines as well as for obtaining blood culture specimens

v. Evaluate fluid status during febrile episodes; assess intake and output to include fluid lost via perspiration; assess skin turgor and mucous membranes

vi. Institute antibiotic therapy as ordered; dilute medication adequately to diminish vein irritation; administer each antibiotic separately; establish an administration schedule to maximize pharmacologic effects and minimize side effects of therapy; assess for superinfections that may occur with long-term antibiotic use; recognize that oral antibiotics are often not efficacious to the degree needed by these patients

vii. Exercise care when using hypothermia (shivering increases metabolism, produces heat, and may increase intracranial pressure, which predisposes to intracranial bleeding in thrombocytopenic patients)

b. Institute good handwashing with antiseptic solution for all persons in contact with patient

c. Place patient in private room

d. Limit the number of visitors

e. Screen visitors and hospital staff with colds or potentially communicable illnesses

f. Provide meticulous perianal care to avoid perirectal abscess

g. Routinely culture common sources of contamination (e.g., bathtubs, respiratory therapy equipment)

h. Avoid invasive procedures to the greatest extent possible (e.g., venipunctures, urinary catheters, enemas, rectal suppositories)

i. Teach patient necessary personal hygiene techniques (e.g., handwashing, pulmonary hygiene)

j. Administer granulocytes as ordered
   i. See preparation for blood product administration in section on potential for hemorrhage (p. 713)
   ii. Usually available only at bone marrow transplant centers
   iii. Each granulocyte suspension contains 200 to 300 ml; does not cause increase in WBC count; increases marginal pool (at tissue level—responsible for phagocytosis) rather than circulating pool

4. **Evaluation of nursing care**
   a. Asymptomatic for infection
   b. WBC count is within normal limits

Altered Nutrition: Less than body requirements related to disease or treatment

1. **Assessment for defining characteristics**
   a. Loss of weight with adequate food intake
   b. Reported inadequate food intake
   c. Weakness of muscles required for swallowing or mastication
   d. Sore, inflamed buccal cavity
   e. Reported altered taste sensation
   f. Lack of interest in food; anorexia
   g. Early satiety
2. **Expected outcomes**
   a. Maintains weight, then gradually increases within range of ideal
   b. Consumes well-balanced, high-caloric diet
   c. Adequate intake of nutrients needed for red blood cell production
3. **Nursing interventions**
   a. In collaboration with patient, establish a range of optimal weight outcomes as well as a dietary plan
   b. Teach and monitor use of food diary
   c. Encourage oral hygiene four times a day or after meals to enhance taste and tolerance of food
   d. Precede meals with antacids or other agents as ordered to reduce gastric distress
4. **Evaluation of nursing care**
   a. Consumes four to six small meals daily
   b. Increases amount of dietary supplement consumed
   c. Weight stabilizes
   d. Weight increases to optimal level

Altered Comfort: Pain

1. **Assessment for defining characteristics**
   a. Verbalizes experiencing pain
   b. Physical or social withdrawal
   c. Altered ability to continue previous activities
   d. Anorexia; weight changes
   e. Changes in sleep patterns
   f. Guarded movement
   g. Facial expressions of pain (e.g., eyes lack luster, grimacing)
   h. Narrowed focus of attention (e.g., unable to concentrate, preoccupation with discomfort)
   i. Muscle tension
   j. Autonomic responses indicative of pain (e.g., perspiration, hypotension, tachycardia)
2. **Expected outcomes**
   a. Pain does not exceed a tolerable level
   b. Demonstrates knowledge of measures that influence comfort

    c. Supplements analgesia with relaxation and other pain-reduction strategies

3. **Nursing interventions**
   a. Teach pain-reduction strategies
      i. Knowledge of analgesia, both narcotic and nonnarcotic agents
      ii. Encourage use of a flow sheet to monitor pain, what precipitates it, what relieves it, and response to intervention: adjust medication administration accordingly
      iii. Teach relaxation, guided imagery, and diversional activity techniques
   b. Administer analgesia to control pain
4. **Evaluation of nursing care**
   a. Patient expresses adequate level of comfort
   b. Patient is knowledgeable regarding what exacerbates pain and how to relieve pain
   c. Patient is able to sleep for 3 to 4 hours without being awakened by pain
   d. Involved in activities of daily living to the greatest extent possible

Potential for Ineffective Coping: Family or Individual

1. **Assessment for defining characteristics**
   a. Patient expresses concern about personal or significant others' responses to patient's illness
   b. Patient or significant others express lack of knowledge regarding the patient's illness that interferes with interactions
      i. Unsatisfactory supportive behaviors
      ii. Limited communication
      iii. Excessive protective behavior
2. **Expected outcomes**
   a. Develops adequate understanding of situation
   b. Experiences greater comfort relating with patient and significant others
3. **Nursing interventions**
   a. Provide information to patient and significant others
   b. Discuss common reactions to changes in health; encourage expression of feelings
   c. Encourage patient to discuss needs with significant others and vice versa
   d. Assist patient and significant others to identify changes in relationships provoked by alterations in health
   e. Encourage significant others to be involved in patient care to the extent they are able
4. **Evaluation of nursing care**
   a. Demonstrates understanding of health situation and requests additional information as needed

b. Displays less anxiety during interactions
c. Seeks assistance in ongoing resolution of important issues
d. Significant others participate in care of patient to the extent that is comfortable for both patient and significant others

Potential for Anticipatory Grieving, Patient and Significant Others

1. **Assessment for defining characteristics**
   a. Potential loss of significant object or other
   b. Evidence of distress over potential loss
      i. Denial
      ii. Guilt
      iii. Anger
      iv. Fear
   c. Changes in eating habits
   d. Altered sleep pattern
   e. Altered activity level
   f. Change in libido
   g. Altered communication process
2. **Expected outcome:** constructive progression of anticipatory grief work
3. **Nursing interventions**
   a. Encourage verbalizing perceptions and feelings regarding possible loss
   b. Base therapeutic approach on understanding of past problem-solving efforts and prior experiences with loss as well as socioeconomic status, education, culture, and religion
   c. Assist patient and significant others to realize that an unpredictable, cyclic pattern of emotions is common during anticipatory grief
   d. Convey that each member of the family unit may respond to loss in their own unique way, with different members experiencing different emotions at different times
4. **Evaluation of nursing care**
   a. Able to discuss anticipated loss
   b. Identifies and seeks assistance appropriately from resources
   c. Significant others demonstrate ability to continue to meet their own needs
   d. Demonstrates evidence of mutual decision making regarding the anticipated loss
   e. Demonstrates the ability to continue interpersonal relationships in a constructive fashion

Potential for Hemorrhage related to disease and treatment

1. **Assessment for defining characteristics**
   a. See actual or potential fluid volume deficit (p. 702)
   b. Hypotension
   c. Tachycardia

  d. Hematuria
  e. Spontaneous bleeding from any site
  f. Presence of petechiae, purpura, ecchymoses, or hematomas
  g. Reduced cardiac output
  h. Diminished mental status

2. **Expected outcomes**
  a. Maintains heart rate, respirations, and blood pressure within an acceptable range of normal
  b. No evidence of gross or occult bleeding, including absence of central nervous system bleeding
  c. Receives required blood product support with appropriate intervention if transfusion reaction occurs
  d. Maintains adequate urine output (>30 ml/hr)

3. **Nursing interventions**
  a. Evaluate mucous membranes and skin each shift (epistaxis, petechiae, ecchymoses, hematoma)
  b. Hematest all excretions and observe for blood in emesis, sputum, feces, urine, nasogastric drainage, wound drainage
  c. Assess CBC and platelet count daily or more frequently if ordered
  d. Measure all blood loss; weigh blood-soaked linen and dressings, count sanitary napkins
  e. Assess for retinal hemorrhage (visual impairment)
  f. Do not administer aspirin or aspirin-containing products owing to their effect on platelets
  g. Control active bleeding with ice, packing, or direct pressure
  h. Reduce chance of central nervous system hemorrhage by preventing rise in intracranial pressure
   i. Teach patient to avoid Valsalva maneuver
   ii. Administer stool softeners as ordered
   iii. Teach patient to cough, sneeze, and blow nose gently
   iv. Prevent shivering
   v. Evaluate mental status for alterations
  i. If the patient is on chemotherapeutic agents that are toxic to the bladder
   i. Force fluids to 3000 ml daily if cardiovascular compromise does not contraindicate
   ii. Avoid ingesting substances that may irritate the epithelium of the bladder (coffee, tea, ETOH, tobacco, spices such as pepper and curry)
   iii. Encourage frequent voiding (about every 2 hours)
  j. Administer blood products as ordered
   i. Differentiate among purposes of transfusion therapy
    (a) Facilitate oxygen transport (RBCs)
    (b) Expand volume (whole blood, plasma, albumin)

    (c) Replace proteins (fresh frozen plasma [FFP], albumin, plasma protein fraction)

    (d) Replace coagulation factors (FFP, cryoprecipitate, fresh whole blood)

    (e) Replace platelets (platelet concentrate, perhaps fresh whole blood)

 ii. Distinguish among various types of blood and blood products

    (a) Citrate-phosphate-dextrose (CPD) whole blood

       (1) Volume—about 500 ml/unit

       (2) Contents—if fresh, provides all components including platelets and coagulation factors; otherwise, RBCs and volume

       (3) Large volume is a drawback—it takes 12 to 24 hours before hemoglobin and hematocrit rise; initially hemoglobin increases 0.5 g/dl/unit and hematocrit elevates 1% to 2%/unit; 24 hours after administration, hemoglobin will have increased 1.0 g/dl/unit and hematocrit 2% to 3%/unit (as extra volume is eliminated via the kidneys)

       (4) Infusion time—2 to 4 hours; may split units (divide units into smaller packets if infusion is sluggish)

       (5) Possible complications

          a) Hepatitis

          b) Transmission of human immunodeficiency virus (HIV)

          c) Volume overload

          d) Infusion of excess potassium and sodium

          e) Infusion of anticoagulant (citrate)

    (b) Packed red blood cells

       (1) Volume—200 to 250 ml/unit

       (2) Contents—RBCs

       (3) Replaces twice the amount of hemoglobin as the same amount of whole blood

          a) Hemoglobin and hematocrit therefore rise faster than with whole blood replacement; hemoglobin rises about 1 g/dl/unit; hematocrit rises 2% to 3%/unit; no further change in hemoglobin/hematocrit values after 24 hours

          b) Oxygen-carrying capacity is improved significantly

       (4) Indicated in anemia, slow blood loss, and congestive heart failure

       (5) Less risk of volume overload

    (c) Fresh frozen plasma (FFP)

       (1) Volume—200 to 250 ml/unit

       (2) Contents—all clotting factors except platelets

        (3) Takes 20 minutes to thaw; is frozen to preserve factors V and VIII; stored at $-30°$ C; good for 1 year

    (d) Platelet concentrate

        (1) Volume—35 to 50 ml/unit

        (2) Storage

            a) Can be stored at room temperature for up to 3 days; bag should be agitated periodically

            b) In facilities where usage level high, storage at $4°$ C is deemed desirable to better preserve platelet function; platelets so stored must be used within 24 hours

        (3) Expect platelets to increase about $10,000/unit/m^2$; failure to rise as expected may be due to fever, sepsis, splenomegaly, or disseminated intravascular coagulation. Alloimmunization will also prevent increases in platelet count. Donor compatibility may be necessary

        (4) Infusion considerations

            a) Use a hemorepellent needle and special tubing (closed system)

            b) Give by direct IV push at rate of 30 to 60 ml/min

            c) When giving multiple units, may "pool" several bags into one

            d) May need order to premedicate with acetaminophen or diphenhydramine hydrochloride (Benadryl) to reduce minor symptoms of reaction

    (e) Cryoprecipitate

        (1) Volume of 10 to 20 ml/bag (coagulopathies such as disseminated intravascular coagulation may require approximately 30 such bags)

        (2) Contents—factors VIII, fibrinogen, and XIII

        (3) Should be used as soon as possible after thawing

        (4) Indicated in hemophilia A, von Willebrand's disease, and disseminated intravascular coagulation

    (f) Leukocyte-poor and washed, frozen RBCs

        (1) Special preparatory methods to remove WBCs and protein from RBCs as a means to decrease febrile reactions

        (2) Indicated for patients who received multiple transfusions and developed reactions (i.e., chronic dialysis patients)

        (3) Similar effect can be achieved by using 20 μm filters

    (g) Volume expanders

        (1) Albumin and plasma protein fraction (Plasmanate)—chemically processed pooled plasma; treated with heat to kill hepatitis virus

       a) Usually given in 250 to 500-ml increments in cases of shock

       b) Solution is hyperosmolar and acts by moving water from extravascular space to intravascular space; should not be used in dehydrated patients

       c) Indicated for plasma volume expansion in shock, hypoproteinemia, cerebral edema, and burns (reduces liquid and sodium losses and prevents hemoconcentration)

    (2) Salt-poor albumin

       a) Usually given in 50 to 100-ml increments

       b) Indicated in hypoproteinemia and hypovolemia

iii. Prepare for blood product administration

  (a) Needle size

    (1) At least 20 gauge to preclude hemolysis if infused under pressure

    (2) Do not use pulmonary artery catheter (too small)

  (b) Solution

    (1) Only normal saline—D_5W causes hemolysis secondary to hypotonicity; lactated Ringer's solution causes agglutination secondary to the calcium

    (2) Do not infuse anything concurrently with blood (i.e., through the same line)

  (c) Filter

    (1) Use the correct filter with all blood products

    (2) Most filters can be used for administering 2 to 4 units

    (3) Where appropriate, fill the drip chamber above the filter to "cushion" the blood element as it drops

  (d) Storage—platelets may be stored at room temperature; all other elements must be stored only in the blood bank or in the operating room refrigerator

  (e) Use warming device when needed (e.g., when exchange transfusing a newborn; when administering to patients with cold agglutinins or patients who are hypothermic postoperatively; when giving large amounts of blood)

iv. Monitor patient responses to blood products according to institution's policy

  (a) Correctly identify patient and product prior to initiating transfusion (errors account for over 90% of transfusion reactions)

  (b) Vital signs—before transfusion, 15 minutes after initiating, and on completion

  (c) Observation—especially attentive during initial 15 minutes

v. Monitor for/promptly manage transfusion reactions

      (a) Major types

          (1) Febrile—most common

          (2) Hemolytic

          (3) Bacterial

          (4) Allergic (if severe, anaphylactic)

          (5) Circulatory overload

      (b) Symptoms vary with type of reaction—all should be reported to blood bank and physicians. May include

          (1) General

              a) Hives

              b) Chills

              c) Fever

              d) Facial flush

          (2) Cardiovascular

              a) Palpitations

              b) Tachycardia

              c) Chest pain

          (3) Pulmonary

              a) Shortness of breath

              b) Rales

              c) Wheezing

          (4) Neurologic

              a) Headaches

              b) Altered level of consciousness

          (5) Gastrointestinal—nausea and vomiting

          (6) Genitourinary—flank pain

      (c) Nursing responsibilities

          (1) Stop transfusion—keep intravenous line open with normal saline; change intravenous tubing; keep blood administration set attached to blood bag

          (2) Call physician

          (3) Call blood bank

          (4) Complete transfusion reaction report

          (5) Procure necessary blood and urine specimens for analysis

          (6) Monitor vital signs, especially blood pressure and urine output

          (7) Definitive therapy will be prescribed by physician

          (8) Be alert for delayed hemolytic reactions that can occur up to 3 days after transfusion

4. Evaluation of nursing care

   a. CBC and platelet values within acceptable limits

   b. Vital signs within normal limits for patient

   c. Excretions hematest negative

   d. Blood products administered without incidents

PATIENT HEALTH PROBLEMS

Red Cell Disorders

Sickle Cell Disease

1. **Pathophysiology**
   a. An HbS gene is inherited from each parent; thus RBCs lack HbA
   b. When oxygen level falls, HbS RBCs assume various crescent shapes (e.g., sickle shapes)
   c. Erythrostasis occurs when sickled RBCs become trapped in small vessels
   d. Further sickling and increased blood viscosity result from deoxygenation and reduced pH
   e. Cycle develops as deoxygenation and reduced pH are perpetuated, leading to more sickling
   f. The cells are hemolyzed when the body recognizes their abnormal structure
   g. Sickled RBCs form solid masses that occlude blood vessels, thus leading to thrombosis, ischemia, and infarction
   h. When stasis resolves, a portion of RBCs released into free circulation will be more sensitive to mechanical trauma, even normal trauma experienced during circulation
2. **Etiology or precipitating factors:** a serious, chronic, hereditary (autosomal recessive), hemolytic disease, occurring almost exclusively in blacks; manifests after 6 months of age when fetal hemoglobin is replaced with HbS
3. **Nursing assessment data base**
   a. Nursing history
      i. Subjective
         (a) Increased susceptibility to infection
         (b) Aching joints, especially in hands and feet (dactylitis)
         (c) Sudden, severe abdominal pain
         (d) Chest pain
      ii. Objective
         (a) Family history of blood disorders
         (b) Retarded development of secondary sex characteristics
         (c) Severe hemolytic anemia due to accelerated hemolysis, with all concomitant signs and symptoms
         (d) Bony deformities
         (e) Leg ulcers in 75% of adults
   b. Nursing examination of patient
      i. Inspection
         (a) Impaired growth and development; failure to thrive

      (b) Retarded development of secondary sex characteristics

      (c) Bony deformities

      (d) Leg ulcers

  ii. Palpation: joint pain

 iii. Auscultation: cardiomegaly—cardiac signs resemble mitral stenosis or mitral regurgitation; peripheral signs resemble aortic insufficiency

c. Diagnostic study findings

  i. Laboratory

      (a) CBC—reflects hemolytic anemia

        (1) Hemoglobin, hematocrit, RBC count—reduced

        (2) RBC indices—normal

        (3) Platelets—may be elevated

      (b) Reticulocyte count—elevated

      (c) Serum iron—normal or elevated

      (d) Total iron binding capacity (TIBC)—normal or reduced

      (e) Bilirubin—elevated

      (f) ESR—extremely elevated

      (g) HbS in erythrocytes—it is important to distinguish sickle cell trait from the disease; sickle cell prep and Sickledex will be positive in both the trait and the disease; hemoglobin electrophoresis will show 100% HbS with the disease and 50% HbS/50% HbA with the trait; peripheral smear will show sickle cells with the disease (but will be normal with the trait)

      (h) Impaired ability to concentrate urine

  ii. Radiologic

      (a) Intravenous pyelogram (IVP) shows increased renal medullary blood flow and dilated tortuous medullary blood vessels

      (b) Bone x-ray films show increased density or aseptic necrosis secondary to infarction (skull—radial striation; vertebral bodies—osteoporosis)

4. **Nursing diagnoses:** see Commonly Encountered Nursing Diagnoses, p. 700

a. Activity intolerance related to disease or treatment

b. Potential for impaired gas exchange related to anemia, hemoglobin abnormalities, or blood loss

c. Potential for impaired skin integrity related to activity intolerance, disease, or treatment

d. Anxiety related to disease, hospitalization, or treatment

e. Potential for infection related to disease

f. Altered comfort: pain

g. Potential for ineffective coping: family or patient

Anemias: This is a simplistic classification and overview. It is important to remember that anemia is a clinical *sign*, not a disease entity

1. **Pathophysiology:** reduced hemoglobin concentration of varying etiologies affects blood's oxygen-carrying capacity. Pathophysiologic effects are related to tissue hypoxia and compensatory mechanisms that try to maintain adequate oxygen delivery to meet cellular needs

   a. Oxyhemoglobin dissociation curve shifts right, thus facilitating removal of more oxygen by tissues at same partial pressure of oxygen

   b. Blood is redistributed: it moves from tissues that have abundant blood supply but low oxygen need (skin, kidneys) to tissues that have high oxygen requirements (myocardium, brain, muscles)

   c. As severity of anemia increases, cardiac output must increase to meet oxygen demands of tissues

   d. Rate of erythrocyte production increases 4 to 5 days after tissue hypoxemia increases erythropoietin production

2. **Etiology or precipitating factors**

   a. Blood loss: may be acute or chronic

      i. Gastrointestinal tract

      ii. Menorrhagia

      iii. Trauma

      iv. Blood vessel rupture

   b. Decreased erythrocyte production

      i. Decreased hemoglobin synthesis

         (a) Iron deficiency

         (b) Decreased globin synthesis (thalassemias)

         (c) Decreased porphyrin—lead poisoning, sideroblastic anemia

      ii. Nuclear-cytoplasmic defect (DNA)

         (a) Vitamin B_{12} deficiency (pernicious anemia)

         (b) Folate deficiency

      iii. Decreased RBC precursors

         (a) Hypoplastic anemia

         (b) Marrow infiltration (leukemia, lymphoma)

         (c) Chronic disease

   c. Increased destruction

      i. Intrinsic to erythrocytes

         (a) Abnormal hemoglobins—HbS (sickle cell anemia)

         (b) Defective metabolic enzymes

            (1) Pyruvate kinase deficiency

            (2) G6PD deficiency

         (c) Membrane abnormalities

            (1) Hereditary spherocytosis

            (2) Hereditary elliptocytosis

            (3) Alpha-beta lipoproteinemias

            (4) Paroxysmal nocturnal hemoglobinuria (PNH)

      ii. Extrinsic to erythrocytes

        (a) Physical

          (1) Prosthetic heart valves

          (2) Extracorporeal circulation

          (3) Abnormally small blood vessels

        (b) Antibodies

          (1) Autoregulation

          (2) Drug-related

        (c) Infectious agents and toxins

          (1) Malaria

          (2) Clostridia

3. Nursing assessment data base

  a. Nursing history

    i. Subjective

      (a) Fatigue and weakness

      (b) Visual changes

      (c) Palpitations

      (d) Anorexia

      (e) Nausea, vomiting

      (f) Pruritus

      (g) Tinnitus

      (h) Menorrhagia

      (i) Headache

      (j) Vertigo

      (k) Bone tenderness, especially sternum

      (l) Joint pain

     (m) Sensitivity to cold

      (n) Chest pain

      (o) Dyspnea

    ii. Objective

      (a) Previous treatment for anemia

      (b) Use of drugs or exposure to toxins that could precipitate anemia

      (c) Underlying causes that could precipitate anemia (e.g., chronic liver disease or uremia)

      (d) Pallor

      (e) Jaundice

      (f) Smooth tongue

      (g) Melenic or hematochezic stools

      (h) Hematuria

      (i) Irritability

      (j) Confusion

      (k) Depression

      (l) Weight loss

      (m) Intermittent claudication

      (n) Congestive heart failure

      (o) Dietary history of iron deficiency, folic acid deficiency, and/or vitamin B_{12} deficiency

b. Nursing examination of patient

  i. Inspection

      (a) Jaundice (including icteric sclera and conjunctivae)

      (b) Spider angiomas

      (c) Retinal hemorrhages

      (d) Smooth tongue

      (e) Glossitis

      (f) Hematuria

      (g) Melenic or hematochezic stools

      (h) Weight loss

      (i) Tachypnea

      (j) Orthopnea

  ii. Palpation

      (a) Bone tenderness, especially sternal

      (b) Joint pain

      (c) Hepatosplenomegaly

  iii. Percussion: Hepatosplenomegaly

  iv. Auscultation

      (a) Tachycardia

      (b) Increased pulse pressure

      (c) Systolic murmurs

  v. Cardiopulmonary examination can help to establish severity of anemia

      (a) Mild

        (1) Palpitations

        (2) Exertional dyspnea

      (b) Moderate

        (1) Increased palpitations

        (2) Dyspnea at rest

      (c) Severe

        (1) Tachycardia

        (2) Increased pulse pressure

        (3) Systolic murmurs

        (4) Intermittent claudication

        (5) Angina

        (6) Congestive heart failure

        (7) Tachypnea

        (8) Orthopnea

c. Diagnostic study findings

  i. Laboratory (actual values will vary depending on the specific type of anemia)

(a) CBC
   (1) RBCs—reduced
   (2) Hemoglobin—reduced; severity classification as follows
      a) Mild—10 to 14 g/dl
      b) Moderate—6 to 10 g/dl
      c) Severe—less than 6 g/dl
   (3) Hematocrit—reduced
   (4) RBC indices (MCV, MCH, MCHC)—varied
(b) Morphologic classification
   (1) Normocytic—MCV 80 to 100 fl
   (2) Macrocytic—MCV >100 fl
   (3) Microcytic—MCV <80 fl
(c) Additional clinical studies—all have variable values depending on nature of anemia: reticulocyte count, ESR, bilirubin, TIBC, serum iron
(d) Platelet count—varies; may increase after hemorrhage
(e) Assays to facilitate classification
   (1) Vitamin B_{12}—absorption decreased
   (2) Folate—decreased
(f) Stool guaiac test—may be positive when anemia is due to blood loss

  ii. Radiologic: upper and lower gastrointestinal series may be positive during current or recent active bleeding

 iii. Special: if indicated by classification
   (a) Bone marrow—is hypercellular in pernicious anemia; contains a large number of erythrocyte precursors with a characteristic megaloblastic pattern
   (b) Gastric analysis—neutral pH and no titratable acidity in patients with pernicious anemia

4. Nursing diagnoses: see Commonly Encountered Nursing Diagnoses for details except for the last diagnosis listed
   a. Activity intolerance related to disease
   b. Potential for impaired gas exchange related to anemia, hemoglobin abnormalities, or blood loss
   c. Altered nutrition; less than body requirements related to disease
   d. Potential for ineffective coping, family or individual
   e. Potential for fluid volume deficit related to blood loss
   f. Potential for injury related to altered tactile sensory perception
      i. Assessment for defining characteristics: reported or measured change in peripheral sensory perception
      ii. Expected outcomes: will not experience thermal injuries
      iii. Nursing interventions
         (a) Avoid using hot-water bottles or mechanical heating devices for complaints of cold or chilling

        (b) Provide warmth with extra clothing, such as socks, and blankets

    iv. Evaluation of nursing care

        (a) Avoidance of thermal injuries

        (b) Patient expresses comfort in regard to body temperature

Polycythemia

1. Pathophysiology

  a. Erythrocytes are produced in greater than usual numbers by various mechanisms (see below)

  b. Hemoglobin rises above normal

  c. Blood volume and viscosity are greatly increased, which may impair circulation; organs and tissues may be congested with blood

2. Etiology or precipitating factors

  a. Primary polycythemia (polycythemia vera)

    i. Unknown etiology: perhaps caused by an intrinsic cell defect, one of the myeloproliferative syndromes

    ii. Insidious onset (usually after age 50): vacillating, chronic course

    iii. Hematologic picture involves increased WBCs and platelets as well as RBCs

  b. Secondary polycythemia

    i. Results from hypoxia: hypoxia stimulates erythropoietin in the kidney, augmenting RBC production

    ii. Really a physiologic response to compensate for hypoxia (alveolar hypoventilation, defective oxygen transport, cardiovascular or pulmonary disease, high altitude)

    NOTE: This discussion will focus on polycythemia vera

3. Nursing assessment data base

  a. Nursing history

    i. Subjective

      (a) Epistaxis

      (b) Gingival bleeding

      (c) Pruritus, especially after bathing

      (d) Intermittent claudication (rare)

      (e) Sensation of fullness

      (f) Belching

      (g) Gas pains

      (h) Headache

      (i) Lassitude

      (j) Vertigo

      (k) Giddiness

      (l) Transient syncope

      (m) Insomnia

      (n) Weakness

    (o) Paresthesias in fingers
    (p) Exertional dyspnea
   ii. Objective
    (a) Ecchymoses
    (b) Hypertension
    (c) Venous thromboses
    (d) Peptic ulcers
    (e) Hemorrhage
    (f) Infections
    (g) Vaginal and uterine bleeding
    (h) Gout
  b. Nursing examination of patient
   i. Inspection
    (a) Facial plethora
    (b) Ecchymoses
    (c) Hyperemic conjunctivae
    (d) Vaginal or uterine bleeding
   ii. Palpation
    (a) Hepatomegaly
    (b) Splenomegaly
   iii. Percussion
    (a) Hepatomegaly
    (b) Splenomegaly
   iv. Auscultation: hypertension
  c. Diagnostic study findings
   i. Laboratory
    (a) CBC—elevated hemoglobin and RBCs; elevated WBCs, elevated platelets (latter two for polycythemia vera only)
    (b) Leukocyte alkaline phosphatase—elevated in polycythemia vera
    (c) Uric acid—elevated in polycythemia vera
    (d) Vitamin B_{12}—elevated in polycythemia vera
    (e) Po_2—may be depressed in secondary polycythemia
   ii. Bone marrow (for polycythemia vera): diagnostic by showing hypercellularity of RBCs, WBCs, and platelets
4. Nursing diagnoses: see Commonly Encountered Nursing Diagnoses, p. 700
 a. Activity intolerance related to disease
 b. Altered comfort; pain

White Cell Disorders

Neutropenia: Actually a clinical sign, not a pathologic condition
1. Pathophysiology

a. Leukopenia: decrease in all WBC elements

b. Granulocytopenia: reduction in all granulocytes; often actually refers to neutropenia since this is the major phagocytic cell of the granulocyte series

c. Neutropenia: absolute neutrophil count of less than 1500/µl, thus reducing phagocytic ability and predisposing to infection

2. **Etiology or precipitating factors**

  a. Acute infections

   i. Bacterial: typhoid, paratyphoid, tularemia

   ii. Viral: yellow fever, infectious hepatitis, measles, influenza, chickenpox, rubella, HTLV III

   iii. Rickettsia: Rocky Mountain spotted fever

   iv. Protozoal: malaria

   v. Fungal: aspergillosis, pneumocystis

  b. Overwhelming infections—miliary tuberculosis, septicemia

  c. Physical agents, chemicals, drugs

   i. Marrow hypoplasia in all recipients: ionizing radiation, benzene, nitrogen mustard, antimetabolites (e.g., folic acid antagonists, purine and pyrimidine analogues), vinblastine, colchicine

   ii. Occasional neutropenia if patient is hypersensitive: phenothiazines, sulfonamides, antithyroid drugs, anticonvulsants, antihistamines, tranquilizers

  d. Certain diseases and conditions

   i. Due to decreased or ineffective production (pernicious anemia; aplastic anemia), paroxysmal nocturnal hemoglobinuria

   ii. Due to increased utilization, destruction, or sequestration (cirrhosis with splenomegaly, lupus erythematosus, hemodialysis)

  e. Cachexia and debilitated states such as alcohol abuse

  f. Anaphylaxis and early stages of reaction to foreign protein

3. **Nursing assessment data base**

  a. Nursing history

   i. Subjective: extreme fatigue and weakness

   ii. Objective

    (a) Fever (other signs of infection will probably be absent due to reduced phagocytic response)

    (b) Chills

    (c) Ulcerative lesions of mouth

    (d) Tachycardia

    (e) Sore throat and dysphagia (if bacteria invade oral and pharyngeal mucosa)

    (f) Cough

    (g) Change in color of sputum

    (h) Burning on urination

  b. Nursing examination of patient

      i. Inspection
        (a) Ulcerative mouth lesions
        (b) Skin flushed
        (c) Yellow or green sputum
     ii. Palpation: skin warm to touch
    iii. Auscultation: tachycardia
  c. Diagnostic study findings
      i. Leukopenia: decrease in total WBCs below 5000/μl
     ii. Neutropenia: absolute neutrophil count less than 1500/μl— count of less than 500/μl puts the patient at severe risk for infection
    iii. Peripheral smear to assess if immature granulocytes are present
    iv. Bone marrow aspiration and biopsy

4. Nursing diagnoses: see Commonly Encountered Nursing Diagnoses, p. 700
  a. Potential for infection related to disease
  b. Potential for impaired skin integrity related to activity intolerance or disease
  c. Potential for impaired oral mucous membrane related to disease
  d. Potential for impaired tissue integrity related to interventions
  e. Anxiety related to disease or hospitalization
  f. Potential for anticipatory grieving, patient or significant others

Leukemia: A general term used to describe various hematologic neoplasms affecting the bone marrow, lymph nodes, and spleen, characterized by unregulated proliferation of WBCs. The disease usually follows a progressive course that is eventually fatal, although the patient may live for decades with some types. Classification as either acute or chronic leukemia is based on the maturity and type of cell involved. It is important to have some understanding of the specific types of leukemia because of their different presentations and outcomes. Therefore, in addition to a general overview, the four major types of leukemia—acute lymphoblastic (ALL), acute nonlymphoblastic (ANLL), chronic lymphocytic (CLL), and chronic granulocytic (CGL or CML)—will be discussed separately

1. Pathophysiology
  a. Although cause is not yet entirely understood, most leukemias are believed to be due to malignant clonal expansion of precursor forms of mature WBCs or impaired maturation of WBCs
  b. Whereas normal cells lose their mitotic ability as they mature, leukemic cells retain their ability to divide and fail to mature and differentiate
  c. The increased number of leukemic cells infiltrate organs to include the central nervous system
  d. Bone marrow is crowded with leukemic cells thus suppressing pro-

duction of regular elements, which may lead to anemia, granulocy-topenia, and thrombocytopenia

2. **Etiology or precipitating factors:** exact etiology is unknown but certain contributing factors may include
   a. Exposure to large doses of ionizing radiation
   b. Various chemical agents (e.g., benzene)
   c. Hypoplastic bone marrow
   d. Immunologic deficiencies
   e. Prior use of certain antineoplastic medications or radiation to treat malignant disorders
3. **Nursing assessment data base:** see specific type of leukemia
4. **Nursing diagnoses:** see Commonly Encountered Nursing Diagnoses, p. 700
   a. Potential for infection related to disease or treatment
   b. Potential for hemorrhage related to disease or treatment
   c. Potential for impaired skin integrity related to activity intolerance, disease, or treatment
   d. Potential for impaired tissue integrity related to interventions
   e. Potential for impaired oral mucous membrane integrity related to treatment, disease, nausea, vomiting, or anorexia
   f. Potential for fluid volume deficit related to nausea, vomiting, or fever
   g. Activity intolerance related to disease or treatment
   h. Anxiety related to disease, hospitalization, or treatment
   i. Altered nutrition, less than body requirements related to treatment
   j. Altered comfort, pain
   k. Potential for ineffective coping, family or individual
   l. Anticipatory grieving: patient or significant others

Acute Lymphoblastic Leukemia (ALL): Accounts for 80% of childhood leukemia; abrupt onset, usually before age 14 and infrequent beyond age 20, with rapid progression; response to treatment is usually good. There is a 95% chance of an initial remission, and 50% to 60% of patients younger than age 15 achieve a 5-year survival. In the French-American-British (FAB) classification system, ALL is differentiated into three subtypes (L-1 to L-3)

1. **Pathophysiology**
   a. Proliferation of immature lymphocytes in bone marrow
   b. Prognosis
      i. 90% long-term survival in children
      ii. <50% long-term survival in adults
2. **Etiology or precipitating factors:** see section on Leukemia, above
3. **Nursing assessment data base**
   a. Nursing history
      i. Subjective

     (a) Fatigue and malaise

     (b) Bone and joint pain

     (c) Headache

  ii. Objective

     (a) Fever

     (b) Chills

     (c) Bleeding (bruising, petechiae, gingiva, epistaxis)

     (d) Mouth sores

     (e) Increased intracranial pressure

     (f) Testicular involvement in males

  b. Nursing examination of patient

    i. Inspection: evidence of bleeding

    ii. Palpation

     (a) Hepatosplenomegaly

     (b) Generalized lymphadenopathy

   iii. Percussion: hepatosplenomegaly

  c. Diagnostic study findings

    i. Laboratory

     (a) WBC—elevated in 60% of patients. Even if normal or low, peripheral smear shows blasts (malignant early lymphocytic precursors)

     (b) RBCs decreased—anemia

     (c) Thrombocytopenia

     (d) Elevated uric acid levels

    ii. Special: bone marrow is hypercellular, with over half of cells being blast cells; not necessary if blasts are present in blood as they disappear from blood prior to resolving from marrow

4. Nursing diagnoses: see Leukemia, p. 725

Acute Nonlymphoblastic Leukemia (ANLL): Accounts for 80% of adult leukemia; previously known as acute myeloblastic or granuloblastic leukemia (AML, AGL). Patients live only 2 to 3 months without treatment; may not appear seriously ill at first; onset may be abrupt or progressive. Affects persons as young as 20, but incidence increases with advancing age. In the FAB system, there are six subtypes (M-1 to M-6) of ANLL. About 70% of those treated experience a remission lasting 6 months to 2 years

1. Pathophysiology

  a. Uncontrolled proliferation of myeloblasts, the granulocytic precursors, with hyperplasia of bone marrow and spleen

  b. Prognosis

    i. Complete remission achieved in about 65% of patients

    ii. Overall survival at 2 years is 15% to 20%

2. Etiology or precipitating factors: see section on Leukemia, p. 725

3. Nursing assessment data base

a. Nursing history
   i. Subjective
      (a) Fatigue and weakness
      (b) Headache
   ii. Objective
      (a) Fever
      (b) Chills
      (c) Bleeding
      (d) Infection
      (e) Anemia
      (f) Mouth sores
b. Nursing examination of patient
   i. Inspection
      (a) Evidence of bleeding
      (b) Tachypnea
   ii. Palpation
      (a) Sternal tenderness
      (b) Minimal hepatomegaly
      (c) Minimal lymphadenopathy
   iii. Percussion: minimal hepatomegaly
   iv. Auscultation: tachycardia
c. Diagnostic study findings
   i. Laboratory
      (a) WBCs—can range from low to very high (i.e., 200,000/µl); blasts are present in normal or low counts. Classic myeloblasts contain Auer rods; Phi bodies are more common and unique to ANLL
      (b) Anemia—often severe
      (c) Platelet count very low unless disease is discovered very early
      (d) Uric acid levels elevated
   ii. Bone marrow is usually markedly hypercellular because normal elements are replaced by diffuse proliferation of immature granulocytes (mostly myeloblasts) and some atypical differentiated cells
4. **Nursing diagnoses:** see section on Leukemia, p. 725

Chronic Lymphocytic Leukemia (CLL): Male predominance—2:1; rare below age 30 with most patients in the 50 to 70 year age range; gradual onset with 25% of patients asymptomatic; often found during examination for an unrelated disease
1. **Pathophysiology**
   a. Disorder of B lymphocytes; therefore normal antibody response is depressed

    b. Excessive number of small abnormal mature-appearing lymphocytes in blood and bone marrow

    c. Due to unchecked growth of a malignant clone of lymphocytes

    d. Lymphocytes accumulate in tissues and organs but do not produce detectable functional damage

2. Etiology or precipitating factors: see section on Leukemia, p. 725

3. Nursing assessment data base

    a. Nursing history

        i. Subjective

            (a) Chronic fatigue

            (b) Anorexia

        ii. Objective

            (a) Anemia—late finding, poor prognostic indicator

            (b) Thrombocytopenia—late finding, poor prognostic indicator

    b. Nursing examination of patient: lymphadenopathy is main finding

    c. Diagnostic study findings

        i. Laboratory

            (a) Persistent lymphocytosis: >15,000/µl absolute lymphocytes

            (b) Mild anemia as disease progresses

            (c) Mild thrombocytopenia as disease progresses

        ii. Bone marrow contains more lymphocytes than normal (>30%)

4. Nursing diagnoses: see section on Leukemia, p. 725

Chronic Myeloid Leukemia (CML): Also called chronic granulocytic leukemia (CGL): predominantly found in adults aged 25 to 60; patient may be asymptomatic at first, but symptoms develop as disease progresses; median survival regardless of treatment is about 3 years

1. Pathophysiology

    a. A stem cell precursor of RBCs, WBCs, and platelets undergoes mutation

    b. An excessive development of neoplastic granulocytes in bone marrow replaces normal WBCs and RBCs

    c. These granulocytes move into peripheral blood in significant numbers

    d. All stages of cells (immature to mature) are found in bone marrow and peripheral blood, but mature cells are dominant peripherally

2. Etiology or precipitating factors: see section on Leukemia, p. 725

3. Nursing assessment data base

    a. Nursing history

        i. Subjective

            (a) Fatigue and weakness

            (b) Bone pain

            (c) Heat intolerance

        ii. Objective

        (a) Fever

        (b) Weight loss

  b. Nursing examination of patient

     i. Palpation

        (a) Sternal tenderness

        (b) Massive splenomegaly

     ii. Percussion: massive splenomegaly

  c. Diagnostic study findings

     i. Laboratory

        (a) Leukocytes—increased granulocytes (generally 20,000/μl); decreased or normal monocytes, normal lymphocytes

        (b) Anemia—usually mild

        (c) Platelet count—early in disease, thrombocytosis; late in disease, thrombocytopenia

        (d) Philadelphia chromosome seen in 90% of patients with this disease—only disease in which it is present

     ii. Bone marrow: hypercellular with an increased myeloid–erythroid ratio

4. Nursing diagnoses: see section on Leukemia, p. 725

Multiple Myeloma: A neoplastic disorder of plasma cells. The median age at diagnosis is 60, and it is rare in persons younger than 40. It usually begins with an asymptomatic period during which ESR is elevated, M protein (an immunoglobulin secreted by malignant plasma cells) is present in serum electrophoresis, or there may be unexplained proteinuria

1. Pathophysiology

  a. Neoplastic plasma cells produce abnormal immunoglobulins (myeloma or M protein), thus diminishing body defenses

  b. In more advanced states, proliferation of myeloma cells causes diffuse osteoporosis as protein destroys bone

     i. Lytic bone lesions are best seen in radiographs of skull, vertebrae, and ribs: lead to pathologic fractures

     ii. Hypercalcemia also accompanies advanced disease because of the calcium mobilized during bone destruction

     iii. Vertebral destruction may lead to collapse of vertebrae with ensuing compression of spinal cord, nerve roots, or spinal nerves (cord compression is a medical emergency)

     iv. Renal failure may develop from

        (a) Damage to the renal tubules by myeloma (Bence Jones) protein

        (b) High uric acid levels that result from increased plasma cell turnover

  c. Hypercalcemia and excessive amounts of circulating protein may lead to kidney obstruction and renal failure

d. Tumor cells within the bone marrow cause anemia, leukopenia, and thrombocytopenia
2. **Etiology or precipitating factors:** abnormal expansion of a malignant plasma cell clone
3. **Nursing assessment data base**
   a. Nursing history
      i. Subjective
         (a) Weakness
         (b) Skeletal pain—prominent manifestation when patients become symptomatic
         (c) Anorexia
      ii. Objective
         (a) Recurrent infections
         (b) Weight loss
         (c) Confusion
         (d) Coma
   b. Nursing examination of patient
   c. Diagnostic study findings
      i. Laboratory
         (a) Increased ESR
         (b) Moderate to severe anemia
         (c) WBCs—normal, occasionally low
         (d) Platelets—normal, occasionally low
         (e) Hyperuricemia
         (f) Hypercalcemia
         (g) Elevated serum creatinine, low creatinine clearance
         (h) Sudden, high elevation in serum and urine protein electrophoresis for M protein, the immunoglobulin secreted by malignant plasma cells
         (i) Positive urine for Bence Jones protein, a portion of the immunoglobulin molecule
      ii. Radiologic: osteolytic skeletal lesions, especially seen in skull, vertebrae, and ribs
      iii. Bone marrow shows increased plasma cells and abnormal forms
4. **Nursing diagnoses:** see Commonly Encountered Nursing Diagnoses for details except for the last diagnosis listed
   a. Potential for infection related to disease or treatment
   b. Potential for impaired skin integrity related to activity intolerance, disease, or treatment
   c. Altered nutrition less than body requirements related to disease or treatment
   d. Potential for fluid volume deficit related to nausea, vomiting, or fever
   e. Anxiety related to disease, hospitalization, or treatment
   f. Altered comfort, pain related to skeletal involvement

g. Potential for ineffective coping, family or individual

h. Anticipatory grieving, patient and significant others

i. Impaired physical mobility

    i. Assessment for defining characteristics

        (a) Inability to move purposefully in bed, to transfer, or to ambulate

        (b) Extreme pain with movement due to pathologic fractures, which can be brought on by sneezing, coughing, and other common occurrences

    ii. Expected outcome

        (a) Diminished pathologic fractures

        (b) Maintains mobility to the greatest extent possible

    iii. Nursing interventions

        (a) Increase patient knowledge regarding pathologic fractures

        (b) Educate patient regarding transfer techniques that minimize strain on bones

        (c) Assist patient to turn and move cautiously

        (d) Provide analgesic and nonanalgesic intervention to relieve pain

        (e) Use back brace when walking to support vertebrae and reduce chance of vertebral fracture

    iv. Evaluation of nursing care

        (a) Pathologic fractures are minimized

        (b) Patient retains maximal mobility

        (c) Pain is adequately controlled

Lymphomas

1. **Pathophysiology:** hyperplasia of lymphoreticular tissues destroys the normal lymph node structure

   a. Probably originates in lymph nodes and spreads along adjacent lymphatics to ultimately infiltrate other organs

   b. These neoplasms can be differentiated by histopathologic appearance, different patterns of development, and immunologic methods

   c. Classification: helpful in predicting patterns of presentation and dissemination; also has predictive value in terms of sites of involvement, tendency to remain localized, treatment, and prognosis

      i. Hodgkin's lymphomas (characterized by Reed-Sternberg cells, malignant histiocytes)

        (a) Seen in persons aged 18 to 35 and those older than 50

        (b) 3:2 male-female predominance

        (c) Histologic classification

           (1) Lymphocytic predominant (16%)

           (2) Nodular sclerosis (35%)

           (3) Mixed cellularity (33%)

        (4) Lymphocyte depletion (16%)
- ii. Non-Hodgkin's lymphoma
  - (a) Median age at onset is 50 years
  - (b) Classification is in transition; one current prototype was proposed by Luke and Collins
    - (1) Seventy per cent of these lymphomas originate from B cells
    - (2) Most are follicular center cell lymphomas
    - (3) Additional concerns are whether cells are large or small and appear cleaved or noncleaved
- d. Staging: determines extent of disease and dictates therapy; based on symptoms and location and node involvement
  - i. Classification by symptoms
    - (a) A—asymptomatic
    - (b) B—symptomatic for certain general symptoms
      - (1) Unexplained weight loss of greater than 10% body weight over 6 months
      - (2) Unexplained fever with temperature above 100.4° F (38° C)
      - (3) Night sweats
  - ii. Staging by extent of disease involvement
    - (a) Stage I—one node group involved
    - (b) Stage II—more than two nodal areas of involvement on same side of diaphragm
    - (c) Stage III—disease involves both sides of diaphragm
    - (d) Stage IV—disease has spread to visceral organs outside lymphatic system
  - iii. Important in terms of prognostic and treatment implications
    - (a) In Hodgkin's disease, stages I and II are usually treated with radiation therapy and 95% of the patients are cured
    - (b) In Hodgkin's disease, stage II-A is treated with both radiotherapy and chemotherapy
    - (c) Some stage III-B and IV disease can be cured with chemotherapy. Use of radiotherapy in these stages is controversial
  - iv. Exploratory laparotomy is often a part of staging procedure
    - (a) Deep lymph nodes can be examined (i.e., retroperitoneal nodes)
    - (b) Splenectomy is often done to examine for evidence of disease involvement
  - v. Staging as a predictive guide is important because statistical chances for cure are greater in patients with more restricted disease. When other problems develop, they may be treated quite aggressively.
- **2. Etiology or precipitating factors:** viruses have been implicated

3. **Nursing assessment data base**
   a. Nursing history
      i. Subjective
         (a) Dysphagia
         (b) Night sweats
         (c) Pain with alcohol ingestion
         (d) Chills
         (e) Pruritus
      ii. Objective
         (a) Mediastinal involvement results in cough, dyspnea, stridor
         (b) Weight loss
         (c) Fever
   b. Nursing examination of patient
      i. Palpation
         (a) Lymphadenopathy—discrete and movable nodes that are also painless (unless nerves are involved) and nontender (usually cervical, axillary, and inguinal)
         (b) Splenomegaly—especially in Hodgkin's lymphoma
         (c) Palpable liver
      ii. Percussion
         (a) Splenomegaly
         (b) Hepatomegaly
      iii. Auscultation: tachycardia
   c. Diagnostic study findings
      i. Laboratory
         (a) Slight leukocytosis
         (b) Anemia—mild
         (c) Lymphopenia
         (d) Presence of Reed Sternberg cells in Hodgkin's lymphoma (an abnormal histiocyte that is diagnostic)
      ii. Radiologic
         (a) Chest radiographs may reveal mediastinal or hilar node involvement
         (b) Bone scans may show involvement of skeletal system
         (c) Lymphangiography may show extent of involvement of lymphatic system
      iii. Bone marrow: not characteristic and rarely helpful
      iv. Excisional lymph node biopsy: offers definitive means to diagnose Hodgkin's disease
4. **Nursing diagnoses:** see Commonly Encountered Nursing Diagnoses, p. 700
   a. Potential for infection related to disease or treatment
   b. Potential for hemorrhage related to treatment
   c. Altered nutrition, less than body requirements related to disease and treatment

   d. Activity intolerance related to disease or treatment
   e. Potential for impaired skin integrity related to activity intolerance, disease, or treatment
   f. Potential for impaired tissue integrity related to interventions
   g. Potential for fluid volume deficit related to nausea, vomiting, or fever
   h. Anxiety related to disease, hospitalization, or treatment
   i. Altered comfort, pain
   j. Potential for ineffective coping, family or patient
   k. Anticipatory grieving, patient or significant others

Immune System Disorders

Anaphylaxis: An exaggerated form of hypersensitivity that occurs within 1 to 20 minutes after introduction of the antigenic agent
1. **Pathophysiology**
   a. Following sensitizing exposure to allergen, subsequent contacts with antigen activate an antibody-mediated reaction
   b. Bronchospasm follows release of histamine, which has potent effect on smooth muscles of bronchioles and small blood vessels
   c. As a result of vasodilation and increased vascular permeability, plasma leaves vascular space, resulting in vessel collapse and interstitial edema. Hypovolemia, resulting from loss of large amounts of fluid from intravascular space, leads to hypotension, shock, and circulatory compromise
2. **Etiology or precipitating factors**
   a. Drugs, especially penicillin
   b. Sera
   c. Insect stings, especially from bees and wasps
   d. Injected diagnostic reagents—intradermal skin tests, dyes, local anesthetics
   e. Blood products
3. **Nursing assessment data base**
   a. Nursing history
      i. Subjective
         (a) Arthralgia
         (b) Generalized feeling of fear that increases with progressive difficulty in breathing and stridor
         (c) Palpitations
      ii. Objective: any existing allergic conditions
   b. Nursing examination of patient
      i. Inspection
         (a) Collapse
         (b) Urticaria or other rashes

(c) Facial edema

(d) Cyanosis

ii. Palpation

(a) Lymphadenopathy

(b) Fever

(c) Facial edema

iii. Auscultation

(a) Profound hypotension

(b) Wheezing

c. Diagnostic study findings: anaphylaxis is diagnosed on the basis of history and symptoms; following incident, however, it is important to evaluate exact etiology in order to prevent recurrences

4. **Nursing diagnoses:** see Commonly Encountered Nursing Diagnoses for details except for the last diagnosis listed

a. Anxiety

b. Potential fluid volume deficit

c. Ineffective breathing pattern

i. Assessment for defining characteristics

(a) Dyspnea

(b) Tachypnea

(c) Cyanosis

(d) Change in depth of respirations

ii. Expected outcomes

(a) Maintains normal, unassisted respirations

(b) Cyanosis resolves

iii. Nursing intervention: monitor respirations

iv. Evaluation of nursing care: respirations sustained at normal rate and depth to support ventilation

Human Immunodeficiency Virus (HIV): Also known as human T cell lymphotropic virus type III (HTLV III); the viral infection that leads to acquired immune deficiency syndrome (AIDS). AIDS is just one late manifestation of this infective process

1. **Pathophysiology**

a. HIV is a T-cell retrovirus

i. Retrovirus is a piece of RNA that invades T_4 (helper) cells; T_4 cells have been called the "quarterback" of the immune system

ii. The retrovirus uses DNA from T_4 cells to reproduce itself, thus contributing to the eventual destruction of T_4 cells

iii. The destruction of T_4 cells creates an imbalance in the ratio of T_4 to T_8 (suppressor) cells; suppressor cells turn off the immune response when it is no longer needed

iv. The decline of T_4 cells gives rise to a general decline in immune functioning

b. Disease course

      i. Incubation period of 6 months to 5 years, with an average of 2 years

     ii. Infected persons may remain asymptomatic before clinical signs develop; they can nevertheless transmit the virus; it remains unknown as to why disease progresses slowly

  c. Walter Reed classification: based on status according to six criteria—HIV antibody and/or virus; chronic lymphadenopathy; T_4 cell count; delayed hypersensitivity; thrush; opportunistic infection. Each stage is characterized by essential criteria as well as laboratory evidence of HIV infection

      i. WR 0: exposure to HIV; negative for HIV

     ii. WR 1: onset of acute infection; positive for HIV

    iii. WR 2: chronic lymphadenopathy; positive for HIV

    iv. WR 3: subclinical immune dysfunction; T_4 count <400 cells/mm³; positive for HIV

     v. WR 4: continued subclinical immune dysfunction; asymptomatic defects in delayed hypersensitivity; positive for HIV

    vi. WR 5: skin and mucous membrane immune defects; complete failure of delayed hypersensitivity response (anergy) or when thrush (an oral fungal disease) and persistent viral and fungal infections of the skin and mucous membranes develop (herpes simplex virus, *Candida albicans*, oral hairy leukoplakia); positive for HIV

   vii. WR 6: systemic immune deficiency (actual diagnosis of AIDS can be made at this point); opportunistic infections develop (infections due to malfunctioning of the immune system)

      (a) *Pneumocystis carinii* pneumonia (PCP)

      (b) Cytomegalovirus (CMV)

      (c) Kaposi's sarcoma—but this manifestation alone is not evidence of WR stage 6 disease

      (d) Toxoplasmosis

      (e) Chronic cryptosporidiosis

      (f) Histoplasmosis

2. Etiology or precipitating factors

  a. The disease syndrome AIDS was identified in 1981; the retrovirus contributing to the progressive deterioration of the immune system, with AIDS being one late manifestation of the process, was identified in 1983

  b. HIV is the highly infectious virus that initiates the immune deficiency syndrome

  c. Prevalence has taken on epidemic proportions and created a major public health crisis

  d. Mode of transmitting the virus

      i. Intimate sexual contact

      (a) Predominantly homosexual/bisexual men

(b) Also heterosexuals of both genders who have sexual contact with persons infected with HIV
  ii. Blood contamination
    (a) Sharing virus-contaminated drug paraphenalia
    (b) Through contaminated blood transfusions
    (c) Through antihemophiliac products derived from blood elements
  iii. From mother to fetus or mother to breast-feeding infant
  e. While HIV has been found in body fluids other than blood and semen (i.e., saliva, tears), transmission through these modes has not been established
  f. It is not yet understood as to what differentiates persons in regard to susceptibility to AIDS and why one person develops AIDS while another harbors the virus (a condition known as AIDS-related complex [ARC])

3. Nursing assessment data base
  a. Nursing history
    i. Subjective
      (a) Male homosexual
      (b) Intravenous drug abuse
      (c) Recipient of blood transfusion
      (d) Fatigue
      (e) Night sweats
    ii. Objective
      (a) Lymphadenopathy
      (b) Weight loss
      (c) Recurring viral infections—upper respiratory tract infections, influenza, shingles
      (d) Fever
      (e) Hemophilia
      (f) Possibly Kaposi's sarcoma
      (g) Diarrhea
  b. Nursing examination of patient
    i. Inspection
      (a) Weight loss
      (b) Diarrhea
    ii. Palpation
      (a) Lymphadenopathy
      (b) Warm skin
  c. Diagnostic study findings: no single test is diagnostic of AIDS; also must consider stage of disease
    i. Laboratory
      (a) Serum antibody test for HIV—confirmed positive test means antibodies have developed secondary to exposure

to virus; it neither means the person is currently harboring the virus nor that he or she has AIDS

    (b) Lymphocyte count—lymphopenia

        (1) Primarily from reduced T_4 counts and reversed T_4/T_8 ratio

        (2) Immunoglobulins are elevated, but humoral antibody response is impaired

    (c) Increased serum levels of immune substances (i.e., acid-labile alpha interferon, HLA-DR5)

  ii. Skin tests: defective or complete failure of delayed hypersensitivity reactions (reflects functional impairment of T lymphocytes)

4. **Nursing diagnoses:** see Commonly Encountered Nursing Diagnoses for details except for the last diagnosis listed

  a. Potential for infection related to disease

  b. Potential for impaired gas exchange related to disease

  c. Activity intolerance related to disease

  d. Potential for impaired skin integrity related to activity intolerance

  e. Potential for impaired tissue integrity related to interventions

  f. Potential for impaired oral mucous membrane integrity related to disease

  g. Potential for fluid volume deficit related to fever

  h. Anxiety related to disease or hospitalization

  i. Altered nutrition, less than body requirements related to disease

  j. Potential for ineffective coping, significant other or patient

  k. Potential for anticipatory grieving: patient or significant other

  l. Potential for infection, health care providers

    i. Assessment for defining characteristics: development of any signs or symptoms of HIV

    ii. Expected outcomes: care providers remain free from infection

    iii. Nursing interventions (to minimize exposure to infectious secretions, although the risk of acquiring HIV while rendering care is <1%)

      (a) Follow same protective measures used with hepatitis B

      (b) Consider all body secretions, especially blood, as potentially infectious

        (1) Wash hands before and after patient contact

        (2) Wear gloves, either vinyl or latex, for anticipated contact with blood or body fluid to include performing venipunctures and other vascular access procedures; change gloves between patients

        (3) Wear gowns, goggles, or masks when there might be splatter from blood or body fluids (e.g., bronchoscopies, tracheal suctioning, operative procedures, deliveries)

(4) Also wear masks when patients with HIV are actively coughing until tuberculosis has been ruled out

(5) HIV is not airborne; therefore private rooms are necessary only when dictated by coexisting conditions (e.g., tuberculosis, inability to control body fluids, disseminated herpes zoster)

(c) Dispose of needles and other sharp instruments in a puncture-resistant container; do not resheath or break needle; keep needle containers as close to the area of use as possible

(d) Handle all specimens from all patients with care

(e) Double bag all linen and label as infectious

(f) Use a 1:10 dilution of household bleach to decontaminate surfaces that have been in contact with blood or body fluids from any patient; use paper towels to clean the surface and dispose of the towels as infectious waste; also decontaminate shower floors and bathtubs after use

(g) Thoroughly wash all equipment that has been in contact with the patient's blood or body secretions; then sterilize or use high-level disinfection

Bleeding and Clotting Disorders

Disseminated Intravascular Coagulation (DIC): A serious bleeding disorder resulting from accelerated normal clotting with a subsequent decrease in clotting factors and platelets

1. Pathophysiology

a. Abundant intravascular thrombin is produced that both converts fibrinogen to a fibrin clot and enhances platelet aggregation

b. Naturally occurring antithrombins, which inhibit thrombin, are inactivated by plasmin

c. Ultimately, as clots are lysed and clotting factors are destroyed, blood loses its ability to clot

d. A stable clot, therefore, cannot be formed at injury sites, thus predisposing patient to hemorrhage

2. Etiology or precipitating factors

a. An abnormal syndrome that is always secondary to another process

b. Disorders in which DIC may be triggered include

   i. Shock

  ii. Obstetric complications

     (a) Abruptio placentae

     (b) Retained dead fetus

     (c) Amniotic fluid embolism

     (d) Septic abortion

    iii. Hemolytic processes
       (a) Transfusion of mismatched blood
       (b) Acute hemolysis with infection or immunologic disorders
    iv. Tissue damage
       (a) Extensive burns and trauma
       (b) Rejection of transplants
       (c) Postoperative damage, especially following extracorporeal circulation
       (d) Heat stroke
       (e) Severe head injury
    v. Neoplastic disorders
    vi. Fat and pulmonary embolism
    vii. Snake bites
    viii. Acute anoxia
    ix. Necrotizing enterocolitis
    x. Infections secondary to virus, rickettsia, protozoa

3. Nursing assessment data base
  a. Nursing history
    i. Subjective: existence of underlying disease that may predispose patient to DIC
    ii. Objective
       (a) Bleeding in a patient with no previous bleeding history—severity may vary from mild oozing at venipuncture sites to significant hemorrhage from all orifices (latter is most common)
       (b) Signs and symptoms (occult to overt bleeding)
          (1) Skin—petechiae, ecchymoses, purpura, hematoma
          (2) Head—gingival bleeding, epistaxis
          (3) Genitourinary—hematuria
          (4) Gastrointestinal—hematemesis, hematochezia, melena, increased abdominal girth (from deep hemorrhages)
          (5) Neurologic—headache, altered level of consciousness, numb legs (deep retroperitoneal hemorrhages may compress the lateral spinal nerves)
          (6) Cardiovascular—tachycardia, orthopnea, hypotension, hypoxemia
  b. Nursing examination of patient
  c. Diagnostic study findings
    i. Laboratory
       (a) Screening
          (1) Prothrombin time—prolonged
          (2) Partial thromboplastin time—prolonged
          (3) Thromboplastin time—increased
          (4) Platelet count—diminished

(5) Fibrinogen—decreased
  (b) Definitive studies
    (1) FSPs—elevated
    (2) Protamine sulfate—strongly positive
    (3) Clotting factor analysis—determines which factors are being consumed
4. **Nursing diagnoses:** see Commonly Encountered Nursing Diagnoses
  a. Potential for hemorrhage related to disease
  b. Potential for impaired tissue integrity related to interventions
  c. Potential for impaired oral mucous membrane integrity related to disease
  d. Potential for impaired gas exchange related to blood loss
  e. Decreased cardiac output related to blood loss
  f. Potential for ineffective coping, significant other or patient
  g. Potential for anticipatory grieving, patient or significant other

Select Hereditary Bleeding States

1. **Hemophilias:** sex-linked recessive traits seen almost exclusively in males, but female carriers transmit the disease
2. **Von Willebrand's disease:** an autosomal dominant trait seen in both sexes, characterized by platelet dysfunction as well as low levels of factor VIII
3. **Nursing assessment data base**
  a. Nursing history
    i. Subjective: familial history of bleeding disorders
    ii. Objective
      (a) Begins in childhood
      (b) Slow, persistent, prolonged bleeding from minor injuries and small cuts
      (c) Uncontrollable hemorrhage subsequent to dental extractions or irritation of the gums
      (d) Epistaxis, especially after facial injury
      (e) Hematuria from genitourinary trauma
      (f) Splenic rupture after falling or experiencing abdominal trauma
      (g) Ecchymoses and subcutaneous hematomas (petechiae are rare)
      (h) Neurologic manifestations, usually from nerve compression secondary to hemorrhage
      (i) Bleeding into joints (hemarthrosis) may lead to severe joint deformity, especially in knees, ankles, and elbows; causes permanent crippling
  b. Nursing examination of patient
    i. Inspection

        (a) Evidence of bleeding

        (b) Joint deformities

        (c) Neurologic abnormalities

     ii. Palpation: tender joints

  c. Diagnostic study findings

     i. Laboratory

        (a) Partial thromboplastin time—prolonged

        (b) Factor VIII assay—decrease in hemophilia A; also decreased, but not consistently, in von Willebrand's disease

        (c) Factor IX assay—decrease in hemophilia B

        (d) Platelet adhesiveness and bleeding time—normal with hemophilia A and B; decreased with von Willebrand's disease

     ii. Radiologic: major joint destruction following repeated hemorrhages

4. Nursing diagnoses: see Commonly Encountered Nursing Diagnoses

  a. Potential for hemorrhage related to disease

  b. Potential for impaired skin integrity related to treatment

  c. Potential for impaired tissue integrity related to interventions

  d. Potential for impaired oral mucous membrane integrity related to disease

  e. Anxiety related to disease or hospitalization

  f. Potential for ineffective coping, significant other or patient

  g. Potential for anticipatory grieving: patient or significant other

References

Adamson, J. W.: The polycythemias: Diagnosis and treatment. Hosp. Pract. 18(12):49–57, 1983.

Ahles, T. A.: Psychological approaches to the management of cancer-related pain. Semin. Oncol. Nurs. 1(2):109–115, 1985.

Aledort, L. M.: Current concepts in diagnosis and management of hemophilia. Hosp. Pract. 17(10):77–84, 89–90, 92, 1982.

American Association of Blood Banks, Committee on Standards: Standards for Blood Banks and Transfusion Services. American Association of Blood Banks, Arlington, Va., 1987.

American Association of Blood Banks, Committee on Transfusion Practices: The latest protocols for blood transfusions. Nursing 16(10):34–41, 1986.

Anderson, J. L.: Nursing management of the cancer patient in pain: A review of the literature. Cancer Nurs. 5:33–41, 1982.

Bayuk, L.: Relaxation techniques: An adjunct therapy for cancer patients. Semin. Oncol. Nurs. 1(2):147–150, 1985.

Bellanti, J. A.: Immunology III. W. B. Saunders Co., Philadelphia, 1985.

Bennett, J. M., Catovsky, D., Daniel, M. T., Flandrin, G., Galton, D. A. G., Gralnick, H. R., and Sultan, C.: Proposals for the classification of the acute leukaemias. Br. J. Haematol. 33:451–458, 1976.

Berk, P. D., Goldberg, J. D., Donovan, P. B., Fruchtman, S. M., Berlin, N. I., and Wasserman, L. R.: Therapeutic recommendations in polycythemia vera based on polycythemia vera study group protocols. Semin. Hematol. 23(2):132–143, 1986.

Berkman, S. A.: The spectrum of transfusion reactions. Hosp. Pract. 19(6):205–208, 210–212, 217–219, 1984.

Berkman, S. A., and Rippee, C.: Autoimmune hemolytic anemia: The role of blood transfusion. Hosp. Pract. 19(12):111–112, 114, 118, 121, 127, 1984.

Berry-Opersteny, D., and Heusinkveld, K. B.: Prophylactic antiemetics for chemotherapy-associated nausea and vomiting. Cancer Nurs. 6:117–123, 1983.

Bodey, G. P., Bolivar, R., and Fainstein, V.: Infectious complications in leukemic patients. Semin. Hematol. 19(3):193–226, 1982.

Bonadonna, G., Santoro, A., Viviani, S., and Valagussa, P.: Treatment strategies for Hodgkin's disease. Semin. Hematol. 25(suppl 2):51–57, 1988.

Brandt, B.: A nursing protocol for a client with neutropenia. Oncol. Nurs. Forum 11(2):24–28, 1984.

Burns, C. P., Armitage, J. O., Frey, A. L., Dick, F. R., Jordan, J. E., and Woolson, R. F.: Analysis of the presenting features of adult acute leukemia: The French-American-British classification. Cancer 47:2460–2469, 1981.

Camp, L. D.: Care of the Groshong catheter. Oncol. Nurs. Forum 15:745–749, 1988.

Canellos, G. P.: Introduction: Advances in chemotherapy for Hodgkin's and non-Hodgkin's lymphomas. Semin. Hematol. 25(suppl 2):1, 1988.

Cannistra, S. A., and Griffin, J. D.: Regulation of the production and function of granulocytes and monocytes. Semin. Hematol. 25(3):173–188, 1988.

Catalano, R. B.: Pharmacology of analgesic agents used to treat cancer pain. Semin. Oncol. Nurs. 1(2):126–140, 1985.

Champlin, R., and Gale, R. P.: Bone marrow transplantation for acute leukemia: Recent advances and comparison with alternative therapies. Semin. Hematol. 24(1):55–67, 1987.

Chessells, J. M.: Acute lymphoblastic leukemia. Semin. Hematol. 19(3):155–171, 1982.

Christou, N. V., Meakins, J. L., and Superina, R.: Host defenses, sepsis, and the critically ill patient. In Bartlett, R. H., Whitehouse, W. M., and Turcotte, J. G. (eds.): Life Support Systems in Intensive Care. Year Book Medical Publishers, Chicago, 1984.

Cohen, D. G.: Metabolic complications of induction therapy for leukemia and lymphoma. Cancer Nurs. 6:307–310, 1983.

Conley, C. L.: Anemia: Accurate diagnosis and appropriate therapy. Hosp. Pract. 19(9):57–66, 1984.

Conley, C. L.: Polycythemia vera: Diagnosis and treatment. Hosp. Pract. 22(3):181–185, 189–191, 195–196, 199–200, 205–208, 210, 1987.

Coward, D. D.: Cancer-induced hypercalcemia. Cancer Nurs. 9:125–132, 1986.

Coyle, N.: Symptom management: Pain—an overview of current concepts. Cancer Nurs. 8(suppl 1):44–49, 1985.

Craytor, J. K., and Tass, M. I.: Changing nurses' perceptions of cancer care. Cancer Nurs. 5:43–49, 1982.

Cronenberger, J. H., and Jennette, J. C.: Immunology: Basic Concepts, Diseases, and Laboratory Methods. Appleton & Lange, Norwalk, Conn., 1988.

Curran, J. W., Jaffe, H. W., Hardy, A. M., Morgan, W. M., Selik, R. M., and Dondero, T. J.: Epidemiology of HIV infection and AIDS in the United States. Science 239:610–616, 1988.

Cushman, K. E.: Symptom management: A comprehensive approach to increasing nutritional status in the cancer patient. Semin. Oncol. Nurs. 2(1):30–35, 1986.

Dalton, J. A., Toomey, T., and Workman, M. R.: Pain relief for cancer patients. Cancer Nurs. 11:322–328, 1988.

Darovic, G.: Disseminated intravascular coagulation. Crit. Care Nurs. 2(6):36–37, 41–43, 46, 1982.

Day, H. J., and Rao, A. K.: Evaluation of platelet function. Semin. Hematol. 23(2):89–101, 1986.

DeVita, V. T.: Hematologic malignancies: non-Hodgkin's lymphomas. Hosp. Pract. 21(9):103–111, 116–118, 1986.

Desforges, J. F., and Miller, K. B.: Blast crisis—reversing the direction. N. Engl. J. Med. 315:1478–1479, 1986.

Donovan, M. I.: Nursing assessment of cancer pain. Semin. Oncol. Nurs. 1(2):109–115, 1985.

Donovan, M. I., and Dillon, P.: Incidence and characteristics of pain in a sample of hospitalized cancer patients. Cancer Nurs. 10:85–92, 1987.

Dudjak, L. A.: Radiation therapy nursing care record: A tool for documentation. Oncol. Nurs. Forum 15:763–777, 1988.

Eilers, J., Berger, A. M., and Petersen, M. C.: Development, testing, and application of the oral assessment guide. Oncol. Nurs. Forum 15:325–330, 1988.

Eisenstaedt, R.: Blood component therapy in the treatment of platelet disorders. Semin. Hematol. 23(1):1–7, 1986.

Ellerhorst-Ryan, J. M.: Complications of the myeloproliferative system: Infection and sepsis. Semin. Oncol. Nurs. 1(4):237–243, 1987.

Fanslow, J.: Attitudes of nurses toward cancer and cancer therapies. Oncol. Nurs. Forum 12:43–47, 1985.

Flaherty, A. M.: Symptom management: Nausea and vomiting. Cancer Nurs. 8(suppl 1):36–38, 1985.

Foley, K. M.: The treatment of cancer pain. N. Engl. J. Med. 313:84–95, 1985.

Foon, K. A., and Gale, R. P.: Staging and therapy of chronic lymphocytic leukemia. Semin. Hematol. 24(4):264–274, 1987.

Foon, K. A., Gale, R. P., and Todd, R. F.: Recent advances in the immunologic classification of leukemia. Semin. Hematol. 23(2):257–283, 1986.

Freireich, E. J.: Hematologic malignancies: Adult acute leukemia. Hosp. Pract. 21(6):91–94, 98, 104–106, 108, 110, 1986.

Gale, R. P., and Foon, K. A.: Biology of chronic lymphocytic leukemia. Semin. Hematol. 24(4):209–229, 1987.

Gale, R. P., and Foon, K. A.: Therapy of acute myelogenous leukemia. Semin. Hematol. 24(1):40–54, 1987.

Gale, R. P., and Quinn, S. J.: The management of acute leukemias. Clin. Adv. Oncol. Nurs. 1(2):1–7, 1989.

Gallucci, B. B.: The immune system and cancer. Oncol. Nurs. Forum 14(suppl 6):3–12, 1987.

Goldman, J. M., and Lu, D-P.: New approaches in chronic granulocytic leukemia: Origin, prognosis, and treatment. Semin. Hematol. 19(4):241–256, 1982.

Greenberg, A. G., and Peskin, G. W.: Blood, salt, and water: Recent advances. In Bartlett, R. H., Whitehouse, W. M., and Turcotte, J. G. (eds.): Life Support Systems in Intensive Care. Year Book Medical Publishers, Chicago, 1984.

Griffin, J.: Nursing care of the immunosuppressed patient in the intensive care unit. Heart Lung 15:179–188, 1986.

Griffin, J. D.: Management of chronic myelogenous leukemia. Semin. Hematol. 23(suppl 1):20–26, 1986.

Griffin, J. P.: Acquired immune deficiency syndrome: A new epidemic. Crit. Care Nurs. 3(2):21–22, 24, 28, 1983.

Griffin, J. P.: The bleeding patient. Nursing 16(6):34–40, 1986.

Griffin, J. P.: Hematology and Immunology: Concepts for Nursing. Appleton-Century-Crofts, Norwalk, Conn., 1986.

Groenwald, S.: Physiology of the immune system. Heart Lung 9:645–650, 1980.

Gurevich, I.: Acquired immunodeficiency syndrome: Realistic concerns and appropriate precautions. Heart Lung 18:107–112, 1989.

Gurevich, I., and Tafuro, P.: The compromised host: Deficit-specific infection and the spectrum of prevention. Cancer Nurs. 9:263–275, 1986.

Haeuber, D., and DiJulio, J. E.: Hemopoietic colony stimulating factors: An overview. Oncol. Nurs. Forum 16:247–255, 1989.

Hallberg, L.: Iron nutrition and food iron fortification. Semin. Hematol. 19(1):31–41, 1982.

Harrington, W. J.: Generalized bleeding. Interpreting clinical findings. Hosp. Pract. 20(1A):75–77, 81, 85–90, 1985.

Hauck, S. L.: Pain: Problem for the person with cancer. Cancer Nurs. 9:66–76, 1986.

Henschel, L.: Fever patterns in the neutropenic patient. Cancer Nurs. 8:301–305, 1985.

Ho, D. D., Pomerantz, R. J., and Kaplan, J. C.: Pathogenesis of infection with human immunodeficiency virus. N. Engl. J. Med. 317:278–286, 1987.

Hoelzer, D., and Gale, R. P.: Acute lymphoblastic leukemia in adults: Recent progress, future directions. Semin. Hematol. 24(1):27–39, 1987.

Howser, D. M., and Meade, C. D.: Hickman catheter care: Developing organized teaching strategies. Cancer Nurs. 10:70–76, 1987.

Huhn, D.: Morphology, cytochemistry, and ultrastructure of leukemic cells with regard to the classification of leukemias. In Theil, E., and Thierfelder, S. (eds.): Recent Results in Cancer Research. Leukemia. Springer-Verlag, Berlin, 1984.

Jacob, S. W., Francone, C. A., and Lossow, W. J.: Structure and Function in Man. W. B. Saunders Co., Philadelphia, 1982.

Jennings, B. M., and Muhlenkamp, A. M.: Systematic misperception: Oncology patients' self-reported affective states and their caregivers' perceptions. Cancer Nurs. 4:485–489, 1981.

Kaszyk, L. K.: Cardiac toxicity associated with cancer therapy. Oncol. Nurs. Forum 13:81–88, 1986.

Koch, P. M.: Thrombocytopenia. Nursing 14(10):54–57, 1984.

Kottra, C.: Infection in the compromised host: An overview. Heart Lung 12:10–14, 1983.

Levy, J. H.: Anaphylactic Reactions in Anesthesia and Intensive Care. Butterworths, Boston, 1986.

Lindsey, A. M.: Building the knowledge base for practice: I. Nausea and vomiting. Oncol. Nurs. Forum 12:49–56, 1985.

Lindsey, A. M.: Building the knowledge base for practice: II. Alopecia, breast self-exam and other human responses. Oncol. Nurs. Forum 12:27–34, 1985.

Linman, J. W.: The myeloproliferative syndromes. Hosp. Pract. 21(4):116A–116E, 116H, 116N–116P, 116S–116T, 116W–116X, 116BB–116CC, 1986.

Lister, T. A., and Rohatiner, A. Z. S.: The treatment of acute myelogenous leukemia in adults. Semin. Hematol. 19(3):172–192, 1982.

Lovejoy, N. C.: The pathophysiology of AIDS. Oncol. Nurs. Forum 15:563–571, 1988.

MacGeorge, L., Steeves, L., and Steeves, R. H.: Comparison of the mixing and reinfusion methods of drawing blood from a Hickman catheter. Oncol. Nurs. Forum 15:335–338, 1988.

Martocchio, B. C.: Family coping: Helping families help themselves. Semin. Oncol. Nurs. 1(4):292–297, 1985.

Mauer, A. M.: Acute lymphoblastic leukemia in a young adult. Hosp. Pract. 22(9):145–150, 155–156, 158–159, 162, 1987.

McConnell, E. A.: Getting the feel of lymph node assessment. Nursing 18(8):54–57, 1988.

McConnell, E. A.: The test of time. Nursing 16(5):47, 1986.

McKenzie, S. B.: Textbook of Hematology. Lea & Febiger, Philadelphia, 1988.

Megliola, B.: Multiple myeloma. Cancer Nurs. 3:209–218, 1980.

Merskey, C.: DIC: Identification and management. Hosp. Pract. 17(12):83–91, 93–94, 1982.

Miller, S. A., Dodd, M., Goodman, M. S., Pluth, N., Ryan, L. S., and Medvec, B. R.: Cancer Chemotherapy: Guidelines and Recommendations for Nursing Education and Practice. Oncology Nursing Society, Pittsburgh, 1984.

Moore, C. L., Erikson, K. A., Yanes, L. B., Franklin, M., and Gonsalves, L.: Nursing care and management of venous access ports. Oncol. Nurs. Forum 13:35–39, 1986.

Nyamathi, A., and van Servellen, G.: Maladaptive coping in the critically ill population with acquired immunodeficiency syndrome: Nursing assessment and treatment. Heart Lung 18:113–120, 1989.

Paice, J. A.: The phenomenon of analgesic tolerance in cancer pain management. Oncol. Nurs. Forum 15:455–460, 1988.

Parades, J. M., and Mitchell, B. S.: Multiple myeloma. Med. Clin. North Am. 64:729–742, 1980.

Peters, C. A. H.: Myths of antiemetic administration. Cancer Nurs. 12:102–106, 1989.

Petrosino, B., Becker, H., and Christian, B.: Infection rates in central venous catheter dressings. Oncol. Nurs. Forum 15:709–717, 1988.

Petton, S.: Easing the complications of chemotherapy. Nursing 14(10):58–63, 1984.

Phillips, A.: Are blood transfusions really safe? Nursing 17(6):63–64, 1987.

Pittiglio, D. H., and Sacher, R. A. (eds.): Clinical Hematology and Fundamentals of Hemostasis. F. A. Davis, Philadelphia, 1987.

Pizzo, P. A.: Combating infections in neutropenic patients. Hosp. Pract. 24(7):93–98, 100, 103–104, 107–108, 110, 1989.

Powles, R., and McElwain, T.: Introduction: Leukemia and lymphoma. Semin. Hematol. 19(3):153–154, 1982.

Querin, J. J., and Stahl, L. D.: Twelve simple, sensible steps for successful blood transfusions. Nursing 13(11):34–44, 1983.

Rankin, M.: Use of drugs for pain with cancer patients. Cancer Nurs. 5:181–190, 1982.

Redfield, R. R., and Burke, D. S.: HIV infection: The clinical picture. Sci. Am. 259(4):90–100, 1988.

Roitt, I.: Essential Immunology, 5th ed. Blackwell Scientific, Boston, 1984.

Rosenberg, S. A.: Hodgkin's disease: No stage beyond cure. Hosp. Pract. 21(8):91–98, 101–102, 104, 107–108, 1986.

Schafer, A. I.: Bleeding disorders: Finding the cause. Hosp. Pract. 19(11):88K–88N, 88S, 88W–88X, 88CC, 88GG–88HH, 1984.

Schnipper, I. M.: Symptom management: Anorexia. Cancer Nurs. 8(suppl 1):33–35, 1985.

Scott, D. W., Donahue, D. C., Mastrovito, R. C., and Hakes, T. B.: Comparative trial of clinical relaxation and an antiemetic drug regimen in reducing chemotherapy-related nausea and vomiting. Cancer Nurs. 9:178–187, 1986.

Sell, S.: Immunology, Immunopathology, and Immunity, 4th ed. Elsevier, New York, 1987.

Shapiro, E. D., Wald, E. R., Nelson, K. A., and Spiegelman, K. N.: Broviac catheter–related bacteremia in oncology patients. Am. J. Dis. Child. 136:679–681, 1982.

Siegrist, C. W., and Jones, J. A.: Disseminated intravascular coagulopathy and nursing implications. Semin. Oncol. Nurs. 1(4):237–243, 1985.

Simonson, G. M.: Caring for patients with acute myelocytic leukemia. Am. J. Nurs. 88:304–309, 1988.

Sokal, J. E., Baccarani, M., Russo, D., and Tura, S.: Staging and prognosis in chronic myelogenous leukemia. Semin. Hematol. 25(1):49–61, 1988.

Steere, A. C., and Mallison, G. F.: Handwashing practices for the prevention of nosocomial infections. Ann. Intern. Med. 83:683–690, 1975.

Strohl, R. A.: The nursing role in radiation oncology: Symptom management of acute and chronic reactions. Oncol. Nurs. Forum 15:429–434, 1988.

Taylor, D. L.: Immune response: Physiology, signs, and symptoms. Nursing 14(5):52–54, 1984.

Thompson, P. D.: Host defenses: Basic physiology and management. In Bartlett, R. H., Whitehouse, W. M., and Turcotte, J. G. (eds.): Life Support Systems in Intensive Care. Year Book Medical Publishers, Chicago, 1984.

Thorne, S.: The family cancer experience. Cancer Nurs. 8:285–291, 1985.

Thorne, S. E.: Helpful and unhelpful communications in cancer care: The patient perspective. Oncol. Nurs. Forum 15:167–172, 1988.

Thorup, O. A. (ed.): Leavell and Thorup's Fundamentals of Clinical Hematology, 5th ed. W. B. Saunders Co., Philadelphia, 1987.

Trester, A. K.: Nursing management of patients receiving cancer chemotherapy. Cancer Nurs. 5:201–210, 1982.

Tringali, C. A.: The needs of family members of cancer patients. Oncol. Nurs. Forum 13:65–70, 1986.

Trotta, P., and Knobf, M. T.: Nursing assessment of symptoms associated with hyperviscosity syndrome. Oncol. Nurs. Forum 14:21–25, 1987.

Wiernik, P. H.: Neutrophil function in infection. Mediguide to Infectious Disease 9(1):1–8, 1989.

Wilkie, D., Lovejoy, N., Dodd, M., and Tesler, M.: Cancer pain control behaviors: Description and correlation with pain intensity. Oncol. Nurs. Forum 15:723–731, 1988.

Williams, W. J., Beutler, E., Erslev, A. J., and Lichtman, M. A. (eds.): Hematology, 3rd ed. McGraw-Hill, New York, 1983.

Woods, N. F., Lewis, F. M., and Ellison, E. S.: Living with cancer: Family experiences. Cancer Nurs. 12:28–33, 1989.

Yasko, J. M. (ed.): Guidelines for Cancer Care: Symptom Management. Reston Publishing Co., Reston, Va., 1983.

Yeomans, A. C.: Rectal infections in acute leukemia. Cancer Nurs. 9:295–300, 1986.

CHAPTER

The Gastrointestinal System

Tess L. Briones, M.S.N., R.N.

PHYSIOLOGIC ANATOMY

Upper Gastrointestinal System (Fig. 7–1)

1. **Oral cavity**
   a. Composed of the lips, cheeks, taste buds, and salivary glands
   b. Prepares the food for absorption by ingestion, mastication (chewing), salivation, and the initial stage of deglutition (swallowing)
   c. Saliva is secreted by the submandibular, parotid, and sublingual salivary glands
   d. Saliva contains large amounts of water and small amounts of sodium chloride, bicarbonate, urea, and a few other solutes (e.g., amylase, mucins)
   e. The average amount of salivary secretion ranges from 1000 to 1500 ml/day
   f. Stimulation of salivary secretion comes from the autonomic nervous system
   g. Swallowing is primarily an involuntary act. The three stages of swallowing (Fig. 7–2) are
      i. Voluntary stage: initiates the swallowing process; the tongue forces the bolus of food into the pharynx
      ii. Pharyngeal stage: an involuntary act that constitutes the passage of food through the pharynx into the esophagus
      iii. Esophageal stage: another involuntary act that promotes passage of food from the esophagus to the stomach

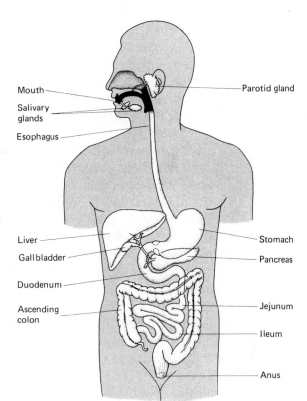

Figure 7–1. The gastrointestinal tract. (From Guyton, A. C.: Textbook of Medical Physiology, 7th ed. W. B. Saunders Co., Philadelphia, 1986.)

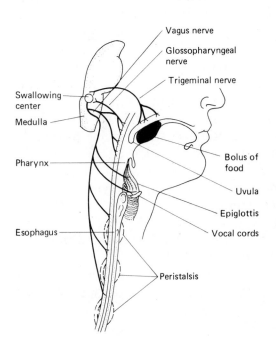

Figure 7–2. The swallowing mechanism. (From Guyton, A. C.: Textbook of Medical Physiology, 7th ed. W. B. Saunders Co., Philadelphia, 1986.)

2. Pharynx

a. Provides for the active movement of food into the esophagus while closing and sealing off the trachea

b. Swallowing receptor areas in pharynx are stimulated when bolus of food is pushed backward in the mouth

c. Divisions of the pharynx

    i. Nasopharynx: has immovable walls that extend from nasal cavity to soft palate, the soft palate is pulled upward and is elevated during swallowing to prevent reflux of food into the nasal cavities

    ii. Oropharynx: has movable walls that extend from soft palate to hyoid bones

    iii. Laryngeal pharynx: extends from hyoid bones to esophagus; this part of the pharynx is pulled upward and anteriorly, causing the epiglottis to swing backward over the superior opening of the larynx, thus preventing the passage of food into the trachea

d. The motor impulses from the swallowing center during the pharyngeal stage of swallowing are transmitted by the trigeminal, glossopharyngeal, vagus, and hypoglossal cranial nerves

3. Esophagus

a. A muscular, pliable tube approximately 10 inches long that provides a passageway for food from the pharynx to the stomach

b. Lies posterior to the trachea and the heart and shares a common fibroelastic membrane with the posterior portion of the trachea

c. Presence of mucus-secreting glands along the length of the tube helps to lubricate the bolus of food passing through

d. Attaches to the stomach below the level of the diaphragm

e. Sphincters

    i. Hypopharyngeal: normally remains closed and is located at the upper part of the esophagus; allows the bolus of food to enter the esophagus (also opens during vomiting)

    ii. Gastroesophageal: normally remains constricted but relaxes when a peristaltic wave is conducted allowing for passage of food to the stomach; located at the junction of the esophagus and the stomach; incomplete closure is referred to as achalasia

f. Achalasia results from damage to or absence of myenteric nerve plexus in the gastroesophageal sphincter

g. Cell layers of the esophagus

    i. Upper third of esophagus: mostly skeletal or striated muscle

    ii. Lower two thirds: mostly smooth muscle

    iii. The outer muscle layer of the esophagus runs longitudinally; the inner muscle layer is positioned transversely around the lumen

iv. Mucosal layer has squamous epithelial cells that lie over the muscle layer

4. **Stomach** (Fig. 7–3)

a. Pear-shaped, hollow, distensible organ that is 10 to 12 inches in length with 4 to 5 inches maximal diameter

i. Proximal part: relaxes to allow for the entrance of food and secretes gastric juice

ii. Distal part: mechanically mixes the food by a churning action and delivers it to the duodenum

b. Rugae: mucosal folds at the inner lining of the stomach, composed of mucosal layer and muscularis mucosa; provide increased surface area and allow for distention

c. Layers of the stomach wall

i. Mucosal: contains the gastric, cardiac, and pyloric glands

ii. Muscularis mucosa: muscle layer that folds the mucosa into rugae

iii. Submucosal: contains loose, connective tissue and elastic fibers, blood vessels, and lymphatics

iv. Mucosal coat: contains three layers that are thin at the fundus and thicker at the antrum; all layers are made up of smooth muscles

d. The stomach occupies the epigastric, umbilical, and left hypochondriac regions of the abdomen

e. Sphincters are responsible for controlling the rate of food passage

i. Cardiac sphincter: located at the opening from the esophagus; another name is gastroesophageal sphincter

ii. Pyloric sphincter: located at the opening into the duodenum

f. Glands of the stomach

i. Cardiac: secretes mucus

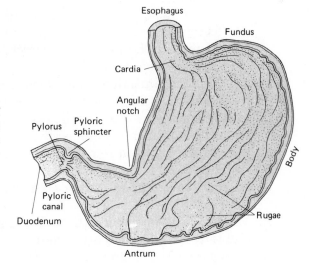

Figure 7–3. Physiologic anatomy of the stomach. (From Guyton, A. C.: Textbook of Medical Physiology, 7th ed. W. B. Saunders Co., Philadelphia, 1986.)

      ii. Fundic: composed of

        (a) Chief cells—secrete pepsinogen, which, in its activated form (pepsin), digests proteins

        (b) Parietal cells—secrete hydrochloric acid and intrinsic factor

g. Gastric secretion

      i. Approximately 1500 to 3000 ml is secreted daily and mixes with the food entering the stomach

      ii. Chyme: a semiliquid mass that is a combination of food and gastric juice (hydrochloric acid, pepsin, mucus, and intrinsic factor)

      iii. Intrinsic factor: a glycoprotein that binds with vitamin B_{12} and makes it available for intestinal absorption

h. Gastric emptying is proportional to the volume of material in it at any given time

      i. Factors that accelerate gastric emptying

        (a) Large volume of liquids

        (b) Anger

        (c) Aggression

        (d) Insulin

      ii. Factors that inhibit gastric emptying

        (a) Fats—most potent inhibition stimulus

        (b) Protein and starch

        (c) Pain

        (d) Sadness and depression

        (e) Hormones from the duodenum

i. Phases of gastric secretion (Fig. 7–4)

      i. Cephalic: prepares the stomach for food and digestion; controlled by the nervous system and initiated by the sight, smell, or thought of food; impulses from the receptors in the retina, taste buds, and the olfactory glands are communicated to the cerebral cortex; motor fibers of the vagus nerve of the stomach stimulate the stomach to secrete gastrin (from the antrum) and hydrochloric acid

      ii. Gastric: initiated when food enters the stomach; food in the stomach initiates local reflexes in the intramural plexus of the stomach; vasovagal reflexes stimulate parasympathetic stimulation to increase the secretion of gastrin

      iii. Intestinal: food remains in the duodenum until it is ready to be absorbed

j. Arterial blood supply to the stomach comes mainly from the celiac artery

k. Venous blood is drained through the gastric veins, which connect to and terminate in the portal vein

l. Nervous system supply to the stomach

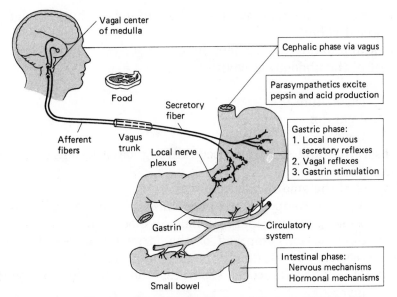

Figure 7–4. Phases of gastric secretion and their regulation. (From Guyton, A. C.: Textbook of Medical Physiology, 7th ed. W. B. Saunders Co., Philadelphia, 1986.)

    i. Intrinsic system: controls the tone of the bowel, rhythmic contractions, and the velocity and excitation of the gut
   ii. Autonomic nervous system: through the parasympathetic branches increases excitation especially in the esophagus, stomach, large intestine, and anal regions

m. Vomiting: propulsion of the contents of the upper gastrointestinal tract and the stomach through the mouth
    i. Coordinated by the vomiting center located in the medulla
   ii. Stimuli that induce vomiting
      (a) Tactile stimulation to the back of the throat
      (b) Increased intracranial pressure
      (c) Intense pain
      (d) Rotating head movements that lead to dizziness
      (e) Anxiety attacks
  iii. Autonomic nervous system discharge that may precede vomiting
      (a) Sweating
      (b) Increased heart rate
      (c) Increased salivation
      (d) Feelings of nausea

Lower Gastrointestinal System

1. Small intestine

a. A portion of the digestive tract that extends from the pylorus to the ileocecal valve
b. It is approximately 12 feet long, coiled, convoluted, and occupies most of the abdominal cavity
c. Divisions
   i. Duodenum
   ii. Jejunum
   iii. Ileum
d. Absorption and secretion occur throughout the length of the small intestine
e. Layers of the small intestinal wall
   i. Mucosa: composed of epithelial and columnar cells, small blood vessels, plasma, nerve cells, and blood cells
   ii. Submucosa: composed of the large blood vessels, connective tissues, nerves, ganglia, and lymphatics
   iii. Muscularis mucosa: separates the mucosal and submucosal layer
   iv. Serosa: composed of an inner circular layer and an outer longitudinal layer; myenteric plexus is interspersed between the two layers
f. Structural features
   i. Villi: finger-like folds of the mucosa that project into the lumen of the intestines and increase the absorptive surface by approximately 600-fold
   ii. Crypts of Lieberkühn: pitlike structures that lie in grooves between the villi and are composed of absorptive cells and mucus-producing goblet cells (Fig. 7–5)
   iii. Peyer's patches: cells that lie in mucosa and submucosa and consist of lymphoid follicles; they play an important role in the immune response of the body because they perform antibody synthesis in some persons
g. Small intestinal motility

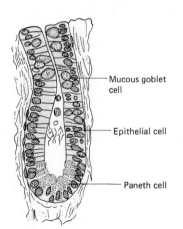

Mucous goblet cell

Epithelial cell

Paneth cell

Figure 7–5. A crypt of Lieberkühn found in all parts of the small intestine between the villi. (From Guyton, A. C.: Textbook of Medical Physiology, 7th ed. W. B. Saunders Co., Philadelphia, 1986.)

i. Mixing contractions or segmentation contractions: localized ring contractions that divide the lumen and its contents into segments, resulting in the mixing of chyme; promotes progressive mixing of the solid food particles with the secretions of the small intestine; the frequency of the segmentation contractions is determined by the basic electrical rhythm (BER)

ii. Propulsive movements or peristaltic movements: weak movements that move the chyme toward the anus; peristaltic activity is greatly increased after a meal

h. Functions

  i. Basic absorption

    (a) Active transport—adenosine triphosphate (ATP) is required as energy source to accomplish this function; substances involved are glucose, protein, sodium, and potassium

    (b) Passive diffusion—movement of molecules from an area of higher concentration to an area of lower concentration; substances involved are water and free fatty acids

    (c) Facilitated diffusion—needs a carrier, but not energy, to move into the cell; substances cannot move against electrochemical gradient; substance involved is fructose

    (d) Non-ionic transport—substances move freely in and out of the cell without energy; substances involved are medications and unconjugated bile salts

    (e) Vitamins are absorbed primarily in the proximal intestine, except for vitamin B_{12}, which is absorbed in the terminal ileum; most vitamins are absorbed by passive diffusion, except for the fat-soluble vitamins, which require bile salts

  ii. Water absorption

    (a) Approximately 8 L of water per day is absorbed by the small intestine into the portal blood by active transport

    (b) Greatest proportion of this absorption occurs in the jejunum

    (c) Rate of absorption is enhanced by glucose and oxygen

  iii. Electrolyte absorption

    (a) Electrolytes are primarily absorbed into the portal blood rather than into the lymphatic system

    (b) Greatest rate of absorption occurs in the proximal portion of the small bowel

    (c) Sodium, chloride, potassium, nitrate, and bicarbonate are more readily absorbed than calcium, magnesium, and sulfate

    (d) Electrolytes are absorbed in all areas of the small intestine

  iv. Iron absorption

    (a) Iron is absorbed in its ferrous form in the duodenum

(b) Occurs by active transport and is facilitated by ascorbic acid

(c) Rate of absorption is extremely slow but increases when iron deficiency exists and decreases when there is an excessive dietary intake of iron

v. Carbohydrate absorption

(a) Carbohydrates are ingested primarily as starches, polysaccharides, and disaccharides

(b) Complex carbohydrates are broken down into monosaccharides or basic sugars by specific enzymes (e.g., amylase, maltase)

(c) The three basic sugars are fructose, glucose, and galactose

(d) There are 4 kcal/g of carbohydrate

(e) Sodium increases cellular permeability to glucose thus enhancing active transport

vi. Protein absorption

(a) Occurs mostly in the duodenum and jejunum

(b) Protein is broken down into amino acids and small peptides

(c) Essential amino acids are lysine, phenylalanine, isoleucine, valine, methionine, leucine, threonine, and tryptophan

(d) There are 4 kcal/g of protein

vii. Fat absorption

(a) Dietary fat or triglycerides are broken down into fatty acids and glycerol by the pancreatic enzymes

(b) Bile salts and fatty acids aggregate to form micelles, which are water soluble

(c) Micelles are absorbed in the jejunum

(d) Triglycerides are transported into the general circulation via the lymphatic system

i. Blood supply to the small intestine comes from the gastroduodenal, the superior pancreaticoduodenal, and celiac arteries; venous drainage is through the superior mesenteric vein, which empties into the portal vein and travels to the liver

i. Physiologic significance of the portal vein system

(a) Partially metabolized products of digestion are brought to the liver sinusoids where hepatocytes complete next stage of metabolism

(b) Liver dysfunction such as cirrhosis causes portal venous hypertension, resulting in ascites and incomplete metabolism of products of digestion

(c) Metabolized products of the liver leave by two separate systems—hepatic duct (drains bile salts, products of drug metabolism and hemoglobin) and hepatic vein (drains blood from portal vein and hepatic artery into the inferior vena cava)

   j. Small intestinal secretion

      i. Stimulated by the presence of chyme in the small intestine and vasoactive intestinal peptides

      ii. Secretions are primarily made up of digestive enzymes (e.g., lipase, amylase, maltase, lactase)

      iii. Intestinal secretion reaches up to 3000 ml/day with a pH of approximately 7.0

2. Large intestine (colon)

   a. Begins with the ending of the ileum at the ileocecal valve called the cecum

   b. Terminates in the rectum and anal canal

   c. Approximately 5 to 6 feet long and 2½ inches in diameter

   d. Parts of the large intestine

      i. Cecum: a cul-de-sac from which the appendix, a relatively nonfunctional pouch, is attached

      ii. Colon is divided into four sections

         (a) Ascending

         (b) Transverse

         (c) Descending

         (d) Sigmoid

      iii. Rectum: extends from sigmoid to anus

   e. Flexures

      i. Hepatic: bend at the junction of the ascending and transverse colon; located at the right upper quadrant of the abdomen

      ii. Splenic: bend at the junction of transverse and descending colon; located at the left upper quadrant of the abdomen

   f. Anal sphincter, external and internal, controls anal opening during fecal elimination

   g. Layers of large intestinal wall

      i. Mucosa: composed of epithelial cells, which are largely responsible for absorption of water and electrolytes

      ii. Submucosa: composed of large blood vessels, nerves, and lymphatics

      iii. Muscular: composed of circular and longitudinal layers

   h. Colonic motility

      i. Factors that enhance motility

         (a) Bacterial enterotoxins (e.g., cholera virus)

         (b) Regional enteritis

         (c) Ulcerative colitis

         (d) Increased bile salts

         (e) Osmotic overload

      ii. Factors that inhibit motility

         (a) Drugs (e.g., morphine)

(b) Low bulk diet

(c) Anticholinergic drugs (e.g., atropine)

i. Colonic functions (Fig. 7–6)

   i. Absorption of water and electrolytes; approximately 1000 ml of water is absorbed per day

   ii. Urea, a metabolic waste product, is broken down into ammonia by the mucosal cells of the colon to conserve nitrogen

   iii. Cellulose is broken down and vitamins (folic acid, vitamin K, riboflavin, nicotinic acid) are synthesized by the help of bacteria

     (a) *Bacteroides fragilis*—main anaerobic bacteria

     (b) *Escherichia coli*—main aerobic bacteria

   iv. Types of colonic movement

     (a) Haustral shuttling—liquid or semiliquid haustral contents are displaced short distances in both directions by apparently random segmental contractions of circular muscle. Contractions are not progressive. Most frequent type of colonic movement in the fasting state

     (b) Segmental and multihaustral propulsion—contents move into neighboring segment of the bowel; net direction is toward the anus. This type of colonic movement increases after eating

     (c) Peristalsis—progressive wave of contraction that pushes the fecal mass ahead at a rate of 1 to 2 cm/min

   v. Fecal elimination (defecation)

     (a) Distention of the wall of the rectum initiates the defecation reflex; mediated primarily by the internal nerve plexus

     (b) Contraction of the rectum, relaxation of the internal and external sphincters, and increased peristaltic activity in the sigmoid colon follows

     (c) Feces is composed of 75% water and 25% solid matter composed of bacteria (30%), fat (10% to 20%), protein (2%

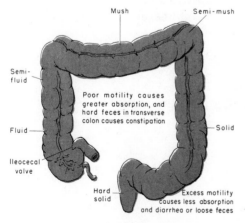

Figure 7–6. Absorptive and storage functions of the large intestine. (From Guyton, A. C.: Textbook of Medical Physiology, 7th ed. W. B. Saunders Co., Philadelphia, 1986.)

to 3%), undigested roughage of food (30%), inorganic matter (10% to 20%), and sloughed epithelial cells
   (d) Urobilin, a derivative of bilirubin, gives feces its brown color

Gastrointestinal Hormones

1. **Gastrin:** secreted in the antrum of the stomach in response to acetylcholine stimulation of the antral cells; effects are
   a. Stimulates secretion of hydrochloric acid by the parietal cells
   b. Stimulates secretion of pepsin by the chief cells
   c. Promotes stomach emptying
2. **Secretin:** secreted in the duodenum in response to acidic gastric juice emptied from the stomach to the pylorus; effects are
   a. Augments the action of cholecystokinin
   b. Stimulates pancreatic and hepatic bicarbonate and water secretion
   c. Mild inhibition on motility of most of the gastrointestinal tract
3. **Cholecystokinin (CCK):** secreted mainly by the jejunum in response to the presence of fatty substance in the intestinal contents; effects are
   a. Increases contractility of the gallbladder
   b. Moderately inhibits stomach motility
   c. Stimulates the secretion of digestive enzymes from the pancreas (e.g., amylase, lipase, trypsin)
4. **Gastric inhibitory peptide (GIP):** secreted by the mucosa of the small intestine in response to fat and carbohydrate in the food; effects are
   a. Decreases the motor activity of the stomach
   b. Slows the emptying of gastric contents into the duodenum
   c. Stimulates the secretion of insulin by the pancreas
5. **Vasoactive intestinal peptide (VIP):** secreted from the small intestine in response to the acidic gastric juice that is emptied into the duodenum; effects are
   a. Main effects are similar to those of secretin
   b. Stimulates the secretion of intestinal juices to decrease the acidity of the chyme
   c. Inhibits gastric secretion

Blood Supply to the Gastrointestinal Tract

1. **Arterial blood supply**
   a. Aorta → abdominal aorta (through aortic arch and thoracic arch) → celiac artery
   b. Branches of the celiac artery
      i. Left gastric: supplies the stomach and the esophagus
      ii. Hepatic branch gives way to right gastric: supplies the stomach
      iii. Gastroduodenal: supplies the stomach and the duodenum

      iv. Cystic: supplies the gallbladder

      v. Splenic: supplies the stomach, spleen, and pancreas

  c. Abdominal aorta → superior and inferior mesenteric arteries

  d. Superior mesenteric artery: supplies the jejunum, ileum, cecum, ascending colon, and part of the transverse colon

  e. Inferior mesenteric artery: supplies the transverse, descending, and sigmoid colon, and the rectum

2. **Venous blood return**

  a. The portal vein collects blood from the entire venous drainage of the gastrointestinal tract to the portal venous system and delivers it to the liver

  b. Branches that bring blood to the portal vein

      i. Gastric: collects blood from the stomach and the esophagus

      ii. Splenic: collects blood from the stomach, esophagus, duodenum, pancreas, and gallbladder

      iii. Superior mesenteric: collects blood from the small intestine, ascending and transverse colon

      iv. Inferior mesenteric: collects blood from the descending and sigmoid colon and the rectum; the inferior mesenteric vein joins with the splenic vein before it drains into the portal vein

  c. The portal vein subdivides into sinusoids in the liver and then unites with branches from the hepatic artery to form the hepatic vein, which empties into the inferior vena cava

Nervous System Innervation of the Gastrointestinal Tract

1. **Extrinsic nerves of the autonomic nervous system:** located outside the wall of the gut

  a. Parasympathetic: arises from the vagus nerve and the sacral nerves

  b. Sympathetic: arises from the vertebral ganglia located on both sides of the vertebral trunk and terminates in all organs of the gut

  c. Parasympathetic stimulation affects the gastrointestinal activity more than the sympathetic

2. **Intrinsic nerves of the autonomic nervous system:** located inside the wall of the gut

  a. This set of nerves is called intramural plexus

  b. Are extensions from the extrinsic nerves

  c. Composed of major and minor networks of plexuses

      i. Major

        (a) Auerbach's plexus—located in the muscular layer

        (b) Meissner's plexus—located in the submucosal layer

      ii. Minor

        (a) Subserosal—located under the serosal layer

        (b) Deep myenteric—located within the muscular layer

        (c) Mucous—found in the villi and glandular cells

Accessory Organs of Digestion

1. **Pancreas**
   a. A fish-shaped retroperitoneal gland that lies behind the duodenum and the spleen
   b. Soft in consistency and has a characteristic lobular appearance with a light yellow and slightly pink coloration
   c. Total length is between 12 and 20 cm, and weight is between 70 and 120 g
   d. Divisions
      i. Head and neck: lie in the C-shaped curve of the duodenum; make up about 30% of the gland
      ii. Body: extends horizontally behind the stomach; accounts for the largest portion of the gland
      iii. Tail: thin, narrow portion that touches the spleen
   e. Duct of Wirsung: main pancreatic duct that travels the length of the organ from left to right
   f. Duct of Santori: accessory pancreatic duct that, when present, enters the duodenum proximal to the duct of Wirsung
   g. Ampulla of Vater: short segment of the pancreas before it enters the duodenum
   h. Sphincter of Oddi: terminal opening of common bile duct located at the entrance in the duodenum
   i. Pancreatic secretions: approximately 1500 to 2000 ml/day with a pH of 8.3; fluid is colorless
      i. Exocrine portion: composed of acinar cells that secrete large volumes of bicarbonate, water, sodium, potassium, and digestive enzymes in response to the presence of chyme in the upper portions of the small intestine; digestive enzymes are
         (a) Trypsin—breaks down amino acids
         (b) Amylase—breaks down complex carbohydrates into simple sugars
         (c) Lipase—breaks down triglycerides into fatty acids and glycerol
         (d) Ribonuclease, deoxyribonuclease—break down nucleic acids into free mononucleotides
      ii. Endocrine portion: the islet of Langerhans, composed of alpha, beta, and delta cells and recently described pancreatic polypeptide (PP) cells
         (a) Alpha cells—secrete glucagon, which is responsible for the breakdown of hepatic glycogen to glucose and of adipose tissue to triglyceride; it also stimulates gluconeogenesis from amino acids
         (b) Beta cells—secrete insulin, which facilitates the utiliza-

tion of glucose by the tissues; the entry of glucose leads to glucose oxidation, fat synthesis, and glycogen oxidation

    (c) Delta cells—secrete a polypeptide called somatostatin, which inhibits insulin, glucagon, and growth hormone secretion

    (d) PP cells—secrete a polypeptide that causes gastrointestinal effects of diarrhea and hypermotility in animals; its exact effect on humans is not clearly understood

  j. Control of pancreatic secretions (Fig. 7–7)

    i. Vagal: parasympathetic stimulation during the cephalic and gastric phases results in the secretion of pancreatic enzymes

    ii. Hormonal: entrance of food in the small intestine stimulates pancreatic secretion by the hormones secretin and cholecystokinin

2. Gallbladder

  a. A saclike organ attached to the inferior portion of the liver

  b. Approximately 7 to 10 cm long and can hold a maximum volume of 40 to 70 ml of bile

  c. Receives bile from the liver that has been diverted from the common bile duct

  d. Divisions

    i. Fundus: lower end of the body

    ii. Body

    iii. Infundibulum

    iv. Neck: joins the body with the cystic duct

  e. Serves as a reservoir for bile from the liver to the intestines

  f. Regulates the flow of bile (through the sphincter of Oddi) and concentrates bile (Fig. 7–8)

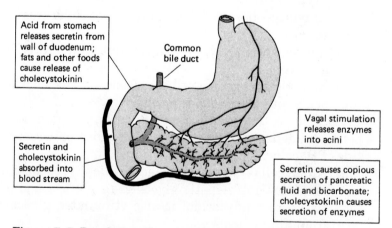

Figure 7–7. Regulation of pancreatic secretion. (From Guyton, A. C.: Textbook of Medical Physiology, 7th ed. W. B. Saunders Co., Philadelphia, 1986.)

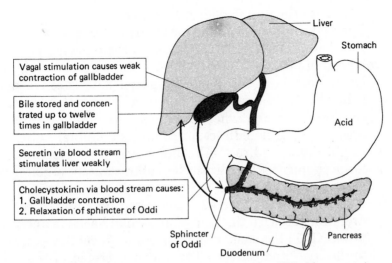

Figure 7–8. Mechanism of liver secretion and gallbladder emptying. (From Guyton, A. C.: Textbook of Medical Physiology, 7th ed. W. B. Saunders Co., Philadelphia, 1986.)

g. Opening of the sphincter of Oddi is regulated by vagal and hormonal stimulation
h. Nerve innervation
    i. Splanchnic nerve
    ii. Right branch of the vagus nerve
    iii. Seventh thoracic segment of the sympathetic nerve
i. Blood supply
    i. Arterial blood supply comes from the hepatic and cystic arteries
    ii. Venous drainage is through the cystic veins
j. Composition of bile
    i. Bile pigments and bile salts: high in cholesterol, some neutral fat, phospholipids, and inorganic salts
    ii. Bile salts: form micelle; responsible for the emulsification of fats
    iii. Majority (80%) of bile salts are reabsorbed in the intestinal tract and returned to the liver; the rest are lost in the feces
    iv. Bilirubin: a major bile pigment that is a breakdown product of hemoglobin
    v. Bile pigments give feces a brown color; absence produces a clay-colored stool
    vi. When the bile ducts are blocked, bile pigments accumulate in the blood and body tissues, producing jaundice
k. Flow of bile
    i. Released by the liver parenchymal cells
    ii. Bile then moves to the canaliculi of the liver
    iii. Flows into the hepatic duct then the cystic duct

      iv. Goes into the gallbladder for storage

      v. Drained from the gallbladder to the cystic duct

      vi. Flows into the common bile duct to the duodenum

  l. Metabolism of bile

      i. Heme portion of the hemoglobin molecule is converted to bilirubin by the reticuloendothelial cells and then released into the blood stream, where it binds with albumin and becomes unconjugated or indirect bilirubin (fat soluble)

      ii. In the liver, indirect bilirubin binds with glucuronic acid to form conjugated or direct bilirubin (water-soluble), which is then excreted into bile

      iii. In the intestinal mucosa, conjugated bilirubin is converted to urobilinogen with the help of intestinal bacteria and is excreted primarily in the stool; a small portion of urobilinogen is recycled to the liver and converted to bile or excreted in the urine

      iv. High concentrations of conjugated bilirubin indicate biliary tract obstruction; high concentrations of unconjugated bilirubin indicate hepatocellular dysfunction; *NOTE:* it is recommended to measure both direct and indirect bilirubin blood levels when jaundice is present to determine its cause

3. Liver

  a. Large glandular organ located in the right upper quadrant of the abdomen that fits snugly against the right inferior diaphragm

  b. Weighs approximately 1½ kg in the adult

  c. Divisions

      i. Right

      ii. Left

      iii. Caudate

      iv. Quadrate

  d. Lobules or sinusoids: functional unit of the liver

  e. Blood supply to the liver is via the hepatic artery and portal vein; an admixture of venous and arterial blood is present in the sinusoids; approximately 1500 ml of blood or 30% of cardiac output is delivered to the liver per minute, making it a large reservoir for blood

  f. Canaliculi: located within the liver lobules; serve as receptacles for bile that is produced by the hepatocytes

  g. Cellular functions of the liver

      i. Kupffer cells: main function is phagocytosis by trapping foreign bodies; it also destroys old erythrocytes and detoxifies toxic substances

      ii. Hepatocytes: secrete bile at a rate of 600 to 1000 ml/day; metabolize carbohydrates, fats, and proteins

      iii. Deaminates amino acids for glucose availability

      iv. Synthesizes amino acids, albumin, globulins, prothrombin, fibrinogen, and other coagulation factors

    v. Stores fat-soluble vitamins, vitamin B_{12}, copper, and iron
    vi. Converts glucose to glycogen, stores it, and breaks it down as needed
    vii. Converts ammonia to urea
    viii. Synthesizes and catabolizes fatty acids and neutral fats to form ketone bodies and acetate; also forms lipoproteins, cholesterol, and phospholipids
    ix. Detoxifies drugs, hormones, and other toxic substances

NURSING ASSESSMENT DATA BASE

Nursing History

1. **Patient health history**
   a. Previous surgery or illness
   b. Nutritional state
   c. Generalized weakness
   d. Easy fatigability
   e. Pain: location, duration, intensity, alleviating and aggravating factors
   f. Weight loss
   g. Difficulty in swallowing
   h. Easy bruising or bleeding
   i. Nausea and vomiting: alleviating and aggravating factors, description of vomitus
   j. Heartburn
   k. Diarrhea/constipation
   l. Darker color of urine
   m. Color of stools
   n. Allergies
2. **Family history**
   a. Carcinoma
   b. Diabetes mellitus
   c. Anemia
   d. Chronic diseases
   e. Pancreatic disease
   f. Hepatitis or exposure to hepatitis
   g. Gastrointestinal-related disease (e.g., peptic ulcer)
3. **Social history**
   a. Alcohol and tobacco use
   b. Cultural food use (e.g., spices, herbs)
   c. Eating habits
   d. Personality type (e.g., tense, stressful)
   e. Occupational history (e.g., exposure to asbestos)
   f. Bowel habits

4. Medication history
   a. Antacids
   b. Laxatives, cathartics
   c. Anticholinergics
   d. Corticosteroids
   e. Antidiarrheal
   f. Antiemetics
   g. Tranquilizers
   h. Sedatives
   i. Antihypertensives
   j. Barbiturates
   k. Antibiotics
   l. Acetylsalicylic acid

Nursing Examination of Patient

1. **Anatomic landmarks:** used to describe the location of tenderness, pain, presence of mass and other abnormal findings
   a. Subcostal margins
   b. Midline of the abdomen
   c. Rectus abdominis muscle
   d. Umbilicus
   e. Costovertebral angle
   f. Symphysis pubis
   g. Poupart's ligaments (inguinal)
   h. Flanks
2. **Quadrants of the abdomen**
   a. Left upper
   b. Right upper
   c. Left lower
   d. Right lower
3. **Inspection**
   a. Symmetry
   b. Contour of the abdomen: flat, rounded, concave, protuberant
   c. Skin: scars, striae, rashes and lesions, visible blood supply, pigmentation, spider angiomata
   d. Umbilicus: contour, signs of inflammation, signs of hernia, eversion, caput medusae (a peculiar appearance in the navel area due to dilatation of the blood vessels from stasis of the cutaneous veins; seen mainly in patients with liver cirrhosis)
   e. Peristalsis: may be visible in thin persons and children
   f. Masses: movable or immovable
   g. Pulsations: aortic pulsation may be visible in the epigastrium
   h. Pubic hair distribution: diamond-shaped in males and triangular-shaped in females

    i. Presence of wounds, fistulas, and/or ostomy

    j. Presence of spider angiomata denoting liver disease

4. Auscultation

  a. Points to remember

    i. Should be done prior to percussion and palpation to avoid alteration of the frequency of bowel sounds

    ii. Listen in all four quadrants and note the location, frequency, and character of bowel sounds and any other abnormal sounds

    iii. Diaphragm of the stethoscope should be placed lightly against the abdominal wall to avoid friction and compression of vessels

    iv. May be necessary to listen for a full 2 to 5 minutes if bowel sounds are hypoactive

  b. Normal bowel sounds

    i. Low-pitched, continuous gurgling sounds

    ii. Present on all four quadrants

    iii. Caused by the basic propulsive movement and the mixing movement of the gastrointestinal tract

  c. Abnormal bowel sounds

    i. Borborygmi: loud gurgles indicating hyperperistalsis; usually occurs before mealtime or when a person is tense or nervous

    ii. Paralytic ileus: absence of bowel sounds; denotes immobile bowel or the presence of peritonitis

    iii. Hypoactive: extreme weakness or infrequency of sounds; usually present after surgery

    iv. Loud, high-pitched bowel sounds that may be accompanied by pain and/or severe cramping and visible peristalsis are usually indicative of intestinal obstruction

    v. Succussion splash: sound caused by increased air and fluid in the stomach as in pyloric obstruction

  d. Other auscultatory findings

    i. Bruit: sound resembling systolic murmur caused by turbulence in the flow of blood through a partially occluded artery. Aortic artery is 2 to 3 cm above the umbilicus in the epigastric area; renal arteries are immediately left and right of midline in the epigastric area; iliac arteries are in the inguinal area

    ii. Venous hum: humming sound heard over the liver area and associated with liver disease or with portal or splenic vein thrombosis

    iii. Friction rub: soft sound associated with respiration; in the spleen area it indicates inflammation or infarction and in the liver area it indicates the presence of tumor

5. Percussion: used to establish the presence of tumor, fluid, and enlargement of solid viscera

    a. Liver: normally dull sounds are present; both upper and lower borders should be examined to detect enlargement

    b. Spleen: normally dull sounds are present

    c. Stomach: normally tympanic sounds are heard when it is empty

    d. Abnormal abdominal sounds

       i. Decreased or absent dullness over the liver area indicates the presence of free air below the diaphragm caused by perforation of a hollow viscus

      ii. Increased tympany of the stomach accompanied by upper abdominal distention indicates gastric dilatation

     iii. Change in percussion from tympany to dullness on inspiration may suggest splenic enlargement

     iv. Shifting dullness from flat to side-lying position indicates the presence of fluid in the abdominal cavity

6. Palpation: one of the most important parts of the abdominal examination

    a. Used to elicit pain or discomfort

    b. Used to determine the change of tone in the abdominal wall

    c. Used to determine firmness and mobility of masses

    d. Used to determine enlargement of an organ

    e. Used to differentiate abdominal wall mass from intra-abdominal mass (Fothergil's test)

    f. Visceral pain: arises from organic lesions or functional disturbance within the abdomen; it is a dull type of pain and poorly localized (e.g., pain of intestinal obstruction)

    g. Somatic pain: involves the nervous system pathways and is characterized by sharp and well-localized pain (e.g., pain of appendicitis)

    h. Rebound tenderness indicates peritoneal inflammation

    i. Involuntary rigidity or spasm indicates peritonitis

    j. Contralateral tenderness (Rovsing's sign): pain on opposite side of palpation and may indicate the presence of appendicitis; commonly seen in children

    k. Enlargement of the liver accompanied by tenderness may indicate hepatitis; without tenderness may indicate cirrhosis

    l. Enlarged, irregular liver may suggest malignancy

    m. Murphy's sign: right upper quadrant pain on inspiration; indicates the presence of cholecystitis

    n. Referred pain: pain is experienced in an area other than the area being palpated

Diagnostic Studies

1. Laboratory findings

    a. Complete blood cell count

    b. Alkaline phosphatase level

    c. Bilirubin level
       i. Serum
      ii. Urine
     iii. Fecal
    d. Serum glutamic oxaloacetic transaminase (SGOT)
    e. Serum glutamic pyruvic transaminase (SGPT)
    f. Lactate dehydrogenase (LDH)
    g. Amylase level
       i. Serum
      ii. Urine
    h. Prothrombin time (PT)
    i. Blood urea nitrogen (BUN)
    j. Stool examination
       i. Occult blood
      ii. Fat
     iii. Protein
     iv. Parasite and ova
    k. Serum calcium level
    l. Serum ammonia level
   m. Serum gastrin level
    n. Serum glucose level
    o. Serum electrolyte profile
    p. Serum albumin level
    q. Total protein level
    r. Serum lipase, cholinesterase level
    s. Serum alpha-fetoprotein: alpha-fetoprotein is excreted in patients with carcinoma
    t. Urobilinogen level
    u. Carcinoembryonic antigen (CEA): an antigen found in the blood of patients with a variety of carcinomas
    v. Albumin/globulin (A/G) ratio

2. Radiologic studies
    a. Cine esophagography
    b. Contrast radiography
    c. Upper gastrointestinal series
    d. Small bowel series
    e. Barium enema or swallow gastrography
    f. Cholangiography
       i. Intravenous
      ii. T-tube
    g. Percutaneous transhepatic cholangiography
    h. Celiac and mesenteric arteriography
    i. Superior and inferior mesenteric angiography
    j. Splenoportography

3. Other diagnostic studies
   a. Noninvasive
      i. Radionuclide imaging
         (a) HIDA scan—hepatobiliary imaging with the use of the HIDA dye
         (b) PAPIDA scan—hepatobiliary imaging with the use of the PAPIDA dye
      ii. Computed tomography (CT) scan
      iii. Ultrasonography
      iv. Gastric cytology
      v. Scans
         (a) Liver
         (b) Spleen
         (c) Pancreas
      vi. Schilling's test: a radioactive vitamin B_{12} absorption test
   b. Invasive
      i. Endoscopy
         (a) Esophageal
         (b) Gastric
         (c) Duodenal
      ii. Biopsy
         (a) Liver
         (b) Rectum
         (c) Esophageal
         (d) Gastric
         (e) Duodenal
         (f) Colon
         (g) Small bowel
      iii. Sigmoidoscopy
      iv. Colonoscopy
      v. Endoscopic retrograde cholangiopancreatography (ERCP)

COMMONLY ENCOUNTERED NURSING DIAGNOSES

Potential for Alteration in Nutrition, less than body requirements, related to nausea/vomiting, dietary intake/restrictions, and increased metabolic needs

1. Assessment for defining characteristics
   a. Body weight less than 80% of ideal body weight
   b. Unplanned weight loss more than 10 lb
   c. Serum albumin less than 3.5 g/dl
   d. Decreased muscle mass

2. Expected outcomes
   a. Maintains body weight
   b. Maintains positive nitrogen balance
3. Nursing interventions
   a. Assess for presence of bowel sounds
   b. Record daily weight
   c. Measure intake and output
   d. Provide frequent oral hygiene
   e. Observe and report indicators of potentially compromised nutritional status (Table 7–1)
   f. Administer enteral/parenteral nutrition as ordered
   g. Administer fat emulsions as ordered
   h. Consult with dietitian regarding patient's food preferences
   i. Administer vitamins as ordered
4. Evaluation of nursing care
   a. Serum albumin 3.5 g/dl or greater
   b. Weight loss less than 10 lb
   c. Body weight greater than 80% of ideal body weight
   d. Maintains adequate muscle mass

Potential for Fluid Volume Deficit related to vomiting, gastric suctioning, third spacing, and hemorrhage. *NOTE:* Third spacing occurs as a result of an imbalance between the osmotic and hydrostatic pressures, causing fluids to shift to the interstitial spaces

1. Assessment for defining characteristics
   a. Hypotension
   b. Tachycardia
   c. Ascites
   d. Decreased urine output
   e. Decreased hemoglobin and hematocrit
   f. Electrolyte imbalance
   g. Decreased filling pressures

Table 7–1. RECOMMENDED MONITORING FREQUENCIES FOR PATIENTS RECEIVING HYPERALIMENTATION

Test	Frequency
Clinical assessment	Daily
Temperature, pulse, and respiratory rate	Every 8 hours
Body weight	Three times/week
Blood: Hb, Hct, WBC, electrolytes, SMA-12	Twice weekly
Triglycerides, cholesterol, PT, serum osmolality	Once weekly
Creatinine clearance, blood culture, blood gases	As necessary
Urine: sugar and ketones, electrolytes	Every 6 hours with diabetic protocol as necessary

Reprinted with permission from Sibbald, W. (ed): Synopsis in Critical Care. © 1988, the Williams & Wilkins Co., Baltimore.

    h. Increased urine osmolality

    i. Decreased serum protein

2. Expected outcomes

    a. Vital signs within normal limits for the patient

    b. Urine output adequate

    c. Normal electrolyte balance

    d. Adequate intake and output

3. Nursing interventions

    a. Assess cardiovascular status by monitoring blood pressure, pulse, and filling pressures (e.g., central venous pressure, pulmonary capillary wedge pressure)

    b. Monitor intake and output

    c. Monitor for electrolyte abnormalities

    d. Replace fluid volume (e.g., blood and blood products, colloids, crystalloids) as ordered

    e. Observe skin turgor and mucous membranes

    f. Assess and monitor gastric drainage

    g. Control bleeding as much as possible

4. Evaluation of nursing care

    a. Skin warm and dry

    b. Blood pressure and pulse within normal limits for the patient

    c. Urine output greater than 30 ml/hr

    d. Absence of alteration in level of consciousness

    e. Balanced intake and output

Potential for Alteration in Bowel Elimination, diarrhea, related to dietary intake and intestinal dysfunction

1. Assessment for defining characteristics

    a. Abdominal cramps

    b. Increased frequency of stools

    c. Rectal pressure

    d. Watery consistency of stools

2. Expected outcomes

    a. Absence of abdominal cramps

    b. Absence of rectal pressure

    c. Change in consistency of stool (e.g., from formed to watery consistency)

3. Nursing interventions

    a. Decrease fiber in the diet

    b. Maintain adequate hydration

    c. Monitor frequency and consistency of stools

    d. Monitor intake and output

    e. Monitor for electrolyte abnormalities

    f. Administer antidiarrheal medication as ordered

    g. Discontinue gastrointestinal stimulants (e.g., tube feedings) as warranted

4. **Evaluation of nursing care**
    a. Normal consistency of stools
    b. Verbalization of the absence of abdominal cramps and rectal pressure

Potential for Alteration in Bowel Elimination, constipation, related to dietary intake, decreased physical activity, use of medications, and metabolic problems

1. **Assessment for defining characteristics**
    a. Decreased frequency of stools
    b. Hard, dry stool
    c. Straining at stool
    d. Pain on defecation
    e. Abdominal distention
    f. Palpable mass on lower abdominal quadrants
2. **Expected outcomes**
    a. Absence of pain on defecation
    b. Absence of straining at stool
    c. Soft, formed stool
    d. Absence of abdominal distention
    e. Resumes normal bowel frequency
3. **Nursing interventions**
    a. Provide for adequate fiber in the diet
    b. Encourage mobility if not contraindicated
    c. Provide for adequate fluid intake
    d. Monitor for electrolyte abnormalities
    e. Provide laxatives and/or enemas as ordered
4. **Evaluation of nursing care**
    a. Absence of abdominal distention and pain on defecation
    b. Absence of straining at stool
    c. Soft, formed stool

Potential Alteration in Comfort related to pain

1. **Assessment for defining characteristics**
    a. Grimacing
    b. Restlessness
    c. Splinting
    d. Decreased respiratory excursion
    e. Verbalization of pain
2. **Expected outcomes**
    a. Relief of pain
    b. Verbalization of reduction of pain

3. **Nursing interventions**
   a. Assess verbal complaints of pain
   b. Assist patient in assuming position of comfort
   c. Provide for comfort measures such as backrubs, relaxation techniques, and biofeedback
   d. Administer analgesics as ordered
4. **Evaluation of nursing care**
   a. Relaxed facial expression
   b. Verbalization of reduction or absence of pain
   c. Able to move freely

PATIENT HEALTH PROBLEMS

Acute Pancreatitis

1. **Pathophysiology**
   a. An inflammatory response of the pancreas to a variety of injuries
   b. Pathologic changes vary from mild edema to extensive hemorrhage, necrosis, and abscess formation
   c. Mortality rate ranges from 5% in its milder form to over 50% with hemorrhagic pancreatitis
   d. The key event seems to be an abnormal activation of the pancreatic proteolytic enzymes—trypsin, chymotrypsin, and elastase—that destroy the tissues in and around the pancreas
   e. There is an increased concentration of phospholipase A, an enzyme that may cause damage to the acinar cell membrane
   f. There is autodigestion of the pancreas by the very enzymes it produces
2. **Etiology or precipitating factors**
   a. Alcohol and biliary disease (gallstones) are the most frequent causes
   b. Other causes
      i. Trauma: blunt and penetrating
      ii. Infections: *Mycoplasma* infection, mumps, infectious mononucleosis, viral hepatitis
      iii. Drugs: thiazides, azathioprine, estrogens, sulfonamides, tetracycline
      iv. Metabolic factors: hyperlipidemia, hyperparathyroidism, hypercalcemia
      v. Heredity
      vi. Ischemia
      vii. Neoplasms
      viii. Operative injury
      ix. More recently pancreatitis has been observed following endoscopy and cardiopulmonary bypass

3. Nursing assessment data base
   a. Nursing history
      i. Subjective findings
         (a) Unrelenting abdominal pain usually located in the epigastrium and periumbilical regions
         (b) Pain often radiates to the chest and back
         (c) Nausea, vomiting, retching, and dry heaves
         (d) Low-grade fever
         (e) Anorexia
         (f) Weakness
         (g) Diarrhea
         (h) Weight loss
         (i) Vague dyspepsia or flatulence
         (j) Abdominal distention
         (k) Diaphoresis
         (l) Jaundice
         (m) Dehydration
         (n) Poorly defined abdominal mass
         (o) In severe cases, mental confusion and agitation, impaired respiratory function, and shock
      ii. Objective findings
         (a) History of gallstones with partial or complete common bile duct obstruction
         (b) History of recent excessive alcohol intake
         (c) Family history of pancreatitis
         (d) Onset of bacterial infection such as mumps or scarlet fever
         (e) History of malignant tumors
         (f) History of abdominal trauma or surgery
         (g) History of erosive connective tissue disease such as Crohn's disease
         (h) Presence of metabolic disorders such as hypercalcemia and hyperlipidemia
         (i) Drug use such as oral contraceptives, corticosteroids, thiazide diuretics, opiates, antihypertensives
         (j) Current pregnancy (third trimester) with shifting of abdominal contents and compression of biliary duct
   b. Nursing examination of patient
      i. Inspection
         (a) Patient may be curled up with both arms over the abdomen to relieve pain
         (b) May be restless, agitated, confused, or apprehensive
         (c) Skin may be pale, cold, mottled, and moist because of fluid shifts, vasoconstriction, and edema
         (d) Jaundice may be mild or pronounced
         (e) Urine may be dark amber or brown and foamy, reflecting the presence of bile

  (f) Grey Turner's sign (blue/green/brown discoloration in the flanks from blood accumulation) or Cullen's sign (similar discoloration around the umbilicus) may be present in hemorrhagic pancreatitis

  (g) Steatorrhea (bulky, pale, foul-smelling stools) may be present

  (h) Abdomen is usually moderately distended

 ii. Auscultation

  (a) Bowel sounds may be decreased or absent

  (b) Basilar crackles may be present because of pleural effusion

  (c) Tachycardia and hypotension may be present in shock states

 iii. Percussion

  (a) Dullness over the pancreas

  (b) Shifting dullness in the presence of ascites

 iv. Palpation

  (a) Upper abdominal guarding is present

  (b) Rebound tenderness is usually present

  (c) Rigidity may or may not be present

c. Diagnostic study findings

 i. Laboratory findings

  (a) Elevated serum amylase and lipase

  (b) Elevated serum bilirubin

  (c) Elevated SGOT, SGPT, LDH, and alkaline phosphatase levels

  (d) Decreased serum protein and albumin

  (e) Decreased serum potassium level due to vomiting

  (f) Elevated triglyceride values

  (g) Decreased serum calcium level

  (h) Elevated hematocrit due to hemoconcentration

  (i) Elevated leukocyte count

  (j) Transient elevations of serum glucose level

  (k) Prolonged prothrombin time may be present

  (l) Elevated urine amylase level

  (m) Increased fat content in the stool

 ii. Radiologic findings

  (a) Upper gastrointestinal series—exhibits evidence of delayed gastric emptying and enlargement of the duodenum due to edema of the head of the pancreas

  (b) Abdominal plain film—may show presence of dilated loop of small bowel ("sentinal loop") adjacent to the pancreas. Calcifications of the pancreas are diagnostic of chronic pancreatitis

  (c) Chest x-ray film may reveal the presence of pleural effusion

      iii. Other diagnostic findings

         (a) Ultrasound may reveal diffuse pancreatic enlargement, pseudocyst, or abscess formation

         (b) CT scan may reveal pancreatic inflammation, pseudocyst, abscess, carcinoma, or obstruction of the biliary tract

         (c) Endoscopy may reveal anomalies of the pancreatic duct. *NOTE:* relatively contraindicated during the acute phase

         (d) Arterial blood gas values may show hypoxemia and hypercapnia reflecting the presence of respiratory insufficiency

         (e) Radionuclide biliary excretion scan (e.g., HIDA scan) may be used to differentiate between alcoholic and biliary pancreatitis if the bilirubin value is less than 10 mg/dl

4. Nursing diagnoses

  a. Potential for injury related to multiple complications such as sepsis, pseudocysts, abscess formation, and pancreatic fistulas

      i. Assessment for defining characteristics

         (a) Elevated temperature

         (b) Worsening abdominal pain

         (c) Persistent fever and leukocytosis

      ii. Expected outcomes

         (a) Afebrile

         (b) Complications are prevented or minimized

      iii. Nursing interventions

         (a) Assess vital signs frequently

         (b) Assess for signs of decreased tissue perfusion such as skin color and temperature

         (c) Monitor hemodynamic pressures if possible

         (d) Monitor cardiac rate and rhythm

         (e) Assess for increased abdominal pain, rigidity/tenderness, and diminished/absent bowel sounds

         (f) Measure abdominal girth and report any increases

         (g) Use aseptic technique when changing dressing and/or invasive lines

         (h) Obtain cultures as ordered

         (i) Monitor clotting studies

         (j) Provide urinary catheter care routinely

         (k) Observe intravenous and drainage tube insertion sites for redness and/or swelling

         (l) Monitor temperature and report developing or persistent elevations

         (m) Prepare for surgical intervention as necessary

         (n) Administer antibiotic as ordered

         (o) Observe urine output for volume and presence of hematuria

    iv. Evaluation of nursing care
      (a) Temperature less than 99° F (37.2° C)
      (b) Cultures negative
      (c) Presence of normal bowel sounds
      (d) Stable abdominal girth measurement
      (e) Absence of redness and tenderness at intravenous and drainage tubes insertion sites
      (f) Absence of hematuria
      (g) Skin warm and dry
      (h) Vital signs within normal limits for the patient
      (i) Urine output greater than 30 ml/hr

b. Potential for injury related to complications such as myocardial infarction, shock, and renal failure (see Chapters 2 and 3 for nursing diagnoses related to these complications)

c. Alteration in nutrition, less than body requirements related to nausea and vomiting, loss of digestive enzymes, anorexia, and increased metabolic needs

    i. Assessment for defining characteristics
      (a) Increase in nausea and vomiting
      (b) Hypermetabolic state
      (c) Hypoactive or absent bowel sounds
      (d) Presence of anorexia

    ii. Expected outcomes
      (a) Positive nitrogen balance
      (b) Weight within normal limits for the patient
      (c) Presence of adequate muscle mass

    iii. Nursing interventions
      (a) Assess presence and character of bowel sounds
      (b) Maintain NPO status and institute nasogastric suctioning during the acute phase
      (c) Obtain daily weights
      (d) Administer antispasmodic and anticholinergic drugs as ordered to reduce gastric and pancreatic secretions
      (e) Administer antacids as ordered to reduce gastric acidity
      (f) Monitor blood glucose levels
      (g) Monitor serum albumin levels
      (h) Administer vitamins as ordered
      (i) Administer hyperalimentation and fat emulsions as ordered
      (j) Provide oral hygiene as frequently as necessary
      (k) Keep nares clean and lubricated with water-soluble lubricant to prevent dryness, irritation and infection
      (l) Begin oral feedings slowly after removal of nasogastric tube

(m) Administer pancreatic enzymes replacement with meals to correct enzyme deficit and to aid in digestion

(n) Correct persistent hyperglycemia with insulin administration

(o) Give nutritional supplements as indicated

iv. Evaluation of nursing care

(a) Will maintain weight within 1 to 2 kg of normal body weight

(b) Serum albumin greater than 3.5 g/dl

(c) Absence of nausea and vomiting

(d) Serum glucose within normal limits

(e) Will maintain adequate muscle mass

(f) Absence of clinical signs of vitamin deficiency

d. Fluid volume deficit and electrolyte imbalance related to nausea and vomiting or nasogastric suctioning, fever and diaphoresis, third spacing, and fluid shifts

i. Assessment for defining characteristics

(a) Presence of nausea and vomiting

(b) Presence of ascites

(c) Presence of nasogastric drainage from suctioning

(d) Presence of hypotension and tachycardia

(e) Decreased urine output

ii. Expected outcomes

(a) Will maintain an adequate fluid balance

(b) Will maintain an adequate circulating blood volume

(c) Serum potassium and serum calcium within normal limits

iii. Nursing interventions

(a) Monitor vital signs and note postural changes in blood pressure

(b) Monitor and record intake and output

(c) Monitor cardiac rate and rhythm

(d) Monitor for electrolyte abnormalities

(e) Monitor filling pressures and report any abnormalities

(f) Infuse intravenous fluids with adequate electrolytes to prevent any deficits

(g) Monitor nasogastric output for amount, character, and color

(h) Administer blood and plasma as ordered to keep circulating volumes adequate

(i) Assess for clinical signs of hypocalcemia such as presence of Chvostek's and Trousseau signs

(j) Monitor hemoglobin and hematocrit for signs of bleeding and dehydration

(k) Assess mucous membranes and skin turgor for signs of dehydration

    iv. Evaluation of nursing care
      (a) Presence of balanced intake and output
      (b) Electrolytes, especially sodium, potassium, and calcium, within normal limits
      (c) Vital signs within normal limits for the patient
      (d) Skin warm and dry
      (e) Skin turgor and mucous membranes normal
      (f) Urine output greater than 30 ml/hr
      (g) Hemoglobin and hematocrit within normal limits

e. Potential alteration in gas exchange related to adult respiratory distress syndrome (ARDS) (complication of pancreatitis): see Chapter 1
    i. Additional assessment for defining characteristics
      (a) Hypoventilation due to abdominal pain
      (b) Elevation of the diaphragm due to ascites
    ii. Additional expected outcomes
      (a) Normal respiratory function
      (b) Arterial blood gases within normal limits for the patient

f. Alteration in comfort: pain related to inflammatory process in the pancreas
    i. Assessment for defining characteristics
      (a) Unrelenting epigastric pain
      (b) Retching
      (c) Tenderness
      (d) Grimacing
    ii. Expected outcome
      (a) Patient will verbalize that he is comfortable
    iii. Nursing interventions
      (a) Assess pain for onset, duration, intensity, and location
      (b) Assist patient in assuming position of comfort
      (c) Use other comfort measures, such as relaxation techniques, biofeedback, and imagery
      (d) Administer drug of choice (meperidine) in a timely manner. *NOTE:* Most opiate narcotics cause spasms of the sphincter of Oddi
      (e) Assess effectiveness of pain medication
      (f) Initiate patient-controlled analgesia as ordered
      (g) Minimize retching
    iv. Evaluation of nursing care
      (a) Verbalizes relief or decrease in pain and/or retching
      (b) Relaxed facial expression
      (c) Demonstrates the use of other pain-relieving techniques
      (d) Able to move without discomfort

Acute Hepatitis

1. **Pathophysiology**
   a. Infectious disease that is viral in origin
   b. Involves inflammation and injury of the liver; necrosis and scarring of the liver
   c. Regeneration of the liver with an increased number of mitotic figures
   d. Reduplication or proliferation of Kupffer cells
   e. Hepatitis A or infectious hepatitis
      i. Rapid onset of symptoms and destruction of liver cells
      ii. Usually affects young adults
      iii. Results most frequently from fecal-oral contamination
      iv. Incubation, following exposure, takes about 2 to 6 weeks before clinical signs are evident
      v. Most frequently seen in crowded, unsanitary living conditions
   f. Hepatitis B or serum hepatitis
      i. Slow onset of symptoms and destruction of liver cells
      ii. Affects all age groups
      iii. High-exposure population are those exposed to the risks of needle contamination
      iv. Has a longer incubation than hepatitis A
   g. Non-A, non-B hepatitis (hepatitis C)
      i. Little is known about this virus
      ii. Symptoms manifested are similar to hepatitis A and hepatitis B
2. **Etiology or precipitating factors**
   a. Viral infections
   b. Intravenous drug use
   c. Alcohol
   d. Shellfish
   e. Contaminated water and food
   f. Contaminated needles
   g. Contaminated blood transfusion
3. **Nursing assessment data base**
   a. Nursing history
      i. Subjective findings
         (a) Nausea and vomiting
         (b) Anorexia
         (c) Weakness
         (d) Dark urine
         (e) Clay-colored stool
         (f) Tenderness in right upper quadrant
         (g) Diarrhea
         (h) Headache
      ii. Objective findings
         (a) Jaundice
         (b) Low-grade fever

        (c) Elevated bilirubin level
        (d) Icteric sclerae

  b. Nursing examination of patient
     i. Inspection
        (a) Jaundice
        (b) Nausea and vomiting
        (c) Icteric sclerae
        (d) Weakness
        (e) Dark, bilirubin-positive urine
        (f) Clay-colored stool
     ii. Palpation
        (a) Hepatomegaly
        (b) Abdominal tenderness especially on right upper quadrant

  c. Diagnostic study findings
     i. Laboratory findings
        (a) Elevated serum bilirubin level
        (b) Elevated SGOT and SGPT levels
        (c) Elevated alkaline phosphatase level
        (d) Presence of bilirubin in the urine
        (e) Elevated LDH level
        (f) Serum antigen/antibody tests positive for hepatitis B virus
        (g) Stool and serology positive for hepatitis A virus
     ii. Other diagnostic findings
        (a) Ultrasound will show marked enlargement of the liver
        (b) Liver biopsy will confirm the extent of hepatic cellular damage

4. Nursing diagnoses
  a. Activity intolerance related to the infectious process
     i. Assessment for defining characteristics
        (a) Malaise
        (b) Easy fatigability
     ii. Expected outcomes
        (a) Maximum activity level
        (b) Absence of fatigue associated with activity
     iii. Nursing interventions
        (a) Maintain bed rest in quiet environment
        (b) Assist patient in assuming position of comfort
        (c) Ambulate with assistance when allowed
        (d) Coordinate care to provide planned periods of rest
        (e) Assist with and teach active and/or perform passive range of motion exercises
     iv. Evaluation of nursing care
        (a) Expressed return of energy
        (b) Maximum activity level increased
  b. Alteration in nutrition related to anorexia

   i. Assessment for defining characteristics
      (a) Decreased appetite
      (b) Nausea and vomiting
      (c) Presence of abdominal pain
  ii. Expected outcomes
      (a) Optimal body weight
      (b) Evidence of good appetite
 iii. Nursing interventions
      (a) Provide ordered diet
      (b) Encourage a high-calorie, high-carbohydrate diet
      (c) Offer small frequent feedings
      (d) Administer antacids and antiemetics as warranted
      (e) Obtain daily weight
      (f) Consult with dietitian and encourage patient to actively participate in choosing foods
  iv. Evaluation of nursing care
      (a) Body weight within 1 to 2 kg of normal
      (b) Adheres to prescribed diet
      (c) Ingests all foods offered
 c. Potential impairment of skin integrity related to deposition of bile salts in the skin
   i. Assessment for defining characteristics
      (a) Pruritus
      (b) Jaundice
      (c) Frequent scratching
  ii. Expected outcomes
      (a) Absence of skin breakdown
      (b) Verbalization of comfort
 iii. Nursing interventions
      (a) Avoid use of soap
      (b) Provide frequent skin care
      (c) Apply lotions and provide shower or bath with baking soda or cornstarch
      (d) Keep patient's fingernails short
      (e) Provide diversional activities
  iv. Evaluation of nursing care
      (a) No evidence of skin breakdown
      (b) Expressed relief of pruritus

Cirrhosis of the Liver

1. **Pathophysiology**
   a. Diffuse destruction and regeneration of liver parenchymal cells
   b. Regeneration causes the liver lobules to be very irregular
   c. Eventually nodular formation occurs in the liver

       d. Secondary to distortion and constriction of lobules, there is increased resistance to portal blood flow
       e. After long periods of damage and scar tissue formation, degeneration and decreased functioning occurs (Fig. 7–9)

2. **Etiology or precipitating factors**
       a. Chronic alcoholism: major cause
       b. Malnutrition
       c. Protein depletion
       d. Hepatitis: causes postnecrotic cirrhosis
       e. Drug toxicity
       f. Biliary obstruction
       g. Metabolic disease
       h. Congestive heart failure: causes cardiac cirrhosis

3. **Nursing assessment data base** (Fig. 7–10)
       a. Nursing history
          i. Subjective findings
             (a) Abdominal pain
             (b) Anorexia
             (c) Weight loss or weight gain
             (d) Weakness
             (e) Fatigue
             (f) Diarrhea/constipation
             (g) Dark urine
             (h) Pruritus
             (i) Decreased urinary output

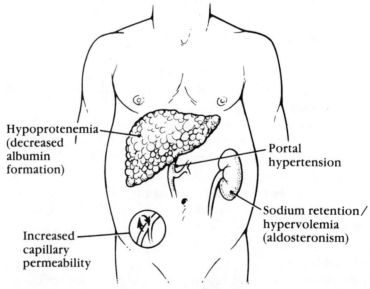

Figure 7–9. Factors contributing to the development of ascites. (From Bullock, B., and Rosendahl, P.: Pathophysiology: Adaptations and Alterations in Function. Little, Brown & Co., Boston, 1986.)

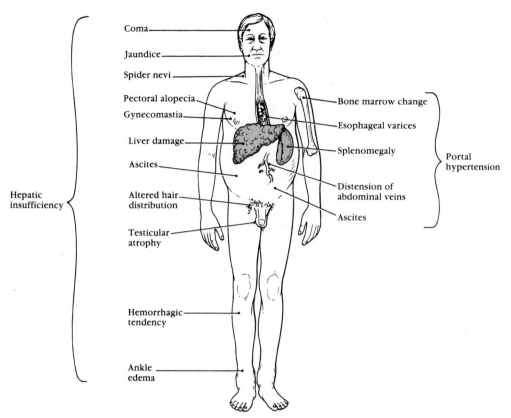

Figure 7–10. Clinical effects of cirrhosis of the liver. (From Bullock, B., and Rosendahl, P.: Pathophysiology: Adaptations and Alterations in Function. Little, Brown & Co., Boston, 1986.)

      ii. Objective findings
          (a) History of substance abuse (especially intravenous drugs)
          (b) History of hepatitis
          (c) Jaundice
          (d) Spider angiomas
          (e) Edema of extremities
          (f) Fetor hepaticus (musty-sweet breath)
          (g) Testicular atrophy
          (h) Altered hair distribution
          (i) History of congestive heart failure
          (j) History of bleeding tendencies
          (k) History of exposure to chemicals and/or anesthetic agents
          (l) History of rheumatic heart disease
   b. Nursing examination of patient
      i. Inspection
          (a) Limited thoracic expansion on respiration secondary to ascites

        (b) Depressed mentation

        (c) Slurred speech

        (d) Personality changes

        (e) Lethargy

        (f) Edema

        (g) Dry skin with poor turgor

        (h) Jaundice

        (i) Pruritus

        (j) Bruising

        (k) Spider angiomata

        (l) Telangiectasis

        (m) Palmar erythema

        (n) Pectoral alopecia

        (o) Gynecomastia

        (p) Oliguria and dark-colored urine

        (q) Asterixis

        (r) Poor nutritional status, including muscle wasting

    ii. Auscultation

        (a) Bowel sounds may be decreased

        (b) Adventitious lung sounds if congestive heart failure is present

   iii. Percussion

        (a) Enlarged liver

        (b) Shifting dullness

    iv. Palpation

        (a) Hepatojugular reflux

        (b) Splenomegaly

        (c) Hepatomegaly

c. Diagnostic study findings

    i. Laboratory findings

        (a) Elevated serum bilirubin

        (b) Elevated SGOT and SGPT

        (c) Elevated alkaline phosphatase

        (d) Decreased serum albumin

        (e) Prolonged prothrombin time

        (f) Elevated BUN

        (g) Elevated serum ammonia

        (h) Decreased fibrinogen level

        (i) Decreased hemoglobin and hematocrit

        (j) Hypokalemia and hyponatremia may be present

        (k) Positive bile in stool

        (l) Urine shows presence of urobilinogen

    ii. Radiologic findings

        (a) Upper gastrointestinal series may reveal esophageal varices

    (b) Endoscopic retrograde cholangiopancreatography (ERCP) may show common bile duct obstruction

    (c) Percutaneous transhepatic portography may show portal hypertension

  iii. Other diagnostic findings

    (a) Ultrasound may show liver destruction

    (b) Liver biopsy will show presence of cirrhosis

    (c) Esophagoscopy may show varices

    (d) Paracentesis will show presence of ascites

    (e) Liver scan may reveal hepatomegaly and splenomegaly

4. Nursing diagnoses

  a. Alteration in nutrition, less than body requirements related to nutrition and metabolism alteration

    i. Assessment for defining characteristics

      (a) Nausea and vomiting

      (b) Impaired carbohydrate metabolism

      (c) Impaired storage of nutrients

      (d) Malabsorption of fats and soluble vitamins

      (e) Anorexia

    ii. Expected outcomes

      (a) Maintains stable muscle mass

      (b) Maintains positive nitrogen balance

      (c) Maintains a stable body weight

    iii. Nursing interventions

      (a) Provide oral care frequently and prior to meals

      (b) Note food intolerances and aversions

      (c) Encourage patient to eat all meals and supplementary feedings

      (d) Provide a diet high in carbohydrates, protein, and calories to aid in the regeneration of liver cells

      (e) Consider small frequent feedings

      (f) Provide vitamin supplements to correct dietary deficiencies

      (g) Consult with dietitian

      (h) Encourage rest periods to conserve energy and decrease metabolic demands

      (i) Administer enteral feedings/hyperalimentation/fat emulsions as ordered

      (j) Obtain daily weights

    iv. Evaluation of nursing care

      (a) Patient's weight within 1 to 2 kg of normal weight

      (b) Adequate muscle mass

      (c) Adheres to diet

      (d) Ingests all or 95% of meals and supplementary feedings

    b. Fluid volume deficit related to changes in osmotic and hydrostatic pressures
        i. Assessment for defining characteristics
            (a) Ascites
            (b) Dry skin
            (c) Poor skin turgor
            (d) Oliguria
       ii. Expected outcomes
            (a) Maintains electrolytes within normal limits
            (b) Maintains stable abdominal girth
            (c) Maintains adequate urine output
      iii. Nursing interventions
            (a) Record intake and output
            (b) Obtain daily weights
            (c) Restrict sodium in the diet
            (d) Observe location and degree of edema and report any changes
            (e) Measure abdominal girth to assess ascites and report any changes
            (f) Administer diuretics as ordered to promote diuresis
            (g) Monitor electrolytes, especially sodium and potassium
            (h) Monitor vital signs and filling pressures
      iv. Evaluation of nursing care
            (a) Urine output greater than 30 ml/hr
            (b) Vital signs within normal limits for the patient
            (c) Stable abdominal girth
            (d) Electrolytes within normal limits
            (e) Balanced intake and output
   c. Impaired skin integrity related to poor nutritional status and deposition of bile salts in the skin
        i. Assessment for defining characteristics
            (a) Edema
            (b) Jaundice
            (c) Pruritus
            (d) Ascites
       ii. Expected outcomes
            (a) Maintains skin integrity
            (b) Absence of pruritus
      iii. Nursing interventions
            (a) Turn every 2 hours and keep off back as much as possible
            (b) Administer antipruritic medications and lotions as ordered
            (c) Keep patient's fingernails short
            (d) Apply powder, talc, or cornstarch
            (e) Avoid the use of soap
            (f) Assess skin for breaks and reddened areas

      (g) Provide range-of-motion exercises as necessary

      (h) Use gentle rubbing or patting of skin for pruritus

      (i) Provide sheepskin, alternating air mattress or egg crate mattress as necessary

    iv. Evaluation of nursing care

      (a) No evidence of skin breakdown

      (b) Expressed skin comfort

d. Ineffective breathing pattern related to impaired mobility and increased pressure under the diaphragm

    i. Assessment for defining characteristics

      (a) Ascites

      (b) Weakness

      (c) Decreased lung expansion

      (d) Tachypnea

    ii. Expected outcomes

      (a) Maintains adequate oxygenation

      (b) Absence of respiratory distress

      (c) Arterial blood gas values normal for the patient

    iii. Nursing interventions

      (a) Place in semi- to high Fowler's position as tolerated

      (b) Encourage use of incentive spirometer to maximize lung aeration

      (c) Monitor respiratory rate, rhythm, and depth and report any changes

      (d) Monitor blood gases and report any abnormalities

      (e) Monitor breath sounds and report any abnormalities

      (f) Assist with paracentesis to relieve pressure on diaphragm

      (g) Administer supplemental oxygen as necessary

      (h) Monitor serial chest x-ray films

    iv. Evaluation of nursing care

      (a) Blood gases within normal limits for the patient

      (b) Breath sounds clear and equal

      (c) Normal respiratory rate and depth

e. Potential alteration in tissue perfusion related to coagulation problems and fluid volume shifts

    i. Assessment for defining characteristics

      (a) Prolonged prothrombin time

      (b) Decreased fibrinogen level

      (c) Decreased clotting factors

      (d) Impaired vitamin K absorption

      (e) Bruising

      (f) Edema

    ii. Expected outcomes

      (a) Absence of bleeding

      (b) Capillary refill within normal limits

    iii. Nursing interventions
        (a) Observe for presence of melena and hematemesis
        (b) Monitor vital signs, hemoglobin, and hematocrit
        (c) Avoid use of razor blades
        (d) Avoid hard-bristled toothbrushes
        (e) Monitor mucous membranes for signs of bleeding
        (f) Counsel patient to avoid straining during bowel movement and forceful nose blowing
        (g) Prepare for endoscopy if bleeding occurs
        (h) Assess location and degree of edema
        (i) Assess capillary refill time
    iv. Evaluation of nursing care
        (a) No evidence of active bleeding
        (b) Decreased degree of edema
        (c) Capillary refill time less than 3 seconds

Hepatic Failure

1. Pathophysiology
    a. With severe hepatic necrosis there is loss of the synthetic and excretory functions of the liver
    b. Exact mechanism of hepatic encephalopathy is not well understood
    c. There is a marked elevation of ammonia levels in the circulatory system due to the liver's inability to conjugate ammonia
    d. There is inadequate production of clotting factors
    e. Presence of secondary dysfunction of other organs including the brain, lungs, kidneys, and pancreas
2. Etiology or precipitating factors
    a. Hepatitis
    b. Wilson's disease
    c. Drugs (e.g., acetaminophen, isoniazid, rifampin, halothane)
    d. Toxins (e.g., alcohol, carbon tetrachloride, *Amanita* mushrooms)
    e. Acute fatty liver of pregnancy
    f. Reye's syndrome
    g. Hepatic ischemia
3. Nursing assessment data base
    a. Nursing history
        i. Subjective findings
            (a) Headache
            (b) Hyperventilation
            (c) Jaundice
        ii. Objective findings
            (a) Personality changes
            (b) Asterixis
            (c) Palmar erythema

       (d) Spider nevi

       (e) Deep rapid respirations

       (f) Bruises

       (g) Testicular atrophy

       (h) Gynecomastia

       (i) Edema

   ii. Auscultation

       (a) Bowel sounds may be decreased

       (b) Presence of crackles on lung auscultation

  iii. Percussion

       (a) Enlarged liver

       (b) Shifting dullness

       (c) Hyperactive reflexes

   iv. Palpation

       (a) Splenomegaly

       (b) Hepatomegaly

 c. Diagnostic study findings

    i. Laboratory findings: same as in cirrhosis

   ii. Radiologic findings: same as in cirrhosis

  iii. Other diagnostic findings

       (a) Electroencephalogram (EEG) shows abnormal and gener-
alized slowing

       (b) Spinal tap shows elevated glutamine

       (c) Positive Babinski's sign

4. Nursing diagnoses

 a. Alteration in thought processes related to increased levels of serum
ammonia

    i. Assessment for defining characteristics

       (a) Elevated serum ammonia level

       (b) Elevated BUN

       (c) Personality changes

       (d) Decreasing levels of consciousness

   ii. Expected outcomes

       (a) Stable and normal level of consciousness

       (b) Serum ammonia level within normal limits

  iii. Nursing interventions

       (a) Monitor neurologic status (e.g., level of consciousness) and
motor ability every 2 hours

       (b) Monitor serum ammonia and potassium levels

       (c) Restrict protein in the diet to prevent increased ammonia
production

       (d) Avoid use of narcotics, sedatives, and tranquilizers as
much as possible

       (e) Provide for a safe environment (e.g., side rails up)

       (f) Administer medications to reduce intestinal ammonia

(e.g., lactulose, neomycin, or kanamycin enemas as ordered)

iv. Evaluation of nursing care

(a) Serum ammonia levels as close to normal as possible

(b) Patient awake, alert, and oriented

b. Other nursing diagnoses same as in liver cirrhosis

Ulcerative Colitis

1. **Pathophysiology**
   a. Diffuse inflammatory intestinal disorder affecting the mucosal lining of the colon and rectum
   b. Purulent exudate and blood are common; chronic inflammation may cause bleeding throughout the mucosa
   c. The bowel fills with a bloody, mucoid secretion that produces crampy pain, rectal urgency, and diarrhea
   d. Colon wall becomes thickened and edematous
   e. Malabsorption is common
   f. There is a significant relationship between ulcerative colitis and cancer of the colon
   g. The disease is characterized by frequent relapses

2. **Etiology or precipitating factors**
   a. Exact etiology unknown
   b. Genetic basis has been suggested: occurs in increased incidence in certain families
   c. Viral infection
   d. Autoimmune nature: plasma in certain persons has been shown to have an antibody to the colonic epithelial cells

3. **Nursing assessment data base**
   a. Nursing history
      i. Subjective findings
         (a) Crampy abdominal pain
         (b) Bloody diarrhea
         (c) Fever
         (d) Anorexia
         (e) Generalized malaise
         (f) Nausea and vomiting
         (g) Tenesmus
      ii. Objective findings
         (a) Weight loss
         (b) Increased peristalsis
         (c) Anemia
         (d) Family history of the disease
   b. Nursing examination of the patient
      i. Inspection

(a) Pale

(b) Facial expression shows evidence of pain

(c) Weight loss

(d) Bloody diarrhea

(e) Nausea and vomiting

ii. Auscultation

(a) Hyperactive bowel sounds

(b) Decreased breath sounds may be present because of pain

iii. Percussion

(a) Increased tympanic sounds in all four quadrants of the abdomen

iv. Palpation

(a) Presence of abdominal tenderness

c. Diagnostic study findings

i. Laboratory findings

(a) Decreased hemoglobin and hematocrit

(b) Leukocytosis

(c) Increased alkaline phosphatase level

(d) Hypokalemia may be present

(e) Hypoalbuminemia

(f) Occult blood in the stool

ii. Radiologic findings

(a) Plain film of the abdomen shows dilated loops of bowel

(b) Barium studies shows location of inflammation

iii. Other diagnostic findings

(a) Colonoscopy—detects lesions in the proximal colon

(b) Sigmoidoscopy—shows site of mucosal inflammation or ulceration

(c) Biopsy—detects type of lesion

4. Nursing diagnoses

a. Alteration in nutrition related to intestinal malabsorption

i. Assessment for defining characteristics

(a) Anorexia

(b) Weight loss

(c) Diarrhea

(d) Generalized malaise

ii. Expected outcomes

(a) Stable body weight

(b) Return of appetite

(c) Maximum energy level

iii. Nursing interventions

(a) Identify foods that are irritating to the gastrointestinal tract

(b) Provide high-calorie, high-protein, low-residue diet low in fats and fibers

(c) Provide supplemental feedings as much as possible

(d) Administer hyperalimentation and fat emulsions as ordered

(e) Obtain daily weights

(f) Administer enteral feedings as ordered

(g) Encourage patient to eat slowly, chew well, and take small bites

(h) Consult with dietitian for patient's food preferences

(i) Monitor serum albumin

   iv. Evaluation of nursing care

(a) Body weight within 1 to 2 g of normal weight

(b) Weight loss less than 10 lb

(c) Stable body mass

(d) Serum albumin greater than 3.5 g/dl

 b. Potential for fluid volume deficit related to diarrhea (see p. 771)

   i. Additional nursing interventions

(a) Assess stool for presence of blood

(b) Monitor hemoglobin and hematocrit

(c) Avoid rectal temperatures

   ii. Additional evaluation of nursing care

(a) Vital signs within normal limits for the patient

(b) Hemoglobin and hematocrit within normal limits for the patient

 c. Alteration in bowel elimination related to diarrhea (see p. 772)

   i. Additional nursing intervention

(a) Monitor stools for occult blood

(b) Prepare for surgery (e.g., colectomy, ileostomy, Hartman's procedure) as indicated

   ii. Additional evaluation of nursing care

(a) Absence of complications (e.g., toxic megacolon, perforation, intestinal obstruction)

 d. Alteration in comfort related to abdominal cramps (see p. 773)

   i. Additional nursing intervention

(a) Avoid use of opiates since it may precipitate toxic megacolon

Regional Enteritis (Crohn's Disease)

1. **Pathophysiology** (Fig. 7–11)

 a. Recurrent, nonspecific inflammation of the entire intestine, usually the terminal ileum, involving the mucosa and surrounding musculature

 b. Deep fissure formation is present in the intestinal wall

 c. Bowel becomes congested, thickened, and rigid, with adhesions involving the peri-intestinal fat

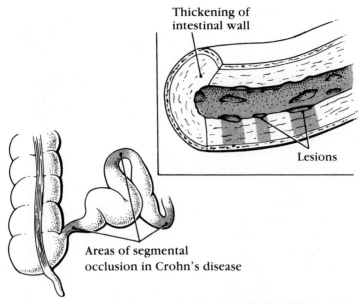

Figure 7–11. Schematic appearance of Crohn's disease showing segmental areas of occlusion and transmural involvement of the intestinal wall. (From Bullock, B., and Rosendahl, P.: Pathophysiology: Adaptations and Alterations in Function. Little, Brown & Co., Boston, 1986.)

d. Dilatation of the lymphatic channels and lymphoid deposits are seen in all levels of bowel involvement
e. Inflammatory changes cause functional disruption of the mucosa (Table 7–2)
f. Fluid imbalances occur when large segments of ileum are affected
g. Stricture and fistulas predispose the intestines to bacterial overgrowth and abscess formation
h. Incidence of the disease is slightly higher in Jews
i. Onset is most common between the ages of 15 and 20

Table 7–2. MAJOR DIFFERENCES BETWEEN ULCERATIVE COLITIS AND CROHN'S DISEASE

	Ulcerative Colitis	**Crohn's Disease**
Extent of Disease	Mucosa	Entire wall
Ulceration	Extensive, superficial	Patchy, deep
Mesentery	Normal	Thickened
Lymph Nodes	Normal	Diseased
Granulomata	Absent	Present (25% to 75%)
Distribution	Symmetric	Eccentric
"Skip" Areas	Never	Common
Diseased Rectum	Always	10% to 20%
Small Intestine Disease	Never	Usual
Results of Surgery	Cure	Frequent recurrence

Reprinted with permission from Bullock, B., and Rosendahl, P. (eds): Pathophysiology: Adaptations and Alterations in Function. Little, Brown & Co., Boston, 1986.

2. **Etiology or precipitating factors**
   a. Exact etiology unknown
   b. Familial predisposition to the disease
   c. Stress
   d. Personality factors (e.g., depression and dependency)
3. **Nursing assessment data base**
   a. Nursing history
       i. Subjective findings
           (a) Diarrhea
           (b) Crampy abdominal pain, especially on the right lower quadrant
           (c) Malaise
           (d) Nausea and vomiting
           (e) Bloody stool
       ii. Objective findings
           (a) Weight loss
           (b) Dependent personality
   b. Nursing examination of patient
       i. Inspection
           (a) Weight loss
           (b) Malaise
           (c) Bloody stool
           (d) Diarrhea
           (e) Nausea and vomiting
       ii. Auscultation
           (a) Hyperperistalsis
           (b) Decreased breath sounds because of pain
       iii. Percussion
           (a) Increased tympanic sounds
       iv. Palpation
           (a) Presence of abdominal tenderness
   c. Diagnostic study findings
       i. Laboratory findings: same as in ulcerative colitis
       ii. Radiologic findings
           (a) "String sign" present on plain film of the abdomen: irregularly narrowed distal ileum
           (b) Barium studies may show intestinal obstruction
       iii. Other diagnostic findings: same as in ulcerative colitis
4. **Nursing diagnoses**
   a. Potential for infection related to the presence of intestinal fistulae
       i. Assessment for defining characteristics
           (a) Elevated temperature
           (b) Poor nutritional state
           (c) Decreased mobility

    ii. Expected outcomes
       (a) Patient will be normothermic
       (b) Presence of negative blood cultures
   iii. Nursing interventions
       (a) Assess vital signs, including temperature
       (b) Assess degree of abdominal pain and report any increased intensity and persistent pain
       (c) Assess stool for presence of pus
       (d) Avoid gas-forming foods
       (e) Administer nutritional supplements as needed
       (f) Administer pain medications to prevent debilitating pain
       (g) Observe universal precautions in handling stools and other secretions
       (h) Administer corticosteroids (e.g., sulfasalazine [Azulfadine]) and antibiotics as ordered
       (i) Prepare for surgical intervention (e.g., continent ileostomy [Koch's pouch]) as indicated
       (j) Obtain and monitor daily weights
   iv. Evaluation of nursing care
       (a) Negative blood cultures
       (b) Temperature maintained below 99° F
       (c) Vital signs within normal limits for the patient
       (d) Absence of pus in the stool
       (e) Stable body weight
  b. Other nursing diagnoses: same as in ulcerative colitis

Toxic Megacolon

1. Pathophysiology
  a. Contractility of the intestinal wall is lost and massive dilatation of the large colon results
  b. Associated with ulcerative colitis
2. Etiology or precipitating factors
  a. Barium enema given during a severe period of diarrhea
  b. Opiates given to patients with ulcerative colitis
  c. Use of anticholinergic agents
  d. Hypokalemia
3. Nursing assessment data base
  a. Nursing history
    i. Subjective findings
       (a) Severe abdominal pain
       (b) Increase in gas formation
       (c) Sudden decrease in the number of stools
    ii. Objective findings
       (a) Severe abdominal distention

(b) Hypoactive or absent bowel sounds
(c) Fever
(d) Tachycardia
(e) Bloody diarrhea
(f) Glucocytosis
   b. Nursing examination of patient
      i. Inspection
         (a) Abdominal distention
         (b) Bloody diarrhea
         (c) Decrease in the number of stools
      ii. Auscultation
         (a) Hypoactive or absent bowel sounds
         (b) Tachycardia
      iii. Percussion
         (a) Increased tympany
      iv. Palpation
         (a) Presence of abdominal pain
   c. Diagnostic findings
      i. Laboratory findings: same as in ulcerative colitis
      ii. Radiologic findings
         (a) Plain film of the abdomen shows dilated loops of bowel
      iii. Other diagnostic studies
         (a) Colonoscopy—shows the level of the lesion
         (b) Biopsy—shows the type of lesion

4. **Nursing diagnoses**
   a. Alteration in comfort related to severe abdominal pain (see p. 773)
      i. Additional nursing interventions
         (a) Avoid use of opiates and anticholinergics
         (b) Initiate intestinal decompression
   b. Fluid volume deficit: related to intestinal decompression and NPO status (see p. 771)
   c. Potential for infection related to perforation
      i. Assessment for defining characteristics
         (a) Elevated temperature
         (b) Elevated leukocyte count
         (c) Abdominal guarding
         (d) Severe abdominal pain
      ii. Expected outcomes
         (a) Patient will be normothermic
         (b) Absence of abdominal guarding
         (c) Leukocyte count within normal limits for the patient
      iii. Nursing interventions
         (a) Assess for signs of perforation or impending perforation
         (b) Administer antibiotics as ordered
         (c) Monitor leukocyte count

(d) Monitor bowel sounds

(e) Measure abdominal girth

(f) Observe stools for increase in the presence of blood

(g) Prepare patient for surgical intervention (e.g., bowel resection)

iv. Evaluation of nursing care

(a) Temperature within normal limits

(b) Leukocyte count within normal limits for the patient

(c) Absence of signs of perforation (e.g., guarding, increasing abdominal girth)

Bowel Infarction

1. **Pathophysiology**
   a. Decreased blood flow to the major mesenteric vessels (celiac, superior, and inferior mesenteric arteries) causes vasoconstriction and vasospasm, leading to hypertonic and contracted bowel with mucosal ulceration
   b. When spasm subsides there is bowel musculature fatigue because of its inability to receive essential nutrients and oxygen
   c. The bowel becomes inert, edematous, and cyanotic, usually with a large accumulation of intraluminal fluid
   d. Full thickness necrosis occurs
   e. As gangrenous changes advance and intraluminal pressure increases, perforation occurs
   f. Peritonitis or local abscess formation results
2. **Etiology or precipitating factors**
   a. Mural thrombosis in the post–myocardial infarction period
   b. Dislodged cholesterol plaques in the aorta
   c. Emboli formed in patients with endocarditis or atrial fibrillation
   d. Decreased cardiac output states
   e. Arteriosclerosis
   f. Thromboangiitis obliterans
   g. Hypercoagulable states (e.g., polycythemia, postsplenectomy)
   h. Cirrhosis of the liver
   i. Intra-abdominal suppuration (e.g., appendicitis, pelvic abscess)
3. **Nursing assessment data base**
   a. Nursing history
      i. Subjective findings
         (a) Acute abdominal pain
         (b) Bloody diarrhea
         (c) Vomiting
         (d) Urgent bowel movements
         (e) Weight loss
      ii. Objective findings

(a) History of atrial fibrillation

(b) History of myocardial infarction

(c) Signs of shock (e.g., tachycardia, hypotension)

b. Nursing examination of patient

   i. Inspection

      (a) Pallor

      (b) Tachycardia

      (c) Abdominal distention

      (d) Respirations usually shallow because of pain

      (e) May be curled up because of intense abdominal pain

   ii. Auscultation

      (a) Bowel sounds may be absent or hypoactive

      (b) Breath sounds may be decreased because of shallow respirations

      (c) Hypotension

   iii. Percussion

      (a) Hyperresonance may be present especially if paralytic ileus occurs

      (b) Absence of dullness in liver area may denote presence of free air in abdomen

   iv. Palpation

      (a) Abdominal tenderness present

      (b) Guarding and rigidity may be present

c. Diagnostic study findings

   i. Laboratory findings

      (a) Leukocytosis

      (b) Elevated serum phosphate level

      (c) Urine may show elevated phosphate level

      (d) Elevated hematocrit and serum osmolality

      (e) Presence of blood in the stool

   ii. Radiologic findings

      (a) Angiography—shows location of infarction

      (b) Plain film of the abdomen shows dilated loops of bowel with air fluid levels

      (c) Barium studies show location of infarction

   iii. Other diagnostic findings

      (a) Sigmoidoscopy may reveal dusky, ischemic bowel

      (b) Arterial blood gas studies may show metabolic acidosis

      (c) Doppler ultrasonic blood flow detection shows level of infarction

4. Nursing diagnoses

a. Potential for infection related to peritonitis or abscess formation

   i. Assessment for defining characteristics

      (a) Elevated temperature

      (b) Guarding and rigidity of the abdomen

    (c) Decreased nutritional state

    (d) Absence of bowel sounds

  ii. Expected outcomes

    (a) Blood cultures negative

    (b) Patient will be normothermic

 iii. Nursing interventions

    (a) Assess vital signs, including temperature

    (b) Measure abdominal girth and report any increases

    (c) Assess bowel sounds

    (d) Provide adequate nutrition

    (e) Monitor leukocyte count and report any elevation

    (f) Obtain blood cultures as ordered

    (g) Observe universal precautions in handling blood and body fluids

    (h) Obtain daily weights

    (i) Administer broad-spectrum antibiotics as ordered

 iv. Evaluation of nursing care

    (a) Normal blood culture

    (b) Leukocyte count within normal limits

    (c) Temperature below 99° F (37.2° C)

    (d) Stable body weight

    (e) Stable abdominal girth

b. Alteration in nutrition, less than body requirements related to malabsorption and vomiting

  i. Assessment for defining characteristics

    (a) Anorexia

    (b) Vomiting

    (c) Presence of abdominal pain

    (d) Reported inadequate food intake less than Recommended Daily Allowance (RDA)

  ii. Expected outcomes

    (a) Stable body weight

    (b) Positive nitrogen balance

    (c) Reduction in abdominal pain

 iii. Nursing interventions

    (a) Assess bowel sounds

    (b) Measure abdominal girth and report any increases

    (c) Promote bowel rest or maintain NPO

    (d) Administer hyperalimentation and fat emulsions as ordered

    (e) Administer IV fluids with electrolytes and vitamins as ordered

    (f) Obtain daily weights

    (g) Monitor caloric intake

    (h) Administer pain medications

      (i) Provide frequent oral hygiene

      (j) Monitor electrolytes and glucose

      (k) Eliminate noxious sight/smell from environment

  iv. Evaluation of nursing care

      (a) Body weight within 1 to 2 kg of normal weight

      (b) Electrolytes within normal limits for the patient

      (c) Stable abdominal girth

      (d) Caloric intake as close to the RDA as possible

      (e) No evidence of vitamin deficiency

c. Alteration in comfort related to acute abdominal pain (see p. 773)

  i. Additional nursing interventions

      (a) Use patient-controlled analgesia for pain control as ordered

      (b) Provide a restful and quiet environment

      (c) Provide other strategies to augment pain relief (e.g., imagery, biofeedback, relaxation techniques, diversional activities)

d. Alteration in tissue perfusion related to the shock state

  i. Assessment for defining characteristics

      (a) Cold and clammy skin

      (b) Pallor

      (c) Delayed capillary refill time

      (d) Decreased urine output

      (e) Hypotension

      (f) History of thrombosis

      (g) Tachycardia

  ii. Expected outcomes

      (a) Vital signs within normal limits for the patient

      (b) Capillary refill normal

      (c) Warm, dry skin

      (d) Urine output within normal limits

  iii. Nursing interventions

      (a) Monitor vital signs

      (b) Monitor filling pressures

      (c) Monitor capillary refill time

      (d) Assess skin temperature and integrity

      (e) Vigorous correction of fluid deficits (e.g., crystalloids and colloids as ordered)

      (f) Administer vasoactive agents (e.g., dopamine) as ordered to augment cardiac output

      (g) Monitor serial blood gases for presence of acidosis

      (h) Prepare for early surgical management as indicated (e.g., bowel resection, embolectomy, revascularization grafts)

      (i) Monitor intake and output

(j) Administer prostaglandins to help improve tissue perfusion and reduce severity of tissue damage

    iv. Evaluation of nursing care

        (a) Urine output greater than 30 ml/hr

        (b) Vital signs within normal limits for the patient

        (c) Capillary refill time less than 3 seconds

        (d) Skin warm and dry

Abdominal Trauma

1. **Pathophysiology**
   a. Any patient with injury from the nipple line to mid thigh is considered to have abdominal trauma
   b. Abdominal trauma occurs less frequently than musculoskeletal trauma or head injuries
   c. Intra-abdominal trauma is seldom a single organ injury
   d. Abdominal trauma varies according to the nature of the wounding agent and the force with which it is applied
   e. Two major types of abdominal trauma are penetrating and blunt trauma
      i. High-velocity penetrating trauma causes extensive destruction of the tissue that it comes in contact with and a severe associated blast effect on the surrounding tissues
      ii. Effects of blunt trauma can be due to direct injury, severe crushing force between two objects, acceleration/deceleration, shearing, or twisting
2. **Etiology or precipitating factors**
   a. Penetrating trauma
      i. Knife wound
      ii. Ice picks
      iii. Sharpened wood or metal objects
      iv. Gunshot wound
      v. Impalement wound
   b. Blunt trauma
      i. Falls
      ii. Traffic accidents
      iii. Sports injuries
3. **Nursing assessment data base**
   a. Nursing history
      i. Subjective findings
         (a) Pain
         (b) Abdominal tenderness
         (c) Referred pain
      ii. Objective findings
         (a) Cullen's sign

          (b) Grey Turner's sign

          (c) Hematoma

          (d) Coopernail sign—ecchymosis of scrotum or labia

          (e) Seatbelt marks

          (f) Entrance and exit wounds

          (g) Pallor

          (h) History of alcohol or drug use

          (i) Mechanism of injury

b. Nursing examination of patient

  i. Inspection

      (a) Pale, cold, clammy skin

      (b) Abdominal distention

      (c) Presence of obvious wounds

      (d) Presence of discoloration, hematoma and frank bleeding

      (e) Presence of impalement of foreign object

      (f) Respiratory difficulty

  ii. Auscultation

      (a) Tachycardia

      (b) Hypotension

      (c) Diminished or absent breath sounds—listen on all four quadrants

      (d) Bruit may be present

  iii. Percussion

      (a) Dullness may be present, which indicates fluid in the abdomen

      (b) Hyperresonance may be present, which indicates perforation of a viscus

  iv. Palpation

      (a) Abdominal tenderness

      (b) Rebound tenderness may be present

      (c) Guarding of the abdomen may be present

      (d) Diminished or absent femoral pulses may be present

c. Diagnostic study findings

  i. Laboratory findings

      (a) Decreased hemoglobin and hematocrit

      (b) Elevated alcohol level

      (c) Positive drug screen

      (d) Urinalysis may show hematuria

      (e) Serum amylase level may be elevated

      (f) Elevated leukocyte count may be present

  ii. Radiologic findings

      (a) Plain film of the abdomen may show loss of psoas shadow, suggesting retroperitoneal hemorrhage

      (b) Chest x-ray film may show fractured ribs and/or presence of free air

        (c) Arteriography—to detect fistulas and aneurysms especially with penetrating trauma

  iii. Other diagnostic findings

        (a) Liver and spleen scan to rule out injury

        (b) Intravenous pyelography (IVP) if blood is present in urine

        (c) CT scan—to assess urologic or retroperitoneal injuries and solid viscera damage

        (d) Peritoneal lavage—may show presence of blood, bile, and/or fecal matter (Fig. 7–12*A* and *B*)

        (e) Rectal examination may show presence of blood

4. Nursing diagnoses

  a. Potential for infection related to breakdown of skin barrier

    i. Assessment for defining characteristics

        (a) Presence of blood or fecal matter in peritoneal fluid

        (b) Presence of obvious wounds

        (c) Impalement injuries with rusty, dirty objects

        (d) Environmental exposure of destroyed tissue

    ii. Expected outcomes

        (a) Negative blood culture

        (b) Patient will be normothermic

        (c) Leukocyte count normal

        (d) Absence of peritoneal signs

   iii. Nursing interventions

        (a) Assess vital signs including temperature

        (b) Monitor abdominal girth

        (c) Observe for presence of peritoneal signs (e.g., abdominal distention, guarding, rigidity, tenderness)

        (d) Monitor leukocyte count

        (e) Maintain strict aseptic technique in caring for abdominal wounds

        (f) Maintain sterility of drains (e.g., Penrose, Jackson-Pratt)

        (g) Obtain blood cultures as ordered

        (h) Observe universal precautions in handling blood and wound secretions

        (i) Monitor bowel sounds closely

    iv. Evaluation of nursing care

        (a) Temperature below 99° F (37.2° C)

        (b) Negative blood cultures

        (c) Absence of redness, pus, and tenderness on wound site

        (d) Leukocyte count within normal limits

        (e) Absence of peritoneal signs

  b. Potential alteration in nutrition, less than body requirements related to gastrointestinal injury

    i. Assessment for defining characteristics

        (a) Weight loss

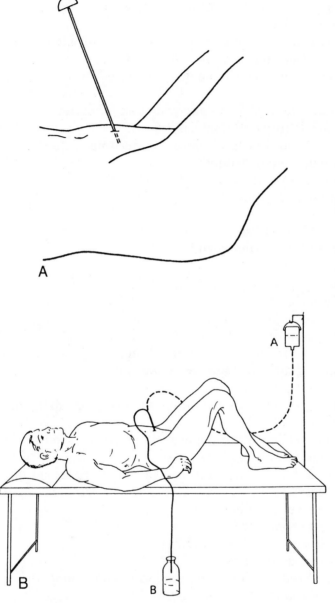

Figure 7–12. Peritoneal dialysis. *A*. A midline insertion is made in the skin 3 to 4 cm below the umbilicus, and the peritoneal dialysis catheter is inserted in the direction of the pelvic cavity after direct visualization and opening of the peritoneum. Bladder must be empty.

B. Lavage fluid is infused with bottle in position A. Bottle is then placed below the patient (B), and siphon effect returns diagnostic fluid from the peritoneal cavity. (From Sibbald W, ed.: Synopsis of Critical Care. © 1988; the Williams & Wilkins Co., Baltimore.)

(b) Presence of nasogastric tube

(c) Decreased or absent bowel sounds

(d) Pain

(e) Intake less than RDA

ii. Expected outcomes

(a) Stable body weight

(b) Positive nitrogen balance

(c) Adequate muscle mass

iii. Nursing interventions

(a) Monitor nasogastric output for color, amount, and odor of drainage

(b) Provide frequent oral and nasal hygiene

(c) Measure abdominal girth

(d) Monitor presence or absence of bowel sounds

(e) Administer hyperalimentation and fat emulsions as ordered

(f) Obtain daily weight

(g) Monitor electrolytes, including glucose level

(h) Provide vitamin supplements to prevent deficiency

(i) Monitor serum albumin

(j) Monitor caloric intake

iv. Evaluation of nursing care

(a) Serum albumin level greater than 3.5 g/dl

(b) Body weight within 1 to 2 kg of normal

(c) Adequate muscle mass

(d) Caloric intake adequate for needs

(e) Electrolytes within normal limits

(f) No evidence of vitamin deficiency

c. Fluid volume deficit related to loss of blood or fluid shifts secondary to traumatic injury

i. Assessment for defining characteristics

(a) Tachycardia

(b) Hypotension

(c) Evidence of frank or occult bleeding

(d) Hematoma

(e) Presence of blood in the urine

(f) Presence of blood in the peritoneum

ii. Expected outcomes

(a) Adequate fluid balance

(b) Electrolytes within normal limits

iii. Nursing interventions

(a) Maintain accurate intake and output

(b) Monitor serum electrolytes, BUN, and creatinine

(c) Vigorous fluid administration of colloids and crystalloids

(d) Monitor vital signs

   (e) Monitor tissue perfusion (e.g., skin temperature, capillary refill time)

   (f) Measure urine specific gravity

   (g) Apply MAST suit as indicated

   (h) Monitor abdominal girth for any increases

  iv. Evaluation of nursing care

   (a) Balanced intake and output

   (b) Urine output greater than 30 ml/hr

   (c) Skin warm and dry

   (d) Vital signs within normal limits for the patient

 d. Potential ineffective breathing pattern related to pain and/or upper abdominal trauma

  i. Assessment for defining characteristics

   (a) Shallow respirations

   (b) Decreased breath sounds

   (c) Pain

   (d) Anxiety

  ii. Expected outcomes

   (a) Maximum lung expansion

   (b) Maintains adequate oxygenation

  iii. Nursing interventions

   (a) Maintain on semi-Fowler's position if not contraindicated

   (b) Monitor breath sounds

   (c) Monitor serial arterial blood gas studies

   (d) Observe lung expansion

   (e) Observe respiratory rate, rhythm, and depth

   (f) Provide supplemental oxygen as indicated

   (g) Provide the use of incentive spirometer to allow for maximum lung aeration

   (h) Administer pain medications to prevent splinting

   (i) Obtain serial chest x-ray films as ordered

   (j) Establish adequate airway

  iv. Evaluation of nursing care

   (a) Arterial blood gases within normal limits for the patient

   (b) Breath sounds equal and normal

   (c) Chest expansion symmetrical and full

   (d) Chest x-ray films show no infiltrates

   (e) Adequate tidal volume

 e. Alteration in comfort related to pain (see p. 773)

  i. Additional nursing interventions

   (a) Assess type, location, and severity of pain

   (b) Provide planned rest periods

   (c) Administer pain medications with caution

   (d) Prepare for surgery (e.g., laparotomy) as indicated

   (e) Provide a quiet restful environment

f. Anxiety/fear related to severity of illness
   i. Assessment for defining characteristics
      (a) Apprehension
      (b) Worried facial expression
      (c) Tremors
      (d) Aggressive behavior
      (e) Withdrawal behavior
      (f) Repeatedly asking the same questions
   ii. Expected outcomes
      (a) Decreased anxiety level
      (b) Demonstrates effective coping skills
   iii. Nursing interventions
      (a) Assess present coping behaviors
      (b) Encourage and allow time for verbalization of feelings
      (c) Explain all treatments and procedures
      (d) Identify support systems and family dynamics
      (e) Assist with and teach relaxation techniques
      (f) Assess anxiety level
      (g) Maintain calm and safe environment
      (h) Encourage participation in care
   iv. Evaluation of nursing care
      (a) Patient will express concerns and feelings
      (b) Demonstrates decreased level of anxiety (e.g., able to relax, decreased agitation)
      (c) Demonstrates effective coping skills (e.g., use of relaxation techniques)

Esophageal Carcinoma

1. **Pathophysiology**
   a. About 10% of malignancies of the gastrointestinal tract arise in the esophagus
   b. Patients are usually asymptomatic until the malignancy is surgically unresectable
   c. Usually occurs after the age of 50, and more than 80% occurs in males
   d. Squamous cell is the most common morphologic form
   e. There is a strong correlation with both heavy alcohol intake and cigarette smoking
   f. Malignancy may grow around the esophagus, causing impingement of the cylindrical tube
   g. Greatest percentage of tumors are located in the middle and lower third of the esophagus
2. **Etiology or precipitating factors**
   a. Heavy alcohol intake

  b. Cigarette smoking

  c. Idiopathic

3. Nursing assessment data base

  a. Nursing history

    i. Subjective findings

      (a) Dysphagia progressing from mild to severe

      (b) Eructation

      (c) Pain

      (d) Hiccups

      (e) Regurgitation after eating

      (f) Generalized malaise

      (g) Feeling of fullness

      (h) Hoarseness

    ii. Objective findings

      (a) Dehydration

      (b) Foul breath

      (c) Weight loss

  b. Nursing examination of patient

    i. Inspection

      (a) Increased salivation and mucus formation

      (b) Weight loss

      (c) Dehydration

      (d) Regurgitation after eating

      (e) Generalized malaise

      (f) Hiccups

    ii. Auscultation

      (a) Bowel sounds normal

      (b) Decreased breath sounds may be present

    iii. Percussion

      (a) Dullness on upper lung area may be present

      (b) Tympanic sounds on abdomen

    iv. Palpation

      (a) Hepatomegaly may be present

      (b) Splenomegaly may be present

  c. Diagnostic study findings

    i. Laboratory findings

      (a) Complete blood cell count—baseline values

      (b) Electrolytes—baseline values

      (c) Liver function test may be abnormal

    ii. Radiologic findings

      (a) Chest x-ray film—to show the location of the tumor

      (b) Barium studies—to rule out metastasis

    iii. Other diagnostic findings

      (a) Bronchoscopy will show location of tumor

      (b) CT scan will confirm diagnosis and show location of tumor

(c) Biopsy may be helpful in further defining the type of tumor

(d) Arterial blood gas studies will rule out hypoxia

4. Nursing diagnoses

a. Alteration in nutrition, less than body requirements related to dysphagia (see p. 770)

   i. Additional assessment findings

      (a) Postprandial regurgitation

      (b) Difficulty in swallowing

      (c) Continuous hiccups

   ii. Additional nursing interventions

      (a) Assess patient's ability to swallow liquid and solid food to prevent aspiration pneumonia

      (b) Assist with feedings as needed

      (c) Provide oral care as frequently as possible

   iii. Additional evaluation of nursing care

      (a) Absence of signs of aspiration

b. Ineffective breathing pattern related to esophageal obstruction

   i. Assessment for defining characteristics

      (a) Hoarseness

      (b) Decreased breath sounds

      (c) Coughing

      (d) Inability to swallow saliva or mucus

   ii. Expected outcomes

      (a) Normal breath sounds

      (b) Absence of respiratory distress

   iii. Nursing interventions

      (a) Monitor breath sounds

      (b) Keep head of bed elevated if not contraindicated

      (c) Monitor vital signs

      (d) Perform tracheal suctioning techniques as needed

      (e) Provide incentive spirometry to promote maximum lung aeration

      (f) Monitor arterial blood gases for signs of hypoxia

      (g) Monitor respirations for rate, rhythm, and depth

   iv. Evaluation of nursing care

      (a) Chest expansion symmetrical

      (b) Lungs clear

      (c) Arterial blood gas values within normal limits for the patient

      (d) Tidal volume adequate

c. Alteration in comfort related to pain (see p. 773)

   i. Additional assessment for defining characteristics

      (a) Difficulty in swallowing

      (b) Hiccups

    ii. Additional expected outcome
        (a) Absence of hiccups
  d. Anxiety/fear related to poor prognosis
        i. Assessment for defining characteristics
            (a) Restlessness
            (b) Agitation
            (c) Short attention span
            (d) Worried facial expression
            (e) Withdrawn behavior
       ii. Expected outcomes
            (a) Verbalization of fears and concerns
            (b) Uses effective coping mechanisms
      iii. Nursing interventions
            (a) Assess availability of support systems
            (b) Assess family dynamics
            (c) Develop means of communication if patient has difficulty
                speaking
            (d) Assess patient's coping behaviors
            (e) Allow time to verbalize fears and concerns
            (f) Provide a calm and safe environment
            (g) Explain all procedures
            (h) Recommend outside support groups (e.g., American Cancer
                Society)
       iv. Evaluation of nursing care
            (a) Able to verbalize concerns and fears
            (b) Demonstrates decreased level of anxiety (e.g., decreased
                agitation)
            (c) Uses effective coping skills (e.g., able to relax)

Gastric Carcinoma

1. **Pathophysiology**
   a. Ninety to 99% of all malignancies of the stomach are classified as
      carcinomas
   b. Incidence of this malignancy has been declining steadily over the
      past decade in the United States but is increasing elsewhere
   c. Highest incidence is reported in Iceland, Japan, and Finland
   d. Survival rates are poor, with less than 10% of those affected surviv-
      ing for 5 years after diagnosis
   e. Carcinoma most commonly occurs in the pyloric segment and along
      the lesser curvature of the stomach
   f. There are no early definitive signs of the disease process
   g. Large masses and/or polypoid tumors may grow and cause obstruc-
      tion of the pyloric outlet
   h. Ulceration may occur, exhibiting a shaggy, necrotic-appearing base

i. Some degree of thickening of the stomach wall may be present

2. **Etiology or precipitating factors**
   a. Diet especially those high in nitrates
   b. Genetic or familial predisposition
   c. High incidence seen in blood type A
   d. Atrophic gastritis
   e. Polyps of the stomach
3. **Nursing assessment data base**
   a. Nursing history
       i. Subjective findings
          (a) Abdominal pain
          (b) Anorexia
          (c) Vomiting
          (d) Change in bowel habits
          (e) Malaise/fatigue
          (f) Eructation
      ii. Objective findings
          (a) Occult blood in stool
          (b) Pallor
          (c) Frank bleeding may be present
          (d) Family history of carcinoma
   b. Nursing examination of patient
       i. Inspection
          (a) Pallor
          (b) Generalized weakness
          (c) Blood in the stool
          (d) Weight loss
      ii. Auscultation
          (a) Hyperactive or hypoactive bowel sounds
          (b) Breath sounds may be decreased because of pain
     iii. Percussion
          (a) Dullness may be present in the epigastric area
          (b) Liver may be enlarged
      iv. Palpation
          (a) Hepatomegaly may be present
          (b) Splenomegaly may be present
          (c) Abdominal tenderness
   c. Diagnostic study findings
       i. Laboratory findings
          (a) Decreased hematocrit
          (b) Decreased serum albumin level
          (c) Occult blood in the stool
      ii. Radiologic findings
          (a) Plain film of the abdomen will reveal the location of the tumor

        (b) Upper gastrointestinal series will show the location and size of the tumor

        (c) Barium studies will also show the size and location of tumor

   iii. Other diagnostic findings

        (a) Gastric analysis may show decreased production of hydrochloric acid

        (b) Biopsy and cytology will reveal the type of tumor

4. Nursing diagnoses

  a. Alteration in nutrition related to nausea and vomiting (see p. 770)

    i. Additional assessment for defining characteristics

        (a) Eructation

        (b) Feeling of fullness with small amounts of food

    ii. Additional expected outcome

        (a) Absence of eructation

   iii. Additional nursing intervention

        (a) Identify foods that cause gastrointestinal discomfort

  b. Alteration in comfort related to pain (see p. 773)

  c. Potential anticipatory grieving related to poor prognosis

    i. Assessment for defining characteristics

        (a) Anger

        (b) Withdrawal behavior

        (c) Denial

        (d) Expression of distress

    ii. Expected outcomes

        (a) Verbalizes feeling of grief

        (b) Maintains constructive interpersonal relationships

   iii. Nursing interventions

        (a) Assess present coping styles and interdependence in relationships with others

        (b) Encourage verbalization of feelings

        (c) Provide realistic reassurance

        (d) Allow more time for family/significant others to visit

        (e) Offer hope realistically

        (f) Provide a supportive environment

        (g) Avoid confrontation

        (h) Allow for use of defense mechanisms to cope with potential loss

        (i) Recommend outside support groups (e.g., American Cancer Society)

   iv. Evaluation of nursing care

        (a) Discusses thoughts and feelings related to anticipated loss

        (b) Verbalizes need for information

        (c) Able to meet self-care needs

(d) Maintains constructive interpersonal relationships

(e) Participates in decision-making regarding own care

d. Powerlessness related to poor prognosis

  i. Assessment for defining characteristics

    (a) Verbal expression of having no control over outcome of the disease

    (b) Depression

    (c) Dependence on others

    (d) Passive behavior

    (e) Reluctance to express feelings

  ii. Expected outcomes

    (a) Able to verbalize feelings

    (b) Engages in problem-solving behavior

  iii. Nursing interventions

    (a) Encourage the patient and allow time to verbalize feelings of concern

    (b) Maintain a calm and confident attitude

    (c) Reinforce patient's right to ask questions

    (d) Help patient to be aware of aspects of care that are patient controlled

    (e) Provide for privacy needs of patient

    (f) Engage patient in decision making as much as possible (e.g., bathing, treatment schedule)

    (g) Involve family/significant others in the plan of care

    (h) Consider individual locus of control (external and internal) when planning care

    (i) Explain all treatments and procedures

    (j) Provide for patient teaching

  iv. Evaluation of nursing care

    (a) Engages in problem-solving behavior

    (b) Identifies situation in which powerlessness is felt

    (c) Participates in health care decision making

    (d) Verbalizes increased sense of control

Carcinoma of the Colon

1. Pathophysiology

a. Accounts for about 20% of all deaths due to cancer in the United States

b. Occurs in all age groups but highest incidence is reported at the fifth, sixth, and seventh decades of life

c. Incidence is greatest in northwest Europe and North America and lowest in South America, Africa, and Asia

d. Carcinoma of the small intestine: malignancy is most commonly found in the lower duodenum and the lower ileum

e. Carcinoma of the large intestine: a slow-growing malignancy most frequently found in the cecum, lower ascending, and sigmoid colon

f. Tumors cause obstruction and may lead to abscess formation and peritonitis

2. **Etiology or precipitating factors**
   a. Polyposis of the colon
   b. Familial tendencies
   c. Dietary factors (e.g., low fiber content, presence of animal fat)

3. **Nursing assessment data base**
   a. Nursing history
      i. Subjective findings
         (a) Diarrhea and constipation
         (b) Weakness
         (c) Generalized malaise
         (d) Melena
         (e) Pain
         (f) Nausea and vomiting
         (g) Anorexia
         (h) Alteration in bowel habits
      ii. Objective findings
         (a) Family history of carcinoma
         (b) Rectal bleeding
   b. Nursing examination of patient
      i. Inspection
         (a) Weight loss
         (b) Generalized weakness
         (c) Nausea and vomiting
         (d) Rectal bleeding
         (e) Tarry stool
      ii. Auscultation
         (a) Hyperactive bowel sounds
         (b) Breath sounds may be decreased
      iii. Percussion
         (a) Dullness on tumor site
         (b) Liver may be enlarged
      iv. Palpation
         (a) Presence of palpable mass
         (b) Abdominal tenderness
   c. Diagnostic study findings
      i. Laboratory findings
         (a) Carcinoembryonic antigen (CEA)
         (b) Decreased hemoglobin and hematocrit
         (c) Electrolytes—baseline values
         (d) Liver function tests—elevated
      ii. Radiologic findings

    (a) Upper gastrointestinal series will show location of the tumor and also show presence of obstruction

    (b) Plain film of the abdomen will show location of tumor; if obstruction is present it will show large amounts of gas in the colon

  iii. Other diagnostic findings

    (a) Sigmoidoscopy will show location of tumor

    (b) Colonoscopy will also show location of tumor

    (c) Biopsy will determine the type of tumor

4. **Nursing diagnoses:** same as in gastric carcinoma

Peptic Ulcers

1. **Pathophysiology** (Fig. 7–13)

  a. A group of ulcerative conditions of the gastrointestinal tract that result from an acid–pepsin imbalance

  b. Develops when the aggressive proteolytic activities of the gastric secretions are greater than their normal protective activities

  c. Vascular occlusion of small nutrient vessels in the mucosa or submucosa of the gastrointestinal tract causes localized necrosis and subsequent ulcer formation

  d. Gastric ulceration is due to a break in the mucosal barrier, allowing backwash of hydrochloric acid

  e. Duodenal ulcers are due to increased amounts of hydrochloric acid in the duodenum

  f. Most frequent site for peptic ulcers is the pyloric region of the duodenum

  g. Duodenal ulcers comprise 80% of all peptic ulcers

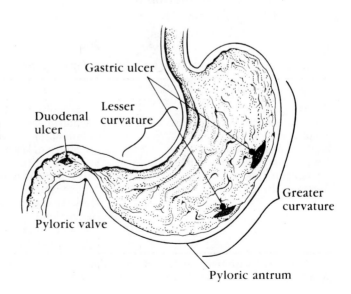

Figure 7–13. Common locations for gastric and duodenal ulcers. (From Bullock, B., and Rosendahl, P.: Pathophysiology: Adaptations and Alterations in Function. Little, Brown & Co., Boston, 1986.)

h. There is a high incidence of malignancy associated with gastric ulcers

i. Gastric ulcers are more likely to bleed than duodenal ulcers

2. Etiology or precipitating factors (Table 7–3)
   a. Gastritis
   b. Stress
   c. Aspirin ingestion
   d. Alcoholism
   e. Smoking
   f. Chemotherapy or radiation therapy
   g. Endocrine factors (e.g., corticosteroids, estrogen)
   h. Familial tendency
   i. Caffeine

3. Nursing assessment data base
   a. Nursing history
      i. Subjective findings
         (a) Epigastric pain
         (b) Nausea and vomiting
         (c) Weight loss
         (d) Pain–food–relief pattern for duodenal ulcers
         (e) Heartburn
      ii. Objective findings
         (a) Bleeding
         (b) History of smoking
         (c) History of chronic aspirin intake
         (d) History of taking corticosteroids and/or birth control pills
         (e) History of alcohol abuse
         (f) History of heavy caffeine intake
   b. Nursing examination of patient
      i. Inspection
         (a) Weight loss

Table 7–3. MOST COMMON CAUSES OF GASTROINTESTINAL HEMORRHAGE

Upper Gastrointestinal Bleeding	Lower Gastrointestinal Bleeding
Erosive gastritis	Diverticulitis
Peptic ulcer: gastric, duodenal	Neoplasm: carcinoma, polyp
Esophageal varices	Inflammatory bowel disease: ulcerative colitis, Crohn's disease
Mallory-Weiss syndrome	
Neoplasms: carcinoma, lymphoma, leiomyoma, polyps	Ischemic colitis
	Arteriovenous malformation
Aortointestinal fistula	Angiodysplasia
	Meckel's diverticulum
	Hemorrhoids
	Aortointestinal fistula
	Upper gastrointestinal lesion

Reprinted with permission from Sibbald, W. (ed): Synopsis of Critical Care. © 1988, the Williams & Wilkins Co., Baltimore.

(b) Bleeding

(c) Nausea and vomiting

(d) Regurgitation

(e) Pallor

 ii. Auscultation

(a) Hyperactive bowel sounds

(b) Decreased breath sounds may be present

 iii. Percussion

(a) Normal tympanic sounds

(b) Dullness may be present on epigastric area

 iv. Palpation

(a) Abdominal tenderness

(b) Guarding may be present if patient is bleeding

c. Diagnostic study findings

 i. Laboratory findings

(a) Decreased hemoglobin and hematocrit

(b) Guaiac-positive stool

(c) Electrolytes—baseline values

(d) Gastric analysis will reveal increased production of gastric juice by the parietal cells

 ii. Radiologic findings

(a) Chest x-ray film will show free air under the diaphragm for bleeding ulcers

(b) Barium studies done for differential diagnosis

 iii. Other diagnostic studies

(a) Endoscopy will show location of the ulcer

(b) Biopsy to rule out carcinoma

(c) Gastrin level elevated in gastric ulcer but normal with duodenal ulcer

4. Nursing diagnoses

a. Alteration in nutrition, less than body requirements related to nausea and vomiting (see p. 770)

 i. Additional nursing interventions

(a) Assess medication history (e.g., corticosteroids, aspirin)

(b) Maintain a nonstressful environment

(c) Provide small frequent feedings

(d) Administer antacids as ordered

(e) Administer histamine H_2-blockers (e.g., cimetidine, ranitidine) as ordered

(f) Avoid foods that irritate the gastrointestinal tract

(g) Administer sucralfate (Carafate) as ordered

(h) Assess patient's nutritional status (e.g., present diet, eating habits, foods precipitating and relieving pain)

 ii. Additional evaluation of nursing care

(a) Decreased incidence of heartburn

b. Potential for fluid volume deficit related to upper gastrointestinal tract bleeding
  i. Assessment for defining characteristics
    (a) Poor skin turgor
    (b) Hypotension
    (c) Tachycardia
    (d) Weakness
    (e) Decreased urine output
    (f) Decreased filling pressures
  ii. Expected outcomes
    (a) Maintains fluid volume at an acceptable level
    (b) No active bleeding present
    (c) Maintains normal electrolyte balance
  iii. Nursing interventions
    (a) Monitor vital signs
    (b) Monitor hemoglobin and hematocrit
    (c) Monitor filling pressures (e.g., central venous, pulmonary capillary wedge, pulmonary artery)
    (d) Maintain nasogastric tube and monitor output and report frank bleeding
    (e) Maintain accurate intake and output
    (f) Monitor cardiac rate and rhythm
    (g) Maintain the patient on NPO
    (h) Provide frequent oral care
    (i) Administer fluid with electrolytes, colloids, and blood as ordered
    (j) Administer vasopressors as ordered
    (k) Administer prostaglandins to patients on aspirin to prevent mucosal injury as ordered
    (l) Prepare patient for surgery as indicated (e.g., gastrectomy, pyloroplasty, vagotomy)
  iv. Evaluation of nursing care
    (a) Balanced intake and output
    (b) Electrolytes within normal limits
    (c) Hemoglobin and hematocrit normal
    (d) No active bleeding
    (e) Absence of blood in the stool
    (f) Vital signs within normal limits for the patient
    (g) Nasogastric tube output negative for blood
    (h) Filling pressures within normal limits for the patient
c. Anxiety related to fear of the unknown
  i. Assessment for defining characteristics
    (a) Agitation
    (b) Worried facial expression
    (c) Restlessness

       (d) Demanding behavior

       (e) Repeatedly asking the same question

    ii. Expected outcomes

       (a) Demonstrates reduced anxiety level

       (b) Demonstrates effective coping

  iii. Nursing interventions

       (a) Explain all procedures including all rationales

       (b) Assess present coping skills and identify successful ones

       (c) Maintain a safe and quiet environment

       (d) Assess level of anxiety

       (e) Encourage patient and allow time to verbalize fears and concerns

       (f) Provide for diversional activities and relaxation techniques

       (g) Allow more time for family/significant others to visit

  iv. Evaluation of nursing care

       (a) Decreased restlessness

       (b) Able to meet self-care needs

       (c) Demonstrates relaxation techniques

       (d) Verbalizes fears and concerns

Esophageal Varices

1. **Pathophysiology**
   a. Obstruction to blood flow through the liver results in increased pressure in the portal venous system
   b. Portal hypertension results; veins becomes dilated and tortuous especially in the submucosa of the lower esophagus
   c. Collateral channels develop around the high pressure areas
   d. Irritation from gastric acidity, alcohol, and spasmodic vomiting can cause the varices to bleed
   e. Approximately one third to one half of patients with varices eventually bleed
2. **Etiology or precipitating factors**
   a. Cirrhosis of the liver
   b. Portal venous thrombosis
   c. Congenital hepatic fibrosis
   d. Schistosomiasis
   e. Hepatic venous outflow obstruction
   f. Circulatory abnormalities in splenic vein or superior vena cava
3. **Nursing assessment data base**
   a. Nursing history
      i. Subjective findings
         (a) Pain
         (b) Hematemesis

        (c) Anxiety

        (d) Melena

        (e) Tarry stools

    ii. Objective findings

        (a) Jaundice

        (b) Abdominal distention

        (c) History of previous gastrointestinal hemorrhage

        (d) History of heavy alcohol intake

        (e) Travel history in a place where water and food may be contaminated

b. Nursing examination of patient

    i. Inspection

        (a) Hematemesis

        (b) Melena

        (c) Pallor

        (d) Jaundice

        (e) Restlessness/disorientation

        (f) Abdominal distention

    ii. Auscultation

        (a) Bowel sounds may be hyperactive

        (b) Tachycardia

        (c) Hypotension

    iii. Percussion

        (a) Enlarged liver

        (b) Dullness may be present

    iv. Palpation

        (a) Hepatomegaly

        (b) Splenomegaly

        (c) Tenderness may be present

c. Diagnostic study findings

    i. Laboratory findings

        (a) Decreased hemoglobin and hematocrit

        (b) Leukocyte count may be elevated

        (c) BUN elevated

        (d) Electrolytes—baseline values

        (e) Serum sodium level may be elevated

        (f) Coagulation profile may be abnormal

        (g) Serum ammonia level may be elevated

        (h) Liver function test results may be abnormal

        (i) Guaiac-positive stools

    ii. Radiologic findings

        (a) Angiogram shows tortuous vessels in the portal venous system

        (b) Chest x-ray film—baseline value

    iii. Other diagnostic findings

(a) Endoscopy—to locate and sometimes treat the varices

(b) Arterial blood gases—may show metabolic acidosis

4. Nursing diagnoses

a. Potential alteration in cardiac output related to hemorrhage

   i. Assessment for defining characteristics

     (a) Pallor of skin and mucous membranes

     (b) Tachycardia

     (c) Hypotension

     (d) Cold, clammy skin

     (e) Decreased urine output

   ii. Expected outcomes

     (a) Maintains a higher than normal cardiac output because of the hyperdynamic state that exists in patients with esophageal varices

     (b) Vital signs within normal limits

     (c) Absence of active bleeding

   iii. Nursing interventions

     (a) Monitor vital signs

     (b) Monitor hemodynamic pressures

     (c) Maintain accurate intake and output

     (d) Monitor hemoglobin and hematocrit

     (e) Perform nasogastric lavage with sterile saline

     (f) Administer intravenous pitressin as ordered

     (g) Administer fluids and electrolytes as ordered

     (h) Assist with insertion of Sengstaken-Blakemore tube as indicated

     (i) Keep the patient NPO

     (j) Assess all emesis and stools for presence of blood

     (k) Prepare patient and assist in injection sclerotherapy as indicated

     (l) Observe for signs of respiratory distress while Sengstaken-Blakemore tube in place

   iv. Evaluation of nursing care

     (a) Urine output greater than 30 ml/hr

     (b) Absence of bleeding as seen through the nasogastric tube, stools, and emesis

     (c) Hemoglobin and hematocrit normal

     (d) Skin warm and dry

b. Potential alteration in tissue perfusion related to bleeding varices

   i. Assessment for defining characteristics

     (a) Hypotension

     (b) Cold, clammy skin

     (c) Bradycardia

     (d) Decreased level of consciousness

        (e) Decreased urine output

        (f) Pallor

   ii. Expected outcomes

        (a) Balanced intake and output

        (b) Absence of metabolic acidosis

        (c) Maintains adequate tissue perfusion

  iii. Nursing interventions

        (a) Monitor vital signs

        (b) Maintain accurate intake and output

        (c) Monitor and report any changes in level of consciousness

        (d) Monitor capillary refill time

        (e) Monitor electrolytes

        (f) Provide supplemental oxygen as needed

        (g) Monitor arterial blood gases

        (h) Palpate peripheral pulses at least every 4 hours for quality

   iv. Evaluation of nursing care

        (a) Skin warm and dry

        (b) Capillary refill less than 3 seconds

        (c) Urine output greater than 30 ml/hr

        (d) Arterial blood gas values within normal limits for the patient

        (e) Peripheral pulses strong and regular

        (f) Maintains alertness

        (g) Absence of acidosis

 c. Potential ineffective individual coping related to disease process

    i. Assessment for defining characteristics

        (a) Verbal manipulation

        (b) Fear

        (c) Guilt

        (d) Anxiety

        (e) History of excessive alcohol use

   ii. Expected outcomes

        (a) Demonstrates adequate understanding of situation

        (b) Demonstrates effective coping skills

  iii. Nursing interventions

        (a) Explain all procedures and rationales

        (b) Maintain patient privacy

        (c) Assess patient and family coping styles

        (d) Encourage patient and allow time to verbalize concerns

        (e) Explain essential life-style changes (e.g., drinking habits) to prevent progression of the disease

        (f) Provide adequate and correct information to patient and family

        (g) Encourage patient and family to have a realistic perspective

        (h) Refer to outside support groups (e.g., Alcoholics Anony-
mous or social worker)

        (i) Assess family dynamics

    iv. Evaluation of nursing care

        (a) Verbalizes need for more information

        (b) Demonstrates decreased level of anxiety (e.g., able to relax)

        (c) Participates in meeting self-care needs

        (d) Seeks help in adjusting to changes in life style

        (e) States plan to adhere to medical regimen

  d. Other nursing diagnoses same as in peptic ulcers

Acute Abdomen

1. **Pathophysiology**
   a. The term denotes a surgical condition with a sudden, unexpected onset of abdominal pain requiring prompt decision-making and surgical intervention
   b. Many specific conditions are responsible for acute abdomen and they share the capacity to contaminate the peritoneal cavity suddenly with septic material
   c. Diagnosis depends primarily on accurate history and the correct interpretation of physical findings
   d. Successful management of acute abdomen depends on establishing a high probability of peritonitis
2. **Conditions that could cause acute abdomen**
   a. Perforated appendix
   b. Perforated peptic ulcer
   c. Perforated gallbladder
   d. Perforated diverticulum
   e. Diverticulitis with peritonitis
   f. Foreign body perforation
   g. Perforated gastrointestinal malignancy
   h. Penetrating abdominal trauma
   i. Ruptured ectopic pregnancy
   j. Bowel obstruction with necrosis or perforation
   k. Ruptured abdominal aortic aneurysm
3. **Nursing assessment data base**
   a. Nursing history
      i. Subjective findings
        (a) Persistent, severe abdominal pain
        (b) Nausea and vomiting
        (c) Referred pain
        (d) Anorexia
        (e) Inability to pass stool or flatus

      (f) Generalized weakness

      (g) Thirst

   ii. Objective findings

      (a) History of peptic ulcer

      (b) Previous abdominal surgery

      (c) Motor vehicle accident

      (d) Obvious abdominal trauma

      (e) History of gallbladder disease

      (f) Pregnancy

      (g) History of excessive alcohol intake

b. Nursing examination of patient

   i. Inspection

      (a) Abdominal distention

      (b) Jaundice

      (c) Elevated temperature

      (d) Pallor

      (e) Hiccups may be present if diaphragmatic peritoneum is irritated

      (f) Respirations may be shallow and rapid

   ii. Auscultation

      (a) Tachycardia

      (b) Hypotension

      (c) Breath sounds may be decreased

      (d) Bowel sounds usually absent

      (e) Loud, high-pitched bowel sounds may be present in intestinal obstruction

   iii. Percussion

      (a) Hyperresonance may be noted

      (b) Loss of dullness over liver area may be present

   iv. Palpation

      (a) Rigidity and guarding

      (b) Abdominal tenderness (rebound tenderness may also be present)

c. Diagnostic study findings

   i. Laboratory findings

      (a) Elevated leukocyte count

      (b) Erythrocyte count may be increased, indicating hemoconcentration

      (c) Serum protein/albumin level may be decreased secondary to fluid shifts

      (d) Serum amylase level usually elevated

   ii. Radiologic findings

      (a) Chest x-ray film—baseline value

      (b) Plain film of the abdomen may show distention of bowel or presence of free air

  iii. Other diagnostic findings
   (a) Arterial blood gas values may show metabolic acidosis
   (b) Paracentesis may contain blood, pus, or bile
4. **Nursing diagnoses**
 a. Potential for infection related to organisms that contaminate the peritoneal cavity
  i. Assessment for defining characteristics
   (a) Elevated temperature
   (b) Trauma
   (c) Rupture of viscus
  ii. Expected outcomes
   (a) Negative blood cultures
   (b) Afebrile
   (c) Leukocyte count within normal limits for the patient
  iii. Nursing interventions
   (a) Monitor vital signs including temperature
   (b) Obtain blood cultures as ordered
   (c) Administer antibiotics (e.g., cephalosporins, aminoglycosides) as ordered
   (d) Observe universal precautions
   (e) Monitor leukocyte count
   (f) Maintain adequate nutrition
   (g) Prepare for surgical intervention
  iv. Evaluation of nursing care
   (a) Leukocyte count within normal limits for the patient
   (b) Temperature below 99° F (37.2° C)
   (c) Presence of negative blood cultures
   (d) Vital signs within normal limits for the patient
 b. Alteration in nutrition, less than body requirements related to surgical abdomen
  i. Assessment for defining characteristics
   (a) Weight loss
   (b) Abdominal pain
   (c) NPO state
   (d) Increased metabolic state
  ii. Expected outcomes
   (a) Positive nitrogen balance
   (b) Adequate muscle mass
   (c) Stable body weight
  iii. Nursing interventions
   (a) Administer fluids with electrolytes and vitamins ordered
   (b) Administer hyperalimentation and fat emulsions as ordered
   (c) Obtain daily weights
   (d) Provide oral care as frequently as possible

(e) Monitor electrolyte levels

(f) Monitor serum albumin level

(g) Maintain NPO

iv. Evaluation of nursing care

(a) Serum albumin level greater than 3.5 g/dl

(b) Body weight within 1 to 2 kg of normal

(c) Electrolyte levels within normal limits for the patient

(d) No evidence of vitamin deficiency

c. Fluid volume deficit related to fluid shifts (see p. 771)

i. Additional assessment for defining characteristics

(a) Presence of peritonitis

ii. Additional nursing interventions

(a) Observe skin/mucous membranes for dryness

(b) Monitor urine specific gravity

(c) Measure abdominal girth and report any increases

iii. Additional evaluation of nursing care

(a) Stable abdominal girth

d. Alteration in comfort related to pain (see p. 773)

i. Additional assessment for defining characteristics

(a) Abdominal guarding and rigidity

(b) Restlessness

ii. Additional nursing intervention

(a) Prepare for surgery as indicated

Pancreatic Cancer

1. **Pathophysiology**

a. Pancreatic cancer occurs most commonly in the late middle years of life, peaking in the sixth decade, and affects men more often than women

b. Patients do not seek medical attention during the early course of the disease because symptoms are usually vague and nonspecific

c. This delay results in the advanced progression of the disease by the time of diagnosis

d. The overall survival rate of patients with pancreatic adenocarcinoma is less than 1%

e. Seventy percent of pancreatic cancer is located at the head of the gland

f. Whipple procedure has remained the classic operation for pancreatic cancer since it was first performed in 1935

g. The procedure consists of duodenectomy with gastrojejunostomy, partial or total pancreatectomy, choledochojejunostomy, and splenectomy

h. Another name for Whipple procedure is pancreatoduodenectomy

2. **Etiology or precipitating factors**
   a. Smoking
   b. Consumption of alcoholic beverages
   c. Consumption of fat
   d. Disease of the gallbladder
   e. Disease of the extrahepatic bile duct
3. **Nursing assessment data base**
   a. Nursing history
      i. Subjective findings
         (a) Pain
         (b) Weight loss
         (c) Anorexia
         (d) Generalized malaise
         (e) Nausea and vomiting
      ii. Objective findings
         (a) Jaundice
         (b) History of alcohol intake
         (c) History of smoking
         (d) History of gallbladder disease
         (e) History of excessive fat intake in the diet
   b. Nursing examination of patient
      i. Inspection
         (a) Jaundice
         (b) Cachexia
         (c) Fever
         (d) Weakness
         (e) Steatorrhea
         (f) Nausea and vomiting
         (g) Scaphoid abdomen
      ii. Auscultation
         (a) Bowel sounds may be decreased or absent
         (b) Hypotension may be present
      iii. Percussion
         (a) Enlargement of the liver
         (b) Hyperresonance may be present
         (c) Dullness may be present over the epigastric area
      iv. Palpation
         (a) Hepatomegaly
         (b) Splenomegaly
         (c) Palpable mass may be present over the epigastric area
         (d) Distended gallbladder
   c. Diagnostic study findings
      i. Laboratory findings
         (a) Hyperglycemia
         (b) Elevated serum lipase level

          (c) Elevated alkaline phosphatase level

          (d) Elevated serum bilirubin level

          (e) Elevated SGOT level

          (f) Decreased hemoglobin and hematocrit

          (g) Elevated carcinoembryonic antigen (CEA)

    ii. Radiologic findings

          (a) Abdominal angiography may show encasement of the major arteries or veins by tumor or increased vascularity of abnormal vessels in the tumor area

          (b) Chest x-ray film—baseline value

          (c) Endoscopic retrograde cholangiopancreatography (ERCP) shows the caliber of the biliary and pancreatic ducts and may reveal areas of cancer in the duodenal wall

    iii. Other diagnostic findings

          (a) CT scan will confirm the presence of tumor

          (b) Biopsy will show the type of tumor

          (c) Secretin and cholecystokinin tests may show abnormal secretion of these hormones

4. Nursing diagnoses

  a. Potential for infection related to surgical procedure

    i. Assessment for defining characteristics

          (a) Presence of peritoneal signs (e.g., guarding and rigidity of the abdomen, paralytic ileus)

          (b) Fever

          (c) Positive blood culture

          (d) Hypermetabolic state

    ii. Expected outcomes

          (a) Absence of peritonitis

          (b) Absence of pancreatic fistula

          (c) Negative blood cultures

    iii. Nursing interventions

          (a) Monitor vital signs, including temperature

          (b) Obtain blood cultures as ordered

          (c) Monitor bowel sounds and report persistent absence

          (d) Use aseptic technique in dressing changes

          (e) Observe universal precautions

          (f) Measure abdominal girth and report any increases

          (g) Observe surgical incision site for redness, swelling, tenderness, and increased drainage

          (h) Maintain patency of nasogastric tube and report color and amount of drainage

          (i) Administer antibiotics as ordered

          (j) Maintain wound drains (e.g., Penrose, Jackson-Pratt)

    iv. Evaluation of nursing care

          (a) Negative blood cultures

   (b) Temperature below 99° F (37.2° C)
   (c) No redness, swelling, or increased drainage noted at incision site
   (d) Leukocyte count within normal limits for the patient
   (e) Stable abdominal girth
   (f) Vital signs within normal limits for the patient
b. Alteration in nutrition, less than body requirements related to altered metabolism (see p. 770)
   i. Additional assessment for defining characteristics
      (a) Cachexia
      (b) Hypermetabolic state (post surgery)
   ii. Additional nursing interventions
      (a) Maintain NPO
      (b) Monitor serum glucose level
   iii. Additional evaluation of nursing care
      (a) Blood sugar level within normal limits for the patient
      (b) Electrolytes within normal limits for the patient
      (c) No evidence of vitamin deficiency
c. Impaired skin integrity related to surgery
   i. Assessment for defining characteristics
      (a) Skin disruption (surgical incision)
      (b) Immobility
      (c) Debilitated state
      (d) Presence of drains
      (e) Altered pigmentation (jaundice)
   ii. Expected outcomes
      (a) Maintain skin integrity
      (b) No further disruption of skin tissue (e.g., dehiscence, evisceration). *NOTE:* Surgical wounds have the greatest potential for dehiscence, fistula formation, and evisceration between postoperative days 5 and 12
   iii. Nursing interventions
      (a) Keep skin clean and dry
      (b) Turn as frequently as possible and keep off back as much as possible
      (c) Consult with enterostomal therapist to control caustic drainage from surgical wound
      (d) Use Montgomery straps to stabilize dressing
      (e) Maintain adequate nutrition
      (f) Avoid the use of soap to prevent further dryness of the skin
      (g) Apply lotion and gentle massage to stimulate circulation
      (h) Monitor wound site for signs of irritation (e.g., redness and slow healing)

     (i) Observe wound for evidence of dehiscence or fistula formation (e.g., presence of any kind of drainage where previously wound has been dry and skin intact)

  iv. Evaluation of nursing care

     (a) Absence of decubiti

     (b) Normal healing of tissues at incision site (e.g., granulation, scar formation)

     (c) No further skin breakdown

d. Potential for impairment of gas exchange related to the postoperative course

  i. Assessment for defining characteristics

     (a) Anxiety

     (b) Restlessness

     (c) Presence of crackles on lung fields

     (d) Decreased breath sounds

     (e) Hypoxemia

  ii. Expected outcomes

     (a) Arterial blood gas values within normal limits for patient

     (b) Absence of adventitious breath sounds

  iii. Nursing interventions

     (a) Monitor lung sounds

     (b) Monitor arterial blood gas values

     (c) Monitor serial chest x-ray films

     (d) Encourage deep breathing and coughing exercises

     (e) Provide incentive spirometer to maximize aeration of the lungs

     (f) Observe lung expansion

     (g) Provide supplemental oxygen as needed

     (h) Administer pain medications to prevent splinting

  iv. Evaluation of nursing care

     (a) Lungs clear

     (b) Chest expansion symmetric and full

     (c) Chest x-ray film shows no infiltrates

     (d) Arterial blood gas values within normal limits for patient

e. Fluid volume deficit related to fluid shifts (see p. 771)

f. Alteration in comfort related to pain (see p. 773)

  i. Additional nursing intervention

     (a) Administer patient-controlled analgesia as indicated

References

Alexander, P., Schuman, E., and Vetto, R.: Perforation of the colon in the immunocompromised patient. Am. J. Surg. 151:557–561, 1986.

Bagg, A. M.: Whipple's procedure: Nursing guidelines. Crit. Care Nurse 8:34–45, 1988.

Bihari, D.: Acute liver failure. Clin. Anesth. 3:973–997, 1985.

Bihari, D., Gimson, A., Lindridge, J., et al.: Lactic acidosis in fulminant hepatic failure: Aspects of pathogenesis and prognosis. J. Hepatol. 1:405–416, 1985.

Bihari, D., Gimson, A., Waterson, M., Mellon, P., and Williams, R.: Tissue hypoxia during fulminant hepatic failure. Crit. Care Med. 13:1034–1039, 1985.

Bihari, D., Gimson, A., and Williams, R.: Cardiovascular, pulmonary and renal complications of fulminant hepatic failure. Semin. Liver Dis. 6:119–128, 1986.

Bismuth, H., Samuel, D., Gugenheim, J., et al.: Emergency liver transplantation for fulminant hepatitis. Ann. Intern. Med. 107:337–341, 1987.

Boey, J., Choi, S., Alagaratnam, T., et al.: Risk stratification in perforated duodenal ulcers: A prospective validation of predictive factors. Ann. Surg. 205:22–26, 1987.

Brayton, D., and Norris, W.: Intussusception in adults. Am. J. Surg. 88:32–43, 1954.

Briones, T.: Nursing care plan for the patient with acute gastrointestinal bleeding. Crit. Care Nurse 4:22–24, 1984.

Bullock, B., and Rosendahl, P.: Pathophysiology: Adaptations and Alterations in Function. Little, Brown & Co., Boston, 1984.

Butterworth, G. F., Guguere, J. F., Michaud, J., et al.: Ammonia: Key factor in the pathogenesis of hepatic encephalopathy. Neurochem. Pathol. 6:1–12, 1986.

Cello, J., Grendell, J., Crass, R., Weber, T., and Trunkey, D.: Endoscopic sclerotherapy versus portocaval shunt in patients with severe cirrhosis and acute variceal hemorrhage. N. Engl. J. Med. 316:11–15, 1987.

Ceneviva, R., de Castro, E., Silva, J., et al.: Simple suture with or without proximal gastric vagotomy for perforated duodenal ulcer. Br. J. Surg. 73:427–430, 1986.

Classen, M.: Endoscopic papillectomy: New indications, short- and long-term results. Clin. Gastroenterol. 15:446–457, 1986.

Cohen, M.: Aspirin-induced gastroduodenal injury and its prevention by prostaglandins. Postgrad. Med. J. 64(suppl. 1):12–14, 1988.

Conomy, J. P., and Swash, M.: Reversible decerebrate and decorticate postures in hepatic coma. N. Engl. J. Med. 278:876–879, 1986.

Debas, H., and Mulholland, M.: New horizons in the pharmacologic management of peptic ulceration. Am. J. Surg. 151:422–430, 1986.

Dickson, R., Evans, L., Koff, R., et al.: Who's a liver transplant candidate? Patient Care 21:83–87, 1987.

Dietel, M., and To, T.: Major intestinal complications of radiotherapy: Management and nutrition. Arch. Surg. 122:1421–1424, 1987.

Eckhauser, M.: Endoscopic laser vaporization of obstructing left colonic cancer to avoid decompression colostomy. Gastrointest. Endosc. 33:105–106, 1987.

Ede, R. J., Gimson, A. E., Bihari, D., et al.: Controlled hyperventilation in the prevention of cerebral edema in fulminant hepatic failure. J. Hepatol. 2:43–51, 1986.

Fabian, T., Mangiante, E., et al.: A prospective study of 91 patients undergoing both computerized tomography and peritoneal lavage following blunt abdominal trauma. J. Trauma. 26:602–608, 1986.

Fain, J. A., and Amato-Vealy, E.: Acute pancreatitis: A gastrointestinal emergency. Crit. Care Nurse 8:47–60, 1988.

Fazio, V.: Regional enteritis: Indications for surgery and operative strategy. Surg. Clin. North Am. 63:27–48, 1983.

Felice, P., Trowbridge, P., and Ferrara, J.: Evolving changes in the pathogenesis and treatment of the perforated gallbladder. Am. J. Surg. 149:466–472, 1985.

Finley, R.: Nutritional support of the critically ill patient. In Sibbald, W. (ed.): Synopsis of Critical Care, 3rd ed. Williams & Wilkins, Baltimore, 1988.

Flancbaum, L., Dauterive, A., and Cox, E.: Splenic conservation after multiple trauma in adults. Surg. Gynecol. Obstet. 162:469–473, 1986.

Girvan, D.: Abdominal trauma. In Sibbald, W. (ed.): Synopsis of Critical Care, 3rd ed. Williams & Wilkins, Baltimore, 1988.

Girvan, D.: Acute gastrointestinal hemorrhage. In Sibbald, W. (ed.): Synopsis of Critical Care, 3rd ed. Williams & Wilkins, Baltimore, 1988.

Given, B. A., and Simmons, S. J.: Gastroenterology in Clinical Nursing. C. V. Mosby, St. Louis, 1984.

Grozman, R.: Drug therapy of portal hypertension. Am. J. Gastroenterol. 82:107–113, 1987.

Guarner, F., Hughes, R., Gimson, A., et al.: Renal function in fulminant hepatic failure: Hemodynamics and renal prostaglandins. Gut 28:1643–1647, 1987.

Guyton, A. C.: Textbook of Medical Physiology, 7th ed. W. B. Saunders, Philadelphia, 1986.

Hall, J.: Liver transplantation: Postoperative care. Nurs. Times 1:59–62, 1984.

Harwood, C. H., and Cook, C. V.: Cyclosporine in transplantation. Heart Lung. 14:529–539, 1985.

Holder, W., Jr.: Intestinal obstruction. Gastroenterol. Clin. North Am. 17:317–339, 1988.

Jordan, P. H., Jr., and Morrow, C.: Perforated peptic ulcer. Surg. Clin. North Am. 68:315–329, 1988.

Joseph, P., Bizer, L., Sprayregen, S., et al.: Percutaneous transhepatic biliary drainage: Results and complications in 81 patients. JAMA 255:2763, 1986.

Kaplun, L., Weissman, H., Rosenblatt, R., et al.: The early diagnosis of common bile duct obstruction using cholescintigraphy. JAMA 254:2431, 1985.

Keifhaber, P., Huber, F., and Keifhaber, K.: Palliative and preoperative endoscopic neodymium-YAG laser treatment of colorectal cancer. Endoscopy 19:43–46, 1987.

Keith, J. S.: Hepatic failure: Etiologies, manifestations, and management. Crit. Care Nurse 5:60–86, 1985.

Keithley, J. K.: Infection and the malnourished patient. Heart Lung 12:23–27, 1983.

Kelly, J. P., and Roper, C. L.: Causes and management of esophageal perforation. Hosp. Physician 19:79–88, 1983.

Laing, F.: Diagnostic evaluation of patients with suspected cholecystitis. Surg. Clin. North Am. 64:3–22, 1984.

Lemoyne, M., and Jeejeebhoy, K.: Total parenteral nutrition in the critically ill patient. Chest 89:568–575, 1986.

Long, J., III, Wilmore, D., Mason, A., Jr., et al.: The effect of carbohydrate and fat intake on nitrogen excretion during total intravenous feedings. Ann. Surg. 185:417–422, 1977.

Jygidakis, N., and Brummelkamp, W.: The significance of intrabiliary pressure in acute cholangitis. Surg. Gynecol. Obstet. 161:465, 1985.

Martin, D., and Tweedle, D.: Endoscopic management of common duct stones without cholecystectomy. Br. J. Surg. 74:209–211, 1987.

Mason, P.: Abdominal trauma. In Cardona, V., et al. (eds.): Trauma Nursing: From Resuscitation through Rehabilitation. W. B. Saunders Co., Philadelphia, 1988.

McCormick, T., Kennedy, H., Salisbury, J., Simms, J., Triger, D., and Johnson, A.: Implications of sclerotherapy program for the medical and surgical care of bleeding in portal hypertension. Surg. Gynecol. Obstet. 161:557–562, 1985.

Miller, H. D.: Liver transplantation: Postoperative ICU care. Crit. Care Nurse 8:19–31, 1988.

Miller, T. A.: Emergencies in acid-peptic disease. Gastroenterol. Clin. North Am. 17:303–315, 1988.

Moriyasu, F., Tamada, T., Miyake, T., Nakamura, T., and Uchino, H.: Ultrasonic Doppler duplex study of hemodynamic changes from portosystemic shunt operation. Ann. Surg. 205:151–156, 1987.

Munoz, S. J., and Maddrey, W. C.: Major complications of acute and chronic liver disease. Gastroenterol. Clin. North Am. 17:265–283, 1988.

Petroianu, A.: Treatment of portal hypertension by subtotal splenectomy and central splenorenal shunt. Postgrad. Med. J. 64:38–41, 1988.

Pohlman, T.: Diverticulitis. Gastroenterol. Clin. North Am. 17:357–379, 1988.

Sabesin, S., and Williams, J.: Current status of liver transplantation. Hosp. Pract. 22:75–86, 1987.

Sarles, H., Sanowski, R., and Talbert, G.: Course and complications of endoscopic variceal sclerotherapy. Am. J. Gastroenterol. 80:595–599, 1985.

Sax, H., Talamini, M., and Fischer, J.: Clinical use of branched-chain amino acids in liver disease, sepsis, trauma and burns. Arch. Surg. 121:358–366, 1986.

Schiller, K.: Endoscopy in the management of upper gastrointestinal disease. Postgrad. Med. J. 64(suppl. 1):25–26, 1988.

Sherk, J., McCort, J., and Oakes, D.: Computed tomography in thoracoabdominal trauma. J. Trauma. 24:1015–1021, 1984.

Siegel, J., and Yatto, R.: Hydrostatic balloon catheters: A new dimension of therapeutic endoscopy. Endoscopy 16:231–236, 1984.

Sievert, W., and Vakil, N.: Emergencies of the biliary tract. Gastroenterol. Clin. North Am. 17:245–263, 1988.

Smith, S. L.: Liver transplantation: Implications for critical care. Heart Lung 14:617–626, 1985.

Teres, J., Baroni, R., Bordas, J., Visa, J., Pera, C., and Rodes, J.: Randomized trial of portocaval shunt, stapling transection, and endoscopic sclerotherapy in uncontrolled variceal bleeding. J. Hepatol. 4:159–167, 1987.

Warren, W., Galambos, J., Riepe, S., et al.: Distal splenorenal shunt versus endoscopic sclerotherapy for long-term management of variceal bleeding. Ann. Surg. 203:454–462, 1986.

Wienceh, R., and Wilson, R.: Abdominal venous injuries. J. Trauma. 26:771–778, 1986.

Willis, B. L., Thompson, L. F., and Howard, J. C.: Esophageal perforation: A nursing diagnosis approach. Crit. Care Nurse 8:20–30, 1988.

Zenilman, M., and Becker, J.: Emergencies in inflammatory bowel disease. Gastroenterol. Clin. North Am. 17:387–405, 1988.

CHAPTER

Psychosocial Aspects

John L. Carty, R.N., D.N.S.

Perception

INTRODUCTION

Perception: The experience of sensory input, that is, all stimuli experienced through sight, hearing, touch, taste, and smell
1. **Discussion**
   a. Perceptions are regulated by invisible filters that allow some perceptions to make an impression on a person and others to be kept out of a person's awareness
   b. The filters regulating the degree of impact that the person experiences depend on
      i. The meaning the stimuli have for the person at a given moment
      ii. How the person feels about himself at a given moment (i.e., weak or strong, overwhelmed or in control, peaceful or agitated)
      iii. The unfulfilled needs operating in a person when he experiences the stimuli
   c. Perceptions lead to thoughts and often to feelings. A person's thoughts and feelings influence the way in which he receives the next perception
   d. Therefore, two persons who experience the same event may perceive it very differently and may have different thoughts and feelings about the shared experience. Perceptions are unique to each individual

2. Example

A nurse meeting a stranger in a social context may meet the stranger's gaze while being introduced. Little attention may actually be paid to the person's eyes. When the same nurse meets the gaze of a patient in a critical care unit, the nurse may note pupil reactivity while looking at the patient's eyes. The nurse's perceptual filters allow the nurse to screen out certain information about "eyes" in the first instance, because of the particular meaning the nurse gives to the information in the professional setting

NURSING ASSESSMENT DATA BASE

Nursing History

1. Medical diagnosis and/or type of surgery
2. Whether the medical diagnosis has a social stigma, such as suicide attempt, acquired immunodeficiency syndrome, or a disfiguring type of surgery
3. The person has the ability to hear, see, and talk
4. On consciousness-altering chemicals either before or after admission (prescribed or nonprescribed)
5. Availability of significant other support

Nursing Examination of Patient

1. Note whether the patient is under the influence of central or peripheral anesthetics
2. Assess the presence of perceptual- or sensory-altering equipment or dressings such as ventilator, eye patch, or arm or leg restraints
3. Check for abnormal physiologic parameters, such as fluid volume, electrolytes, and air exchange

COMMONLY ENCOUNTERED NURSING DIAGNOSIS

Sensory-perceptual Alterations

1. **Assessment for defining characteristics**
   a. Ask "What is it like for you now . . . (having this illness, having had this surgery, being in these surroundings, having your spouse in the hospital)?"
   b. Listen for remarks disclosing self-perception
   c. Clarify the remarks if you see the need. Say something like "I think

if I were in your shoes, I might feel a little . . . (unsure, helpless, sorry, afraid, worried)"
   d. Alterations of emotional responses such as extremes of emotional responses, anger, or laughter in inappropriate situations
   e. Decreased ability to concentrate
   f. Altered communication patterns
   g. Changes in usual response to stimuli
2. **Expected outcomes**
   a. Explores environment: asks questions, what, who, when, where, how
   b. Seeks to experience things/events for self
   c. Asks reality-oriented questions about treatment, condition
   d. Expresses positive feelings about self
   e. Expresses situation-appropriate emotions and behavior: when happy, laughs; when afraid, states he is afraid and asks appropriate questions about fearful situation
3. **Nursing interventions**
   a. Rapport-building begins during assessment, validating/clarifying data. Process itself shows concern and increases closeness
   b. Validate and reinforce accurate perceptions and positive self-worth by providing clear, concise information and an attitude of caring and concern
   c. Focus on strengths rather than limitations
   d. Take time to validate perceptions: when giving information about a treatment/procedure have patient tell you in his own words what you have said
   e. Always forewarn patient before giving a treatment or doing a procedure (set the stage before doing anything)
4. **Evaluation of nursing care**
   a. Positive perceptions of situation/self
   b. Questions or requests are made in a positive mode
   c. A more positive perception of situation and self as reflected in the patient's assertive rather than aggressive approach to fulfilling needs
   d. Emotional response is appropriate to situation

Self-Concept

INTRODUCTION

Self-concept: All that one can identify as being characteristic of oneself. The components of self-concept are those things one believes about oneself based on past experiences and present experiences currently being confronted

1. **Discussion**
   a. Self-concept is formed over time in the context of others and in the presence of the beliefs, values, and norms of the culture. It consists of what one *believes* others think of one (not to be confused with what others may *actually* think of one) in light of one's own beliefs and value system
   b. Self-concept is always seeking consistency: one is continually attempting to find information to reinforce one's beliefs about oneself, even if those beliefs are negative or incorrect
   c. When one's self-concept is threatened, one will fight to hold on to one's beliefs about oneself
   d. One behaves in a manner that is consistent with one's self-concept: in a way that demonstrates one's beliefs about oneself
   e. The state of one's self-concept is one of the most important influences on behavior
   f. The more positive one feels about oneself, the more comfortable one will feel, and the more open one will be to new perceptions and new information
2. **Example**
   A 20-year-old man was admitted to ICU for observation after a one-car accident. This accident occurred on a clear evening with good visibility on a straight section of road in good weather conditions. There is some question of suicidal attempt. The patient is unresponsive to questions or requests of staff. He repeats at intervals, "I can't win; nothing good ever happens to me; my parents don't want me; my girlfriend left me." "You think I am a loser, too." Despite much encouragement the patient relates that everyone sees him as a loser.

NURSING ASSESSMENT DATA BASE

Nursing History

1. Review chart for medical concerns
2. Talk to significant others such as family, friends, and/or patient's co-workers
3. Assess whether patient received any state of consciousness-altering drugs (prescribed or nonprescribed)
4. Physical disability or disfigurement

Nursing Examination of Patient

1. Assess the physiologic parameters
2. Ask the same type of questions as used when assessing perceptions
3. Determine whether patient passively accepts or resists procedures
4. Note specific remarks and/or attitude toward self

COMMONLY ENCOUNTERED NURSING DIAGNOSIS

Self-concept Disturbance

1. **Assessment for defining characteristics**
   a. Listen for self-disclosing remarks concerning himself as individual, worker, and opinion giver and what he sees happening to himself
   b. Listen for consistent self-devaluating remarks
   c. Inability to see himself in positive terms
   d. Believes others see him as worthless and/or bad
   e. Poor eye contact
   f. Extremely aggressive behavior, demanding angry voice
   g. Overemphasis on powerfulness and achievements
2. **Expected outcomes**
   a. Initiates conversations, questions procedures, and listens
   b. Responds in a positive manner to suggestions and explanations for procedures
   c. Body posture and facial features are relaxed
   d. Participates in own treatment
   e. Able to make decisions about timing of care ("I need my pain medication before morning care")
   f. More assertive rather than aggressive
   g. Emotions/behavior appropriate to situation
3. **Nursing interventions**
   a. Note changes in self-concept by comparing original assessment with present assessment of self-concept
   b. Use interpersonal interaction with patient to build rapport and obtain clear, concise information
   c. Reinforce positives, show interest in subjects initiated by patient such as his work, family, hobbies, and expressed opinions
   d. Explain procedures and treatment. Encourage questions and give clear, concise responses
   e. Allow and encourage patient to make decisions about his care within safe medical and nursing care (i.e., "I want pain medication before the treatment." "Wake me when my visitors arrive")
   f. Encourage and listen to both positive and negative opinions/remarks of patient
   g. Use comfort measures (e.g., back rub, arm massage) to increase touch, thus accomplishing physical relaxation and acceptance of patient
   h. Demonstrate acceptance of patient as a worthwhile person
   i. Give honest praise; avoid false hope
   j. Initiate personal grooming measures (e.g., washing face, combing

hair, and brushing teeth) and encourage patient to undertake these things within his physical limits
4. **Evaluation of nursing care**
   a. Spontaneously initiates conversation, questions procedure, and listens positively with responses such as "How is that going to help me?" rather than "Is that going to hurt? What's it going to do to me?"
   b. Increasingly initiates and participates in own treatment
   c. Exhibits decreased passiveness and/or aggressiveness with concomitant increase in assertiveness
   d. Body posture and facial expression indicate sense of relaxation such as relaxed muscles (less rigid), face relaxed, maybe a smile, eyes bright, and acknowledges activity around him

Self-Esteem

INTRODUCTION

Self-esteem: Feelings one has about oneself—one's perceived self-worth. As such, it is a part of self-concept
1. **Discussion**
   a. Self-esteem is based on one's personal goals measured against one's perceived successes, in interaction with the beliefs and values of the culture/society
   b. Self-esteem is derived from a comparison between the strengths one believes one possesses and the limitations one believes one possesses
   c. The amount of self-esteem one enjoys influences the manner in which one behaves. The impact is seen through demonstrations of self-confidence and the level of comfort with oneself
   d. When one's self-concept is raised, one's self-esteem is enhanced, and a greater degree of comfort is experienced
2. **Examples**
   A 40-year-old woman with a healthy self-concept and a high level of self-esteem has a total mastectomy because of malignancy. She is seen reacting with spontaneous signs of grief but does not report feelings of helplessness or devastation. She appears to be able to maintain herself and to find sufficient strength to cope with the situation, much as she remembers having done with previous painful situations. She is overheard remarking to a doctor in the ICU: "I'm what you call a survivor. I've gotten through some pretty difficult times in my life, and I guess I've got what it takes to deal with this one too, but I'm scared about how long it well take for me to feel well enough to take care of my teenagers again."

A 15-year-old boy steals a car and subsequently is involved in a two-car collision. Because of his multiple injuries, he is admitted to an ICU for observation. While in the unit, he constantly complains about his care, the poor quality of food, and the fact that he is "with all these sickees." He repeatedly states his beliefs that the "nurses are mean" and "my parents don't like me anyway." He refuses to cooperate in having vital signs taken and yells out rather than using his call light. The night he spends in the unit is obviously difficult for him and he is unable to sleep. A night nurse spends some time with him and begins to explore his behavior to try to find out what he is feeling and to see if she can be of assistance. She finds that the boy feels ashamed because he has "caused trouble" for his family twice during the past year. He views himself as "a rotten kid—just like my father said I was." The boy acts the role of a rotten kid

NURSING ASSESSMENT DATA BASE

Nursing History

1. Use the same assessment material as self-concept. At the same time you assess self-concept you are assessing self-esteem
2. Availability of family or significant others' support
3. The medical diagnosis and prognosis
4. Impaired senses: unable to speak, unable to see; touch is impaired by bandages/restraints
5. Assess whether there is disfigurement or physical disability

Nursing Examination of Patient

1. Assess whether the patient sees himself as adequate or inadequate in the present situation
2. Note self-devaluation remarks
3. Note negative responses, such as, "I'll never get out of here, no one cares about me, nothing will help me."
4. Assess whether patient is passive, and never questions what is being done to him

COMMONLY ENCOUNTERED NURSING DIAGNOSIS

Self-concept, Disturbances in Self-esteem

1. Assessment for defining characteristics
   a. Inability to accept positive reinforcement
   b. Very passive, will not participate in own care

    c. Poor eye contact

    d. Responses to questions are limited: one or two words or turns head and eyes away

    e. Does not initiate personal grooming or ask for help with personal hygiene

    f. Describes self in negative terms

2. Expected outcomes

    a. Participates in own care

    b. Initiates personal hygiene care or initiates request for personal hygiene care

    c. Requests explanation of procedures before initiated

    d. Increase in positive remarks about himself in this situation

    e. Asks for medication when needed, such as pain medication before some procedure

    f. Initiates conversations with staff and others

3. Nursing interventions

    a. Convey acceptance of the patient as a worthwhile person

    b. Build rapport with interventions

    c. Encourage patient to initiate self-care or to request care when needed

    d. Give positive reinforcement for accomplishments but do not give false praise

    e. Zero in on patient's strengths rather than limitations

    f. Encourage patient to become involved in decision-making about own care

4. Evaluation of nursing care

    a. Demonstrates by words/behavior positive self-worth

    b. Perceives himself as adequate in present situation

    c. Expresses both limitations and strengths about himself: "Not knowing scares me. Please tell me what is planned for me today."

    d. Participates in own care within physical limitations

    e. Emotions are appropriate to the situation

Needs

INTRODUCTION

Needs: A person's perceived physical and psychosocial requirements for developing, maintaining, and enhancing himself

1. Discussion

    a. Maslow (1968) has categorized human needs according to the following levels (the first level being the most basic)

        i. Physiologic

        ii. Safety and security

       iii. Love and belonging

       iv. Self-esteem

        v. Self-actualization

  b. Need satisfaction progresses from basic needs to higher level needs: one does not become preoccupied with meeting higher level needs until basic needs are satisfied

  c. Unfulfilled needs are constantly operating in humans and influences their behavior. A person consistently strives to fulfill perceived needs in an ongoing dynamic process throughout the life cycle. The influence of needs on behavior is sometimes a conscious process and at other times unconscious. In other words, one is sometimes aware of one's unfulfilled needs and at other times unaware of them. Even when one does not recognize one's unfulfilled needs, those needs continue to influence one's behavior

  d. The greatest human need is to perceive the self as an adequate person

  e. Major life changes (e.g., illness) may necessitate a refocusing of energies to meet a more basic need

2. Example

A young man purchases a motorcycle to help him act out his wish to be daring. Analyzing his conversation concerning how he thinks he will look to his girlfriend when he picks her up on his cycle, one can hypothesize that he is attempting to meet his need for belonging and for self-esteem at the time of purchase. Within 3 weeks he suffers an accident in which he sustains a crushed chest, internal bleeding, and a concussion. In the ICU his energies become intensely focused on all the apparatus to which he is attached for survival and treatment. His need level has apparently reverted to physiologic and safety requirements

NURSING ASSESSMENT DATA BASE

Nursing History

1. Medical diagnosis and prognosis
2. Significant other availability
3. Work history
4. Whether illness will influence relationship with family or significant others, ability to work, or ability to take care of self
5. Effect of the patient's physiologic and psychologic condition on sensory ability (sight, taste, hearing, touch)
6. Effect of the patient's physiologic and psychologic condition on self-concept and self-esteem

7. Effect of the patient's physiologic and psychologic condition on communication

Nursing Examination of Patient

1. **Assess physiologic needs** such as airway, nutrition, general physical condition, mobility, and skin integrity
2. **Safety and security needs** such as equipment safety: whether the person sees the equipment as hazardous to physical safety; need for safety measures (bed rails); whether the patient understands function/ sounds of machines, uses of catheters, intravenous lines, etc.
3. **Belonging needs** (love): assess whether patient feels as though he is a number, a diagnosis, or a human being. Listen for questions and requests of patient. Determine whether patient still identifies himself as part of family and community
4. **Self-esteem needs** are assessed under concepts of self-esteem and self-concept
5. **Self-actualization:** listen for self-description in relation to having future, sense of control, and having meaning
6. **Assess whether patient is future-oriented or past-oriented**

COMMONLY ENCOUNTERED NURSING DIAGNOSIS

Need Disturbance

1. **Assessment for defining characteristics**
   a. Threat to self-preservation
   b. Threat to self-concept/self-esteem
   c. Threat to health status
   d. Threat to relationships
   e. Threat to normal role function (as student, as worker, as parent, as spouse)
2. **Expected outcomes**
   a. Able to maintain physiologic self within limits of condition
   b. Patient accepts environment as nonthreatening
   c. Patient sees himself as part of family and community and as a participant in relationships
   d. Views himself as a person with worth and dignity
   e. Talks about himself in future terms: going back to school, back to work, back to family or significant others
3. **Nursing interventions**
   a. Implementation starts at the first meeting and interaction with the patient

   b. Clear, concise information sharing with the patient is a necessary element to meet physiologic needs. For example, use of tracheal tube to allow and enhance breathing needs to be explained. The use of intravenous lines or other modes for nutrients, medication, and fluids is essential for physiologic survival but also needs explanation
   c. Use of all safety measures such as bed rails, and alarms needs to be explained. At the same time, the security needs also should be addressed. Reassurance and optimal meeting of needs along with shared information and a sense of caring expressed by words, touch, and concern will help answer security needs
   d. Self-esteem needs are best answered by showing concern, etc. See section on self-esteem
4. **Evaluation of nursing care**
   a. Physiologic parameters indicate physical needs are being met (e.g., respiratory, nutritional, excretory)
   b. Psychologic parameters (e.g., positive self-esteem, self-concept) indicate psychologic needs are being met
   c. Necessary physical safety and security measures (e.g., bed rails, alarms, monitors) are in place
   d. Love and belonging: patient refers to himself as an important person rather than a diagnosis or number. Patient still identifies himself as part of a family/community. Family's or friends' visits are positive events
   e. Self-esteem: sees self as important and as having value. See section on self-esteem
   f. Self-actualization is future oriented. Takes control of some event such as requesting specific time for medication, bath, or other care

Strengths, Potentials, Limitations

INTRODUCTION

Strengths, Potentials, Limitations: Strengths are perceived as positive attributes believed to be characteristic of oneself or others. Potentials are perceived as latent strengths believed to be characteristic of oneself or others. Limitations are perceived as inadequacies or shortcomings believed to be characteristic of oneself or others
1. **Discussion**
   a. Generally, persons are more aware of their perceived limitations than of their perceived strengths
   b. Often, one desperately attempts to hide the limitations one believes one possesses in an effort to protect one's self-concept and self-esteem

    c. Humans consciously and unconsciously choose the boundaries of their lives through

       i. The strengths they choose to maintain

      ii. The potentials they choose to develop, as well as those they choose not to develop

     iii. The limitations they choose to maintain

    d. Since all humans struggle to maintain the "self" as adequate, focusing on their strengths and potentials (instead of their shortcomings) enables them to feel more competent and to deal more effectively with perceived or actual limitations. Learning and growth also are greatly facilitated by recognizing strengths in oneself and in others

    e. A poor self-concept and self-esteem result from focusing only on one's limitations

2. Example

    A nurse working in a critical care nursery observes a mother anxiously attempting to feed her 4-week-old infant who has just been removed from the incubator. The mother's efforts look awkward, and the infant is crying loudly. The mother says to the nurse: "I feel like a klutz when she cries like this. I want to give her all the love I feel for her, but I'm so uncoordinated!" The nurse responds:"Jenny is awfully lucky to have such a caring mother. I wonder if she would feed more easily if you held her head a little higher. That way she might stop crying and you might better enjoy feeding her." The nurse realistically focuses on the mother's strengths and attempts to assist her in developing her potential as a competent caregiver. The interaction helps to increase the mother's self-concept, facilitates her feelings of adequacy, and enables her to perform in a manner that makes her feel more comfortable

NURSING ASSESSMENT DATA BASE

Nursing History

1. Identification of strengths, potentials, and limitations can be accomplished by interpersonal interaction and validated observations. Other sources of information are records (i.e., nursing history to include work, social, medical, and family history) and information from family and friends
2. Medical diagnosis and prognosis
3. Limitations secondary to condition
4. Condition's influence on sensory organs
5. Availability of family or significant other

Nursing Examination of Patient

1. Patient sees himself as important, being of value
2. History of coping with illness in past
3. Employment history
4. Marital status, availability of friends. Sees himself as important or unimportant to family and friends
5. General state of health
6. Involvement in community, kind of hobbies
7. Presence or absence of positive self-esteem/self-concept

COMMONLY ENCOUNTERED NURSING DIAGNOSIS

Disturbance in Perception, Self-concept, Self-esteem, or Needs

1. **Assessment for defining characteristics**
   a. Alteration of emotional responses (i.e., extremes in emotions, emotions inappropriate to situation)
   b. Condition of patient restricts involvement in relationships, family, community, and work
   c. Degree of independence is limited by condition
   d. Nonparticipation in self-care
   e. Needs not met
2. **Expected outcomes**
   a. Able to identify strengths, potentials, and limitations in a realistic manner
   b. Increased involvement in own care
   c. Increased interest/involvement in relationships, family, and community
   d. Future oriented: talks about returning to school, job, and family
   e. Return to premorbid health
3. **Nursing interventions**
   a. Implementation is started at the time of assessment, when these attributes are identified and should be reinforced
   b. Support identified strengths and enhance potential strengths by verbal and nonverbal encouragement
   c. Note limitations but do not overemphasize them
   d. Allow patient to use already developed coping mechanisms to handle situation
   e. Reinforce outside interests such as family, work, and hobbies
   f. Give honest, timely compliments that will reinforce strengths
   g. Involve patient in own care as much as possible, from as little as nodding of head for "yes" or "no" to actual hands-on care of himself.

Encourage patient's taking charge of own life within physical and safety limits

4. **Evaluation of nursing care**
   a. Identifies strengths, potentials, and limitations realistically
   b. Increased interactions in job, community, and hobbies
   c. Increased interaction with and about family
   d. Increased showing of concern, love, and caring by family and friends
   e. Increased involvement in own care within physical and safety limits

Growth and Development

INTRODUCTION

Growth and Development Problems: Growth and development are those repeated cumulative behaviors frequently exhibited by persons as they confront and deal with issues that typically arise during life stages

1. **Discussion**
   a. Some types of growth seem to occur automatically, whereas others take place through focused effort
   b. Because growth and development processes are constantly operating within a person, they have an influence on behavior
   c. In the ongoing process of evaluating oneself to see if one is adequate, a measuring stick frequently used is one's success in mastering developmental tasks. For example, during adolescence many persons measure their adequacy in part by evaluating their success in forming relationships with members of the opposite sex
   d. If one does not master the developmental tasks of a particular life stage, one will have increased difficulty in mastering the developmental tasks of future stages

2. **Example**
   During a spring break vacation in Florida, a 19-year-old man is involved in a diving accident and is left hemiplegic. While in the ICU, he constantly struggles with being dependent on the nursing staff for many basic needs. He had recently begun to enjoy a great deal of independence while away at college and finds his dependent position in the hospital almost unbearable. The struggle makes him reluctant to ask nurses to assist him when he needs help, and he becomes increasingly irritable, frustrated, demanding, and depressed

NURSING ASSESSMENT DATA BASE

Nursing History

1. Medical diagnosis and prognosis
2. Note prior history of illness
3. Assess prior history of disturbed growth and development
4. Impact of patient's condition on the normal growth and development tasks of his age group

Nursing Examination of Patient

1. Assessment is geared to identifying responses to illness, ICU, and self
2. Note whether patient is fighting equipment such as ventilator, oxygen mask, nasal sponges, or intravenous lines unrelated to physiologic causes
3. Patient withdraws and/or "cringes" when the staff approaches
4. Patient has tears in eyes, is unresponsive (conscious), or pulls away with frightened look
5. Consistently demands pain medication or attention
6. Refuses staff's help or medication
7. Needs for privacy and maintenance of human dignity
8. Patient feels guilty for being ill, blames self or others for illness
9. Patient expresses concerns and fears about illness

COMMONLY ENCOUNTERED NURSING DIAGNOSIS

Growth and Development, Altered

1. **Assessment for defining characteristics**
   a. Altered physical/psychologic growth
   b. Difficulty performing age-normal skills (motor, social, or expressive)
   c. Difficulty in performing self-care and/or self-control activities appropriate for age
   d. Listlessness, decreased responses
2. **Expected outcomes**
   a. Age-appropriate self-care skills
   b. Cooperative with procedures
   c. Age-appropriate expression of feelings/concerns
3. **Nursing interventions**
   a. The assessment phase itself is the first step in the implementation phase
   b. Give clear, concise information about equipment. Frequent interac-

tion at specific times such as: "I'll be back in 15 minutes." Then
   return at said time
   c. Introduce self: "My name is . . . and I'll be caring for you today."
   d. Touch the patient, especially when you are *not* going to adjust or
   change dressing or equipment. Talk in a calm and caring voice
   (softly) before doing any procedure
   e. Encourage verbalization of fears, concerns, or likes and dislikes
   f. Encourage person to take as much control of himself as safe care
   and physical limitations will allow
4. **Evaluation of nursing care**
   a. Increasingly cooperative with procedures
   b. Age-appropriate expression of feelings/concerns (i.e., 6-year-old tearful and frightened; 30-year-old tearful and verbally expressing fears)
   c. Decreasing demand for pain medication
   d. Requests help when needed
   e. Expresses needs in age-appropriate manner: small child cries, adult
   verbally expresses needs

Stress

INTRODUCTION

Stress: The condition that exists in an organism when it meets with stimuli.
Selye (1974) has identified two types of stress: (1) distress—the condition
that exists in an organism when it meets with *noxious* stimuli, that is,
when an individual encounters threatening stimuli, and (2) eustress—the
condition that exists in an organism when it meets with *nonthreatening*
stimuli
1. **Discussion**
   a. Persons may experience the same stressors differently. Stressors that
   may cause distress in one person may evoke eustress in another
   b. Persons respond to stressors differently because their perception of
   the stressful event may be different and they may possess different
   coping abilities
   c. A person experiencing distress feels uncomfortable. The discomfort
   provides the motivation to find a way to deal effectively with the
   stressor so that the discomfort will be decreased
   d. If one perceives oneself as adequate in the face of stressors, self-
   concept is maintained and may even be enhanced; growth is experienced and self-esteem is heightened. One functions out of strength
   e. If one perceives oneself as inadequate in the face of stressors, one
   may use defensive mechanisms (e.g., denial, projection) to mask the

fact that one views one's handling of the stressor as inadequate; however, one will feel overwhelmed and helpless. One functions out of a sense of frustration and helplessness

    f. If one continues to experience oneself as inadequate in the face of stressors for a prolonged period, crisis will result

2. Example

Two critical care nurses begin orientation to a new hospital on the same day. Three weeks after completing orientation, one nurse begins to relax and talk about feeling more comfortable on the unit and about how much she is learning. This nurse has worked in an ICU in the past, knows generally what to expect, and has learned to deal effectively with occupational stressors. She generally finds ways to take allotted breaks with other staff members and to discuss any difficulties she is having in adjusting to the unit. She feels comfortable enough to seek the advice of a clinical specialist in planning care for a very involved patient. The second nurse begins to report feeling nervous, fatigued, overwhelmed, and constantly on the verge of tears or a "blow-up" whenever a patient or colleague asks her to do anything she has not anticipated. This nurse has no previous experience in critical care nursing and has not yet found ways to deal effectively with the stressful stimuli with which she is constantly being bombarded. The life/death atmosphere of urgency within the unit is a constant source of stress

NURSING ASSESSMENT DATA BASE

Nursing History

1. Medical diagnosis and prognosis
2. Significant other availability
3. When appropriate, social/work history
4. Prior illness
5. Condition's impact on sensory organs and communication ability

Nursing Examination of Patient

1. Assessment is based on observation, daily interaction, and patient's response to environment (e.g., ICU, equipment, staff)
2. Remember that any change in a patient's normal environment will affect the patient and can be considered stressful
3. Therefore, by assessing perceptions, self-esteem, self-concept, strengths, potentials, and limitations along with growth and development, the nurse is actually assessing the degree of stress experienced by a patient
4. Assess the patient's perception of self, of situation, and of status of self in situation

5. Assess how the person sees self, whether he feels adequate to cope
6. The patient's interactions emphasize limitations rather than positive attributes
7. Assess what the patient identifies as stressful: remember, stress for one may not be stress for another, or at least not to the same degree
8. Stress expressed by both emotional and physical signs: pulse elevated, blood pressure elevated, respirations elevated, headache, stomachache

COMMONLY ENCOUNTERED NURSING DIAGNOSIS

Stress Level, Alteration

1. **Assessment for defining characteristics**
   a. Hypervigilance or hypovigilance
   b. Impaired ability to make decisions
   c. Impaired problem-solving ability
   d. Feeling uncomfortable with oneself
   e. Feeling inadequate to situation
   f. Increased tension
   g. Increased sense of helplessness and powerlessness
2. **Expected outcomes**
   a. Increased initiation of requests and decision making
   b. Explores environment: asks questions, what, who, when, where, how
   c. Asks reality-oriented questions about condition
   d. Increasingly expresses positive aspects of oneself
   e. More involved in own care
   f. Future oriented, talks about (in realistic terms) return to work, family, community
3. **Nursing interventions**
   a. Implementation starts with assessment by rapport-building, providing sense of concern, and caring
   b. Include frequent interactions; clear, concise information; and timely explanations of equipment, sounds, and sights. Use touch to convey caring
   c. Provide for privacy
   d. Encourage patient to make decisions about his daily care (e.g., time of medication, time of bath, or personal hygiene); thus the patient will feel in control
   e. Decrease amount of noise (e.g., monitor sounds, loud conversation)
4. **Evaluation of nursing care**
   a. Exhibits behavioral signs of decreased stress reaction (e.g., increased initiation of requests, making decisions)

    b. Able to express needs either verbally or nonverbally; able to disagree with staff in positive, constructive manner

    c. Increased ability to express doubts, fears, and concerns to staff

    d. Increased self-esteem/self-concept, along with expression of strengths (e.g., talking about work, hobbies, family)

    e. Increased interaction with family or significant others (i.e., supporting each other)

    f. Physical signs of stress decreasing. Pulse, blood pressure, and respirations no longer rise drastically when monitor sounds are heard or procedures are done

Pain

INTRODUCTION

Pain: A concept denoting the experience of multiple stimuli, all perceived as unpleasant by the person involved. It is a multidimensional perception that has an influence on all aspects of one's life

1. Discussion

    a. Pain is an individual and personal experience. Behavioral expressions of pain are socially and culturally determined. Because of the complexity of pain phenomena, there is no one theory that takes into account all the ramifications. Scientists and clinicians view pain from as many perspectives as there are clinical specialties. However, there appear to be three elements common to most definitions of pain

        i. There is a break in the protective barrier of the person

        ii. It is perceived as a danger signal

        iii. It is an expression of all previous pain experiences

    b. Painful stimuli and their associated responses are composed of both physiologic and psychosocial elements. Humans almost always are born with the physiologic ability to experience pain

    c. It is within the psychosocial realm that one develops behavioral responses to pain. Humans are both blessed and cursed by the fact that they can experience pain and remember it. The moment one experiences an unpleasant (painful) stimulus, it is integrated with memories of previous painful experiences and a response occurs. One responds not only to the immediate painful stimulus but also to the memories of other experiences. In fact, the ability to think and remember allows one to feel discomfort without presently experiencing a physiologically unpleasant stimulus

    d. The meaning one places on an unpleasant sensation is determined by one's beliefs and values within the context of societal beliefs, values, and norms

   e. Pain, like beauty, is in the eye of the beholder. It is whatever the person experiencing it says it is, whenever it is being experienced

2. Example

A 48-year-old man has been admitted for the fourth time to the ICU with chest pain and shortness of breath. Four months ago, he experienced a myocardial infarction with residual heart damage. The patient describes events prior to admission as follows: "I started to breathe more rapidly, felt dizzy, light-headed, and faint with increasing chest pain. I felt like this while I was driving to a job interview." While the nurse is talking to the patient he reports that he is becoming more nervous and anxious. His breathing becomes more rapid and he mentions that his dizziness is more pronounced. The following diagnosis is made: angina (normal for this patient) and hyperventilation secondary to anxiety. The patient's past memories of the heart attack and feelings of anxiety about the job interview are expressed behaviorally as hyperventilation and its sequelae. He perceives his symptoms of hyperventilation as chest "pain" and associates it with a heart attack

NURSING ASSESSMENT DATA BASE

Nursing History

1. Prior history of painful conditions/situation
2. Medical diagnosis and prognosis
3. Duration of this episode of pain
4. Whether painfulness interferes with work, social interaction, or family relationships
5. Amount and kind of pain medication being taken and history of pain medication use
6. Whether family or significant others have had a painful condition in the past
7. Obtain good pain history to include, but not be limited to, the following: accidents, broken bones, operations, and how the patient coped with the pain (by laughing, crying, ignoring, overuse of medications, or screaming or by appropriate use of medications or by combination of above)
8. Pain history will give information as to what pain means and how patient copes with pain

Nursing Examination of Patient

1. Assessment aimed at identifying what the patient is experiencing and what it means to the patient

2. Determine what these painful situations mean to the patient: pain is a normal response, I am critically hurt, I am dying
3. Assess the degree of pain felt: use scale of 1 to 10, with 1 being the least severe and 10 being the most severe
4. Determine location and description of pain
5. Assess whether pain medications have been adequate for controlling the pain

COMMONLY ENCOUNTERED NURSING DIAGNOSIS

Comfort, Altered: Pain

1. **Assessment for defining characteristics**
   a. Communication (verbal or nonverbal) of pain description
   b. Guarding behavior; protective
   c. Self-focusing
   d. Narrowed focus (withdrawal from social contact, impaired perception and thought process)
   e. Restless, moaning, crying, pacing
   f. Eyes lack luster, grimacing
   g. Muscle tone may be flaccid to rigid
2. **Expected outcomes**
   a. Experiencing periods of activity/rest
   b. Reports increased periods of uninterrupted sleep at night
   c. Increased participation in own treatment within physical limitations
   d. Decreased signs of anxiety
   e. Exhibits increased self-esteem/self-concept
   f. Periods of being pain free
3. **Nursing interventions**
   a. Assessment is starting point of pain plan: shows concern and caring
   b. When appropriate, use and reinforce familiar modes of coping with pain
   c. Give clear, concise information about pain. For example, postoperative incisional pain does not mean sutures have broken or person is dying
   d. Reassure patient that when he says "I am in pain," you believe it
   e. Use touch whenever possible; perform frequent and consistent checks for pain relief
   f. Whenever possible, administer pain medication routinely, rather than only as needed
4. **Evaluation of nursing care**
   a. Patient participates in own treatment within physical limitations
   b. Obtains pain relief

    c. Expresses concerns and fears about pain
    d. Requests for pain medication decrease
    e. Decreased signs of anxiety
    f. Increased interactions with family or significant others
    g. Increased positive self-esteem, self-concept

Interpersonal Communication

INTRODUCTION

Interpersonal Communication: A dynamic process involving verbal and nonverbal means of conveying and receiving information

1. **Discussion**
   a. One of the most important aspects of interpersonal communication is that one *cannot* not communicate. Interpersonal interactions means that every word (spoken or written), movement, facial expression, and body posture convey information. This begins the circular process of communication
   b. The receiver accepts information conveyed through the words, gestures, facial expressions, and postures of the sender and assigns meaning to that information. The meaning assigned is understood in context of the situation and in light of the beliefs, values, knowledge, and self-concepts of both sender and receiver. The meaning and significance of the information influences how the receiver responds. The response is based on the meaning the receiver has given the information. The sender then receives the response
   c. The response may not be what the sender desired to know, and a breakdown in communication could result. This can be forestalled by verification (i.e., verifying the information received and its meaning with the sender). Verification can be accomplished in a variety of ways (e.g., directly questioning, restating, and reflecting the information received). Through verification, the receiver and sender both achieve a clearer understanding of the information conveyed. In order to accomplish effective communication, it is not necessary to agree with what another says—only that both parties understand that which is communicated

2. **Example**
   A 26-year-old man is admitted to the ICU after an automobile accident. His medical diagnoses are three fractured fingers of the right hand, no internal abdominal injuries, no closed head injury, and trauma to the throat requiring a tracheostomy. The patient, a pianist by profession, is oriented and alert. The nurse says, "How

are you?" The patient stares at his right hand, which is wrapped in bandages and elevated. The nurse observes the patient's staring, shares with him the meaning she assigned to his behavior, and attempts to verify it by saying, "Does this mean that you are having pain in your hand?" The patient clarifies his meaning by shaking his head to signify "no" and points to his right hand with his left hand. He opens and closes his left hand. The nurse now shares her perception and thoughts about the patient's new behavior by asking, "Are you saying that you have no pain, but you want to know about being able to move your right hand?" The patient verifies for the nurse by nodding his head to signify "yes"

NURSING ASSESSMENT DATA BASE

Nursing History

1. Assessment of communication begins at first interaction with patient
2. Review chart, talk to family or significant other to gain understanding of how patient normally communicates
3. Determine whether the patient's condition alters ability to communicate
4. Assess whether patient and staff speak same language (i.e., staff speaks English, patient speaks only Polish)
5. Identify if a prior condition affects the patient's ability to communicate (i.e., mentally retarded, born unable to speak, uses sign language)

Nursing Examination of Patient

1. Assessing the communication process involves at least two persons (e.g., health care provider and health care receiver)
2. Assess nonverbal and verbal communication by validating the meaning of what you (staff) perceive and what the patient may perceive. In other words, you assess the meaning of nonverbal and verbal communication
3. By assessing the preceding concepts of perception, self-esteem, self-concept, and others, you begin the assessment of interpersonal communication
4. Evaluate the congruence between nonverbal clues and verbal responses, for example, "I am fine" at same time face is white, body rigid. The incongruence between verbal and nonverbal communication gives clues on how the patient really feels (i.e., feels scared, self-esteem/self-concept threatened, feels alone, decreased trust, and feelings of weakness)
5. Identify not only verbalized needs but also nonverbalized needs
6. Identify staff needs to assess how they are being perceived

COMMONLY ENCOUNTERED NURSING DIAGNOSIS

Communication, Impaired

1. **Assessment for defining characteristics**
   a. Unable to speak dominant language
   b. Does not or cannot speak
   c. Medical condition affects ability to communicate
   d. Chronic condition (mental retardation) affects communication
   e. Incongruence between verbal communication and nonverbal communication (e.g., patient smiles with body rigid, no eye contact)
2. **Expected outcomes**
   a. Responds to relevant stimuli
   b. Demonstrates congruent verbal and nonverbal communication
   c. Listens actively
   d. Asks for and receives feedback
   e. Spontaneously initiates communication
   f. Demonstrates a positive self-esteem
3. **Nursing interventions**
   a. When the assessment process is initiated in a positive manner, enhancement of interpersonal communication is part of that process
   b. For the health care provider there must be congruence between their verbal and nonverbal communication before trust can be initiated and enhanced
   c. Give clear, concise information with adequate time allowed for clarification by the patient
   d. Visit patient frequently to check status and needs, not just to check equipment. Use touch and facial expressions of warmth and concern along with words
   e. Clarify your own perceptions. Ask questions; do not assume
   f. Use all modes of communication if unable to use verbal route, such as written, sign language, eye blinks, or any other mode that will foster the link between health care provider and health care receiver. Trust is enhanced, therefore compliance and communication are increased
   g. Clarify any misperceptions
4. **Evaluation of nursing care**
   a. Patient responds willingly
   b. Congruence exists between verbal and nonverbal modes of communication
   c. Patient becomes involved in own care within physical limitations
   d. Questions for clarification increase in a positive sense
   e. Compliance with treatment increases
   f. Trust increases
   g. Self-esteem/self-concept increases

Body Image

INTRODUCTION

Body Image: The concept of one's own body. It is formed through an accumulation of all perceptions, information, and feelings incorporated about one's body as different and apart from all others

1. **Discussion**
   a. One is not born with a body image. The concept of body is built slowly over a period of time as an integral part of one's growth and development. Body image is an essential component of the self-concept and as such is grounded in interactions occurring between persons and their environment
   b. Like self-concept, body image reflects sociocultural beliefs and values. Body image evolves in a dynamic, everchanging process that incorporates not only one's body but also devices attached to it (e.g., clothes, rings, watches, dialysis machine, pacemaker). It is more than a portrait in the mind: it is the *significance* attached to the structures and functions of the body that is truly important
   c. Body image is social in nature, yet is individually experienced. If a person experiences a positive body image, then self-concept and self-esteem are likely to be influenced favorably. Conversely, a negative body image could lead to a less than favorable self-concept and self-esteem. Changes in body image influence a person's perception of consequential events

2. **Example**
   A 33-year-old woman with a bilateral mastectomy has experienced an altered body image. She perceives herself as less than whole and less feminine. Her changed body image has affected her self-concept. She complains that when she is alone with her husband, he seems nervous and afraid to touch her. Her perception is that he no longer "cares for me or finds me desirable." She feels repulsive. The woman's altered body image influences her perception of her husband's attitude toward her

NURSING ASSESSMENT DATA BASE

Nursing History

1. Verbally responds to actual or perceived changes in body structure/function
2. Nonverbally by behavior responds to perceived or actual change in structure/function

3. Medical condition's impact on body image
4. Medical condition's influence on the patient's ability to work, socialize, or relate to family or significant other

Nursing Examination of Patient

1. Assessing body image is started when assessments of self-concept and self-esteem are done
2. Observe the impact of any invasive procedures such as intravenous lines, cutdowns, or central lines on body image
3. Listen to how patient describes and perceives the machines (e.g., monitors, ventilators). Determine whether these machines infringe on body image. *EXAMPLE:* Cardiac monitor is incorporated into body image or ventilator becomes extension of lungs—necessary for life. Does the patient have names for machines or does he just state "that machine?"
4. Assess need for privacy: covering of culturally defined private parts (e.g., breasts, genitals). If they are not covered, body image is impinged on and self-esteem/self-concept is threatened
5. Identify areas of body most important to patient (e.g., hands of the pianist, legs of the runner, general mobility of the young adult or teenager). Disturbance in body image is sorely affected when these areas are affected. There is increased stress, anxiety, fear, and anger, with decreased self-concept/self-esteem
6. Determine how patient perceives himself and his body in this situation (e.g., distorted, feeling apart, weak, and/or unhappy)

COMMONLY ENCOUNTERED NURSING DIAGNOSIS

Self-concept, Disturbance in: Body Image

1. **Assessment for defining characteristics**
   a. Verbal response to actual or perceived change in structure and/or function
   b. Nonverbal response to actual or perceived change in structure and/or function
   c. Does not look at actual/perceived structural/functional body change area
   d. Does not touch actual/perceived structural/functional body change area
   e. Body boundaries are extended to environment (e.g., ventilator, bedside stand)
   f. Feelings of hopelessness, helplessness, and powerlessness

2. **Expected outcomes**
   a. Demonstrates improved self-care practices
   b. Able to talk about and focus on affected area
   c. Facial expression/body posture reflects sense of relaxation
   d. Age-appropriate expression of feelings about perceived or actual change in structure/function
   e. Decreased apprehension about equipment and procedure
   f. More assertive in questions about procedures and future care
3. **Nursing interventions**
   a. Encourage patient to participate in own care (i.e., dressing changes, personal hygiene)
   b. Provide positive appropriate encouragement, avoid false praise
   c. Help set realistic goals
   d. Object of plan is to maintain body image in at least a premorbid status with improvement when possible
   e. Provide adequate time (when possible) for discussion with patient about any invasive procedure (e.g., "This catheter will enhance your ability to return to health, and it will allow us (staff) to monitor and respond to your needs more rapidly and effectively")
   f. Explain clearly and concisely what each machine will do and what the different sounds, lights, and functions of the machines signify
   g. Reassurance that a staff member will be available frequently to make sure everything functions correctly
4. **Evaluation of nursing care**
   a. Patient's perception of self reflects feelings of being in control of body and/or still liking one's self (body image)
   b. Demonstrates less resistance to procedures such as intravenous lines or central lines
   c. Decreased apprehension regarding machines (i.e., decreased frequency of call button, decreased anger and anxiety)
   d. Increased requests for information about procedures and machines and their effect on body

Human Sexuality

INTRODUCTION

Human Sexuality: A developmental process encompassing a blend of the physiologic aspects of genetic sex and the psychosocial aspects, which include gender identity, sexual behavior, and sexual attitudes or values. Sexuality is part of one's self-concept, embodying how one sees oneself as a sexual being

1. **Discussion**
   a. The interaction between the psyche and the soma is nowhere more evident than in the area of sexuality, where perception, self-concept, self-esteem, body image, and personal values combine with basic mechanisms of physiologic functioning in a complex system. Although the genetic sex of an infant is determined by chromosomal factors before birth, the psychosocial impact on gender identity becomes predominant after birth. The concept of sexuality, or more specifically the psychosocial aspect of sexuality, primarily involves the quality of a person's interactions with significant others throughout the life cycle. One's gender identity, sexual behaviors, and sexual attitudes and values are integrated into the fabric of one's self-concept. Sexuality is so closely interwoven with the self-concept that a perceived threat to the self-concept can have an impact on one's sexuality, which is expressed in both physiologic and psychosocial realms
   b. For different reasons, sexuality is as important to a 70-year-old person as it is to a 20-year-old person. Younger persons often are concerned about their sexual attractiveness as well as their ability to reproduce. Older persons usually are concerned with feeling like a sexual being and being perceived by others as such
   c. A perceived threat to the self within a critical care environment has an effect on sexuality. The effects can be expressed in a variety of symptomatic behaviors (e.g., depression or anger, a sense of loss, sexual aggressiveness, noncompliance, or demands on others). Such behavior can result in decreased self-esteem, influencing the person's perception of events occurring in the environment

2. **Example**
   A 37-year-old man is admitted to the hospital with chest pain and shortness of breath. Laboratory studies confirm that he has suffered a myocardial infarction. The patient married for the second time 18 months ago. His wife is 27 years old, and they have two children from her previous marriage. The patient appears to be apprehensive, restless, and withdrawn, and these symptoms seem to increase after his wife's visit. He discusses his apprehensiveness with a nurse after his wife's visit. The patient says: "Things won't be like they have been. I won't be able to support my family now." He then grimaces and quickly looks away. The nurse says, "Is there something wrong right now?" The patient replies, "I'm just thinking about my wife. Because of my heart attack, I won't be able to be the husband she's known. She's younger than me and can have almost any guy she wants." The myocardial infarction is a threat to the patient's self-concept, self-esteem, body image, and sexual identity

NURSING ASSESSMENT DATA BASE

Nursing History

1. Medical condition's physiologic impact on the sexuality of the patient: is there a change in the function or structure of the physical sexual characteristics?
2. Patient's medical condition impacts on the gender identity, sexual behavior, and/or sexual attitudes: does the patient perceive his medical condition affecting his sexual relationship with significant other?
3. Assess contact between patient and significant other: do they touch hands or use soft touches on arms, shoulder, or cheek?

Nursing Examination of Patient

1. See assessment of self-concept, self-esteem, and body image
2. Assess how this situation will affect sexual identity and/or function
3. Determine whether patient saw self as attractive or unattractive before this illness/accident. Identify changes this patient sees now
4. Evaluate whether patient feels comfortable with own self identity (male/female) and role identity
5. Assess how this patient reinforces sexual identity: use of clothes, perfumes, reproductive ability, anatomic features, strong-muscled, or soft/warm, etc.

COMMONLY ENCOUNTERED NURSING DIAGNOSIS

Human Sexuality, Altered Patterns

1. **Assessment for defining characteristics**
   a. Actual or perceived limitations imposed by condition and/or therapy
   b. Seeking behavior for confirmation of desirability
   c. Changes of interest in oneself and others
   d. Extreme bashfulness or, on the other hand, exhibitionistic behavior
   e. Speaks of oneself as negative and undesirable
2. **Expected outcomes**
   a. Increased attention to personal grooming (e.g., hair combed, shaved, perfume used, requests use of mirror, dentures in when possible)
   b. Takes time to perform personal grooming before seeing significant others
   c. Appropriate use of privacy
   d. Emotional responses are appropriate to questions and procedures that relate to sexuality

e. Patient asks questions about medical condition in relation to self-esteem, self-concept, and body image

3. **Nursing interventions**
   a. Reinforce identified strengths
   b. Address patient as patient desires (i.e., Mr., Mrs., Miss, Ms., John, Mary)
   c. Use touch when talking to patient or doing treatments
   d. Provide equipment and time for personal hygiene: hair combing, shaving, and/or both
   e. Provide privacy: cover culturally defined private parts
   f. Reinforce sexual identity modes used in part by the patient and reinforce other modes of being male/female
   g. Clarify with the patient any uncertainties regarding terminology being used: medical terms or slang or street terms that may have several meanings

4. **Evaluation of nursing care**
   a. Identifies self with words or actions that reinforce sexual identity
   b. Requests equipment for enhancing personal appearance (e.g., comb, makeup, after-shave, perfume)
   c. Requests privacy by verbal or nonverbal questions
   d. Increases interaction with special friends and/or family
   e. Shows increased self-concept/self-esteem with increased emphasis on strengths rather than limitations

Family

INTRODUCTION

Family: A social group with culturally determined characteristics, which include economic cooperation, reproduction, and the rearing and socialization of children. It is an interacting and transacting group in relation to the larger society

1. **Discussion**
   a. The family is the conveyor of the beliefs, values, norms, and roles of society. The entire family participates in the socialization process of its members. A child must acquire an immense amount of traditional knowledge and skill and must learn to subject some natural inborn impulses to the discipline prescribed by society before being accepted as an adult member. One of the immutable facts about the family is that it is a primary building block of all societies
   b. Within the family, norms are found, usually modeled after those of the larger society, which prescribe role-appropriate behaviors for

family members—each member has a role. The family usually acts to support and protect its members, both collectively and individually. It is the primary support agency for its members

c. Like individuals, families attempt to maintain a steady state. Any perceived threat to the family's function or structure causes it to feel anxious and to close ranks

d. If one family member is in an ICU, other members attempt to assume the role-behavior of the absent member. If a family feels the threat of losing one of its members, it mobilizes to defend against the loss

e. A patient in an ICU may experience a biologic crisis, and at the same time his family may undergo a psychologic crisis. The provision of effective care for a patient necessarily involves extending care to available family members

2. **Example**

Mr. B. is a 36-year-old married man with three children: two boys, aged 9 and 12, and a 10-year-old girl. He is admitted to the ICU with renal and liver impairment secondary to cancer. During the first week of hospitalization, Mrs. B. is present nearly all day every day. She looks tired and behaves as if she were quite anxious. During the second week of hospitalization, Mrs. B. visits less frequently and has dark circles under her eyes. Her behavior appears increasingly agitated, except when with her husband: when talking to him and holding his hand, she seems to relax considerably. While talking to a nurse, Mrs. B. starts to cry and tremble, saying, "We try to carry on, but it's so hard. My oldest son tries to be his father for the other children, and when I am not home my daughter cooks. But it is so hard."

NURSING ASSESSMENT DATA BASE

Nursing History

1. Impact of medical diagnosis/prognosis on family interaction
2. When family visits, assess family interactions
3. Family members are available for support of patient
4. Identify the patient's role in family (i.e., brother, sister, mother, father, husband, wife, financial supporter, homemaker, son, or daughter)
5. Note significant others' description of the patient
6. Assess whether the medical condition is acute, chronic, temporary, or permanent
7. Review medication's impact on patient's sexual function or perceived sexual function

Nursing Examination of Patient

1. Assess role and status of patient in family
2. Observe the members relating to each other: warmly, with physical sharing of feelings, or reserved, with very little physical demonstration
3. Identify the modes of communication within the family: verbal or nonverbal (i.e., believe what I do, not what I say)
4. Determine who will fill role of hospitalized person within family
5. Identify what expectations the patient has of family members
6. Identify what expectations the family has of the patient
7. Determine the identified strengths within the family (i.e., good communication, strong loving/caring feelings, willingness to give to the other, decision making shared)
8. Identify family resources and needs

COMMONLY ENCOUNTERED NURSING DIAGNOSIS

Family Processes, Altered

1. **Assessment for defining characteristics**
   a. Family system unable to meet physical needs of its members
   b. Family system unable to meet emotional needs of its members
   c. Rigidity in function and roles
   d. Inability to express or accept feelings of members
   e. Inability of family members to relate to each other
   f. Family inability to adapt to change or to deal with traumatic experience constructively
2. **Expected outcomes**
   a. Demonstrates role congruence (acts age, cries when hurt, smiles when happy)
   b. Demonstrates clear communication
   c. Demonstrates constructive interaction
   d. Future oriented: talks about returning to previous family role
   e. Patient and family communicate with each other
   f. Patient involved in own care
   g. Expresses positive feelings about himself
3. **Nursing interventions**
   a. Support efforts to clarify the what, who, when, and where among the interactions of family
   b. Identify positive behaviors of family members
   c. Reinforce role and status of patient in family
   d. Support family with encouragement and clear, concise information; mobilize family support resources; maintain frequent contact with family

    e. Maintain and reinforce communication between family and patient and staff

    f. Clarify for family and patient what they should expect in the hospital

    g. Reinforce identified family and patient strengths

4. Evaluation of nursing care

    a. The patient sees himself as a viable part of the family

    b. The family and the patient communicate and support each other

    c. Compliance and actual participation of patient in own care increases

    d. Family able to express needs and concerns

    e. Patient able to express needs and concerns about self and family

    f. Decrease in projecting blame on staff and others for family member's problems and patient's lack of improvement

The Critical Care Environment

INTRODUCTION

Critical Care Environment: The sum of interactions among all persons, objects, and circumstances that affect the well-being of patients in an ICU. The ICU environment is strange and unknown to patients and their families, therefore it is stressful

1. Discussion

    a. Stressors within the critical care environment that have an impact on patients include machines, the noise level, spatial structures, persons' preconceived ideas, human interactions, thwarted needs and desires, and volumes of decisions. Interactions that occur within this environment are significant in that they regulate the amount of distress as well as the amount of support experienced by persons, in addition to the amount of control each has over the environment

    b. In order to deal with the ever-changing demands of the environment, those present use a variety of coping mechanisms to assist them with their struggles to feel adequate. If a patient's coping mechanisms fail to provide sufficient protection, the environment is usually perceived as overwhelming and dysfunctional behavior can result

    c. Dysfunctional behavior is commonly seen in the following ways

        i. Among patients: by demanding and acutely aggressive behavior, as well as by withdrawn behavior

        ii. Among family members: by repetition of questions or statements, putting blame on nurses, and making unrealistic demands on staff, as well as by withdrawn behavior

        iii. Among staff: by rashes of errors, avoiding patients, other staff members, or family members; increased feelings of competitiveness; and emotional lability "for no apparent reason"

2. **Example**

A 37-year-old man is admitted to the CCU with diagnosis of myocardial infarction. He has chest pain and shortness of breath. On the third day after admission, the patient appears apprehensive and restless, jumping at all noises and whenever he is touched. He continuously handles his monitor leads and is unable to sleep for more than 2 hours at a time. When an alarm goes off anywhere in the unit he becomes ashen, and he pushes the call button every couple of minutes. He repeatedly asks the nurses for reassurance that he will not die, and nothing the nurses do satisfies him. The nurses' reactions become characterized by irritation, as they grow weary of his demands for their time and attention. As the days wear on, the staff increasingly avoids the patient who becomes increasingly symptomatic

NURSING ASSESSMENT DATA BASE

Nursing History

1. Note history of being in critical care environment before
2. If "yes," what was the medical condition and how long was patient in critical care
3. Whether the patient is married, separated, or single and lives with spouse, family, or alone
4. Patient's occupation or previous work history
5. Patient's expected length of stay in critical care
6. Whether medical condition is life threatening, permanently dysfunctional, or has long-term limitations on function
7. Whether the patient's medical condition and its treatment influence physiologic parameters (volume overload or depletion, cardiovascular function, neurologic function, metabolic function) and could influence psychosocial function

Nursing Examination of Patient

1. Assessment is aimed at identifying, clarifying, and making known what the environment is all about
2. Assess the meaning to the patient of the machines, noise, lights, spatial structure, and interactions within this strange environment
3. Assess the preconceived ideas held by the patient and family members about the ICU
4. Assess impact of ICU on the patient and family. Use previously assessed concepts

5. Assess orientation to person, time, and place
6. Assess patient's perception of self (i.e., speaks of self in negative terms, not future oriented)

COMMONLY ENCOUNTERED NURSING DIAGNOSIS

Psychosocial Impact of the Critical Care Environment, Disturbance

1. **Assessment for defining characteristics**
   a. Increased tension, apprehension, fearfulness
   b. Increased alertness, aggressive behavior, or increased withdrawal
   c. Verbal expressions of having no control or influence over situation
   d. Verbal expressions of having no control over self-care
   e. Dysfunctional interaction with peers, family, and/or staff
   f. Increased blaming behavior
   g. Sleep pattern disturbance with jittery movements
2. **Expected outcomes**
   a. Less tense, more relaxed in bed
   b. Behavior more assertive rather than aggressive
   c. Verbally expresses feelings of being in control
   d. Involved in own care
   e. Periods of sleep and wakefulness within normal limits: at least 2 hours of uninterrupted sleep
3. **Nursing interventions**
   a. Clarification of information about ICU is essential, even if the patient is unable to respond. Each procedure should be explained to the patient and whenever possible to the family
   b. Clarify functions and purpose of machines and the significance of the noise and lights
   c. Correct and clarify perceptions of ICU: "not a place to die, but a special place to enhance life"
   d. Support, reinforce, and enhance positive factors identified earlier
   e. Involve family in patient's treatment/care
   f. Encourage questions and information sharing
   g. Provide familiar objects (locate nearby): bathrobe, pictures, watch
4. **Evaluation of nursing care**
   a. Decreases use of call light
   b. Demonstrates decreased anxiety with increased ability to rest and sleep
   c. Exhibits less anger or withdrawal
   d. More patient and family participation in care
   e. Demonstrates increased compliance
   f. More communication with family and self

Crisis

INTRODUCTION

Crisis: The state of feeling overwhelmed by stressors and struggling unsuccessfully to cope with the situation. It involves an attempt to regain equilibrium. Crisis is not all illness; it is an opportunity for growth

1. **Discussion**
   a. Like stress, crisis is a matter of perception. Events that trigger crisis in one person may not do so in another
   b. Crisis usually lasts from 4 to 6 weeks and is characteristically self-limiting. The reason for this is related to the fact that humans become depleted of energy after enduring significant distress over a prolonged period. They then begin to adapt to the crisis in order to recoup their energies
   c. There are two identified types of crisis commonly experienced
      i. Situational: derived from a particular set of circumstances that occasion major changes in a person's life (e.g., role change, illness, divorce, death)
      ii. Maturational: derived from difficulties in mastering developmental tasks associated with life stages (e.g., going to school, puberty, middle age, involutional changes)
   d. Crisis is part of normal growth and development
   e. Whether the crisis is experienced by critical care nurses, their patients, or the patients' families, four observable phases can be distinguished. Fink (1967) has identified these as follows
      i. Shock: one perceives a threat to existing familiar structures, views reality as overwhelming, and experiences anxiety, helplessness, and thought disorganization
      ii. Defensive retreat: one attempts to maintain one's usual structures; tries to avoid reality by wishful thinking, denial, or repression; and experiences indifference or euphoria, *except* when challenged. Challenge makes one angry and resistant to change, because one is defensively reorganizing one's thoughts
      iii. Acknowledgment: one gives up the existing, familiar structures; faces reality; and feels depressed. One may experience apathy, agitation, bitterness, mourning, high anxiety, or suicidal thoughts if the stressor is too overwhelming. The thought process is disorganized owing to a reorganization in light of altered perceptions of reality
      iv. Adaptation and change: one establishes a new structure, feels a renewed sense of self-worth, engages in new reality testing,

and experiences a gradual increase in satisfaction. The thought process is reorganized in light of present resources and abilities

f. The outcomes of crisis fall into three categories
   i. Some persons break down under the stress and never learn to cope with the traumatic change
   ii. Others experience the crisis and emerge from it about the same as they were before
   iii. Others learn about themselves and their ability to handle new situations and emerge feeling stronger and with increased self-esteem

g. Persons in crisis are more open than usual to help

NURSING ASSESSMENT DATA BASE

Nursing History

1. Note length of present illness
2. Diagnosis/prognosis of medical condition
3. History of person being in critical care before
4. Assess whether this is a situational or maturational crisis (i.e., is this a young teenager who is struggling with independence versus dependence or is this a 70-year old who has been diagnosed with a critical illness)
5. Note supports available: family, co-workers, friends

Nursing Examination of Patient

1. Identify what the patient perceives as stressful
2. Distinguish whether this crisis is situational, maturational, or a combination of both
3. Assess behavior: responses demonstrating reaction, whether verbal or nonverbal (crying, withdrawal, inappropriate laughter, denial, anger, fear, frequent use of call bell/light, constant need for attention)
4. Determine when crisis situation started, how long the patient has been in crisis, where the patient is in the crisis: shock, retreat, acknowledgment, or adaptation
5. Identify what kind of coping mechanisms were used in past crisis situations that helped the patient handle crisis
6. Evaluate what strengths this patient has and whether perceptions are realistic
7. Determine what sociocultural supports are available

COMMONLY ENCOUNTERED NURSING DIAGNOSIS

Crisis, Altered Response to Stress

1. **Assessment for defining characteristics**
   a. Inability to cope with stress situation
   b. Inappropriate use of defense mechanisms
   c. Increased tension, apprehension, withdrawal
   d. Extremes of emotional responses from euphoria to depths of depression
   e. Feels overwhelmed, anxious, and helpless as if in a state of shock
   f. Thought patterns disorganized
   g. Decision-making ability altered or inability to make any decision
   h. Focuses only on crisis situation: has tunnel vision in that only the perceived crisis is of concern

2. **Expected outcomes**
   a. Able to identify the crisis situation in realistic terms
   b. Learns about self and develops the ability to handle new situation
   c. Self-esteem increased
   d. Able to mobilize coping resources

3. **Nursing interventions**
   a. Assist patient in sharing ideas and feelings by asking questions and listening
   b. Share with patient in crisis your own perceptions of what is happening. Validate your perceptions with patient
   c. Help patient to identify and clarify problem; help correct distortions
   d. Help patient identify coping mechanisms. Give support while patient is trying these mechanisms
   e. Mobilize, as necessary, community resources
   f. Involve patient in performing constructive tasks that can be successfully completed. This will enhance self-concept/self-esteem and influence perceptions
   g. Assist patient in identifying alternative solutions. It is important to encourage patient to develop or decide which alternative approaches to use
   h. Reinforce strengths identified

4. **Evaluation of nursing care**
   a. Exhibits fewer crisis behaviors
   b. Expresses decrease in feeling overwhelmed
   c. Uses denial less often
   d. Increased ability to make decisions
   e. Increased self-concept/self-esteem
   f. Increased participation in own care
   g. Increased feelings of being in control

Fear/Anxiety

INTRODUCTION

Fear/Anxiety: Unpleasant feeling states, precipitated by perceived threats to the self and manifested by psychophysiologic symptoms

1. **Discussion**
   a. The psychophysiologic symptoms of fear and of anxiety are indistinguishable from each other. Commonly identified symptoms are increased heart rate, increased muscular tension, trembling, increased startle response, perspiration, sinking feeling in stomach, dry mouth and throat, feelings of faintness, nausea, fatigue, restlessness, appetite changes, insomnia or increased sleep, nightmares, speech pattern changes, and meaningless gestures. Each of these symptoms can be experienced as normal, everyday feelings at a low intensity level. Some are adaptive in nature, such as
      i. Increased heart rate and respiratory exchange, which results in increased oxygen and blood supply to muscles
      ii. Increased oxygen supply, which enhances mental alertness
   b. Adaptive functions enable the person to be in peak condition to respond more effectively to stress
   c. When the symptoms of fear and anxiety reach a certain level of intensity, they cease being adaptive and become maladaptive. When one perceives that one's symptoms are becoming harmful, one begins to channel energies toward achievement of a steady state. This process decreases the amount of energy available to cope with incoming stimuli, and increased anxiety and fear may result. One feels vulnerable and cannot experience oneself as safe
   d. Critical care nurses often encounter patients who are unable to sleep because of fear related to illness or to the unfamiliarity of their surroundings. The longer patients are unable to sleep, the greater the fear and anxiety become. When fear and anxiety increase, other symptoms are demonstrated (e.g., confusion, restlessness, irritability, and signs of aggression). Patients experience themselves as threatened and may behave in noncompliant ways. They may even hallucinate or speak from a delusional frame of reference
   e. When assessing patients who are experiencing high levels of fear and anxiety, the nurse will want to ascertain
      i. What they are experiencing, and what is the perceived threat
      ii. What in the environment can be modified to decrease the sense of threat
      iii. What support resources (from within patients as well as externally) are available to help decrease their fear and anxiety
      iv. What identified needs for help can be met by the nursing staff

NURSING ASSESSMENT DATA BASE

Nursing History

1. Identify diagnosis and prognosis of medical condition
2. Medical condition's impact on patient's ability to communicate
3. Note length of patient's illness
4. History of being in critical care before
5. Identify available support systems
6. Determine whether patient is able to speak the dominant language

Nursing Examination of Patient

1. Monitor vital signs (manifestations of fear and anxiety are increased heart rate, increased muscular tension, increased startle response, sinking feeling, etc.)
2. Assess behavior: look for increased crying, feelings of unrealness, irritability, aggressiveness, urge to run and hide, change in sleeping patterns, and nightmares
3. Explore what the patient is experiencing, what the perceived threat is
4. Determine what resources could be mobilized to decrease feelings of fear/anxiety
5. Evaluate what the patient's needs are
6. Determine what in the environment can be modified to decrease the sense of threat

COMMONLY ENCOUNTERED NURSING DIAGNOSIS

Fear/Anxiety

1. **Assessment for defining characteristics**
   a. Increased tension, apprehension
   b. Increased helplessness
   c. Decreased self-assurance, increased feelings of inadequacy
   d. Sympathetic stimulation: cardiovascular excitation, superficial vasoconstriction, pupil dilation
   e. Focus on perceived object of fear or unknown source of anxiety
2. **Expected outcomes**
   a. Demonstrates decreased level of anxiety as evidenced by decreased tension, apprehension, restlessness
   b. Ability to talk about fear/anxiety
   c. Demonstrates effective coping skills as evidenced by increased ability to problem solve and ability to meet self-care needs

    d. Verbalizes increased psychological comfort and coping skills

    e. Experiences a restful sleep

3. **Nursing interventions**

    a. Deal with distorted perception; provide information to reduce distortion

    b. Avoid surprises; tell patient what to expect

    c. Include patient in planning of care

    d. Maintain calm and safe environment; decrease stimuli; reassure patient

    e. Assist patient to identify those coping mechanisms that were successful in decreasing fear/anxiety

    f. Teach relaxation techniques

    g. Involve family or significant other in patient's care

4. **Evaluation of nursing care**

    a. Decrease in fear/anxiety-induced behavior

    b. Able to share fears and anxious feelings

    c. Increased feelings of being in control of self as ascertained from patient's words and actions

    d. More interaction with family and staff

Loneliness

INTRODUCTION

Loneliness: Uncomfortable feelings of alienation caused by separation from significant relationships, events, and objects—painful aloneness

1. **Discussion**

    a. Loneliness often accompanies major life changes in which some familiar structures are lost. Illness and hospitalization are prime precipitators of feelings of loneliness

    b. Everyone experiences loneliness at times, but for some it is a characteristic way of life

    c. When attempting to assist someone who is lonely, the goal is to facilitate the person's sense of relatedness to

        i. His body

        ii. His psyche

        iii. Significant others

        iv. Familiar events

        v. Yourself, the nurse

    d. This goal can be accomplished through interventions, such as

        i. Encouraging patients and family members to participate in their care, when appropriate, and to ask questions

ii. Initiating and facilitating discussion about patients' pain/surgery/illness, feelings about self/visitors/environment/cherished possessions, and other topics of importance to them

iii. Allowing patients to get to know you, insofar as it seems helpful in enabling them to relate to the caregivers on whom they are dependent

iv. Relating on a person-to-person basis that fosters personalized care

e. Promoting relationships, providing familiar activities, and permitting patients to have objects that hold positive meaning for them are the focus of intervention

f. It is important to remember, however, that the nurse can only be a facilitator when working with those who feel lonely. If, during your intervention, patients refuse to relate to others, or feel too angry or depressed to focus on familiar (usually comforting) activities, they must make their own choice as to what to do to help themselves feel more comfortable

g. Patients will make choices based on their self-concept, self-esteem, and need levels at the time. It is not helpful for the nurse to attempt to coerce them into feigning interest when they clearly are not interested: coercion makes them feel more alienated, and thus more lonely

NURSING ASSESSMENT DATA BASE

Nursing History

1. Identify major life events that have happened recently (i.e., job loss, divorce, illness)
2. Determine impact of patient's medical condition and/or treatment on his ability to respond to stimuli
3. Determine whether the patient's medical condition and/or treatment influences his ability to communicate (i.e., pain medication, tranquilizers)
4. Significant others' availability for support
5. Medical condition is disfiguring or perceived to be disfiguring
6. Identify influence of medical condition on future social, work, and/or family functions

Nursing Examination of Patient

1. Assess what major life changes have happened lately (hospitalization, divorce, death, etc.)
2. Assess perception of patient to hospitalization: what the individual perceives as being lost

3. Assess what resources patient has: strengths, coping mechanisms that helped in the past to deal with loneliness
4. Assess what family, friend, or community resources are available to fill needs

COMMONLY ENCOUNTERED NURSING DIAGNOSIS

Loneliness, Sense of Alienation

1. **Assessment for defining characteristics**
   a. Uncommunicative, withdrawn: no eye contact
   b. Seeks to be alone
   c. Expresses feelings of aloneness
   d. Absence of supportive significant other: family, friends, co-worker
   e. Sad, dull affect
   f. Observed use of unsuccessful social interaction behaviors
2. **Expected outcomes**
   a. Demonstrates a trusting relationship by expressing feelings of loneliness, distrust, and sense of self
   b. Initiates conversations and focuses on others rather than himself
   c. Involved in own care
   d. Asks questions about treatment
   e. Talks to significant others about himself in relation to family, work, and other social situations
   f. Expresses feelings of being in control
3. **Nursing interventions**
   a. Encourage patient and family members to participate in own care when appropriate
   b. Initiate and facilitate discussion about patient's pain/surgery/illness, feelings about self/visitors/environment/cherished possessions, and other topics of importance to patient
   c. Relate on a person-to-person basis that fosters personalized care
   d. Facilitate patient's sense of relatedness to his body, his psyche, significant others, familiar events or objects, and staff
   e. Encourage patient's involvement in own care and making decisions about own care
4. **Evaluation of nursing care**
   a. Talks about feelings, asks questions related to body responses to situation
   b. Family and patient are increasing communication and are more supportive and involved with treatments
   c. Expresses future orientation: whether it is 1 hour or 5 years in the future
   d. Increased sense of belonging with enhanced self-esteem

e. Involved in deciding time sequence of care (i.e., when medication is given, when visitors can come in)

Powerlessness

INTRODUCTION

Powerlessness: A perceived lack of control over the outcome of a specific situation

1. **Discussion**
    a. Powerlessness derives from the belief that, no matter how one behaves, one is unable to influence the outcome of a situation
    b. In the process of concluding that one is incapable of effecting a desired change, one attempts to solve problems in as many ways as one can. However, one consistently runs up against obstacles, and all efforts to bring about a desired outcome are ineffective
    c. As this process is repeated, one begins to feel frustrated, inadequate, hopeless, angry, and depressed
    d. In the critical care environment, all parties are capable of experiencing themselves as powerless: patients, family members, and staff
    e. In order to counteract the powerlessness phenomenon, one must believe that one is able to behave in ways that will make a difference in the resulting outcome
    f. In an effort to help those who feel powerless, a nurse might consider the following interventions
        i. Assist them to redefine goals that they are unable to accomplish, in the hope that they will consider shorter, more attainable goals
        ii. Assist them to identify ways in which they can be effective in given situations: help them to focus on ways in which they can be powerful, if they choose
        iii. Help them by giving information they need in order to be effective in given situations
        iv. Support them by attempting to understand their feelings of impotence when they express them
    g. It is helpful to remember that the nurse cannot take away another's feelings of powerlessness, since they grow out of a person's life situation, and one cannot change another person's life. However, patients themselves can work with inner strengths to discover new meaning in life and to solve problems by determining ways in which they can be effective in influencing desired changes

   h. A nurse can be helpful by displaying a caring presence, by actively listening, and by using empathy. The nurse can provide feedback in relation to knowledge gaps, strengths, or confusions that are expressed by patients and can let them know that their emotional pain is recognized

   i. It does no good to tell patients how to solve their problems; this only reinforces their view of themselves as inadequate and adds to their feelings of powerlessness

NURSING ASSESSMENT DATA BASE

Nursing History

1. Medical condition's influence on sense of independence and self-control
2. Medical treatment's influence on independence and self-control
3. Identify patient's strengths (i.e., whether the patient has a job, goes to school, is married, or single parent)
4. Assess patient's ability to speak the dominant language
5. History of illness or dependence on medication or medical equipment for control of illness
6. Availability of significant others for support

Nursing Examination of Patient

1. Assess the patient's perception of self in this situation (i.e., everything is so strange here, everyone takes care of me, they tell me what and when to take medicines)
2. Assessment of perception, self-concept/self-esteem, body image, and loneliness will provide clues to the patient's feelings of powerlessness
3. Observe nonverbal and verbal behavior for signs of depression, anger, hopelessness, and/or resignation
4. Assess communication ability, language, and influence of equipment/medication/condition on ability to communicate
5. Does patient verbalize or behave as if out of control (e.g., never questions treatment)
6. Patient withdrawn in bed, eyes closed or eyes darting around, body rigid

COMMONLY ENCOUNTERED NURSING DIAGNOSIS

Powerlessness

1. **Assessment for defining characteristics**
   a. Verbal expressions of having no control or influence over situation
   b. Verbal expressions of having no control over self-care

c. Verbal expressions of having no control or influence over outcome

d. Reluctance to express true feelings, fearing alienation from care-givers

e. Self-depreciating remarks

2. **Expected outcomes**

a. Verbalizes increased feelings of self-control

b. Involved in self-care

c. Future oriented

d. Makes appropriate decisions about own care

e. Verbalizes increased self-concept/self-esteem

3. **Nursing interventions**

a. A plan aimed at enhancing the patient can make a difference in outcomes

b. Assist the patient to redefine goals into obtainable size; stress "realistic goals"

c. Assist the patient to identify and use concrete ways to be effective in specific situations. This will enhance sense of being in control

d. Involve in own care within physical limitations

e. Take time to listen and hear what is said about feelings of power-lessness/being out of control

f. Identify and reinforce strengths. Encourage sharing of positives (i.e., successes the patient has had)

g. Be empathetic; put yourself in the patient's place. Acknowledge you hear his pain

h. Allow the patient to find a solution. Staff can be the guide by exploring alternatives, reinforcing strengths, and encouraging participation

4. **Evaluation of nursing care**

a. Makes decisions affecting himself

b. Is able to say "no"

c. Is more involved in own care within physical limitations

d. Makes requests for information to make decisions (e.g., "I need to know how this procedure will affect my ability to work")

e. Verbalizes positive feelings about self; self-concept/self-esteem increasing

Sensory Overload

INTRODUCTION

Sensory Overload: Repeated multisensory experiences that occur with greater intensity than is normally experienced by a person. Often, the excessive stimuli are experienced suddenly. Sometimes, they are not understood by the person but rather are perceived simply as bothersome, mean-ingless experiences. In general, excessive sensory stimuli are caused by an onslaught of unfamiliar, uncomfortable, unexpected stimulation

1. **Discussion**
   a. Sensory stimuli are stressors. Since ICUs are areas of excessive sensory stimuli for patients, family members, and staff, stress levels are excessively high. Patients frequently tend to act out high stress levels by creating a noisy environment, which perhaps relieves some of the tension for those creating the noise
   b. However, the increased noise level creates new stressors for all in the environment, adding to the sensory stimuli
   c. Along with auditory stimuli, the ICU hosts a myriad of visual, tactile, olfactory, and gustatory stimuli 24 hours a day, which are absorbed by those in the environment. Family members and staff are able to change the types and patterns of stimuli to which they are exposed by routinely leaving the critical care area. Patients, of course, are continually subjected to high levels of stimulation for as long as they are housed on the unit. *All* who encounter this environ-ment are prone to experience sensory overload
   d. Some common symptoms of sensory overload include confusion, restlessness to the point of agitation, anger, and sometimes halluci-nations
   e. In attempting to prevent or minimize sensory overload, the nurse could
      i. Assess the noise level on the unit, particularly at the bedside of patients, since it is here that many noise-producing mechan-ical devices are located (e.g., the bellows of ventilators and the alarm mechanism of cardiac monitors)
      ii. Assess the visual intensity generated by the unit lighting
      iii. Assess the environment for malodorous stimuli
      iv. Assess each patient's level and type of gustatory stimuli
      v. Assess how staff and family members touch individual patients and the amount of pain experienced by each patient
      vi. Implement modifications that seem appropriate regarding
         (a) Noise levels—attending particularly to the intensity of conversational tones used by staff members, the position-ing of noisy machinery in relation to the head of each patient; and loud, banging noises caused by dropped equip-ment, bedpan hoppers in need of repair, mishandled food trays, and messengers delivering supplies
         (b) Visual intensity—monitoring the light intensity on the unit to ensure that the environment is as safe and com-fortable as possible and attempting to simulate natural light cycles from morning to night

    (c) Environmental odors—using air deodorizers and disposing of malodorous substances appropriately

    (d) Gustatory stimuli—assisting patients with mouth care when needed and offering palatable fluids and foods as appropriate

    (e) Tactile communication—each time the nurse makes physical contact with patients the nurse should be aware of the message one may convey through touching. This can be accomplished by appropriate gentleness as a nurse turns patients, changes dressings, administers injections, gives baths and back rubs, and provides hair care. When a nurse becomes aware of the amount of invasive tactile stimulation experienced by patients, the method of evaluating their need for pain medication may change. Administering pain medication effectively greatly helps to decrease tactile overload

NURSING ASSESSMENT DATA BASE

Nursing History

1. Medical diagnosis/prognosis has influence on sensory organs: eyes, ears, touch, taste
2. History of being in critical care before
3. Medications' influence on perception of sensory stimuli
4. Availability of significant others: spouse, parents, friends, co-workers

Nursing Examination of Patient

1. Assess indicators of sensory overload such as
   a. Confusion
   b. Restlessness
   c. Agitation
   d. Anger
   e. Hallucinations, delusions
   f. Increased startle response
   g. No response at all/withdrawn
2. Appraise the noise/light level of unit, specifically at bedside
3. Assess the environment for malodorous stimuli
4. Evaluate patient's level and type of gustatory stimuli
5. Observe how staff and family touch the patient. Assess what comes in contact with patient (e.g., bed clothes, intravenous and central lines, hoses, leads from monitor)

6. Evaluate pain routinely and frequently
7. Assess sleep pattern, amount of time awake/asleep, and pattern of awake/sleep cycle

COMMONLY ENCOUNTERED NURSING DIAGNOSIS

Sensory Overload

1. **Assessment for defining characteristics**
   a. Confusion/disoriented in time, place, and person
   b. Restlessness to point of agitation
   c. Anger, irritability
   d. Possibly hallucinations
   e. Anxiety/fear
   f. Mood swings
   g. Poor concentration
2. **Expected outcomes**
   a. Oriented to person, time, place
   b. Decreased anxiety/fear
   c. Mood swings decreased/more stable mood
   d. Concentration increases
   e. Sleep/awake cycle improved
   f. More relaxed
3. **Nursing interventions**
   a. Assist the patient to screen out unrelated stimuli
      i. Dim hall or outside room lights and patient's room lights
      ii. Avoid banging equipment
      iii. Turn monitor alarms as low as possible
      iv. Provide soft music, if possible
      v. Provide pictures of quiet scenes
      vi. When giving information, do so slowly, quietly, clearly, and unhurriedly
      vii. Explain what noise and lights on machines mean
      viii. Get rid of odors
   b. Use gentle touch, backrubs, etc.
   c. Control pain by positioning, turning, and medication
4. **Evaluation of nursing care**
   a. Decreased confusion
   b. Decreased restlessness
   c. Decreased agitation
   d. Decreased anger
   e. Body more relaxed
   f. Decreased complaints of discomfort or pain
   g. Increased appropriate interactions

Sensory Deprivation

INTRODUCTION

Sensory Deprivation: The opposite of sensory overload—it denotes a lack of sensory input or a lack of variety, intensity, or perceived meaning of sensory stimulation

1. **Discussion**
   a. Since most critical care patients are immobile, they are generally confined to a limited space in a machine-oriented, totally unfamiliar environment. They often experience consciousness-altering drugs that numb sensory receptors. Sometimes the nature of their illness reduces sensitivity to stimuli. At other times, technical assists are so complex as to require much time and attention from caregivers, perhaps more than are focused on the patient. All these factors predispose critical care patients to sensory deprivation
   b. The goal of nursing interventions aimed toward preventing or eliminating sensory deprivation is to provide sensory stimuli that patients can experience and find meaningful, in order to facilitate their relatedness to themselves and the unfamiliar world in which they find themselves
   c. Communicating through meaningful touch and conversation is one way in which a nurse can assist patients to increase their ability to relate, thereby decreasing sensory deprivation. Encouraging family members to provide familiar personal items when possible is also helpful, as is the presence of loved ones
   d. Usual symptoms of sensory deprivation can mimic symptoms of sensory overload, including lethargy
   e. To distinguish between sensory hunger and sensory overload, the nurse must carefully assess the types and amounts of sensory stimuli experienced by individual patients and make judgments based on the data collected
   f. In general, sensory alterations are caused by a variety of factors found within the ICU. Some common factors include
      i. Abnormal physiologic conditions
      ii. Ingestion of drugs
      iii. Prolonged experience of pain
      iv. Lack of familiar persons and objects
      v. Fear
      vi. Lack of understanding about one's condition
      vii. Sleep deprivation caused by interrupted sleep cycles that deny a person opportunity to adequately restore depleted energy supplies

g. Effective nursing interventions involving sensory deprivation and overload are crucial for the protection of patients' compromised health states

NURSING ASSESSMENT DATA BASE

Nursing History

1. Whether patient's condition requires isolation
2. Whether sense organs are influenced by medication
3. History of being in critical care unit in past
4. Past hospitalizations
5. Patient's marital status, age, education
6. Work history: computer operator, laborer, machinist, lawyer, housewife, student
7. Availability of significant others
8. Interaction between patient and significant others

Nursing Examination of Patient

1. Assessment can be carried out simultaneously with sensory overload assessment
2. In addition, assess whether medications being given can disturb sensory receptors
3. Evaluate physiologic impact of condition on sensory receptors (e.g., tumors that cause blindness, deafness, or paralysis)
4. Monitor laboratory studies, such as blood gas analysis that could impact on sensory receptors
5. Assess time spent with the patient, whether there are interactions, and quality of interactions
6. Observe sleep pattern changes
7. Evaluate possibility of developing a routine (i.e., regular times for treatments and regular time for rest)

COMMONLY ENCOUNTERED NURSING DIAGNOSIS

Sensory Deprivation

1. Assessment for defining characteristics
   a. Disoriented to person, place, and time
   b. Changes in behavior pattern
   c. Daydreaming
   d. Noncompliance
   e. Lethargy/withdrawal

f. Decreased concentration

g. Difficulty interacting with staff and significant others

2. **Expected outcomes**

a. Increased compliance with treatments

b. Able to verbalize concerns and questions

c. More assertive

d. Sleep/awake pattern more normal

e. Able to relax/less agitated

f. Oriented to person, time, and place

g. Reality oriented

3. **Nursing interventions**

a. Plan is aimed at preventing or eliminating sensory deprivation: to provide sensory stimuli that can be experienced fully by the patient

b. Increase communication. Use touch or any other method (writing, sign language, pictures)

c. Have family bring personal items of special meaning to patient such as family pictures, letters

d. Use music or tape of family members' voices. Have family tape messages or favorite music for person to play

e. Frequent verbal interaction by primary caregiver to enhance rapport-building. This will give predictability to environment

4. **Evaluation of nursing care**

a. Exhibits decreased agitation and more compliance with treatment

b. Increases involvement in own needs and treatment

c. Increases interactions with staff and/or family

d. Demonstrates fewer extremes in emotions such as anger, crying, and sadness

Addiction

INTRODUCTION

Addiction: Dependence on a chemical substance outside the self that is perceived by the person as being necessary for self-maintenance and for the self to feel complete (i.e., adequate)

1. **Discussion**

a. The addiction phenomenon is a maladaptive effort to help the self feel adequate. The process is considered maladaptive because the end result involves the person in spending time and energy numbing the self, so that spontaneous growth-producing doubts, fears, and stressors are not experienced or dealt with constructively. Growth does not take place, and the person stagnates

b. When a nurse encounters addicts in the ICU it is important to remember the following
   i. If patients are still under the influence of the addictive substance, their perceptions of reality will be altered
   ii. Patients' self-concept and self-esteem will be threatened because they do not have access to that which they believe will make them complete; they probably feel incomplete and desperate for the substance
   iii. There is usually some concern on the part of addicts regarding how others will view them, so that self-concept and self-esteem are again threatened
   iv. While withdrawing from the substance, patients will be acutely reactive to physical and emotional stimuli
c. In attempting to deal effectively with addicts, the nurse should remember that they may feel threatened. Their behavior, therefore, may reflect a strong need to defend themselves by keeping persons at a comfortable distance
d. Distancing maneuvers include withdrawal behavior as well as those actions that tend to push others away by evoking feelings of anger, frustration, repulsion, or fear
e. The nurse will not want to make addicted patients feel even more threatened (which would occasion further acting-out behavior) and so might consider the following
   i. Attempting to understand their suffering and concerns
   ii. Communicating in a straightforward manner (e.g., if patients' behavior is disruptive to the nurse or to the unit, telling them so and requesting that they behave in a specifically different manner)
   iii. Assisting patients to feel secure on the unit by providing simple, clear explanations regarding what is happening to them
   iv. Avoiding power struggles and arguments by approaching conflicts from the perspective of understanding patients' feelings about the issues and making clear statements about how the nurse views the situation
f. In general, communicating that the nurse cares about addicted patients and wants to be of help during this difficult time is an important factor in establishing a helping relationship. At times, attempts to help will include insisting that patients do things they may not want to do

NURSING ASSESSMENT DATA BASE

Nursing History

1. Identify substance patient is addicted to

2. Length of time addicted to substance
3. History of being treated for addiction in past
4. Time the last dose (hit) of substance taken
5. Patient's normal withdrawal behavior (i.e., agitated, combative, withdrawn, physiologic problems)
6. Availability of significant others

Nursing Examination of Patient

1. Determine what substance the patient is addicted to and how much is required to satisfy addiction
2. Evaluate the effect of substance on perceptions and how it makes the patient feel
3. Determine the last time the substance was taken. What happens to patient when he stops taking this substance? (Patient or family can probably give this information)
4. Evaluate whether behavioral responses are part of withdrawal
5. Observe staff's reaction to addicted patient
6. Assess what resources are available for short- and long-term help with addiction

COMMONLY ENCOUNTERED NURSING DIAGNOSIS

Addiction

1. **Assessment for defining characteristics**
   a. Perceptions of reality are altered
   b. Self-concept/self-esteem may be threatened because patient is unable to obtain addictive substance
   c. There is a craving for addictive substance
   d. Physically nervous, anxious, shaky, tremors, sweating
   e. Altered physical and psychologic response to stimuli (i.e., hyperreaction or hyporeaction)
   f. Unable to sleep or unable to stay awake, restlessness
2. **Expected outcomes**
   a. Patient oriented to person, time, and place
   b. Self-concept/self-esteem less threatened
   c. Reactions are more stable
   d. Patient verbalizes less craving for substance
   e. Verbalizes feelings about himself and addictive problem
   f. Begin verbalizing need to get help for addiction problem
3. **Nursing interventions**
   a. Do not be judgmental. Addicts are very sensitive to others' acceptance and/or judgment

    b. Decrease as much as possible physical and emotional stimuli during withdrawal. (Addicts are very sensitive to stimuli during this period)

    c. Communicate in a straightforward manner without judgmental statements

    d. Avoid power struggles and arguments by approaching conflicts from the perspective of understanding the patient's feelings and making clear staff's own views of situation

    e. Mobilize resources for short- and long-term help for the addict

    f. Take care of physiologic needs; during withdrawal keep close watch on vital signs and other parameters

4. Evaluation of nursing care

    a. Physical signs of withdrawal decreasing (e.g., pupils not dilated or pinpoint, decreasing sweating and/or muscle tension)

    b. Less anger and hostility expressed

    c. Increased ability to express needs without self-depreciation

    d. Some increase in self-esteem/self-concept

    e. Increase in treatment participation

    f. Seeking help with addiction (community resources being used)

Suicidal Phenomenon

INTRODUCTION

Suicidal Phenomenon: Suicide is an active or passive self-destructive act that results from a perceived, overwhelming threat to oneself

1. Discussion

    a. Everyone at one time or another has suicidal thoughts. These can be as casual as a morning wish to cancel the day owing to lack of interest, which one generally would not act on because less drastic coping mechanisms can effectively handle the situation

    b. Every case of self-destructive behavior involves the pressure of a phenomenologically unbearable threat to oneself. Other less drastic and less destructive coping mechanisms no longer are experienced as effective in handling the perceived overwhelming threat. Suicide, therefore, is the ultimate attempt to deal with this threat, is considered, and sometimes is acted on. In a sense, suicidal behavior is seen as an escape from, rather than a movement toward, something

    c. A suicidal person experiences many emotions (e.g., despair, guilt, shame, dependency, hopelessness, weariness, boredom, depression). There is a point at which despair becomes overwhelming and unbearable. For some, there is a sense that life is just not worth living anymore—it no longer has meaning. Others feel that someone does not want them around or that their individual problems can never be resolved

d. In providing nursing services to patients who have attempted suicide, nurses should be aware of the following common characteristics of the suicidal phenomenon

    i. The acute crisis period or high lethality time is of short duration: it can be counted in hours or days

    ii. Suicidal patients are usually ambivalent about dying. At the same time at which they plan suicide, they have fantasies of rescue

    iii. Persons who talk about it commit suicide, as well as those who do not talk about it

    iv. Suicidal persons usually give clues about their intentions

    v. Suicidal behavior has no racial, social, religious, cultural, or economic boundaries

    vi. Suicide has no characteristic genetic qualities; however, its incidence is greater in families in which there have been previous suicides

    vii. Suicidal behavior does not necessarily mean that the person is mentally ill; in some cases, suicide is viewed as a logical last step by one who is overwhelmed with stress

    viii. Most important, directly asking a person about suicidal intent will *not* cause suicide

e. In addition to *knowing* about suicide, one must also be aware of one's own feelings about it. Dealing with suicidal persons can raise fears and reactions within caregivers (e.g., anger, anxiety about one's own suicidal thoughts, dislike/resentment toward those who have attempted suicide, a wish to avoid the suicidal person in favor of other patients whose conditions do not appear to be self-inflicted, and doubts about one's ability to care for them). It is easier to care for suicidal patients if one is able to understand why they attempted suicide

NURSING ASSESSMENT DATA BASE

Nursing History

1. History of previous suicide attempts
2. Degree of threat to life by suicide attempts
3. Methods used to attempt suicide: gun, pills, gas, car accident, starving, burning self
4. History of significant other's successful completion of suicide (i.e., brother, sister, mother, father, best friend)
5. Assess presence of other medical conditions such as AIDS, cancer, disfigurements

Nursing Examination of Patient

1. Assessment is aimed at gathering information that will identify why suicide attempt, what was used, where attempt was made, and what is the psychological condition at the present moment
2. Determine what major life changes have happened recently. (This is what the patient perceives as a major change, such as job loss, loss of status, divorce, death, etc.)
3. Identify strengths such as good health, hard worker, caring person, good work history, community involvement, etc.
4. Assess where suicide attempt was made: in a public place or in privacy. This will give clue to seriousness of the attempt
5. Specify what was used (e.g., 10 aspirin, 40 Valium, knife, gun, or rope). This will give clue as to lethality
6. Identify what close friend and/or family member is available
7. Estimate what resources are available for help
8. Evaluate the emotional state at present: tearful, angry, despondent, sad, depressed, euphoric, or withdrawn

COMMONLY ENCOUNTERED NURSING DIAGNOSIS

Suicidal Behavior

1. **Defining characteristics**
   a. Cognitive or emotional difficulties
   b. See common characteristics of suicidal phenomenon (pp. 891)
2. **Expected outcomes**
   a. Verbalizes need for help
   b. No additional attempts of suicide
   c. Verbalizes positive feelings about oneself
   d. Able to communicate with significant others
   e. Verbalizes desire to recover
   f. Future oriented
3. **Nursing interventions**
   a. Accept the suicidal behavior as logical from the patient's point of view. Do not pass judgment
   b. Reinforce patient's self-esteem by interacting in such a manner as to accord dignity
   c. Use all communication modes (verbal and nonverbal) in an attempt to understand how the patient perceives world and self
   d. Reinforce positive aspects (strengths) of patient's self-concept
   e. Do not place or leave dangerous objects near bedside (e.g., medication, razors)

f. Assist patient to reestablish supportive relationships with those whom he chooses

g. Support significant others so they can support the patient

h. Avoid power struggles with the person when there is noncompliance or belligerent behavior

i. Be aware of and deal with your own fears, feelings, and conflicts related to suicide

4. **Evaluation of nursing care**

a. Communicates needs and concerns

b. Makes no further suicide attempts

c. Cooperates with treatment

d. Communicates with significant others

e. Asks for help from mental health resources or other suicide resources

f. Future oriented in discussions

g. Verbalizations are congruent with nonverbal behavior

The Dying Process and Death

INTRODUCTION

Dying Process and Death: Dying is a psychophysiologic process that evokes many stresses and crises and that ultimately terminates in death for the dying and in suffering for significant survivors; death is the antithesis of life

1. **Discussion**

a. Death is not amenable to change or intervention. It incorporates the greatest loss

b. The dying process is part of the life cycle. When one is conscious of this process, the threat of death unleashes the primordial feelings of hopelessness, helplessness, and abandonment. The fear of the unknown in death evokes fears of the unknown, of annihilation of self, of being, and of identity

c. The dying process imposes a two-fold burden

   i. Intrapsychic stress: preparing oneself for death

   ii. Interpersonal stress: preparing oneself for death in relation to significant others, while simultaneously preparing those others to be survivors

d. This two-fold task evokes a pervasive state of grief about the impending death and anger about one's impotence. The anger can be directed toward God, loved ones, or caregivers. In addition, dying persons may experience anxiety related to fear of pain, loss of identity, loneliness and abandonment, powerlessness, fear of the unknown, and fear of annihilation

e. Elisabeth Kubler-Ross (1969) has described five psychologic stages of the dying process

   i. Denial or isolation: "no, not me"

   ii. Anger, rage, envy, resentment: "why me?"

   iii. Bargaining: "if you will . . . then I will"

   iv. Depression: "what's the use?"

   v. Acceptance: the final resting stage before the long journey

f. Some who are inexperienced in working with the dying may expect patients to follow the exact sequence described above. In reality, the dying process may include all the stages (although some never get beyond the denial stage), but the stages shift, depending on what the person experiences. A person may fluctuate from depression to anger or may revert to the denial stage once again

g. Providing care for the dying may evoke strong emotions in caregivers: anger, frustration, or dislike. These reactions may result in a desire to avoid dying patients or their families. Likewise, being with a dying loved one may evoke strong emotions in family members and may cause them to be less and less available as the process continues. The dying process predisposes persons to a sense of abandonment

h. Because psychologic states are complicated clusters of intellectual and affective factors that occur in the context of persons' perception of their world and of themselves in the world, it is important to remember two principles: denial and hope

   i. *Denial can be an important coping mechanism for enabling persons to maintain some control over the most threatening of situations.* Denial can make it possible for them to block out information with which they cannot successfully cope and to begin to deal with reality in smaller, more manageable segments

      (a) Because denial operates protectively in persons on the verge of crises, it is important for the nurse to respond to dying patients by

         (1) Listening to find out their perception of their situation

         (2) Showing acceptance whenever they are found to be in the dying process

         (3) Not encouraging false beliefs

         (4) Attempting to understand why they are behaving as they are

      (b) Examples

         (1) A man who suffered a life-threatening myocardial infarction 2 days ago says: "I think I'm well enough to go home now." The nurse responds: "I'm trying to

appreciate how badly you want to go home, but it wouldn't be beneficial for you now because of your illness"

    (2) A 64-year-old, recently retired woman has been diagnosed as having cancer and told that she will probably live another 6 months. She tells a nurse that she plans to buy a new Mercedes, "even though it will probably take me three years to pay for it." The nurse responds: "I can hear how much you want to own that car. I hope you will be able to do it"

  ii. *Hope is usually present throughout the dying process in some degree.* Hope, a belief in the desirability of survival, is usually found in persons demonstrating a healthy self-concept and self-esteem but can be lost when persons are unable to act on their own behalf and must submit to the influence of others

    (a) To a large extent, denial and hope are necessary for a person to experience the dying process with some control. Denial provides a sorely needed locus of control over the primordial feelings unleashed during that process. Hope is the core of strength needed to withstand the pain, suffering, fears, and conflicts encountered throughout the process

i. In order to provide quality care to dying patients, it is helpful for nurses to be aware of the following

  i. Through caring for the dying, the nurse is often made aware of the dying process. All the fears, feelings, and conflicts demonstrated in dying patients are also evoked in the nurse, which in turn evokes the nurse's coping mechanisms. It is essential that nurses be aware of and accept their own fears about dying

  ii. Like all other kinds of nursing assessments, the assessment of dying patients is aimed at achieving an understanding of the needs of the patient and of family members. This can be accomplished by ascertaining the following

    (a) Perception of their situation and the feelings being expressed

    (b) Family perception of situation and the feelings being expressed

    (c) The strengths and supports used by the patient and family to help them cope with the stress

    (d) Needs the patient wishes to have met, and the most appropriate persons to meet those needs

    (e) Whether body image and sexual identity are significantly affected; whether intervention can be designed to reaffirm these identities

    (f) Whether loneliness and powerlessness are causing the

dying process to be more painful than is necessary; whether these factors can be altered through interventions

   j. The goal of intervention is to respond effectively to the patient's identified needs for help. Because dying is an individual experience, the nurse will want to respond to the needs identified at a given point in time. The following are suggested interventions for the stages identified by Kubler-Ross

      i. During the denial stage

        (a) Attempt to have someone stay with dying patient for a time

        (b) Take cues for conversation from the patient

        (c) Listen (one need not attempt to provide solutions to the questions raised, unless specifically requested to do so)

        (d) Respond to patients by sharing your reactions when you think it might be helpful to them or their families

        (e) Provide opportunities for continued communication

      ii. During the anger stage

        (a) Allow patients to express their feelings to you and to ask: "Why me?"

        (b) Remember that you need not attempt to answer that unanswerable question

        (c) Try to remember that the anger patients are expressing is not directed at you personally but rather toward that which you represent (continued life) and toward their own painful situation

     iii. During the bargaining stage

        (a) Find out what kind of help patients need to complete their unfinished business

        (b) Try to make time just to be with dying persons and to listen

     iv. During the depression stage, patients mourn all that they are losing. One can help by

        (a) Not interrupting the grieving process

        (b) Supporting patients in their grief

        (c) Sharing your feelings of sadness appropriately, if you feel sad

     v. During the acceptance stage, the issue of letting go of dying persons arises. One can be helpful by

        (a) Not deserting them

        (b) Respecting their acceptance of death

        (c) Assisting the family with their letting go of someone whom they love by listening and by intervening in areas in which the family feels that it needs help

  k. Providing comfort measures for dying patients is reported to be a most important nursing intervention, for the sake of both the patient and the family. Effective verbal and nonverbal communication is essential to evaluate the need for the following

    i. Adequate medication for control of pain

    ii. Frequent mouth care

    iii. Positioning for comfort

    iv. Allowing family members to visit more frequently when the patient desires closer contact with loved ones

    v. Supporting the family's involvement in providing comfort measures for the dying person

l. Providing nursing care for dying patients can be one of the most rewarding experiences, if critical care nurses are knowledgeable about and prepared to confront the dying process themselves. Knowing that one may experience the ups and downs of the grieving cycle along with a few dying patients helps to diminish the fear of getting involved. Recognizing personal strengths and limitations helps to prevent burnout. Realizing that one will ultimately learn more about life and about oneself while working with dying patients helps one to take advantage of opportunities for growth

NURSING ASSESSMENT DATA BASE

Nursing History

1. Length of time diagnosed with terminal illness
2. Whether physician has discussed diagnosis and prognosis with patient
3. Whether physician has discussed diagnosis and prognosis with significant others
4. The medical plan of care: curative oriented, pain control, return home to die, to hospice
5. Supports available to patient and significant others
6. Financial consideration that would require other resources be brought into situation (social work)

Nursing Examination of Patient

1. Assessment is aimed at achieving and understanding the needs of the individual and of family members so that the dying process can be influenced in a positive manner
2. Using Kubler-Ross' stages, determine where the patient is in the dying process. Remember, these are only guidelines to help understand behavior
3. Assess how the person perceives the situation: what feelings are being expressed
4. Evaluate how the family or significant others perceive the situation: what feelings are they expressing

5. Identify what strengths and supports the patient and family are using to help cope
6. Appraise what needs the patient and family want met: who can meet these needs (chaplain, mental health worker, etc.)
7. Determine if body image/sexuality is significantly affected
8. Evaluate whether loneliness and powerlessness are causing the dying process to be more painful
9. Assess what comfort measures can be used: pain control, positioning, warmth and caring, community resources
10. Assess where the caregiver is in coping with concerns and fears of own death

COMMONLY ENCOUNTERED NURSING DIAGNOSIS

Dying Process and Death

1. **Defining characteristics**
   a. Medically diagnosed with terminal illness
   b. Verbal expression of distress at loss
   c. Denial of loss
   d. Anger, sorrow, crying
   e. Alterations in sleep patterns
   f. Alterations in eating habits
   g. Alterations in dream patterns
   h. Labile affect
   i. Interference with life functions
2. **Expected outcomes**
   a. The dying process is positively influenced
   b. Pain controlled
   c. Patient able to share fears and concerns
   d. Patient able to communicate with significant others
   e. Needed and available resources initiated for support of family
   f. Significant others are able to find support with staff or clergy or other resources
3. **Nursing interventions**
   a. Goal is to respond effectively to the patient's and family's needs
   b. Following are suggested interventions based on Kubler-Ross' stages (pp. 896)
   c. Continue to show respect for and maintain dignity of the patient. Provide good personal hygiene (shaves, hair done, clean clothes)
   d. Involve all available resources in assisting the patient and family. Encourage communication and allow person to make decisions
   e. Maintain good pain control with regularly ordered pain medication

rather than as needed. Use frequent mouth care, positioning, and more frequent family visits. Support the family so family can support their loved one

f. Nursing staff needs to realize where they are in terms of coping with death themselves and that they can experience the ups and downs of the grieving cycle. Also they should recognize their strengths, share concerns and feelings with co-workers

4. **Evaluation of nursing care**

   a. Evaluation is not based on whether the disease or disorder was cured but rather that the dying process was positively influenced
   b. Was the patient able to share fears and concerns
   c. Was pain under control? Was the patient comfortable
   d. Was communication between patient/family accomplished
   e. Were resources initiated to support the family during the dying process and after death
   f. Were the staff able to share their feelings among themselves

The Nurse's Coping With Critical Care

Since nurses who work in critical care environments are exposed to the same environmental stressors as are patients and family members, one can expect similar emotional reactions to occur in staff over a prolonged period. Nurses are subject to additional stresses: responsibility for knowing how to respond appropriately to patients' medical and emotional crises and desiring to be viewed by peers as competent practitioners. The nurse's position in the administrative structure is sometimes a source of further distress. All of this can lead to exhaustion if the nurse is not able to develop effective ways to deal with the distress.

It is helpful for nurses to remember that they are effective in the work setting to the degree that their own needs are met and in accordance with the level of self-esteem experienced at a given moment.

To help promote self-esteem and to provide mechanisms for discharging distress, nurses may find it useful to

1. Identify their reasons for choosing the critical care setting for practice
2. Identify their strengths as critical care nurses
3. Identify their own individual professional potentials (goals)
4. Identify their limitations as critical care nurses
5. Routinely identify the effect critical care nursing is perceived to have on them individually
6. Develop peer relationships that allow them to feel safe enough to be comfortable in the critical care setting
7. Develop peer relationships that promote open communication (exchang-

ing ideas, complaining, sharing difficult and positive experiences, resolving conflicts)
8. Use formal and informal multidisciplinary clinical care conferences
9. Use staff groups facilitated by a mental health resource person
10. Devise work plans that allow for sharing responsibilities as needed
11. Use break and meal times to replenish energy levels constructively
12. Use moments alone when feeling overwhelmed by excessive stimuli
13. Develop a relationship with supervisors that promotes open communication
14. Use supports available outside the critical care unit (e.g., clinical nurse experts, in-service personnel, staff clergy)
15. Routinely schedule participation in continuing education events
16. Develop sources of support and areas of enrichment outside their professional lives

It is suggested that nurses use the critical care environment in such a way that an area be established for staff use only, out of view of patients and family members.

Satir (1972) relates a story from her childhood that seems appropriate for critical care nurses. When she was growing up on a farm, the family water supply was located outside in the yard. Every time the water bucket was empty, someone had to go to the well to refill it. So, too, nurses working in high stress areas must go out and "refill" themselves when they feel empty and unable to give anymore. We hope you may always be "refilled!"

References

Allen, M.L., Jackson, D., and Younger, S.: Closing the communication gap between physicians and nurses in the intensive care unit setting. Heart Lung 9:836–840, 1980.

Ashworth, P.: Technology and machines—bad masters but good servants. Intens. Care Nurse 3:19–27, 1987.

Aquilera, D.C., and Messick, J.: Crisis Intervention: Theory and Methodology. C.V. Mosby Co., St. Louis, 1980.

Ballard, K.S.: Identification of environmental stressors for patients in a surgical intensive care unit. Issues Ment. Health Nurs. Jan–Jun:89–108, 1981.

Bandman, E.L.: The dilemma of life and death: Should we let them die? Nurs. Forum 17:118–132, 1978.

Barrie-Shevlin, P.: Maintaining sensory balance for the critically ill patient. Nursing 4:597–601, 1987.

Bechervaise, M.D.: The riddle of communication: I. Nurs. Times 75:1434–1436, 1979.

Benson, H.: The relaxation response. Psychiatry 37:37–46, 1974.

Berni, R., and Fordyce, W.E.: Behavior Modification and the Nursing Process. C.V. Mosby Co., St. Louis, 1973.

Bibbings, J.: The stress of working in intensive care: A look at the research. Nursing 3:567–570, 1987.

Billie, D.A.: The role of body image in patient compliance and education. Heart Lung 6:143–148, 1977.

Bozett, F.W., and Gibbons, R.: The nursing management of families in the critical care setting. Crit. Care Update 2:22–27, 1983.

Brissett, D.: Toward a clarification of self-esteem. Psychiatry 35:255–263, 1972.

Bugental, J.: The listening eye. J. Hum. Psychol. 16:55–65, 1976.

Caldwell, T., and Weiner, M.F.: Stresses and coping in ICU nursing. Gen. Hosp. Psychiatry 6:119–127, 1981.

Calhoun, G., and Perrin, M.: Management, motivation and conflict. Top. Clin. Nurs. 1:71–80, 1979.

Carnevale, F.A., Annibale, F., Grenier, A., Guy, E., and Ottoni, L.: Nursing in the I.C.U.: Stress without distress? Can. Crit. Care Nurs. J. Mar–Apr:16–18, 1987.

Cassem, N.H.: Treating the person confronting death. In Nicholi, A.M. (ed.): The Harvard Guide to Modern Psychiatry. Harvard University Press, Cambridge, Mass., 1978.

Chapman, R.C.: Role of anxiety in acute pain. Pain Overview, pp. 6–13, 1980.

Clifford, C.: Patients, relatives and nurses in a technological environment. Intens. Care Nurse 2:67–72, 1986.

Cohe, C., Levin, E., Whitly, J., et al.: Brief sexual counseling during cardiac rehabilitation. Heart Lung 8:124–129, 1979.

Collins, V.J.: Ethical considerations in therapy for the comatose and dying patient. Heart Lung 8:1084–1088, 1979.

Cooley, G.H.: The Social Self. In Farrell, R., and Swigert, V. (eds.): Social Deviance. J.B. Lippincott Co., Philadelphia, 1975.

Coombs, A., Richards, A.C., and Richards, F.: Perceptual Psychology: A Humanistic Approach to the Study of Persons. Harper & Row, New York, 1976.

Coopersmith, S.: The Antecedents of Self-Esteem. W.H. Freeman Co., San Francisco, 1960.

Corbeil, M.: Nursing process for a patient with a body image disturbance. Nurs. Clin. North Am. 6:155–163, 1971.

Corcoran, L., and Diers, D.: Nursing intensity in cardiac surgical care. Nurs. Manage. 2:80I–80J, 1989.

Costello, A.M.: Supporting the patient with problems related to body image. American Cancer Society Professional Education Publication, 1975.

Crickmore, R.: A review of stress in the intensive care unit. Intens. Care Nurse 3:19–27, 1987.

Daniels, V.: Stress and the I.C.U. Is it for you? Imprint Sep–Oct:32–35, 1987.

Diekstra, R.F., Stubbie, L.T., and Willemsteyn, B.: ICU sensory deprivation. Nurs. Success Today 6:21–25, 1986.

Eisendrath, S.J., and Dunkel, J.: Psychological issues in intensive care unit staff. Heart Lung 8:751–758, 1979.

Erikson, E.: Identity and the Life Cycle: Selected Papers. International Universities Press, New York, 1959.

Erikson, E.: Childhood and Society, 2nd ed. W.W. Norton & Co., New York, 1963.

Erikson, E.: Identity, Youth and Crisis. W.W. Norton Co., New York, 1968.

Farberow, N.L., and Shneidman, E.S.: The Cry for Help. McGraw-Hill Book Co., New York, 1961.

Felicetta, J.V., and Sowers, J.R.: Endocrine changes with critical illness. Crit. Care Clinician 10:855–869, 1987.

Fleming, M.L.: The nurse, the family system, and the client. Top. Clin. Nurs. 1:1003, 1979.

Fink, S.L.: Crisis and motivation: A theoretical model. Arch. Phys. Med. Rehabil. 48:592–597, 1967.

Fisher, S., and Cleveland, S.: Personality, body perception, and body image boundary. In Wapner, S., and Warner, H. (eds.): The Body Percept. Random House, New York, 1965.

Fitts, W.: Interpersonal Competence: The Wheel Model. Counselor Recordings and Tests, Nashville, 1970.

Fowler, M.D.: Moral distress and the shortage of critical care nurses. Heart Lung 18:314–315, 1989.

Gardner, D., and Stewart, N.: Staff involvement with families of patients in critical care units. Heart Lung 7:105–110, 1978.

Garfield, C.A.: Psychosocial care of the dying patient. In Patterson, M.E. (ed.): The Living-Dying Process. McGraw-Hill Book Co., New York, 1978.

Garfield, C.A.: Stress and Survival: The Emotional Realities of Life-Threatening Illness. C.V. Mosby C., St. Louis, 1979.

Gentry, W.D., and Parkes, K.R.: Psychologic stress in intensive care unit and non-intensive care unit nursing: A review of the past decade. Heart Lung 11:43–47, 1982.

Gick, R., and Whipple, B.: A holistic view of sexuality: Education for the health professional. Top. Clin. Nurs. 1:91–98, 1980.

Gowan, N.J.: The perceptual world of the intensive care unit: An overview of some environmental considerations in the helping relationship. Heart Lung 8:340–344, 1979.

Green, A.: On the outside, looking in. Am. J. Nurs. 9:1398–1399, 1984.

Guzetta, C.E.: Relationship between stress and learning. Adv. Nurs. Sci. 1:35–49, 1979.

Hague, C.: Caring can damage your health. Intens. Care Nurse 3:28–33, 1987.

Hamachek, D.E.: Encounters with the Self. Holt, Rinehart and Winston, New York, 1971.

Harris, J.S.: Home study program: Stressors and stress in crit. care. Crit. Care Nurs. 4(1):83–87, 1984.

Harrison, M., and Cotanch, P.H.: Pain: Advances and issues in critical care. Nurs. Clin. North Am. 9:691–697, 1987.

Hartl, D.E.: Stress management and the nurse. Adv. Nurs. Sci. 1:91–100, 1979.

Hatten C., Loing, V., McBride, S., et al.: Suicide Assessment and Intervention. Appleton-Century-Crofts, New York, 1977.

Hein, E.C.: Communication in Nursing Practice, 2nd ed. Little, Brown & Co., Boston, 1980.

Hervie, C., Gaillard, M., Martel, S., and Huguenard, P.: Serious suicides: Short and long-term results. Acta Anaesthesiol. Belg. 35:353–359, 1984.

Herzog, B.B., and Herrin, J.T.: Near-death experience in the very young. Crit. Care Med. 12:1074–1075, 1985.

Hill, P.M.: Nursing aspects of pain control in intensive care units. Intens. Care Nurse 1:92–101, 1985.

Hoff, L.A.: People in Crisis: Understanding and Helping. Addison-Wesley Publishing Co., Reading, Mass., 1978.

Hoffman, M., Donckers, S., and Hauser, M.: The effect of nursing intervention on stress factors perceived by patients in a coronary care unit. Heart Lung 7:804–809, 1978.

Hogatt, L., and Spika, B.: The nurse and the terminally ill patient: Some perspectives and projected actions. Omega J. Death Dying 9:255–266, 1978–79.

Hott, R.: Sex and the heart patient: A nursing view. Top. Clin. Nurs. 1:75–84, 1980.

Huckabay, L.M.D., and Jagla, B.: Nurses' stress factors in the intensive care unit. J. Nurs. Admin. 9:21–26, 1979.

Johnson, M.N.: Anxiety/stress and the effects on disclosure between nurses and patients. Adv. Nurs. Sci. 1:1–20, 1979.

Jourard, S.M.: Suicide: Invitation to die. Am. J. Nurs. 70:269, 1970.

Kendal, M.: The Community Health Nurse and Alcohol-related Problems. National Institute of Alcohol Abuse and Alcoholism, Bethesda, Md., June 1978, pp. 25–44.

Kim, M.J., McFarland, G.K., and McLane, A.M.: Pocket Guide to Nursing Diagnosis, 2nd ed. C.V. Mosby Co., St. Louis, 1987.

Kirchling, J.M., and Pierce, P.K.: Nursing and the terminally ill: Beliefs, attitudes, and perceptions of practitioners. Issues Ment. Health Nurs. 4:275–286, 1982.

Kolodny, R.C., Masters, W.H., Johnson, V.E., et al.: Textbook of Human Sexuality for Nurses. Little, Brown & Co., Boston, 1979, pp. 31–78.

Kubler-Ross, E.: On Death and Dying. Macmillan, New York, 1969.

Lammon, C.A.: Reducing family hostility. Dimens. Crit. Care Nurs. 4(1):58–63, 1985.

Lawrence, J.A., and Farr, E.H.: The nurse should consider: Critical care ethical issues. J. Adv. Nurs. 5:223–229, 1982.

Lazarus, R.: Psychological Stress and the Coping Process. McGraw-Hill Book Co., New York, 1966.

Lewis, G.: Nurse-Patient Communication. W.C. Brown Co., Dubuque, Iowa, 1978.

Lief, H., and Payne, T.: Sexuality, knowledge and attitudes. Am. J. Nurs. 75:2026–2029, 1975.

Limandri, B.J., and Boyle, D.W.: Instilling hope. Am. J. Nurs. 1:78–80, 1978.

MacKinnon-Kesler, S.: Maximizing your ICU patient's sensory and perceptual environment. Can. Nurse 5:41–45, 1983.

Maconachy, M.M.: The riddle of communication: I. Nurs. Times 75:1493–1496, 1979.

Maslach, C.: How people cope. Public Welfare Association, Spring, 1978.

Maslow, A.H.: Toward a Psychology of Being. Van Nostrand, Princeton, Mass., 1968.

McCaffery, M.: Pain in the critical care patient. Dimens. Crit. Care Nurs. 4(6):323–325, 1984.

McChoskey, J.C.: How to make the most of body image theory in nursing practice. Nursing 76:68–72, 1976.

McCullougy, W.B.: The postoperative pain-anxiety circuit: A general surgeon's perspective. Pain Overview, pp. 14–19, 1980.

McGonigal, K.S.: The importance of sleep and the sensory environment to critically ill patients. Intens. Care Nurse 2:73–83, 1986.

McLarty, N.: Emotional commitment: How much dare you care? RN 6:42–47, 1980.

Modlin, H.C.: Crisis intervention. J. Cont. Ed. Psychiatry 42:13–22, 1979.

Mohl, P.C., Denny, N.R., Mote, T.A., and Coldwater, C.: Hospital unit stressors for nurses— primary task vs social factors. Psychosomatics 4:366–374, 1982.

Molter, N.C.: Needs of relatives of critically ill patients, a descriptive study. Heart Lung 8:332–339, 1979.

Moritz, D.A.: Understanding anger. Am. J. Nurs. 78:81–83, 1978.

Murphy, G.: Human Potentialities. Basic Books, Inc., New York, 1958.

Murphy, N.: Critical care nurse becomes critical care patient. Nurs. Forum 21:178–183, 1984.

Nash, M.L.: Dignity of person in final phase of life—an exploratory study. Omega J. Death Dying 8:71–80, 1977.

Oakes, A.R.: Near-death events and critical care nursing. Top. Clin. Nurs. 10:61–78, 1981.

Orlando, I.J.: The Dynamic Nurse–Patient Relationship. G.P. Putnam's Sons, New York, 1961.

Oskins, S.L.: Identification of situational stressors and coping methods by intensive care nurses. Heart Lung 8:953–960, 1979.

Otto, H.: The human potentialities of nurses and patients. Nurs. Outlook 13:32–35, 1965.

Otto, H.: New light on human potential. Saturday Review, Dec. 20, 1969, pp. 14–18.

Parad, H.J.: Crisis Intervention: Selected Readings. Family Service Association of America, New York, 1965.

Puksta, N.S.: All about sex—after a coronary. Am. J. Nurs. 77:602–605, 1977.

Rahe, R., and Arthur, R.: Life changes and illness studies. J. Hum. Stress 4:3–15, 1978.

Reichman, W.: The alcoholic stigma—in the eye of the beholder. Alcohol. Dig. 6:5–6, 1977.

Richmond, T., and Craig, M.: Timeout: Facing death in the ICU. Dimens. Crit. Care Nurs. 5(1):41–45, 1985.

Richter, J.M.: Physical symptoms—a signal of distress in the family system. Top. Clin. Nurs. 1:31–40, 1979.

Roberts, S.: Behavioral Concepts and the Critically Ill Patient. Prentice-Hall, Inc., Englewood Cliffs, N.J., 1976.

Robinson, L.: Liaison Nursing: Psychological Approach to Patient Care. F.A. Davis Co., Philadelphia, 1974.

Rogers, B.J., and Mengel, A.: Communicating with families of terminal cancer patients. Top. Clin. Nurs. 1:55–61, 1979.

Rosel, N.: Toward a social theory of dying. Omega J. Death Dying 9:49–55, 1979.

Sanford, S., and Paul, L.: Dying in a hospital intensive care unit: The social significance for the family of the patient. Omega J. Death Dying 8:29–40, 1977.

Satir, V.: Peoplemaking. Science and Behavior Books, Inc., Palo Alto, Calif., 1972.

Satir, V.: Psychology of Self-Esteem. Bantam Books, New York, 1971.

Satterfield, S.B., and Stayton, W.R.: Understanding sexual function and dysfunction. Top. Clin. Nurs. 1:21–32, 1980.

Scalzi, C., and Dracup, K.: Sexual counseling of coronary patients. Heart Lung 7:840–845, 1978.

Seligman, M.E.P.: Submissive death: Giving up on life. Psychol. Today 10:80–85, 1974.

Selye, H.: Stress Without Distress. J.B. Lippincott Co., Philadelphia, 1974.

Selye, H.: The Stress of Life. McGraw-Hill Book Co., New York, 1956.

Shneidman, E.S.: On the Nature of Suicide. Jossey-Bass, San Francisco, 1970.

Shneidman, E.S.: Deaths of Man. Penguin Books, Baltimore, 1973.

Shontz, F.: Body image and its disorders. In Lipowski, Z., Lipsitt, D., and Whybrow, P.P. (eds.): Psychosomatic Medicine. Current Trends and Clinical Applications. Oxford University Press, New York, 1977.

Shubin, S.: Prescription for stress—your stress. Nursing 9:52–55, 1979.

Slater, P.: The Pursuit of Loneliness. Beacon Press, Boston, 1970.

Smith, H.L., Mangelsdorf, K.L., Louderbough, A.W., and Piland, N.F.: Substance abuse among nurses: Types of drugs. Dimens. Crit. Care Nurs. 8:159–168, 1989.

Smith, M.J.T., and Selye, H.: Reducing the negative effects of stress. Am. J. Nurs. 79:1953–1955, 1979.

Soupios, M.A., and Lawry, K.: Stress on personnel working in a critical care unit. Psychiatr. Med. 5:187–198, 1987.

Stern, S.B.: Nursing the patient, not the machines. Am. J. Nurs. 10:1310, 1986.

Stevens, B.J.: A phenomenological approach to understanding suicidal behavior. J. Psychiatr. Nurs. 9:33–35, 1971.

Stewart, J.: Bridges Not Walls. Addison-Wesley, Reading, Mass., 1972.

Stone, L.J., and Church, J.: Childhood and Adolescence—A Psychology of the Growing Person. Random House, New York, 1975.

Summers, S.: Stress in ICU and non-ICU nurses (letter). Nurs. Res. Jul–Aug:236, 1986.

Tierney, E.: Accepting disfigurement when death is the alternative. Am. J. Nurs. 75:2149–2150, 1975.

Ulberg, K.: Burned out: Should a battle-weary nurse endure—or find another job? J. Christ. Nurs. 3:20–21, Summer 1986.

Vaillot, C.: Hope: The restoration of being. Am. J. Nurs 79:268–273, 1970.

Weimer, S.R.: Use of physiological monitoring in crisis interviewing: Intervention in suicidal states. Gen. Hosp. Psychiatry 3:52–55, 1980.

Weiner, M.F., Caldwell, T., and Tyson, J.: Stresses and coping in ICU nursing: Why support groups fail. Gen. Hosp. Psychiatry 6:179–183, 1983.

Wepman, B.: Pain as an interpersonal device. Psychosomatics 20:561–562, 1979.

West, A.M.: Suggestions for health care providers in critical care units (letter). Heart Lung 1:103–104, 1989.

Whitley, M.P., and Willingham, D.: Adding a sexual assessment to the health interview. J. Psychiatr. Nurs. 16:17–27, 1978.

Wise, T.: Sexual difficulties with concurrent physical problems. Psychosomatics 18:56–64, 1977.

Woods, J.R.: Death on a daily basis. Focus Crit. Care 6:50–51, 1984.

Yura, H., and Walsh, M.B.: Human Needs and the Nursing Process. Appleton-Century-Crofts, New York, 1978.

CHAPTER

Legal and Ethical Aspects of Critical Care Nursing

Ginger Schafer Wlody, R.N., M.S., CCRN, FCCM

LEGAL ASPECTS OF CRITICAL CARE NURSING

Law: Sum total of rules/regulations

Sources of Law

1. **The Constitution:** provides the framework of our government
2. **Common law:** court-made law and interpretation of statutes
3. **Statutory law:** written laws enacted by the legislature. Basic rules for society established by the Senate and House of Representatives or the state legislatures
4. **Administrative law:** made by administrative agencies appointed by the executive branch of the government, president, or governors of the states

State Nurse Practice Acts

1. **Purpose is to protect the public**
2. **Statutory laws written by the individual states**
3. **Usually authorize board of nursing to oversee nursing** (by use of regulations)
4. **Scope of practice:** provides guidance for acceptable nursing roles and practices
   a. Nurses are expected to follow nurse practice act and not deviate from usual nursing activities

b. Advanced Nursing Practice: expanded roles for nurses in special positions. Nurses in expanded roles may not be covered by state practice acts. Nurses need to be aware of their state practice act limitations. The duty of nurses in expanded roles differs from that of nurses working under direct supervision in the clinical setting
   i. Nurse practitioners: may write prescriptions in certain states
   ii. Clinical nurse specialists: may be privileged to order tests, perform certain procedures
   iii. Nurse anesthetists: first specialty group to be involved in advanced/expanded practice

Standards of Nursing Care: Any established measure of extent, quality, quantity, or value; an agreed-upon level of performance or a degree of excellence of care that is established. Standards of care, standards of practice, policies, procedures, and performance criteria all establish standards

1. *AACN Standards of Care for the Critically Ill* (1989)
2. *ANA Standards:* ANA has generic standards and also specialty standards (e.g., medical-surgical nursing)
3. **Community/regional standards:** standards prevalent in certain areas of the country, or in specific communities
4. **Hospital/medical center standards:** standards developed by institutions for their staff and patients
5. **Unit practice standards/policies/protocols:** specific standards of care for specific groups or types of patients
6. **Precedent court cases:** standard of "reasonable, prudent nurse" (e.g., what a reasonable, prudent nurse would have done in the same situation)
7. **Specialty organization standards:** standards developed by other nurse specialty organizations (e.g., AORN Standards, Neuroscience Nursing Standards, Emergency Nursing Standards of Care)
8. **Certification in a specialty area:** certification is defined by Steele (1985) as "a means by which a professional organization attests that an individual has attained proficiency in an area of that profession's practice"
   a. Common goal of specialty programs is to promote consumer protection
   b. The certified nurse may be held to a higher standard of practice in the specialty
   c. Critical care certification awarded by the AACN CCRN Certification Program. The main objectives of the CCRN Certification Program are to
      i. Establish the body of knowledge necessary for CCRN certification
      ii. Test, by written examination, the common body of knowledge needed to function effectively in the critical care setting

iii. Recognize professional competence by granting CCRN status to successful candidates

Documentation

1. **Mandated by regulatory agencies**
   a. Federal requirements: related to narcotics, controlled substances, transplantation
   b. National voluntary requirements: Joint Commission on Accreditation of Healthcare Organizations (JCAHO) requirements related to quality assurance activities
   c. State requirements: may exist in specific situations (e.g., related to minors)
   d. Community standard: regional or local standards may include enhanced documentation in specific areas of practice (e.g., epidural medication)
   e. Hospital/medical center requirements
2. **Purposes of documentation of nursing care** in the patient record are to
   a. Plan and evaluate care
   b. Show progress of patient care, treatment and change in condition, and continuity of care and to reflect patient status, appearance, and behavior
   c. Demonstrate use of the nursing process
   d. Reflect nursing observations, interventions, and evaluation
   e. Protect patient: medical record used in litigation
   f. Protect health care professionals and institutions
3. **Documentation requirements**
   a. General requirements
      i. Accurate, factual observations
      ii. Timely documentation: notations and events must be timed
      iii. Reflects patient status and unusual events
      iv. Reflects nursing interventions and evaluation of their effectiveness
      v. Should reflect omissions of care and rationale
      vi. Should reflect that physician was informed of unusual/adverse situations and nature of physician's response
      vii. Should note deviations from standard hospital practice and their rationale
      viii. Should be legible
      ix. Should carefully document method of patient's admission, his condition on admission, discharge planning, and condition on discharge
      x. Should reflect documentation of the nursing process on a continuing basis throughout the hospitalization

b. Specific requirements of Joint Commission on Accreditation of Healthcare Organizations for patient records
    i. Identifying patient information
    ii. Evidence of appropriate informed consent or explanation for its absence
    iii. Medical history
    iv. Report of physical examination
    v. Diagnostic and therapeutic orders
    vi. Observations of patient's condition including patient's progress and nursing notes
    vii. Reports of all procedures and tests and their results
    viii. Conclusions, provisional diagnosis, associated diagnosis, clinical resume, and necropsy report(s)

Informed Consent

1. **Informed consent:** The President's Commission for the Study of Ethical Problems in Medicine and Biomedical and Behavioral Research recommended "that patient and provider collaborate in a continuing process intended to make decisions that will advance the patient's interests both in health (and well-being generally) and in self-determination. Self-determination sometimes called 'autonomy' involves a person forming, revising over time, and pursuing his or her own particular plan of life."
2. **Doctrine of informed consent**
    a. Based on principle of autonomy of persons
    b. Includes right of informed refusal
    c. Obligation of health care provider to provide adequate information to patient regarding
        i. Treatment options
        ii. Risk vs. benefit
        iii. Expected outcomes
    d. Three requisites to informed consent
        i. Patient must have capacity to reason and make judgments (decision-making capacity)
            (a) Competent adults
            (b) Incompetent adults and minors
                (1) Doctrine of substituted judgment—this standard requires that a surrogate attempt to reach the decision that the incapacitated person would make if he were able to choose. As a result, the patient's interest in self-determination is preserved to a certain extent
                (2) Best interest test—this standard rests solely on protection of the patient's welfare. Surrogates often lack guidance for making a substituted judgment because many persons have not given serious thought to how

they would want to be treated under particular circumstances or have failed to tell others their thoughts. In these cases the surrogates try to make a choice for the patient that seeks to implement what is that patient's best interest by reference to more objective, societally shared criteria. Conflict may arise when decision making seems not to take account of a child's best interest

    (3) Individual state requirements for court-appointed guardian/next-of-kin issues

  (c) Competence refers to the ability to make rational decisions about one's life

  (d) Determining whether a patient lacks the capacity to make a decision to forego life-sustaining treatment rests on generally accepted principles for making assessments of decisional incapacity in medical care

  ii. The decision must be made voluntarily and without coercion

  iii. The patient must have a clear understanding of risks/benefits of proposed treatment

e. ANA Code of Ethics: nurses have a special obligation to ensure that the patient receives informed consent: "Each nurse has the obligation to be knowledgeable about moral and legal rights of all clients and to protect and support those rights."

f. The responsibility for informing the patient is the physician's, although in most hospital settings the nurse obtains the signature on the consent form. Lawyers view nurses as merely facilitators of informed consent, whereas nurses see themselves as guardians of informed consent. The trend is to view nurses as sharing some of the physician's responsibility for informed consent if the circumstances warrant. Nurses' advocacy function must be considered

g. Informed refusal

  i. Right of patient to refuse care

  ii. Duty of practitioner to ensure that refusal is based on informed choice

h. Exceptions to informed consent: most hospitals have strict policies that are followed when there is a dire emergency, the patient is unable to give consent, and no relatives/significant others can be reached

Declaring Death: Until recently there were no uniform criteria for declaration of death. The Harvard Criteria referred only to a definition of "irreversible coma"

1. **Brain death:** Uniform Determination of Death Act (UDDA) Guidelines developed by the Presidential Commission for the Study of Ethical Problems in Medicine and Biomedical and Behavioral Research state that "Any individual who has sustained either irreversible cessation of

circulatory and respiratory functions, or irreversible cessation of all functions of the entire brain, including the brain stem, is dead"

   a. A determination of death must be made in accordance with accepted medical standards

   b. UDDA guidelines have been adopted in most states

2. Procedural guidelines for the declaration of death

   a. Triggering a neurologic evaluation: as soon as responsible physician has a reasonable suspicion that an irreversible loss of all brain functions has occurred, he should perform the appropriate tests and procedures to determine patient's neurologic status

   b. Obligation to declare a patient dead: cardiopulmonary criteria for determining death are recognized in all states; when the physician determines that the patient has experienced an irreversible cessation of cardiopulmonary functions, he declares the patient dead

      i. Consent of the surrogate, family, or concerned friends is not required

      ii. Sensitivity to their needs is required, and they should be allowed to obtain a second opinion

   c. Cessation of treatment after a declaration of death: once the declaration of death has been made, all treatment of the patient ordinarily should cease. Exceptions to this might be efforts to use the body or body parts for purposes stated in Uniform Anatomical Gift Act (education, research, advancement of medical or dental science, therapy, transplantation) or if the patient is pregnant and efforts are being made to save the life of the fetus

   d. In cases involving organ donation, health care professionals who make the declaration of death

      i. Should not be members of the organ transplant team

      ii. Should not be a member of the patient's family

      iii. Should not have malpractice charges pending against him related to the case

      iv. Should not have any other special interest in declaration of the patient's death (i.e., stand to inherit under patient's will)

Patient Rights: The rationale surrounding the doctrine of informed consent is that competent adult patients have a right of self-determination, which includes the right to refuse care. These are legal rights that have been established by the courts

1. Right to die: controversial, but has emerged through case law in the individual states and is based on the right to self-determination

2. Right to refuse treatment: refusal of care by a competent and informed adult should be respected even if that refusal leads to serious harm to the person

3. Right to information: related to rights of informed consent and right to self-determination

4. **Right to privacy:** invasion of the right of privacy traditionally has four separate causes—appropriation of name and likeness, intrusion on solitude or seclusion, public disclosure of private facts, and false light in the public eye
5. **Right to confidentiality:** many states have statutorily created a physician–patient privilege that protects physicians from being compelled to testify confidential communications about the patient. Legislation is needed to extend the privilege to nurses, but courts have held that the premise applies by analogy to the nurse–patient relationship

Do Not Resuscitate Orders

1. **A "do not resuscitate order" (DNR)** is a signed order directing that no cardiopulmonary resuscitation efforts are to be undertaken in the event of a cardiac or respiratory arrest
2. **Cardiopulmonary resuscitation (CPR)** refers to an array of interventions undertaken at the time of a cardiac or respiratory arrest to restore pulse and respiration

Advance Directives: A document in which a person gives advance directions about medical care or designates who should make medical decisions for them if he should lose decision-making capacity. There are two types of advance directives: treatment directives and proxy directives (such as durable power of attorney or living will).
1. **Treatment directive:** a written statement prepared by a person directing what forms of medical treatment the person wishes to receive or forego should he be in such medical condition (such as irreversible coma, terminal illness) so as to lack decision-making capacity. A "living will" is one type of treatment directive
2. **Durable power of attorney (DPA):** a person's written designation of another person to act on his behalf, when the designation is authorized by the state's durable power of attorney statute. A durable power of attorney does not terminate under state law (as does a regular power of attorney) when one loses decision-making capacity. Nurses should be familiar with their specific state laws

Good Samaritan Acts

1. **Various states have enacted Good Samaritan Acts** that provide immunity from civil liability for acts or omissions of a person who provides emergency care in good faith at the scene of an accident
2. **According to traditional common law, there is no duty to render assistance to one who needs medical care,** even in emergency situations, unless there is an established care relationship, or the condition can be attributed to the provider's actions

The Legal Process

1. **Professional liability**
   a. Professional negligence: the failure to do what the reasonably prudent nurse would do under similar circumstances. Four elements are necessary for professional negligence action and must be established by the plaintiff
      i. Duty: to act in a reasonable and prudent manner
      ii. Breach: breach of duty occurs when a nurse fails to do what a reasonable, prudent nurse would do under the same or similar circumstances. There may be a breach of a standard of care
      iii. Proximate cause: proof must be introduced that the nurse's conduct was the cause of the injury to the patient
      iv. Damages: proof of actual loss or damage proximately caused by nurse's conduct
   b. Malpractice: professional misconduct, improper discharge of professional duties, or a failure to meet the standard of care by a professional that results in harm to another

ETHICAL ASPECTS OF CRITICAL CARE NURSING
Ethical Principles

1. **Patient autonomy:** refers to self-determination, freedom of choice for competent patient
2. **Justice:** refers to what one deserves, what is just, or what is right. One deserves to be treated fairly and should not be discriminated against on the basis of social contribution or mental capacity
3. **Veracity:** truth-telling, honesty, or integrity
4. **Fidelity:** refers to keeping our "promises" or professional obligations as professional nurses to care for patients to the best of our ability
5. **Beneficence:** refers to doing good for others, being helpful, considerate of others' rights. Beneficence involves removing harmful conditions.
6. **Nonmaleficence:** this is the principle of "do no harm." This principle may conflict with others when treatment decisions are made
7. **Formalism (Immanuel Kant)/deontologic approach:** refers to the "duty" involved; duties are viewed as the basis for morality. Actions are not justified by the consequences alone but by the rightness or wrongness of the act itself
8. **Consequentialism (John Stuart Mill)/teleologic approach:** this theory bases the rightness or wrongness of an action on the consequences of that action. It looks at "outcome" or what the result will be
9. **Utilitarianism:** this approach or theory states that the morally right thing to do is that act that produces the greatest good (for the most people or for society). Utilitarianism is derived from the teleologic approach.

10. **Paternalism:** this approach claims that beneficence should take precedence over autonomy—at least in some cases (e.g., a health care worker makes a decision for a patient saying, "It's in his best interest." The patient is then denied the right to make his own decisions)

Moral Concepts and Theories

1. **Respect for persons:** giving due weight to the welfare and wishes of persons
   a. A person should be treated with caring
   b. A person should not be treated as a means to an end
2. **Justice:** justice is a minimal claim on social order—everyone fundamentally deserves equal respect
   a. Distributive justice: allocation of goods and services
   b. Retributive justice: primarily concerned with punishment for wrongdoing
   c. Procedural justice: focuses on how things are done regardless of final outcome
3. **Values:** the foundation of the seriousness and importance of things; what a person sees as good or bad. Values have different weights or importance. Thinking about values is part of ethical decision making.
   a. Instrumental values: activity valuable only as a means to an end
   b. Final values: values that are valuable in and of themselves
   c. Value conflicts occur when nurses' values are not congruent with patient's, physician's, or family's values
4. **Rights**
   a. Basic human rights
      i. Protect a person from the state (e.g., the Bill of Rights protects one from illegal search and seizure)
      ii. Demand provision of goods/services by the state (i.e., water)
      iii. Are established by systems of law and backed by state
      iv. Moral rights: backed by general opinion of society or culture
      v. Rights involve responsibilities

ANA Ethical Code for Nurses

1. **Based on a belief about the nature of persons, nursing, health, and society**
2. **Provides guidance for conduct and relationships in carrying out nursing responsibilities** that are consistent with ethical obligations of the profession and with high-quality nursing care
3. **Reflects an essential activity of a profession and provides one means for the exercise of professional self-regulation**
4. **Offers general principles to guide and evaluate nursing actions,**

informing both the nurse and the society of the profession's expectations and requirements in ethical matters

5. **Adopted originally in 1950,** revised in 1976 adding intrepretative statements. Latest revision, 1985.
6. **Code statements** include
    a. The nurse provides services with respect for human dignity and the uniqueness of the client, unrestricted by considerations of social or economic status, personal attributes, or the nature of health problems
    b. The nurse safeguards the patient's right to privacy by judiciously protecting information of a confidential nature.
    c. The nurse acts to safeguard the patient and the public when health care and safety are affected by incompetent, unethical, or illegal practice by any person
    d. The nurse assumes responsibility and accountability for individual nursing judgments and actions
    e. The nurse maintains competence in nursing
    f. The nurse exercises informed judgment and uses individual competency and qualifications as criteria in seeking consultation, accepting responsibilities, and delegating nursing activities
    g. The nurse participates in activities that contribute to the ongoing development of the profession's body of knowledge
    h. The nurse participates in the profession's efforts to implement and improve standards of nursing
    i. The nurse participates in the profession's efforts to establish and maintain conditions of employment conducive to high-quality nursing care
    j. The nurse participates in the profession's effort to protect the public from misinformation and misrepresentation and to maintain the integrity of nursing.
    k. The nurse collaborates with members of the health professions and other citizens in promoting community and national efforts to meet the health needs of the public

American Hospital Association: Patient's Bill of Rights

1. **The patient has the right**
    a. To considerate and respectful care
    b. To obtain from the physician information regarding his diagnosis, treatment, and prognosis
    c. To give informed consent before the start of any procedure or treatment
    d. To refuse treatment to the extent permitted by law
    e. To privacy concerning his own medical care program
    f. To confidential communication and records

g. To expect that the hospital will make a reasonable response to a patient's request for service
h. To information regarding the relationship of his hospital to other health and educational institutions as far as his care is concerned
i. To refuse to participate in research projects
j. To expect reasonable continuity of care
k. To examine and question his bill
l. To know the hospital rules and regulations that apply to patients' conduct

Role of the Nurse in Addressing Ethical Issues

1. **Nurse as a moral agent:** morality in the broad sense refers to the search for general action guiding principles
   a. Values clarification for the nurse
      i. Aesthetic considerations
      ii. Demands of etiquette or "proper" behavior
      iii. Our selfish wishes
      iv. Sense of morality (basic values)
      v. Principles of Critical Care Nursing Practice (1981): AACN Position Statement includes
         (a) The critical care nurse respects the rights of patients, families, colleagues, in the promotion or prolongation of life, by individualizing each patient situation
         (b) The critical care nurse identifies the values of patients, families, colleagues and self and incorporates these beliefs and attitudes into situations of ethical dilemmas
         (c) The critical care nurse adheres to the American Nurses' Association (ANA) Code of Ethics with Interpretive Statements
   b. Patient advocacy role: essential component of contemporary nursing practice
      i. Linked with the notation of rights
      ii. Based on the value of human dignity
      iii. Nurses advocate the rights of patients
      iv. Nurses become partisans in conflicts and assume responsibility for presenting rights and interests of patients
      v. Values-based decision model of advocacy: portrays the nurse as helping the patient to discuss the patient's needs and interests and assist the patient to make choices congruent with the patient's values
      vi. Nurses are expected to prevent others from limiting the freedom of the patient
      vii. The advocacy role may produce conflict for the nurse
      viii. AACN Position Statement: Role of the Critical Care Nurse as

Patient Advocate states that as a patient advocate the critical care nurse shall
- (a) Respect and support the right to autonomous informed decision making by the patient or designated surrogate
- (b) Intervene when the best interest of the patient is in question
- (c) Assist the patient to obtain necessary care
- (d) Respect the values, beliefs, and rights of the patient
- (e) Assist patients/designated surrogates in the decision-making process through education and support
- (f) Represent the patient in accordance with the patient's choices
- (g) Support the decisions of the patient/designated surrogate or transfer care to an equally qualified critical care nurse
- (h) Intercede for patients who cannot speak for themselves in situations requiring immediate action
- (i) Monitor and safeguard the quality of care the patient receives
- (j) Act as liaison among the patient, family, and health care professionals

c. Role of nurse in research
   i. AACN Position Statement: Ethics in Critical Care Research
      - (a) Supports conduct of research in manner that assumes that patients give informed consent for study participation
      - (b) Supports conduct of research in manner that ensures patients' rights continue to be safeguarded during conduct of the study
      - (c) Recommends that health care institutions establish formal multidisciplinary peer review boards to ensure that ethical principles that underlie conduct of research are followed when research is conducted
      - (d) Recommends that at least one professional nurse with equal voting rights be a regular member of all multidisciplinary peer review boards, including Institutional Review Boards (IRB)
      - (e) Recommends that nursing administrations establish procedures that ensure communication between the investigator and nurses involved in conducting the study so that adequate information regarding the research and its risks and possible benefits are understood by the critical care nurses who function as caregivers, assist the researcher, are responsible for unit management, or are asked to answer questions of patient participants regarding study participation
      - (f) Recommends that nursing administrations establish

mechanisms for addressing nursing concerns about critical care research

d. Role of the nurse participating in futile care

   i. Critical care nurses frequently care for the hopelessly ill patient

   ii. Withdrawal of medical therapy does not mean withdrawal of nursing care

   iii. The nurse should participate in team/family decisions to withhold or withdraw care

   iv. When the patient is being treated against his will, it is generally the nurse's moral duty to act as patient advocate

   v. It is morally permissible for a nurse to refuse to participate in withdrawing or witholding therapy on grounds of personal beliefs or patient advocacy, as long as a replacement is available and the patient is not abandoned

e. Whistleblowing: Role of the nurse in reporting immoral, illegal, or incompetent behavior with a view to stop it

   i. Reporting incompetence of peers, physicians, subordinates

   ii. ANA Code of Ethics

   iii. State laws

f. Individual ethical dilemmas arise from the current health care environment and are related to

   i. The nursing shortage: deciding priorities in care in accepting and carrying out assignments (e.g., aging population, sicker patients)

   ii. Interference of cost consideration in providing patient care/ maintaining quality (e.g., reimbursement changes, increased use of technology)

   iii. Nurse is bound by license and conscience to provide safe, appropriate care

   iv. Prior to rejection of an assignment the nurse must

     (a) Understand potential consequences

     (b) Document concerns for patient safety

     (c) Document process used to inform management

     (d) Use other strategies, such as joint committees to explore issues and increase recruitment/retention (at a later time)

g. Role of nurse in addressing ethical issues

   i. Assessment: identify the factors affecting the patient, family, and situation

     (a) Separate assumptions from facts

     (b) Clarify unclear items

     (c) Identify who is making decision

     (d) Identify own perspective

   ii. Advocacy: identify and use ethical principles, considering dignity and autonomy of the patient

   iii. Action: define problem, determine strategies, identify alternatives, and formulate and take action to address ethical dilemma within the multidisciplinary context

h. Resources for addressing ethical issues

   i. ANA Code for Nurses

  ii. ANA Social Policy Statement

 iii. ANA Position Statements

    (a) Statement Regarding Risk vs. Responsibility in Providing Nursing Care

    (b) Guidelines for Nurses' Participation and Leadership in Institutional Ethical Review Processes

    (c) Guidelines on Mechanisms Through Which State Nurses' Associations Consider Ethical Issues and Concerns

    (d) Committee on Ethics—Guidelines on Withdrawing or Withholding Food and Fluid

      (1) Discusses whether or not it is morally permissible to ever withhold food/fluids from patients

 iv. AACN Position Statements

    (a) Clarification of Resuscitation Status in Critical Care Settings requires that guidelines must be written denoting levels of resuscitation for each patient within the critical care setting. These guidelines must include the following components

      (1) A system and process for classification of patient resuscitation status

      (2) A mechanism for documentation and review of resuscitation status and the process used to arrive at this decision

      (3) A mechanism for assurance of patient and family rights

      (4) Use of clearly defined terminology

      (5) The critical care nurse will

        a) Ensure quality of patient care regardless of resuscitation status

        b) Review the current resuscitation status daily with the physician

        c) Reflect the resuscitation status in the patient's plan of care

    (b) Required Request and Routine Inquiry: Methods to Improve Organ and Tissue Donation Process

      (1) AACN strongly supports legislation for required request

      (2) AACN strongly recommends that institutions adopt policies that standardize the process of routine inquiry concerning organ and tissue donation

      (3) AACN recommends that the critical care nurse, in

accordance with personal beliefs and values, participates in the development, implementation, and evaluation of the hospital's policy related to required request

(c) Roles and Responsibilities of Critical Care Nurses in Organ and Tissue Transplantation defines the roles/responsibilities related to organ/tissue transplantation and resolves that the critical care nurse shall

(1) Collaborate with health care professionals/families in donor identification and care, the organ and tissue procurement process, and recipient care

(2) Develop knowledge and awareness of personal, professional, cultural, social, religious, and ethical issues related to organ and tissue transplantation

(3) Develop knowledge and awareness of local state and national legislation relevant to organ and tissue transplantation

(4) Provide support needed by families of potential and actual organ and issue donors

(5) Participate in the implementation of standards for care of potential donors, recipients, and families

(6) Participate in the selection process of potential recipients

(7) Participate in endeavors designed to advance the science and art of transplantation nursing

v. Position statement by American College of Emergency Physicians, "Guidelines for DNR Orders in the Prehospital Setting" (1988): statement recommends that a comprehensive "do not resuscitate" policy should be endorsed by the local, regional, or state medical society and that medical treatments limited by a "do not resuscitate" order should be clearly defined, so that these orders could be honored in prehospital care

vi. Institutional Ethics Committees (IECs)

(a) Establishment of IECs

(1) Recommended by President's Commission for the Study of Ethical Problems in Medicine and Biomedical and Behavioral Research

(2) First recommended by court in Karen Quinlan case (1976)

(3) Current trend is toward establishing IECs in other health care institutions (e.g., hospitals)

(b) Purposes of IECs

(1) Initiate educational programs related to ethical dilemmas in health care

(2) Formulate institutional policies and guidelines in sen-

sitive areas (e.g., related to DNR, withholding or withdrawing therapy)

(3) Monitor compliance with those policies

(4) Review/revise policies already in effect

(5) Advise/act as consultants on specific cases

(6) Act as forum for discussing and resolving issues and disagreements regarding treatment issues

(7) Provide emotional support for staff

(c) Membership of IECs

(1) Multidisciplinary

(2) Large enough to represent diverse professional viewpoints

(d) Models/types of committees (Veatch)

(1) Autonomy model—accountable to the competent patient; facilitates decision making by competent patient

(2) Patient benefit model—accountable to incompetent patient; facilitates decision making for incompetent patient

(3) Social justice model—accountable to institutions; considers broad social issues (i.e., hospital policies, health care policy, resource allocation, cost effectiveness)

(e) Confidentiality related to IECs

(1) Of proceedings

(2) Of records

(3) Should be determined by committee at outset

(f) Education and development of IECs

(1) Self-education—communicate with others; attend workshops

(2) Education of others—forums, ethics rounds, clinical discussions

(g) Policy development (i.e., do not resuscitate, case review, nutrition, withdrawal of life support)

(1) Develop and disseminate policies

(2) Educate staff

(3) Monitor compliance

(h) Review of ongoing cases—procedural guidelines should reflect

(1) Optional vs. mandatory consultation

(2) Decision-making authority vs. options

(3) Source of requests for review

(4) Types of problems for consideration

(5) Members' responsibilities

(i) Advantages/disadvantages of IECs

(1) Advantages

       a) Core group of staff knowledgeable regarding ethical issues

       b) Patient is focus of ethical dilemma

       c) Forum for multidisciplinary dialogue related to ethical issues of patient care

       d) Objective body to consult and provide assistance to staff

   (2) Disadvantages

       a) May pose threat to traditional decision-making process

       b) Committee may not be able to remain nonbiased

       c) Committee may become preoccupied with risk management/prevention of litigation

       d) Committee involvement raises potential for loss of patient confidentiality

ETHICAL CONFLICTS IN THE HEALTH CARE ENVIRONMENT

Allocation of Resources/Scarce Resources

1. Organ donation

  a. Donation vs. sale of body parts

  b. Use of anencephalic tissue

  c. Organ procurement/harvesting

  d. Caring for patients in a "suspended state of being" (potential donor)

  e. Uniform Anatomical Gift Act (1968)

     i. "Any individual of sound mind and eighteen years of age or more may give all or any part of his body . . . the gift to take effect upon death"

     ii. In the absence of a gift by the deceased, his relatives, in a stated order of priority (spouse, adult children, parents, siblings) have the power to give away the body or any of its parts

    iii. Recipients are restricted to hospitals, doctors, medical and dental schools, universities, tissue banks, and a specified person in need of treatment. The purposes are restricted to transplantation, therapy, research, education, and the advancement of medical or dental science

     iv. A gift may be made by will or by a card or other document

      v. A gift may be revoked at any time

     vi. A donee may accept or reject a gift

  f. Donor issues

     i. Presumed consent: routine salvage of donor organs when there has been no expressed wish not to donate by the deceased.

Thirteen countries have presumed consent (United States does not have presumed consent)

    ii. Sale of organs by unrelated live donors or by the next of kin after a donor's death is not dealt with by the Uniform Anatomical Gift Act: it is the unwritten code of ethics of transplantation surgeons that prevents the sale of organs

2. **Transplantation**
   a. Sanctity of life in the western world
   b. Cost vs. benefit
   c. Scarcity of organs vs. demand
   d. Number and types of organs transplanted increases every year
      i. Heart
      ii. Lung
      iii. Heart/lung combination
      iv. Pancreas
      v. Joints
      vi. Multiple abdominal organs
      vii. Cornea
      viii. Liver
      ix. Nerves
   e. Issues related to nursing staff may cause ethical conflicts
      i. Death of another makes organ transplantation possible
      ii. Identification of brain death removes hope of survival
      iii. Special meaning of the heart

3. **Technologic imperative:** technologic advances force health care administrators to opt for technology in spite of cost even when there is little hope for survival of individual patients

4. **Transfer/discharge of patients unable to pay** ("patient dumping")

5. **Do not resuscitate (DNR) orders**
   a. Hopelessly ill/right to die
   b. Incompetent patients
      i. Who can decide?
      ii. Principle of substituted judgment
   c. No code/slow code issues

6. **Withdrawal of care**
   a. Legal responsibilities
   b. Ethical responsibilities

7. **Withholding food/fluids vs. forced feeding**
   a. Patients in prolonged coma

8. **Advance directives:** enhance patient autonomy and increase patient involvement in the decision-making process

9. **Euthanasia/assisted suicide**
   a. Legal in Holland
   b. Groups in United States attempting to modify laws

10. **Ethical issues in acquired immunodeficiency syndrome (AIDS)**
    a. There is basic professional ethic that nurses care for patients regardless of their personal attributes or health problems
    b. AIDS challenges that basic ethic: being treated differently than other communicable diseases
    c. Conflicts of patient privacy vs. nurses' safety
    d. Nurses have moral duty to provide care, but is that obligation absolute? Under all circumstances?
    e. ANA has concluded that a nurse's obligation is limited by degree of personal risk
    f. Nurse has moral obligation to provide care if situation meets criteria (ANA Position Statement)
        i. Patient is at significant risk of harm, loss, or damage if nurse does not assist
        ii. Nurse's intervention is directly related to preventing harm
        iii. The benefit the patient gains outweighs any harm the nurse might incur and does not present more than a minimal risk to the nurse

11. **Triage decisions**
    a. Who gets the bed when there are two potential patients and only one bed
    b. Role of the critical care nurse
    c. Role of the unit medical director
    d. AACN Guidelines for Admission/Discharge Criteria in Critical Care
        i. Development of admission/discharge criteria is based on
            (a) Standards for critically ill
            (b) Current unit admission and discharge patterns
            (c) Available resources within the critical care unit
            (d) Number and distribution of critical care beds in the institution
            (e) Institutional occupancy trends
            (f) Data provided by existing measurement tools in the institution (e.g., patient classification tools, severity of illness index)
        ii. That admission/discharge criteria contain or address the following
            (a) Physiologic parameters that define the need for critical care
            (b) Physiologic parameters that define readiness for discharge
            (c) Definition of unit-specific patient population
            (d) Frequency and type of medical evaluation and/or treatment required by the patient's condition
            (e) Frequency and type of critical care nursing assessments and interventions needed by the patient

    (f) Technologic monitoring and intervention only available in the critical care setting

    (g) Requirements by external regulatory bodies

    (h) Institutional policies that mandate or preclude critical care for specific patient populations

    (i) Designation of the health team member(s) accountable for admission/discharge decisions

    (j) A plan for triage when the need exceeds available physical or human resources

    (k) A plan for conflict resolution between health care team members using the admission/discharge criteria

  iii. That the admission/discharge criteria will be approved through appropriate institutional channels and disseminated to all health care team members involved in the process

  iv. That compliance to the admission/discharge process will be regularly monitored and evaluated annually by the multidisciplinary team

Patient Care Dilemmas: Types

1. **Withholding treatment** (e.g., quadriplegic patient with other medical problems such as renal disease requiring dialysis)
2. **Code vs no-code** (e.g., cardiac patient with severe chronic obstructive pulmonary disease who needs ventilator for the rest of his life)
3. **Right to die at home** (e.g., transplantation patient)
4. **Technology vs. cost** (e.g., patient receives single-chambered pacemaker vs. dual chamber)
5. **Nutritional dilemmas** (e.g., withdrawal of food and fluids vs. tube feeding)
6. **Resource allocation/triage decisions** (e.g., who gets the last temporary pacemaker when two need it?)
7. **Technology vs. quality of life decisions** (e.g., left ventricular assist device)
8. **Informed consent** (e.g., patient scheduled for bilateral above-the-knee amputations vs. death)

Use of Technology

1. **Increased use of technology escalates ethical conflicts**
2. **High cost of technology**
   a. Personnel
   b. Equipment
   c. Training
3. **Abuse of technology** (inappropriate use)
4. **Types of technologies in health care**

   a. Devices
      i. Ventilator
      ii. Left ventricular assist device
      iii. Total artificial heart
      iv. Pacemaker (multiple types)
      v. Artificial feeding devices
      vi. Defibrillators (internal/external)
      vii. Insulin pumps
   b. Procedures
      i. Hemodialysis
      ii. Surrogate motherhood (embryonic transplant)
      iii. Genetic engineering
      iv. Artificial insemination
      v. Fetal surgery
      vi. Continuous ambulatory peritoneal dialysis
      vii. Amniocentesis/genetic identification
      viii. Hemofiltration
   c. Organ transplantation

Common Ethical Conflicts in Care of the Critically Ill

1. Autonomy vs. paternalism
   a. Conflicts related to rights of the individual
      i. Informed consent
      ii. Technology vs. quality of life
      iii. Code vs. no-code decisions
2. Justice vs. utilitarianism
   a. Conflicts related to resource allocation and triage decisions
      i. Nutritional dilemmas
      ii. Quality of life decisions
3. Veracity vs. fidelity
   a. Conflicts related to the unique role of the nurse/other health care professionals
      i. Withholding therapy
      ii. Right to die at home
      iii. Truth telling
4. Professional integrity vs. one's own ethical and moral beliefs
   a. Professional vs. personal conflicts
      i. Delivering therapy that goes against one's own moral and ethical beliefs
      ii. Caring for those whose practices we do not accept

Corporate Ethics

1. Setting
   a. Hospital as corporate environment
   b. Individual vs. corporation resulting in ethical conflicts

2. **Types of unethical behaviors** (e.g., changing documentation, charting inaccurate data or information)
3. **Promotion of ethical behavior by the nurse manager**
   a. Recognition that there is a lack of ethical behavior when it occurs
   b. Standards development: use of current standards, ANA Code of Ethics for Nurses, or development of specific standards by the group
   c. Responsibility for ethical behavior belongs to all involved in the patient care environment

References

American Association of Critical-Care Nurses: Role of the Critical Care Nurse as Patient Advocate. AACN, Newport Beach, Calif., 1989.

American Association of Critical-Care Nurses Certification Corporation: CCRN Certification Handbook. AACN, Newport Beach, Calif., 1989.

American Association of Critical-Care Nurses: Guidelines for Admission/Discharge Criteria in Critical Care. AACN, Newport Beach, Calif., 1987.

American Association of Critical-Care Nurses: Roles and Responsibilities of Critical Care Nurses in Organ and Tissue Transplantation. AACN, Newport Beach, Calif., 1986.

American Association of Critical-Care Nurses: Required Request and Routine Inquiry: Methods to Improve the Organ and Tissue Donation Process. AACN, Newport Beach, Calif., 1986.

American Association of Critical-Care Nurses: Clarification of Resuscitation Status in Critical Care Settings. AACN, Newport Beach, Calif., 1985.

American Association of Critical-Care Nurses: Ethics in Critical Care Research. AACN, Newport Beach, Calif., 1985.

American Hospital Association: Patient Bill of Rights. AHA, Chicago, 1978.

American Nurses' Association: Code for Nurses. ANA, Kansas City, Mo., 1976.

Anderson G., and Steinberg, E.: To buy or not to buy: Technology acquisition under prospective payment. N. Engl. J. Med. 311:182–185, 1987.

Barber vs. Superior Court: 147 Cal. App 3d 1006, 1986.

Bartling vs. Superior Court: 163 Cal. App 3d 186, 195, 1984.

Bayer, R., Callahan, D., Fletcher, J., Hodgson, T., Jennings., B., Monsies, D., Sievert, S., and Veatch, R.: The care of the terminally ill: Morality and economics. N. Engl. J. Med. 309:1493–1497, 1983.

Cobbs vs. Grant (1972): 8 Cal 3d 229.

Cullen, D. C., Ferrara, L., Briggs, B., Walker, P., and Gilbert, J.: Survival, hospitalization, charges and followup results in critically ill patients. N. Engl. J. Med. 295:980–987, 1976.

Davis, A.: Helping your staff address ethical dilemmas. J. Nurs. Admin. 12:9–12, 1982.

Eisendrath, S. J., and Jonsen, A. R.: The living will: Help or hindrance? JAMA 249:2054–2058, 1983.

Fiesta, J.: The Law and Liability: A Guide for Nurses, 2nd ed. John Wiley & Sons, New York, 1988.

Fowler, M. D., and Levine-Ariff, J.: Ethics at the Bedside. J.B. Lippincott Co., Philadelphia, 1987.

Gilfix, M., and Raffin, T. A.: Withholding or withdrawing extraordinary life support: Optimizing rights and limiting liability. West. J. Med. 141:387–394, 1984.

Greenspan, A., Kay, H., Berger, B., Greenberg, R., and Gaughan, M. J.: Incidence of unwarranted implantation of permanent cardiac pacemakers in a large medical population. N. Engl. J. Med., 318:158–163, 1988.

Guido, G. W.: Legal aspects of critical care nursing. Crit. Care Currents 5:1–10, 1987.

Guido, G. W.: Legal-ethical dilemmas: The patient's right to die. AACN NTI Proceedings Book. Newport Beach, Calif., 1986.

Guido, G. W.: Assuring informed consent in critical care. AACN NTI Proceedings Book. Newport Beach, Calif., 1985.

Haddad, A.: Ethics: Using principles of beneficence, autonomy to resolve ethical dilemmas in perioperative nursing. AORN J. 46:120–124, 1987.

Harlan, W. R., Chianchiano, D., Himes, K. R., Jesse, M. J., Moore, C., Tarazi, R., Weldon, C. S., Buckwalter, K., Molen, M., and Smith, H.: Ethics of biomedical technology transfer: Committee report on ethics. Circulation 67:942A–946A, 1983.

Hastings Center: Guidelines for the Termination of Life Sustaining Treatment and Care of the Dying. Briarcliff Manor, N.Y., 1987.

Hastings Center: Values, ethics and CBA in health care. In: The Implications of Cost Effectiveness Analysis of Medical Technology, Office of Technology Assessment, Washington, D.C., 1980.

Hoffman, P., and Banja, J.: Exceptions to the right to refuse treatment. AORN J. 54:892–897, 1987.

Jameton, A.: Nursing Practice: The Ethical Issues. Prentice-Hall, Englewood Cliffs, N.J., 1984.

Jonsen, A. R., Siegler, M., and Winslade, W.: Clinical Ethics, 2nd ed. Macmillan Publishing Co., New York, 1986.

Kalisch, B., and Kalisch, P.: An analysis of the source of physician–nurse conflict. In Muff J. (ed.): Socialization, Sexism, and Stereotyping: Women's Issues in Nursing. C.V. Mosby, St. Louis, 1982.

Levine, M.: Bioethics of cancer nursing. J. Rehabil. Nurs. 7:27–30, 1982.

McIntyre, K.: Recent case law and medical life and death decision making. Ala. J. Med. Sci. 8:4–12, 1981.

Murphy, C.: The changing role of nurses in making ethical decisions. Law, Medicine, and Health Care, pp. 173–175, 1984.

Northrop, C., and Kelly, M. E.: Legal Issues in Nursing. C.V. Mosby Co., St. Louis, 1987.

Pohlman, K.J.: Nursing negligence. Focus Crit. Care 16:296–298, 1989.

President's Commission for the Study of Ethical Problems in Medicine and Biomedical and Behavioral Research: Deciding to Forego Life-Sustaining Treatment: Ethical, Medical and Legal Issues in Treatment Decisions. U.S. Government Printing Office, Washington, D.C., 1983.

President's Commission for the Study of Ethical Problems in Medicine and Biomedical and Behavioral Research: Defining death. U.S. Government Printing Office, Washington, D.C., 1981.

Richards, G.: Technology, costs and rationing issues. Hospitals 58:80–81, 1984.

Ruark, J., Raffin, T. A., and the Stanford University Medical Center Committee on Ethics: Initiating and withdrawing life support: Principles and practices in adult medicine. N. Engl. J. Med. 318:25–28, 1985.

Society for the Right to Die: The Living Will. Society for the Right to Die, New York, 1985.

Spingarn, N. D.: Hospitals seek ways to make intensive care more efficient. New York Times, June 5, 1984.

Steele, J. E.: The impact of certification specialty practice. J. Rehabil. Nurs. 10:16–19, 1985.

Veatch, R.: Hospital ethics committees: Is there a role? Hastings Center Report, pp. 22–25, June 1977.

Wanzer, S., Adelstein, J., Cranford, R., Federman, D., Hook, E., Moertal, C., Safar, P., Stone, A., Taussig, H., and Van Eys, J.: The physician's responsibility toward hopelessly ill patients. N. Engl. J. Med. 310:955–959, 1984.

Wlody, G. S., and Smith, S.: Ethical dilemmas in critical care: A proposal for hospital ethics advisory committees. Focus Crit. Care 12:41–46, 1985.

Index

Note: page numbers in *italics* refer to illustrations; page numbers followed by a t refer to tables

A

Abdomen, acute, 825–828
clinical signs of, 825–826
conditions causing, 825
diagnostic studies for, 826–827
fluid volume deficit with, 828
infection with, 827
malnutrition with, 827–828
pain with, 828
pathophysiology of, 825
auscultation of, 767
diagnostic studies of, 768–770
distention of, with spinal cord injury, 403–404
inspection of, 766–767
landmarks of, 766
palpation of, 768
percussion of, 767–768
quadrants of, 766
trauma to, 803–809
anxiety with, 809
clinical signs of, 803–804
diagnostic studies for, 804–805
etiology of, 803
examination of patient with, 804
fluid volume deficit with, 807–808
ineffective breathing with, 808
infection with, 805
malnutrition with, 805, 807
pain with, 808
pathophysiology of, 803
types of, 803
Abdominal reflex, 353, 398t
Abducens nerve, 344
testing of, 351
ABO blood group system, 685–686
Abscess, with bowel infarction, 800–801
Accelerated junctional rhythm, 179
Acetaminophen, for infection, 705–706
toxicity of, 448
acetylcysteine in treatment of, 456

Acetaminophen *(Continued)*
injury due to, 453
laboratory signs of, 451–452
Acetazolamide, action of, 508
Acetylcholine, 144
function of, 331
in neuromuscular transmission, 342, *342*
receptors for, in myasthenia gravis, 442
Acetylcholinesterase, in neuromuscular transmission, 342
Acetylcysteine, 456
Achalasia, 750
Acid-base balance, chloride regulation and, 485
chronic renal failure and, 551
diabetic ketoacidosis and, 655, 659–660
disturbances in, 24–26
drug intoxication and, 455–456
in shock, 302
physiology of, 22–27
buffering in, 22
Henderson-Hasselbach equation and, 22
renal parameter of, 24
respiratory parameter of, 23
terminology used in, 22
renal disease and, 511–512
renal regulation of, 486–488
Acidic liquid, aspiration of, 109–110
Acinus, structure of, 3–4, *4*
Acoustic nerve, 344
neuroma of, 419
testing of, 351–352, 359
Acquired immune deficiency syndrome (AIDS). See also *Human immunodeficiency virus (HIV).*
ethical issues in, 923
etiology of, 736–737
Acromegaly, 420
ACTH, 609
glucocorticoid secretion and, 619
in adrenal insufficiency, 652
pituitary tumor secreting, 420

ACTH *(Continued)*
  secretion and activity of, 614–615
Action potential, in neuromuscular transmission, 342
  of cardiac muscle, *145*, 145–147
  of cardiac pacemaker cells, 146–147, *147*
Addiction, psychosocial aspects of, 887–890
Addison's disease, 651–652
Adenocarcinoma, of lung, 121
Adenosine monophosphate, cyclic (cAMP), hormone action and, 610, *611*
ADH. See *Antidiuretic hormone.*
Admission-discharge criteria, ethical issues in, 923–924
Adrenal crisis, 650–654
  clinical signs of, 651–652
  diagnostic studies of, 652
  etiology of, 650–651
  fluid volume overload with, 652–653
  history and, 651–652
  knowledge deficit with, 653–654
  pathophysiology of, 650
Adrenal glands, 618–621
Adrenergic responses, of body tissues, 621t
Adrenocorticotropic hormone. See *ACTH.*
Adult respiratory distress syndrome, 87–90
  data base for, 89–90
  etiology of, 88–89
  pathophysiology of, 87–88
  with pancreatitis, 780
Advance directives, 911, 922
Afterload, 151
Agitation, with mechanical ventilation, 66
Agnosia, sensory, stroke and, 409
AIDS. See *Acquired immune deficiency syndrome (AIDS).*
Airway, artificial, 48–51. See also *Intubation, endotracheal; Tracheostomy.*
  complications with, 51–54
    physiologic alterations due to, 51
  assessment of, 47
  defense system of, pneumonia and, 105–106
  esophageal obturator, 48
  in status epilepticus, 434
  ineffective clearance of, 47–54, 105, 117
    in asthma, 97
    neurologic abnormalities and, 368–369
    with lung cancer, 124
  nasopharyngeal, 48
  oropharyngeal, 48
Akinetic seizures, 429
Albumin, in blood transfusions, 712–713
Albuminocytologic dissociation, in Guillain-Barré syndrome, 439
Albuterol, for ventilation control, 71
Alcohol, hematologic disorders and, 690, 694
  toxicity of, 447
    clinical signs of, 449
    injury due to, 453
    laboratory signs of, 451
Aldosterone, inhibition by diuretics, 507
  potassium regulation and, 483–484
  secretion and activity of, 619–620
  sodium balance and, 482–483, 488
Alienation, sense of, 878–879

Alkalemia, 22, 488
Alkalosis, 22, 485
Allergic reaction, anaphylactic, 734
  pulmonary abnormalities and, 29, 30
  with thrombolytic agents, 229
Alport's syndrome, 546
Alveolar oxygen tension, 12–13
Alveolar ventilation, 4–7, 19
  formula for, 6
Alveolar-arterial oxygen pressure difference, 13
American Association of Critical Care Nurses, guidelines on admission/discharge of, 923–924
  position on Ethics in Critical Care Research, 916–917
  position on patient advocacy of, 916
  position on values clarification of, 915
  position statements on ethical issues of, 918–919
American Hospital Association, Patient's Bill of Rights of, 914–915
American Nurses Association, Ethical Code for Nurses of, 909, 913–914
  standards of nursing care of, 906
Aminophylline, action of, 508
Amiodarone, action of, 221
Ammonia, serum, in hepatic failure, 791–792
Amrinone, action of, 245–246
Anaphylaxis, 734–735
Anatomic dead space, 2
Anemia, 717–721
  chronic, 513
  cyanosis and, 34
  diagnostic study findings with, 719–720
  etiology of, 717–718
  examination of patient with, 719
  in uremic syndrome, 558
  nursing history for, 718–719
  pathophysiology of, 717
  renal disease and, 512–513
  with acute renal failure, 539–540
  with chronic renal failure, 551–552
Anesthesia, intracranial pressure and, 379
  recovery from, 457–462
    clinical findings with, 457–458
    complications with, 458–461
    laboratory findings in, 458
    nursing interventions in, 459–461
    pathophysiology of, 457
    reversal of action of anesthetic drug and, 460
Aneurysms, abdominal, symptoms of, 291
  aortic, *290*, 290–291
  intracranial, 412–416
    classification of, 413–414
    clinical signs of, 413–414
    etiology of, 412
    nursing diagnoses with, 414–416
    pathophysiology of, 412
  peripheral atherosclerosis and, *290*, 290–291
  signs of, 292
  surgical repair of, 294–296, *295–296*
  thoracic, 290–292
Angina pectoris, 207–223
  cardiac output and tissue perfusion and, 217–223